Eighth Edition

Prentice Hall Nursing Diagnosis Handbook with NIC Interventions and NOC Outcomes

Judith M. Wilkinson, PhD, ARNP
Nurse Educator, Consultant

PEARSON
Prentice
Hall

Upper Saddle River, New Jersey 07458

Library of Congress Cataloging-in-Publication Data

Wilkinson, Judith M.,
  Prentice Hall nursing diagnosis handbook with NIC interventions and NOC outcomes. —
8th ed. / Judith M. Wilkinson.
    p. ; cm.
  Rev. ed. of: Nursing diagnosis handbook with NIC interventions and NOC outcomes. 7th ed.
c2000.
  Includes bibliographical references and index.
  1. Nursing care plans—Handbooks, manuals, etc. 2. Nursing diagnosis—Handbooks,
manuals, etc.
  [DNLM: 1. Nursing Diagnosis—Handbooks. 2. Patient Care Planning—Handbooks.
WY 49 W686p 2005] I. Title: Nursing diagnosis handbook with NIC interventions and NOC
outcomes. II. Wilkinson, Judith M., Nursing diagnosis handbook with NIC interventions and
NOC outcomes. III. Title.
  RT49.W54 2005
  610.73—dc22

                                                                          2003027585

Publisher: Julie Levin Alexander
Executive Assistant & Supervisor:
  Regina Bruno
Editor-in-Chief: Maura Connor
Executive Editor: Barbara Krawiec
Editorial Assistants: Malgorzata
  Jaros-White and Jennifer Dwyer
Director of Manufacturing and Production:
  Bruce Johnson
Managing Editor: Patrick Walsh
Production Liaison: Cathy O'Connell
Production Editor: Penny Walker,
  The GTS Companies/York, PA Campus

Manufacturing Manager: Ilene Sanford
Manufacturing Buyer: Pat Brown
Creative Director: Cheryl Asherman
Senior Design Coordinator: Maria
  Guglielmo Walsh
Cover Designer: Mary Siener
Senior Marketing Manager: Nicole Benson
Channel Marketing Manager: Rachele Strober
Marketing Coordinator: Janet Ryerson
Composition: *The GTS Companies/*
  York, PA Campus
Printer/Binder: Banta/Harrisonburg
Cover Printer: Banta/Harrisonburg

Notice: Care has been taken to confirm the accuracy of information presented in this book.
The authors, editors, and the publisher, however, cannot accept any responsibility for errors
or omissions or for consequences from application of the information in this book and make
no warranty, express or implied, with respect to its contents.
    The authors and publisher have exerted every effort to ensure that drug selections and
dosages set forth in this text are in accord with current recommendations and practice at
time of publication. However, in view of ongoing research, changes in government regulations,
and the constant flow of information relating to drug therapy and drug reactions, the reader is
urged to check the package inserts of all drugs for any change in indications of dosage and for
added warnings and precautions. This is particularly important when the recommended
agent is a new and/or infrequently employed drug.

10 9 8 7 6 5 4 3
ISBN 0-13-049367-

CONTENTS

Plans of Care in Alphabetical Order   1–634

Each plan of care contains the following information:

Taxonomy number
Definition
Defining Characteristics
Related Factors
Risk Factors
Suggestions for Use
Suggested Alternative Diagnoses
NOC Outcomes
Goals/Evaluation Criteria (Examples of NOC and Other)
NIC Interventions
Nursing Activities (NIC and Other)

Clinical Conditions Guide to Nursing Diagnoses and Collaborative Problems   635

PREFACE

Prentice Hall Nursing Diagnosis Handbook with NIC Interventions and NOC Outcomes, 8th edition, is designed to help nurses and students develop individualized patient care plans. The new edition has been expanded to include all nursing diagnoses approved by the North American Nursing Diagnosis Association (NANDA International) for 2003–2004, as well as linkages to current Nursing Outcomes Classification (NOC) and Nursing Interventions Classification (NIC) research-based outcomes and interventions. NANDA International, NOC, and NIC standardized terminology is generally used under those designated headings; exceptions are enclosed in brackets [].

Features
NOC Suggested Outcomes

To facilitate use of a unified nursing language and computerized patient records, each nursing diagnosis lists the suggested outcomes found in *Nursing Diagnoses, Outcomes, & Interventions: NANDA International, NOC, and NIC Linkages* (Johnson, Bulechek, Dochterman, Maas, & Moorhead, 2001). These suggested outcomes are nurse-sensitive, that is, they may be influenced by the nursing care given for a particular NANDA International diagnosis. This text also demonstrates ways to use NOC outcomes, outcome indicators, and measuring scales to state patient goals.

Updated NIC Interventions

NIC interventions have been updated to reflect the continuing work of the Iowa Interventions Project. The interventions given and defined for each nursing diagnosis are those (1) designated by the Nursing Interventions Classification (McCloskey & Bulechek, 2000) as the treatments of choice for that diagnosis, or (2) associated with the outcomes listed in *NANDA International, NOC, and NIC Linkages* (Johnson et al., 2001) for that nursing diagnosis. NIC interventions were developed and linked to the NANDA International categories by a research team using a multimethod process that included the judgments of experts in nursing practice and research.

Inclusion of NIC Nursing Activities

In an effort to further promote use of standardized language, some of the Nursing Activities for each nursing diagnosis are written in NIC language. This helps to illustrate how the NIC activities, as well as the broader NIC interventions, can be used in care planning.

Inclusion of Family, Community, and Collaborative Content

More family- and community-oriented goals have also been included in the Goals/Evaluation Criteria Examples section. More collaborative, family, and community nursing interventions and activities have also been included.

Collaborative Problems

In the Clinical Conditions Guide to Nursing Diagnoses and Collaborative Problems section, each disease or medical condition includes the associated multidisciplinary (collaborative) problems. Appendices D, E, and F contain the most comprehensive listing of multidisciplinary problems available, organized for (1) diseases/pathophysiology, (2) tests and treatments, and (3) surgical treatments.

Other Features

Organized for Easy Use

The book is divided into two main parts: (1) Complete plans of care for each NANDA International nursing diagnosis; and (2) a list of medical, surgical, psychiatric, perinatal, and pediatric conditions, each accompanied by nursing diagnoses and collaborative problems commonly associated with those conditions. This organization allows the nurse to begin the care planning process with either a medical condition or a nursing diagnosis.

Suggestions for Using NANDA International Diagnoses

Author suggestions help to clarify the nursing diagnosis labels and to advise how they can best be used.

Organization of Defining Characteristics

These cues have been alphabetized and categorized as subjective or objective. NANDA International no longer designates major, minor, and critical defining characteristics.

Easy to Individualize

Each plan of care is comprehensive and allows nurses to select specific content according to the patient's condition and situation. Each nursing diagnosis includes related factors or risk factors that make it easy to individualize the care plan to the specific patient situation. Creative nurses will tailor standardized outcomes, interventions, and related and risk factors to meet the needs of each individual patient.

Assessment, Teaching, and Collaborative Nursing Activities

Nursing activities are grouped under the headings: Assessments, Patient/Family Teaching, Collaborative Activities, and Other. This makes it easier to locate a particular activity and helps assure that the nurse considers each type of activity.

Critical Paths

An up-to-date discussion of nursing diagnosis and critical paths is featured, along with an example of a format for a multidisciplinary care plan (critical path).

Care Planning Checklist

A checklist (see perforated flap on back cover) is provided to assist the practitioner in evaluating the finished care plan for completeness and suitability for the client.

Audience

This pocket guide is intended to facilitate care planning for nursing students, staff nurses in a variety of settings, clinical nurse specialists, and staff development instructors.

REVIEWERS

INTRODUCTION

Background

In 1973 the American Nurses Association (ANA) mandated the use of nursing diagnosis. That same year, clinicians, educators, researchers, and theorists from every area of nursing practice came together to offer labels for conditions they had observed in practice. From that beginning, the North American Nursing Diagnosis Association (now NANDA International) was established as the formal body for the promotion, review, and endorsement of the current list of nursing diagnoses used by practicing nurses. The NANDA International membership convenes every 2 years. The current list of more than 150 diagnoses (see inside back cover) will undoubtedly expand as nurses explore the breadth and depth of nursing practice.

As the list of nursing diagnoses expanded, NANDA International developed a classification system to organize them. The current taxonomy (Taxonomy II) is found in Appendix B. Work continues to address a number of issues (e.g., there is some overlapping among the diagnostic labels). NANDA International has been working with the ANA and other organizations to include the NANDA International labels in other classification systems, for example the World Health Organization International Classification of Diseases (ICD). NANDA International diagnosis-related articles are presently indexed in the Cumulative Index of Nursing and Allied Health (CINAHL) and in the National Library of Medicine Medical Metathesaurus for a Unified Medical Language.

The growing use of computerized patient records demands a standardized language for describing patient problems. Nursing diagnosis fulfills that need and helps define the scope of nursing practice by describing conditions the nurse can independently treat. Nursing diagnosis highlights critical thinking and decision making, and provides a consistent and universally understood terminology among nurses working in various settings, including hospitals, ambulatory care clinics, extended care facilities, occupational health facilities, and private practice.

Nursing Process in Relation to Nursing Diagnosis

The nursing process provides a structure for nursing practice—a framework in which nurses use knowledge and skills to express human caring. The nursing process is used continuously when planning and giving nursing care. The nurse considers the patient as the central figure in the plan of care and confirms the appropriateness of all aspects of nursing care by observing the patient's responses.

Assessment (also called data collection) is the initial step in the critical thinking and decision-making that leads to a nursing diagnosis. The nurse uses the definition and defining characteristics of the nursing diagnosis to validate the diagnosis. Once the nursing diagnosis and the related factors or risk factors are determined, the plan of care is created. The nurse selects the relevant patient outcomes, including the patient's perceptions and suggestions for the outcomes, if possible. The nurse next works with the patient to determine which activities will help achieve the stated outcomes. Finally, after implementing the nursing activities, the nurse evaluates the care plan and the patient's progress. Is the nursing diagnosis still appropriate? Has the patient achieved the desired goals? Are the documentation interval and the target date still appropriate and realistic? Are certain interventions no longer needed? The individualized plan of care is revised as needed.

Standards of Care in Relation to Nursing Diagnosis

Nursing diagnosis care planning and standards of care are interrelated. Standards of care are developed for groups of patients about whom generalized predictions can be made. These standards direct a set of common nursing interventions for specific patient groups (e.g., for all patients having a total hip replacement). Where there are written standards of care, nursing diagnosis care planning is not used to communicate routine nursing actions. Instead, it is used for those exceptional patient problems that are not addressed in the standards of care.

Case Management and Critical Paths

Escalating health care costs and the demand for health care reform have brought about a restructuring of traditional practice patterns. Two multidisciplinary clinical systems that have emerged are case management and managed care.

Case Management

Case management is a system in which health care professionals coordinate care for high-risk, complex patient populations. These are the unusual, uncommon cases seen in an agency—patients whose condition changes frequently and unpredictably, and whose needs cannot be addressed by a standardized plan or critical path. The case manager, often an advanced practice nurse, focuses on roles and relationships and provides a well-coordinated care experience for patients and families in all settings in which the patient receives care.

Critical Paths and Managed Care

Managed care is used to standardize practice for the common, most prevalent case types in an agency. For example, case types in a cardiac care unit might be myocardial infarction and cardiac catheterization. Managed care uses a tool called a critical path as a guide for achieving predictable client outcomes within a specified time frame. The critical path is a multidisciplinary plan of care that outlines crucial activities to be performed by nurses, physicians, and other health team members at designated times in order to achieve the desired patient outcomes (see the table on p. xxiv).

In managed care systems, the standardized critical path replaces the traditional nursing care plan for many clients. Some agencies have incorporated nursing diagnoses directly into the critical paths. Others use nursing diagnoses to name variances and develop an individualized plan for achieving revised outcomes. A variance occurs when desired outcomes are not achieved at the specified times.

Nursing Diagnosis Incorporated into Critical Path As an example, when incorporating a nursing diagnosis into a critical path for a client newly diagnosed with insulin-dependent diabetes, the following nursing diagnosis would be a part of the preprinted multidisciplinary care plan:

Ineffective therapeutic regimen management related to limited information and limited practice of skill, as evidenced by verbalization of limited knowledge, inaccurate follow-through of instruction, and inaccurate performance on tests.

Client goals might be that by day 3, the client will recognize signs and symptoms of hypo/hyperglycemia, and by day 5, be able to self-inject the required dose of insulin.

Nursing Diagnosis Used to Name Variance In this system, the critical path for a newly diagnosed insulin-dependent diabetic would not include a nursing diagnosis, but rather would list teaching needs for each day. On day 5, if the patient is unable to meet the outcome of self-injection, this variance would be identified and analyzed. At that point the nursing diagnosis of *Ineffective therapeutic regimen management* related to difficulty mastering psychomotor skill for injections would be used to individualize the nursing care for this patient's variance from the critical path.

Even in organizations using managed care, the nursing process is used to plan and deliver patient care via a multidisciplinary care plan, and nursing diagnoses are valuable in individualizing critical paths to meet unique, individual patient needs. It is vital that today's nurse be well versed in using nursing diagnoses in order to effectively identify and address nursing care issues within the multidisciplinary team.

COMPONENTS OF NURSING
DIAGNOSIS CARE PLANS

This book is organized into two parts: "Plans of Care" and "Clinical Conditions Guide to Nursing Diagnoses and Collaborative Problems." Information regarding these two parts, with some examples of how to use them, follows.

Plans of Care

Each plan of care includes a nursing diagnosis label, the label definition, defining characteristics, related factors or risk factors, suggestions for use, suggested alternative diagnoses, NOC outcomes, client goals, NIC priority interventions, and nursing activities. See the figure on p. xiv.

The nursing diagnosis care plans are organized alphabetically to make the labels easy to locate. The diagnoses are worded in order to set forth the key concept in the first word of the label. For example, *Ineffective denial* is easier to find in an index when it is written as *Denial, ineffective.*

Nursing Diagnosis

The nursing diagnosis is a concise label that describes patient conditions observed in practice. These conditions may be actual or potential problems. Using NANDA International terminology, potential problems are labeled Risk for. Appendix C contains a list of axis descriptors (previously called diagnosis qualifiers) that are used in many of the diagnostic labels (e.g., acute, altered, impaired). Add other qualifying words as needed to make diagnoses precise and descriptive.

Definition

The definition for each nursing diagnosis helps the nurse verify a particular nursing diagnosis. Unless otherwise specified, the definitions in this text were taken from the NANDA International taxonomy.

Defining Characteristics

Defining characteristics are cues that describe patient behavior, either observed by the nurse (objective) or verbalized by the patient and family (subjective). After assessing the patient, nurses organize the defining characteristics into meaningful patterns that alert them to the possibility of a patient problem. Usually, the presence of two or three defining characteristics verifies a nursing diagnosis.

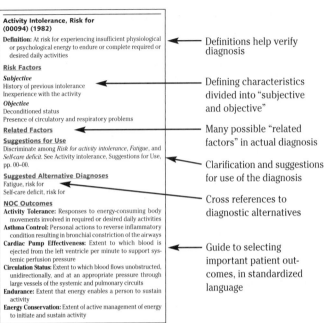

**Activity Intolerance, Risk for
(00094) (1982)**

Definition: At risk for experiencing insufficient physiological
or psychological energy to endure or complete required or
desired daily activities ◀—— Definitions help verify
diagnosis

Risk Factors

Subjective
History of previous intolerance ◀—— Defining characteristics
Inexperience with the activity divided into "subjective
Objective and objective"
Deconditioned status
Presence of circulatory and respiratory problems

Related Factors ◀—— Many possible "related
factors" in actual diagnosis

Suggestions for Use
Discriminate among *Risk for activity intolerance*, *Fatigue*, and
Self-care deficit. See Activity intolerance, Suggestions for Use, ◀—— Clarification and suggestions
pp. 00–00. for use of the diagnosis

Suggested Alternative Diagnoses
Fatigue, risk for
Self-care deficit, risk for ◀—— Cross references to
diagnostic alternatives

NOC Outcomes
Activity Tolerance: Responses to energy-consuming body
movements involved in required or desired daily activities
Asthma Control: Personal actions to reverse inflammatory
condition resulting in bronchial constriction of the airways
Cardiac Pump Effectiveness: Extent to which blood is ◀—— Guide to selecting
ejected from the left ventricle per minute to support sys- important patient out-
temic perfusion pressure comes, in standardized
Circulation Status: Extent to which blood flows unobstructed, language
unidirectionally, and at an appropriate pressure through
large vessels of the systemic and pulmonary circuits
Endurance: Extent that energy enables a person to sustain
activity
Energy Conservation: Extent of active management of energy
to initiate and sustain activity

Goal statements ——▶ **Goals/Evaluation Criteria**
measure progress **Examples Using NOC Language**
• Tolerates usual activity, as demonstrated by: Activity Tolerance, Endurance, Energy Conservation, and Self-Care: ADLs
(and IADLs)
• Demonstrates **Energy Conservation**, as evidenced by the
following indicators (specify 1–5: not at all, to a slight,
moderate, great, or very great extent):
Recognizes energy limitations
Balances activity and rest
Endurance level adequate for activity

Other Examples
Patient will:
• Identify activities or anxiety-producing situations that may
contribute to *Activity intolerance*
• Participate in necessary physical activity with appropriate
increases in heart rate, respiratory rate, and blood pres-
sure, and monitor such patterns within normal limits
• Report freedom from dyspnea, difficulty breathing, and
fatigue with daily activities
• Make lifestyle changes necessary to conserve energy

Guide to selecting the ——▶ **NIC Interventions**
most important nursing **Emotional Support:** Provision of reassurance, acceptance,
interventions in and encouragement during times of stress
standardized language **Energy Management:** Regulation of energy use to treat or
prevent fatigue and optimize function
Exercise Promotion: Strength Training: Facilitating regular
resistive muscle training to maintain or increase muscle
strength

Nursing Activities
Assessments
• Determine the knowledge and recognition of energy limitations by client and significant other
Select from many nursing ——▶ • Monitor energy level and tolerance for activity
activities that help patient • Identify the obstacles to activity
achieve outcomes • Refer to the Activity intolerance diagnosis, p. 00 for other
assessments

Patient/Family Teaching
• Develop a realistic plan for adapting to patient's limitations
• Explore with patient the specific consequences of inactivity
• Instruct patient and family to notify primary care provider
if fatigue is persistent

In this text, all NANDA International defining characteristics have been included. NANDA International no longer designates defining characteristics as major, minor, and critical. This simplification was made in order to support: (1) the development of electronic nursing diagnosis databases, (2) diagnosis development, and (3) classification work.

Related Factors

The related factors imply a connection with the nursing diagnosis. Such factors may be described as related to, antecedent to, associated with, or contributing to the diagnosis. Related factors indicate what should change for the patient to return to optimal health, and therefore help the nurse to select effective nursing interventions. As an example, for the diagnosis *Activity intolerance*, the nursing activities for a patient whose related factor is arrhythmias would be quite different from those needed for a patient whose related factor is chronic pain.

Risk Factors

Risk factors will be found only in the "risk for" (potential) nursing diagnoses. The risk factors are similar to related factors and defining characteristics in the development of the care plan. They describe events and behaviors that put the patient at risk and suggest interventions to protect the patient. As an example, an elderly patient might be diagnosed with *Risk for trauma*, and exhibit the following risk factors: weakness, poor vision, balancing difficulties, slippery floors, and unanchored rugs. As an etiology, this cluster of risk factors suggests the need for interventions to prevent falls.

Suggestions for Use

For problematic labels, clarifying comments are included, along with suggestions for using the diagnosis appropriately or differentiating it from similar diagnoses.

Suggested Alternative Diagnoses

Suggested alternative diagnoses are other nursing diagnoses that may be considered when identifying the patient's problem. If a review of the definition and defining characteristics indicates that they only partially match the patient data, the nurse may consider the suggested alternative diagnoses as options. This is particularly helpful for the nurse unfamiliar with the nuances of each nursing diagnosis.

NOC Outcomes

For each NANDA International diagnosis, this text lists the NOC outcomes links that have been recognized by the ANA (Johnson et al., 2001). NOC outcomes are neutral concepts reflecting patient states or behaviors (e.g., memory, coping, rest). These nurse-sensitive patient outcomes are not goals, but the nurse can use them along with their indicators to set goals for a specific patient. Indicators are more specific behaviors that are used to measure or rate the patient outcome.

Goals/Evaluation Criteria

Each nursing diagnosis also includes examples of patient goals/evaluation criteria that were developed by using NOC outcomes, outcome indicators, and measuring scales. Goals are statements of patient and family behaviors that are measurable or observable. For example, to evaluate a client outcome of Cognitive Orientation, the nurse might use these indicators:

Identifies self (often)
Identifies significant other (sometimes)
Identifies current place (often)

Use as few or as many patient outcomes and sample goals as necessary. If more are needed, refer to the *Nursing Outcomes Classification (NOC)* manual (Johnson, Maas, & Moorhead, 2000).

Patient goals, like all components of the care planning process, are dynamic. Therefore, they change frequently. Specific, individualized patient goal statements are critical because they are used to evaluate patient responses to care and the success of the nursing care plan.

The nurse should be realistic when constructing patient goal statements, because partial behavior change may be the only attainable goal. With shortened length of hospital stay, nurses in the community setting may help patients to achieve goals and outcomes after they are discharged from the hospital. At time of discharge, the nurse may initiate discussion with the patient to determine patient and family goals still requiring completion, with referral to appropriate community resources.

Always specify a target date and documentation interval for patient goals. The target date is the estimated date by which the outcome will be accomplished. The date is flexible and individualized to the patient. The documentation interval designates how often documentation should occur for each outcome. This interval should be determined during initial assessment and may be changed as patient nears completion of a goal. For example, in the care plan for *Fatigue,* the documentation interval for the goal, "Maintains adequate nutrition" could be specified as t.i.d. This would mean that documentation must occur at least three times daily, after meals, until the outcome is accomplished.

NIC Interventions

This text lists NIC interventions from two sources:

1. *NIC Priority Interventions*—NIC categorizes nursing activities using standardized language. Priority interventions are the research-based interventions developed by the Iowa Intervention Project team as the treatments of choice for a particular nursing diagnosis (NIC, 2000). They are the most obvious interventions to effect resolution *of a nursing particular diagnosis*, but this does not mean that they are the only interventions to be used. The priority interventions are shaded in this text.

2. *NIC Major Interventions*—These are the interventions found in *Nursing Diagnoses, Outcomes, & Interventions: NANDA International, NOC, and NIC Linkages* (Johnson et al., 2001). In that book, NOC outcomes were linked to nursing diagnoses, and then NIC interventions were linked to the NOC outcomes. The major interventions are the most obvious interventions for achieving *a particular outcome* and should be considered first (Johnson et al., 2001).

A variety of interventions should always be considered. In NIC terminology, *interventions* are broad, general category labels. These category labels were linked to the NANDA International diagnosis labels through a systematic process drawing upon the judgments of experts in nursing practice and research. They were linked to NOC outcomes using expert opinion and in some instances nursing literature.

Nursing Activities

In NIC terminology, the specific, detailed actions taken by the nurse (e.g., taking vital signs, monitoring intake and output) are called activities. The NIC Priority and Major Interventions direct the nurse to review first the nursing activities related to those interventions. Other specific nursing activities can be found in the *NIC* handbook (McCloskey & Bulechek, 2000). Following is an example of how the NIC priority interventions can guide care planning for the nursing diagnosis *Fatigue:*

1. In the care plan for *Fatigue,* note that the NIC Priority Intervention is Energy Management. The definition of this intervention is shown as: "regulating energy use to treat or prevent fatigue and optimize function."

2. Look in the Nursing Activities section for the specific activities that would accomplish Energy Management—that is, those that specifically focus on regulating energy and treating or preventing fatigue, such as the following examples:

- Plan activities with patient and family that minimize fatigue. Plan may include setting small, realistic, attainable goals for patient that decrease fatigue.
- Encourage patient to report activities that increase fatigue.
- Discuss with patient and family ways to modify home environment to maintain usual activities and to minimize fatigue.
- Teach organization and time management techniques to reduce fatigue (NIC).

3. Finally, review the rest of the nursing activities for *Fatigue*. There may be activities in addition to those for Energy Management that would be helpful, depending on the client's problem etiologies and individual needs.

You will be able to find effective nursing activities to deal with your patient's fatigue by using Steps 1, 2, and 3. However, you may wish to compare your chosen nursing actions to the research-based interventions and activities listed in the 2000 *NIC* handbook (McCloskey & Bulechek, 2000). In the NIC handbook under the intervention label Energy Management, there are other specific nursing activities that accomplish Energy Management. Following are three examples:

- Plan activities for periods when the patient has the most energy
- Encourage an afternoon nap, if appropriate
- Assist patient to schedule rest periods

In addition to the Priority Interventions, the NIC handbook lists other nursing interventions to address *Fatigue,* for example, Exercise Promotion and Sleep Enhancement. The nursing activities for those interventions might also be used.

Nursing orders and activities should address the etiology of the patient's nursing diagnosis. From the activities listed for each care plan, choose those that apply to the patient's condition. Alter standardized nursing activities to make them specific to the patient. In certain instances, "q ___" or "specify plan" is included in the nursing activity as a reminder to individualize the nursing orders. As the patient's condition changes, other activities may be added, changed, or deleted. Frequent updating of this portion of the care plan is essential.

Clinical Conditions Guide to Nursing Diagnoses and Collaborative Problems

The second part of this handbook is organized to help nurses focus their assessments when the patient's medical condition is known but the appropriate nursing diagnoses have not yet been established. In this section, medical, surgical, psychiatric, perinatal, and pediatric conditions are listed with associated collaborative problems and nursing diagnoses.

Nursing Diagnoses

The nursing diagnoses listed are those that most logically occur when the particular medical condition is present. Of course, a patient with one of the medical conditions will not have all of the nursing diagnoses listed. Select only those nursing diagnoses that are confirmed by assessment data. Furthermore, these lists should not be considered exhaustive. It is quite possible that a client with a particular medical condition will have nursing diagnoses that are not on the list. Because they represent unique human responses, nursing diagnoses cannot be predicted on the basis of medical condition alone.

Multidisciplinary (Collaborative) Problems

Multidisciplinary problems, on the other hand, are associated with specific medical conditions. According to Carpenito (1997b), collaborative problems are the physiological complications, associated with a particular medical condition, that nurses cannot treat independently. The nurse's responsibility is to monitor the patient in order to detect the onset of collaborative problems, and to use both physician- and nursing-prescribed interventions to prevent or minimize the complication. Because there are a limited number of physiological complications possible for a particular disease, the same collaborative problems tend to be present any time a particular disease or treatment is present; that is, each disease or treatment has particular complications that are always associated with it.

Before making an individualized nursing diagnosis care plan, the nurse should identify the patient's collaborative problems. These will guide the common assessments and preventive care that all patients with that medical diagnosis should receive, much like a critical pathway. Collaborative problems are included for each condition listed in the Clinical Conditions Guide to Nursing Diagnoses and Collaborative Problems beginning on page 635. Also refer to Appendix D, Multidisciplinary (Collaborative) Problems Associated with Diseases and Other Physiologic Disorders; Appendix E, Multidisciplinary (Collaborative) Problems Associated with Tests and Treatments; and Appendix F, Multidisciplinary (Collaborative) Problems Associated with Surgical Treatments, on pp. 753–762, 763, and 764–765, respectively.

The list of clinical conditions does not include rare disease conditions, so for unusual diseases it may be necessary to refer to a more general title. For example, the patient's medical diagnosis may be scleroderma. Since this condition occurs infrequently, the nurse should look under the general title Autoimmune Disorders and review the nursing diagnoses listed there.

HOW TO CREATE A NURSING DIAGNOSIS CARE PLAN

The following example shows how to use this book to create an individualized care plan for a patient.

Situation: Mrs. B, a 75-year-old female, has been admitted to a surgical unit from the recovery room following a hip pinning. Her history indicates that Mrs. B lives alone in an apartment. Her husband died 10 years ago. She has many friends and is involved in community affairs at the local senior center. She loves to walk and to ride a bicycle. Her current hospital admission is a result of falling off her bicycle. Mrs. B's postoperative medical orders include the following:

Foley catheter to gravity drainage

$D_5 2\%$ NaCl with KCl 20 mEq to be infused over 8 hr

Morphine sulfate 1–2 mg, IV push, q15 minutes until comfortable to a maximum of 10 mg in 1 hr

Morphine sulfate 6–8 mg, IM q3–4h, prn pain

Phenergan 25 mg IM q4–6h, prn nausea

CBC and electrolytes tomorrow in a.m.

Overhead trapeze to bed

Turn patient from back to unaffected side q1–2h

Pressure-reducing mattress overlay to bed to relieve pressure to bony prominences

Ambulate with assistance in am and then qid

Assessment

4:00 pm—The nurse's initial assessment following return from the recovery room indicates that the patient is sleeping comfortably, vital signs are within normal limits, and the operative dressing is dry and intact. Foley catheter is draining clear, amber urine. The IV is infusing at the prescribed rate; skin is warm and dry.

5:30 pm—The nurse enters Mrs. B's room to check her vital signs and finds Mrs. B attempting to climb out of bed "because I have to go to the bathroom." The nurse reminds Mrs. B that she is in the hospital and has a Foley catheter in place. Mrs. B's responses indicate that she is disoriented to place and time.

Diagnosis

From her assessment of Mrs. B., the nurse identifies the cues of altered mobility, disorientation, pain medication, and change in environment. These seem to match the defining characteristics for a nursing diagnosis of *Risk for injury*. In this book the definition of *Risk for injury* is "a state in which the individual is at risk of injury as a result of environmental conditions interacting with the individual's adaptive and defensive resources." The nurse considers suggested alternative diagnoses to see if a better diagnosis can be found. She looks at the definition and defining characteristics for *Disturbed Sensory Perception, Ineffective tissue perfusion, Risk for trauma,* and *Risk for impaired skin integrity.* After reviewing the alternatives, the nurse decides to use the broad nursing diagnosis, *Risk for injury* related to altered mobility, disorientation, pain medication, and change in environment.

NOC Outcomes

In order to focus her goal statements, the nurse begins with the NOC Suggested Outcomes for *Risk for injury:* Parenting (Social Safety), Risk Control, and Safety Behavior (Fall Prevention). After reading the outcome definitions and referring to the *NOC* handbook, the nurse determines that Safety Behavior (Fall Prevention) is probably the only outcome needed for Mrs. B's care plan.

Goals/Evaluation Criteria

Goals: The nurse chooses and modifies the following goals from the listed sample goals and NOC indicators:

Use of restraints as needed (totally adequate)

Agitation and restlessness controlled (moderately adequate)

Patient will avoid physical injury (totally adequate)

The goals are observable and appropriate for Mrs. B's situation. The documentation interval for the goals could be q4h, and the target date could be 1–2 days after surgery, except for the last goal, for which it should be "at all times." The target date should be stated as an actual date (e.g., 1/30). The documentation interval and target date should be reviewed at least daily to evaluate appropriateness.

Evaluation: The nurse would collect data about the first two goals in order to evaluate progress in controlling Mrs. B.'s risk factors. Status of the last goal will indicate whether interventions were successful in preventing the potential problem, Risk for injury.

Nursing Interventions and Activities

Next, the nurse selects nursing interventions. The NIC interventions are: Electronic Fetal Monitoring, Fall Prevention, Labor Induction, Latex Precautions, and Malignant Hyperthermia Precautions. The nurse determines that only Fall Prevention applies to Mrs. B.

The NIC interventions provide direction for choosing nursing activities, but they are general. In order to write individualized nursing orders for Mrs. B., the nurse selects the following from the list of nursing activities:

> Identify characteristics of the environment that may increase potential for falls (NIC).
>
> Reorient patient to reality and immediate environment when necessary.
>
> Place articles within easy reach of patient (NIC).
>
> Provide the dependent patient with a means of summoning help (e.g., bell or call light) when caregiver is not present (NIC).

The listed activities are adequate to address Mrs. B's problem for the present. If they were not, the nurse would have referred to the *NIC* manual for interventions in addition to the priority and major interventions (e.g., Surveillance or Physical Restraint).

All of the aforementioned nursing orders could be part of Mrs. B's care plan. Once an intervention or activity is no longer applicable, the nurse deletes it from the care plan. New activities should be added as needed. This example demonstrates the process used to develop a care plan for one nursing diagnosis. Other nursing diagnoses might also be appropriate for Mrs. B.

Creating a Critical Path

Explained very simply, creating a critical path is a matter of combining the care plans from nursing, medical, and other services, and imposing a timeline upon the combined plan. All care and treatments are shown on the plan, and care is organized by days, weeks, or even hours and minutes, for example:

Day 1	Day 2	Day 3
Outcomes	Outcomes	Outcomes
Nursing orders	Nursing orders	Nursing orders
Medical orders	Medical orders	Medical orders

The timeline of a critical path is different for each institution, depending on the patient population. In some hospitals a hernia repair might mean an overnight stay (and therefore a two-day critical path); in others it might be an outpatient procedure, with the critical path broken up into hourly segments. Therefore, standardized times cannot be given for the interventions on the nursing diagnosis care plans in this book. However, the care plans can be used when creating critical paths, the same as they are used in creating nursing diagnosis care plans.

1. Determine the nursing diagnoses your patient population (e.g., herniorrhaphy patients) typically has pre- and postoperatively—or on day 1, day 2, and so forth. Refer to the Clinical Conditions Guide to Nursing Diagnoses and Collaborative Problems for ideas as needed.

2. Choose patient goals and nursing activities for each day (or hour), just as you would for a traditional nursing care plan. The difference is that instead of a single care plan for a nursing diagnosis, you will have, essentially, a care plan for each day of the patient's stay in the institution. Refer to the following table.

Critical Pathways for Client Following Laparoscopic Cholecystectomy

	Date _____ PREOPERATIVE	Date _____ 1st 24 hr following surgery
Daily outcomes	Client will verbalize understanding of preoperative teaching, including turning ...	Client will • Be afebrile • Have a dry, clean wound with well-approximated. . .
Tests and treatments	CBC Urinalysis Baseline physical assessment	Vital signs and O_2 saturation, neurovascular assessment, dressing, and ...
Knowledge deficit	Orient to room and surroundings. Include family in teaching	Reorient to room and postoperative routine, include family in teaching
Psychosocial	Assess anxiety related to pending surgery	Assess level of anxiety Encourage verbalization ...
Diet	NPO Baseline nutritional assessment	Advance to clear liquids ...
Activity	OOB ad lib until premedicated for surgery	Provide safety precautions Bathroom privileges ...
Medications	NPO except ordered medications	IM or PO analgesics Antibiotics if ordered
Transfer/ discharge plans	Assess discharge plans and support system	Probable discharge within 24 hr of surgery

Nursing Diagnoses— with Outcomes and Interventions

Diagnosis labels, definitions, and defining characteristics are based primarily on the NANDA International taxonomy. The first number following the label is the number of the diagnosis in the NANDA International taxonomy. The second number indicates the year the diagnosis was accepted or revised. Suggested alternative diagnoses are provided for most labels. Consider those if a label does not fit the patient data satisfactorily. The author's discussion and recommendations for using certain diagnoses are identified by the heading Suggestions for Use.

Individualizing Client Goals/Evaluation Criteria

NOC Outcomes and indicators presented under Goals/Evaluation Criteria are quoted verbatim from the Nursing Outcomes Classification (NOC). To help you create goals using standardized language, examples of such goals are given. To individualize these and the Other Examples provided in the text, add patient-specific target dates and evaluation and documentation intervals. If you do not find goals appropriate to your patient, refer to the NOC manual for outcome indicators and scales to develop other goals, as needed. To save space, some indicators have been combined into one goal; however, NOC lists them separately, and they must be evaluated separately.

Individualizing Nursing Activities

NIC Interventions are quoted verbatim from the Nursing Interventions Classification (NIC). The shaded interventions are NIC Priority Interventions for the diagnosis. Selected nursing activities are also written in standardized language. Choose only those activities that address patient problems and etiologies. Individualize nursing activities to meet the unique needs of each patient (e.g., by adding times of and frequencies for nursing activities, including more specific details). If you do not find the exact activities you need, refer to the NIC manual for other interventions and activities.

ACTIVITY INTOLERANCE
(00092) (1982)

Definition: Insufficient physiological or psychological energy to endure or complete required or desired daily activities

Defining Characteristics
Subjective
Exertional discomfort or dyspnea
Verbal report of fatigue or weakness
Objective
Abnormal heart rate or blood pressure in response to activity
ECG changes reflecting arrhythmia or ischemia

Related Factors
Bed rest and immobility
Generalized weakness
Imbalance between oxygen supply and demand
Sedentary lifestyle
NOTE: The preceding factors are from NANDA International. They are secondary to a wide variety of pathophysiologies, including cardiac disease (e.g., congestive heart failure), respiratory disease (e.g., emphysema), renal disease, cancer, anemia, obesity, and infections (e.g., mononucleosis).

Suggestions for Use
Do not use this label unless it is possible to increase the patient's endurance. Use *Activity intolerance* only if the patient reports fatigue or weakness in response to activity. Medical conditions (e.g., heart disease or peripheral arterial disease) often cause *Activity intolerance*. The nurse cannot independently treat medical conditions, so a diagnostic statement such as "*Activity intolerance* related to coronary artery disease" is not useful.

Activity intolerance often creates other problems, such as *Self-care deficit*, *Social isolation*, or *Ineffective breastfeeding*, and you can use it most effectively as the etiology of these other problems. Specify *Activity intolerance* by levels of endurance, as follows (Gordon, 1994, p. 110):

Level I: Walks regular pace on level ground but becomes more short of breath than normal when climbing one or more flights of stairs

Level II: Walks one city block 500 feet on level or climbs one flight of stairs slowly without stopping

Level III: Walks no more than 50 feet on level without stopping and is unable to climb one flight of stairs without stopping

Level IV: Dyspnea and fatigue at rest

The following is an example of such a diagnostic statement: *Self-care deficit (total)* related to Activity intolerance (Level IV).

Suggested Alternative Diagnoses

Fatigue (Activity intolerance is relieved by rest. Fatigue is not.)
Self-care deficit

NOC Outcomes

Activity Tolerance: Responses to energy-consuming body movements involved in required or desired daily activities

Endurance: Extent that energy enables a person to sustain activity

Energy Conservation: Extent of active management of energy to initiate and sustain activity

Self-Care: Activities of Daily Living (ADLs): Ability to perform the most basic physical tasks and personal care activities

Self-Care: Instrumental Activities of Daily Living (IADLs): Ability to perform activities needed to function in the home or community

Goals/Evaluation Criteria

Examples Using NOC Language

- Tolerates usual activity, as demonstrated by Activity Tolerance, Endurance, Energy Conservation, and Self-Care: ADLs (and IADLs)
- Demonstrates **Activity Tolerance**, as evidenced by the following indicators (specify 1–5: extremely compromised to not compromised):
    Oxygen saturation in expected range (IER) in response to activity
    Respiratory effort in response to activity
    Ability to speak while exercising
- Demonstrates **Energy Conservation**, as evidenced by the following indicators (specify 1–5: not at all, to a slight, moderate, great, or very great extent):
    Recognizes energy limitations
    Balances activity and rest
    Endurance level adequate for activity

Other Examples

Patient will:
- Identify activities or anxiety-producing situations that may contribute to activity intolerance

- Participate in necessary physical activity with appropriate increases in heart rate, respiratory rate, and blood pressure, and monitor patterns within normal limits
- Verbalize understanding of need for oxygen, medications, and/or equipment that may increase tolerance for activities
- Perform ADLs with some assistance (e.g., toilets with help ambulating to bathroom)
- Perform home maintenance management with some help (e.g., needs weekly cleaning help)

NIC Interventions

Activity Therapy: Prescription of and assistance with specific physical, cognitive, social, and spiritual activities to increase the range, frequency, or duration of an individual's (or group's) activity

Energy Management: Regulating energy use to treat or prevent fatigue and optimize function

Exercise Promotion: Strength Training: Facilitating regular resistive muscle training to maintain or increase muscle strength

Home Maintenance Assistance: Helping the Patient and Family to maintain the home as a clean, safe, and pleasant place to live

Nutrition Management: Assisting with or providing a balanced dietary intake of foods and fluids

Self-Care Assistance: Assisting another to perform ADLs

Nursing Activities

Assessments

- Assess emotional, social, and spiritual response to activity
- Evaluate patient's motivation and desire to increase activity
- *(NIC) Energy Management:*
  Determine causes of fatigue (e.g., treatments, pain, and medications)
  Monitor cardiorespiratory response to activity (e.g., tachycardia, other dysrhythmias, dyspnea, diaphoresis, pallor, hemodynamic pressures, and respiratory rate)
  Monitor patient's oxygen response (e.g., pulse rate, cardiac rhythm, and respiratory rate) to self-care activities
  Monitor nutritional intake to ensure adequate energy resources
  Monitor and record patient's sleep pattern and number of sleep hours

Patient/Family Teaching

Instruct patient and family in:

- Use of equipment, such as oxygen, during activities
- Use of relaxation techniques (e.g., distraction, visualization) during activities
- *(NIC) Energy Management:*

  Teach patient and significant other techniques of self-care that will minimize oxygen consumption (e.g., self-monitoring and pacing techniques for performance of ADLs)

  Teach activity organization and time management techniques to prevent fatigue

Collaborative Activities

- Administer pain medications prior to activity
- Collaborate with occupational, physical, or recreational therapists to plan and monitor an activity program, as appropriate
- Refer to home health to obtain services of a home care aide, as needed
- Refer to dietitian for meal planning to increase intake of high-energy foods

Other

- Avoid scheduling care activities during rest periods
- Help patient to change position gradually, dangle, sit, stand, and ambulate, as tolerated
- Plan activities with patient and family that promote independence and endurance, for example:

  Encourage alternate periods of rest and activity

  Keep frequently used objects within easy reach

  Provide positive reinforcement for increased activity

  Set small, realistic, attainable goals for patient that increase independence and self-esteem
- Plan care for the infant or child to minimize the oxygen needs of the body:

  Anticipate needs for food, water, comfort, holding, and stimulation, to prevent unnecessary crying

  Avoid environments low in oxygen concentration (e.g., high altitudes, unpressurized airplanes)

  Minimize anxiety and stress

  Prevent hyperthermia and hypothermia

  Prevent infection

  Provide adequate rest

- *(NIC) Energy Management:*
  Assist patient to identify preferences for activity

  Plan activities for periods when the patient has the most energy

  Assist with regular physical activities (e.g., ambulation, transfers, turning, and personal care), as needed

  Limit environmental stimuli (e.g., light and noise) to facilitate relaxation

  Assist patient to self-monitor by developing and using a written record of calorie intake and energy expenditure, as appropriate

---

ACTIVITY INTOLERANCE, RISK FOR
(00094) (1982)

Definition: At risk for experiencing insufficient physiological or psychological energy to endure or complete required or desired daily activities

Risk Factors
Subjective
History of previous intolerance
Inexperience with the activity
Objective
Deconditioned status
Presence of circulatory and respiratory problems

Suggestions for Use
Discriminate among *Risk for activity intolerance*, *Fatigue*, and *Self-care deficit*. See Activity intolerance, Suggestions for Use, pp. 2–3.

Suggested Alternative Diagnoses
Fatigue, risk for
Self-care deficit, risk for

NOC Outcomes
Activity Tolerance: Responses to energy-consuming body movements involved in required or desired daily activities

Asthma Control: Personal actions to reverse inflammatory condition resulting in bronchial constriction of the airways

Cardiac Pump Effectiveness: Extent to which blood is ejected from the left ventricle per minute to support systemic perfusion pressure

Circulation Status: Extent to which blood flows unobstructed, unidirectionally, and at an appropriate pressure through large vessels of the systemic and pulmonary circuits

Endurance: Extent that energy enables a person to sustain activity

Energy Conservation: Extent of active management of energy to initiate and sustain activity

Immobility Consequences: Physiological: Extent of compromise in physiological functioning due to impaired physical mobility

Knowledge: Prescribed Activity: Extent of understanding conveyed about prescribed activity and exercise

Nutritional Status: Energy: Extent to which nutrients provide cellular energy

Pain Level: Severity of reported or demonstrated pain

Respiratory Status: Gas Exchange: Alveolar exchange of CO_2 or O_2 to maintain arterial blood gas concentrations

Respiratory Status: Ventilation: Movement of air in and out of the lungs

Goals/Evaluation Criteria

Examples Using NOC Language

- Tolerates usual activity, as demonstrated by: Activity Tolerance, Endurance, Energy Conservation, and Self-Care: ADLs (and IADLs)
- Demonstrates **Energy Conservation**, as evidenced by the following indicators (specify 1–5: not at all, to a slight, moderate, great, or very great extent):
    Recognizes energy limitations
    Balances activity and rest
    Endurance level adequate for activity

Other Examples

    Patient will:
- Identify activities or anxiety-producing situations that may contribute to *Activity intolerance*
- Participate in necessary physical activity with appropriate increases in heart rate, respiratory rate, and blood pressure, and monitor such patterns within normal limits
- Report freedom from dyspnea, difficulty breathing, and fatigue with daily activities
- Make lifestyle changes necessary to conserve energy

NIC Interventions

Emotional Support: Provision of reassurance, acceptance, and encouragement during times of stress

Energy Management: Regulation of energy use to treat or prevent fatigue and optimize function

Exercise Promotion: Strength Training: Facilitating regular resistive muscle training to maintain or increase muscle strength

Nursing Activities

Assessments

- Determine the knowledge and recognition of energy limitations by client and significant other
- Monitor energy level and tolerance for activity
- Identify the obstacles to activity
- Refer to the Activity intolerance diagnosis, p. 4 for other assessments

Patient/Family Teaching

- Develop a realistic plan for adapting to patient's limitations
- Explore with patient the specific consequences of inactivity
- Instruct patient and family to notify primary care provider if fatigue is persistent
- *(NIC) Energy Management:*

  Teach patient and significant other techniques of self-care that will minimize oxygen consumption (e.g., self-monitoring and pacing techniques for performance of ADLs)

  Teach activity organization and time management techniques to prevent fatigue

Other

- Enlist family in efforts to support and encourage the patient's completion of activities
- Provide decision-making (and other) support during periods of illness or high stress

---

ADAPTIVE CAPACITY: INTRACRANIAL, DECREASED (00049) (1994)

Definition: Intracranial fluid dynamic mechanisms that normally compensate for increases in intracranial volumes are compromised, resulting in repeated disproportionate increases in intracranial pressure (ICP) in response to a variety of noxious and non-noxious stimuli.

Defining Characteristics

Objective

Baseline ICP $\geq$ 10 mmHg

Disproportionate increase in ICP following single environmental or nursing maneuver stimulus

Elevated P_2 ICP waveform

Repeated increases in ICP of $>$ 10 mmHg for more than 5 min following any of a variety of external stimuli

Volume-pressure response test variation (volume-pressure ratio $>$ 2, pressure-volume index $<$ 10)

Wide-amplitude ICP waveform

Related Factors

Brain injuries

Decreased cerebral perfusion pressure $\leq$ 50–60 mmHg

Sustained increase in ICP $\geq$ 10–15 mmHg

Systemic hypotension with intracranial hypertension

Suggestions for Use

This diagnosis requires both medical and nursing interventions. Most of the nursing care will be dictated by agency protocols. Therefore, this diagnosis may be better stated as a collaborative problem (Potential Complication of head injury: Increased ICP).

Suggested Alternative Diagnoses

Tissue perfusion, ineffective (cerebral)

NOC Outcomes

Electrolyte and Acid–Base Balance: Balance of electrolytes and nonelectrolytes in the intracellular and extracellular compartments of the body

Fluid Balance: Balance of water in the intracellular and extracellular compartments of the body

Neurological Status: Extent to which the peripheral and central nervous systems receive, process, and respond to internal and external stimuli

Neurological Status: Consciousness: Extent to which an individual arouses, orients, and attends to the environment

Goals/Evaluation Criteria

NOTE: The following outcomes cannot be produced by independent nursing activities.

Examples Using NOC Language

- Demonstrates increased *Intracranial adaptive capacity*, as demonstrated by Electrolyte and Acid–Base Balance, Fluid Balance, Neurological Status, and Neurological Status: Consciousness
- Demonstrates **Neurological Status**, as evidenced by the following indicators (specify 1–5: extremely, substantially, moderately, mildly, or not compromised):
    - Pupil size and reactivity
    - Seizure activity not present
    - Headaches not present
    - Breathing pattern
    - Neurological status: consciousness
    - Neurological status: cranial sensory/motor function
    - Neurological status: autonomic

Other Examples

- Cerebral perfusion pressure will be ≥ 70 mmHg (in adults)
- ICP will stabilize at four or less episodes of abnormal waveforms in 24 hr

NIC Interventions

Cerebral Edema Management: Limitation of secondary cerebral injury resulting from swelling of brain tissue

Cerebral Perfusion Promotion: Promotion of adequate perfusion and limitation of complications for a patient experiencing or at risk for inadequate cerebral perfusion

Electrolyte Management: Promotion of electrolyte balance and prevention of complications resulting from abnormal or undesired serum electrolyte levels

Fluid-Electrolyte Management: Regulation and prevention of complications from altered fluid or electrolyte levels

Intracranial Pressure (ICP) Monitoring: Measurement and interpretation of patient data to regulate ICP

Neurologic Monitoring: Collection and analysis of patient data to prevent or minimize neurologic complications

Nursing Activities

Assessments

- Monitor ICP and cerebral perfusion pressure (CPP) continuously with alarm settings on
- Monitor neurologic status at regular intervals (e.g., vital signs; pupil size, shape, reaction to light, equality; consciousness/mental

status; response to painful stimuli; ability to follow commands; symmetry of motor response; reflexes such as Babinski, blink, cough, gag)

- Note events that trigger changes in the ICP waveform (e.g., position change, suctioning)
- Determine baseline for vital signs and cardiac rhythm, and monitor for changes during and after activity
- *(NIC) Intracranial Pressure (ICP) Monitoring:*
  Monitor pressure tubing for bubbles
  Monitor amount and rate of cerebrospinal fluid drainage
  Monitor intake and output
  Monitor insertion site for infection
  Monitor temperature and WBC count
  Check patient for nuchal rigidity

Patient/Family Teaching

- Teach caregiver about signs that will indicate increased ICP (e.g., changes in eye coordination, increased seizure activity, restlessness, changes in speech). **NOTE:** Changes are specific to the patient, depending on the disability (e.g., trauma, hydrocephalus) underlying the increased ICP.
- Teach caregiver the specific situations that trigger ICP in the client (e.g., pain, anxiety); discuss appropriate interventions

Collaborative Activities

- Initiate agency protocols for lowering ICP (e.g., plan may include ventriculostomy to drain cerebrospinal fluid)
- Follow protocols to maintain systemic blood pressure adequate to keep CPP at ≥ 70 mmHg
- *(NIC) Intracranial Pressure (ICP) Monitoring:*
  Notify physician for elevated ICP that does not respond to treatment protocols
  Administer pharmacologic agents to maintain ICP within specified range
  Administer antibiotics
  Maintain controlled hyperventilation, as ordered

Other

- Do not use the knee gatch and avoid 90-degree hip flexion
- Stop any activity (e.g., suctioning) that triggers *Decreased intracranial adaptive capacity*
- Limit the duration of procedures and care activities; allow time for baseline ICP to recover between noxious activities such as suctioning

- For patients who are performing Valsalva maneuver, if they can follow directions, instruct them to exhale through their mouths
- Use gentle touching and talking
- Suction only if necessary—not prophylactically
- If suctioning is needed, preoxygenate, do not hyperventilate, and use only one or two catheter passes; administer intratracheal lidocaine, per protocol, to minimize coughing
- Allow family to visit
- *(NIC) Intracranial Pressure (ICP) Monitoring:*
  Calibrate and level the transducer
  Restrain patient, as needed
  Change transducer and flush system
  Change and/or reinforce insertion site dressing, as necessary
  Position the patient with head elevated 30–45 degrees and with neck in a neutral position [support with sand bags, small pillows, and/or rolled towels]
  Minimize environmental stimuli [e.g., noise, painful procedures]
  Space nursing care to minimize ICP elevation
  Maintain systemic arterial pressure within specified range

ADJUSTMENT, IMPAIRED
(00070) (1986, 1998)

Definition: Inability to modify lifestyle and behavior in a manner consistent with a change in health status

Defining Characteristics
Subjective
Denial of health status change
Failure to achieve optimal sense of control
Objective
Demonstration of nonacceptance of health status change
Failure to take actions that would prevent further health problems

Related Factors
Absence of social support for changed beliefs and practices
Disability or health status change requiring change in lifestyle
Failure to intend to change behavior
Intense emotional state
Lack of motivation to change behaviors
Low state of optimism

Multiple stressors

Negative attitudes toward health behavior

Suggestions for Use

This diagnosis is not specific enough to be clinically useful. If you use it, add clarifying phrases (e.g., *Impaired adjustment: Inability to resolve anger over illness*). When possible, use a different diagnostic label that identifies the specific way in which adjustment is impaired (e.g., *Anxiety*, *Ineffective management of therapeutic regimen*).

Suggested Alternative Diagnoses

The following are examples of other diagnoses you might consider. Almost every NANDA International label indicates some type of impaired adjustment.

Coping, ineffective

Grieving, dysfunctional

NOC Outcomes

Acceptance: Health Status: Reconciliation to health circumstances

Compliance Behavior: Actions taken on the basis of professional advice to promote wellness, recovery, and rehabilitation

Coping: Actions to manage stressors that tax an individual's resources

Grief Resolution: Adjustment to actual or impending loss

Health Seeking Behavior: Actions to promote optimal wellness, recovery, and rehabilitation

Participation: Health Care Decisions: Personal involvement in selecting and evaluating health care options

Psychosocial Adjustment: Life Change: Psychosocial adaptation of an individual to a life change

Treatment Behavior: Illness or Injury: Personal actions to palliate or eliminate pathology

Goals/Evaluation Criteria

Examples Using NOC Language

• Demonstrates adjustment to changes in health status as evidenced by Acceptance: Health Status, Compliance Behavior, Coping, Grief Resolution, Health-Seeking Behavior, Participation: Health Care Decisions, Psychosocial Adjustment: Life Change, and Treatment Behavior: Illness or Injury

- Demonstrates **Acceptance: Health Status**, as evidenced by the following indicators (specify 1–5: none, limited, moderate, substantial, or extensive):

   Relinquishment of previous concept of health
   Pursuit of information
   Demonstration of positive self-regard
   Health-related decision making

Other Examples

Patient will:

- Verbalize acceptance of changes in health status
- Verbalize feelings about the required lifestyle and behavior changes
- Begin to make lifestyle and behavior changes
- Identify priorities for own health outcomes
- Demonstrate decreased anxiety and fear in independent activities
- Comply with prescribed treatments

NIC Interventions

Anticipatory Guidance: Preparation of patient for an anticipated developmental and/or situational crisis

Behavior Modification: Promotion of a behavior change

Coping Enhancement: Assisting a patient to adapt to perceived stressors, changes, or threats which interfere with meeting life demands and roles

Counseling: Use of an interactive helping process focusing on the needs, problems, or feelings of the patient and significant others to enhance or support coping, problem solving, and interpersonal relationships

Crisis Intervention: Use of short-term counseling to help the patient cope with a crisis and resume a state of functioning comparable to or better than the precrisis state

Decision-Making Support: Providing information and support for a patient who is making a decision regarding health care

Emotional Support: Provision of reassurance, acceptance, and encouragement during times of stress

Grief Work Facilitation: Assistance with the resolution of a significant loss

Health Education: Developing and providing instruction and learning experiences to facilitate voluntary adaptation of behavior conducive to health in individuals, families, groups, or communities

Health System Guidance: Facilitating a patient's location and use of appropriate health services

Mutual Goal Setting: Collaborating with patient to identify and prioritize care goals, then developing a plan for achieving those goals

Patient Contracting: Negotiating an agreement with a patient that reinforces a specific behavior change

Self-Responsibility Facilitation: Encouraging a patient to assume more responsibility for own behavior

Teaching: Disease Process: Assisting the patient to understand information related to a specific disease process

Values Clarification: Assisting another to clarify her/his own values in order to facilitate effective decision making

Nursing Activities

Assessments

- Assess patient's need for social support
- Assess amount and quality of social support available
- *(NIC) Coping Enhancement:*

    Appraise patient's adjustment to changes in body image, as indicated

    Appraise the impact of the patient's life situation on roles and relationships

    Evaluate the patient's decision-making ability

Collaborative Activities

- Refer patient to community agencies and/or support groups
- Include patient and family in a multidisciplinary conference to establish a plan of care, for example:

    Identify obstacles that hinder lifestyle and behavior changes

    Identify personal strengths that will facilitate goal achievement

    Review necessary lifestyle and behavior changes and select one as an initial goal

Other

- Provide a nonjudgmental environment in which patient and family can share concerns, anxieties, and fears
- *(NIC) Coping Enhancement:*

    Assist the patient to identify available support systems [to learn new ways to cope and to decrease isolation and fear]

    Appraise and discuss alternative responses to situation

AIRWAY CLEARANCE, INEFFECTIVE
(00031) (1980, 1996, 1998)

Definition: Inability to clear secretions or obstructions from the respiratory tract to maintain a clear airway

Defining Characteristics

Subjective
Dyspnea

Objective
Adventitious breath sounds (e.g., rales, crackles, rhonchi, wheezes)
Changes in respiratory rate and rhythm
Ineffective or absent cough
Cyanosis
Difficulty vocalizing
Diminished breath sounds
Orthopnea
Restlessness
Sputum
Wide-eyed [look]

Related Factors

Environmental: Smoking, smoke inhalation, secondhand smoke
Obstructed Airway: Airway spasm, retained secretions, excessive mucus, presence of artificial airway, foreign body in airway, secretions in the bronchi, exudate in the alveoli
Physiological: Neuromuscular dysfunction, hyperplasia of the bronchial walls, chronic obstructive pulmonary disease, infection, asthma, allergic airways, trauma

Suggestions for Use

Use the key defining characteristics in Table 1 to discriminate carefully among this label and the two alternative respiratory diagnoses. If cough and gag reflexes are ineffective or absent secondary to anesthesia, use *Risk for aspiration* instead of *Ineffective airway clearance* in order to focus on preventing aspiration rather than teaching effective coughing.

Table 1

Nursing Diagnosis	Present	Not Present
Impaired Gas Exchange	Abnormal blood gases Hypoxia Changes in mental status	Ineffective cough Cough
Ineffective Breathing Pattern	"Appearance" of the patient's breathing: nasal flaring, use of accessory muscles, pursed lip breathing	Tachycardia, restlessness Ineffective cough
	Abnormal blood gases	Obstruction or aspiration
Ineffective Airway Clearance	Cough, ineffective cough	Abnormal blood gases
	Changes in rate or depth of respirations Usual cause is increased or tenacious secretions or obstruction (e.g., aspiration)	

Suggested Alternative Diagnoses

Aspiration, risk for
Breathing pattern, ineffective
Gas exchange, impaired

NOC Outcomes

Aspiration Control: Personal actions to prevent the passage of fluid and solid particles into the lung

Respiratory Status: Airway Patency: Extent to which the tracheobronchial passages remain open

Respiratory Status: Gas Exchange: Alveolar exchange of CO_2 or O_2 to maintain arterial blood gas concentration

Respiratory Status: Ventilation: Movement of air in and out of the lungs

Goals/Evaluation Criteria

Examples Using NOC Language

- Demonstrates effective airway clearance, as evidenced by Aspiration Control; and Respiratory Status: Airway Patency, Gas Exchange and Ventilation not compromised,
- Demonstrates **Respiratory Status: Gas Exchange**, as evidenced by the following indicators (specify 1–5: extremely, substantially, moderately, mildly, or not compromised):

  Ease of breathing

  Restlessness, cyanosis, and dyspnea not present

  O_2 saturation within normal limits

  Chest x-ray findings in expected range

Other Examples

Patient will:
- Have a patent airway
- Expectorate secretions effectively
- Have respiratory rate and rhythm within normal range
- Have pulmonary function within normal limits
- Be able to describe plan for care at home

NIC Interventions

Acid–Base Monitoring: Collection and analysis of patient data to regulate acid–base balance

Airway Management: Facilitation of patency of air passages

Airway Suctioning: Removal of airway secretions by inserting a suction catheter into the patient's oral airway and/or trachea

Aspiration Precautions: Prevention or minimization of risk factors in the patient at risk for aspiration

Cough Enhancement: Promotion of deep inhalation by the patient with subsequent generation of high intrathoracic pressures and compression of underlying lung parenchyma for the forceful expulsion of air

Oxygen Therapy: Administration of oxygen and monitoring of its effectiveness

Positioning: Deliberative placement of the patient or a body part to promote physiological and psychological well-being

Respiratory Monitoring: Collection and analysis of patient data to ensure airway patency and adequate gas exchange

Ventilation Assistance: Promotion of an optimal spontaneous breathing pattern that maximizes oxygen and carbon dioxide exchange in the lungs

Nursing Activities

Assessments

- Assess and document the following:
    Effectiveness of oxygen administration and other treatments
    Effectiveness of prescribed medications
    Trends in arterial blood gases
- Auscultate anterior and posterior chest for decreased or absent ventilation and presence of adventitious sounds
- *(NIC) Airway Suctioning:*
    Determine the need for oral or tracheal suctioning
    Monitor patient's oxygen status (SaO_2 and SvO_2 levels) and hemodynamic status (MAP [mean arterial pressure] level and cardiac rhythms) immediately before, during, and after suctioning
    Note type and amount of secretions obtained

Patient/Family Teaching

- Explain proper use of supportive equipment (e.g., oxygen, suction, spirometer, inhalers, intermittent positive pressure breathing,)
- Inform patient and family that smoking is prohibited in room
- Instruct patient and family in plan for care at home (e.g., medications, hydration, nebulization, equipment, postural drainage, signs and symptoms of complications, community resources)
- Instruct patient in coughing and deep-breathing techniques to facilitate removal of secretions
- Teach patient and family the significance of changes in sputum, such as color, character, amount, and odor
- *(NIC) Airway Suctioning:* Instruct the patient and/or family how to suction the airway, as appropriate

Collaborative Activities

- Confer with respiratory therapist, as needed
- Consult with physician concerning need for percussion or supportive equipment
- Administer humidified air and oxygen according to agency policies
- Perform or assist with aerosol, ultrasonic nebulizer, and other pulmonary treatments according to agency policies and protocols
- Notify physician of abnormal blood gases

Other

- Encourage physical activity to promote movement of secretions
- If patient unable to ambulate, turn patient from side to side at least q2h
- Inform patient before initiating procedures, to lower anxiety and increase sense of control
- Suction the naso- and oropharynx to remove secretions q _____
- Perform endotracheal or nasotracheal suctioning, as appropriate. (Hyperoxygenate with Ambu bag before and after suctioning endotracheal tube or tracheostomy.)
- Maintain adequate hydration to decrease viscosity of secretions

ANXIETY
(00146) (1973, 1982, 1998)

Definition: Vague, uneasy feeling of discomfort or dread accompanied by an autonomic response (the source often nonspecific or unknown to the individual); a feeling of apprehension caused by anticipation of danger. It is an alerting signal that warns of impending danger and enables the individual to take measures to deal with the threat.

Defining Characteristics

Behavioral

Diminished productivity
Expressed concerns due to change in life events
Extraneous movement (e.g., foot shuffling, hand/arm movements)
Fidgeting
Glancing about
Insomnia
Poor eye contact
Restlessness
Scanning and vigilance

Affective

Anguish
Anxious
Apprehension
Distressed
Fearful
Feelings of inadequacy
Focus on self

Increased wariness
Irritability
Jittery
Overexcited
Painful and persistent increased helplessness
Rattled
Regretful
Scared
Uncertainty
Worried

Physiological

Insomnia
Shakiness
Trembling or hand tremors
Voice quivering

Parasympathetic

Abdominal pain
Decreased blood pressure
Decreased pulse
Diarrhea
Faintness
Fatigue
Nausea
Sleep disturbance
Tingling in extremities
Urinary frequency
Urinary hesitancy
Urinary urgency

Sympathetic

Anorexia
Cardiovascular excitation
Dry mouth
Facial flushing
Facial tension
Heart pounding
Increased blood pressure
Increased perspiration
Increased pulse
Increased reflexes
Increased respiration
Increased tension
Pupil dilation

Respiratory difficulties
Superficial vasoconstriction
Twitching
Weakness

Cognitive

Awareness of physiologic symptoms
Blocking of thought
Confusion
Decreased perceptual field
Difficulty concentrating
Diminished ability to problem solve
Diminished learning ability
Expressed concerns due to changes in life events
Fear of unspecific consequences
Focus on self
Forgetfulness
Impaired attention
Preoccupation
Rumination
Tendency to blame others

Related Factors

Exposure to toxins
Familial association/heredity
Interpersonal transmission and contagion
Situational and maturational crises
Stress
Substance abuse
Threat of death
Threat to or change in economic status
Threat to or change in role status or function
Threat to or change in environment
Threat to or change in health status
Threat to or change in interaction patterns
Threat to self-concept
Unconscious conflict about essential values and goals of life
Unmet needs

Suggestions for Use

Anxiety should be differentiated from *Fear* because the nursing actions may be different. When a patient is fearful, the nurse tries to remove the source of the fear or help the patient deal with the specific fear. When a patient is anxious, the nurse helps identify the cause of anxiety; however, when the source of anxiety cannot be identified, the nurse helps the patient explore and express anxious feelings.

Fear and *Anxiety* present diagnostic difficulty because they are not mutually exclusive. A person who is afraid is usually anxious as well. Impending surgery may be the etiology for *Fear*, but most of the feelings about surgery relate to *Anxiety*. Because the etiology (surgery) cannot be changed, nursing interventions should focus on supporting patient coping mechanisms for managing *Anxiety* (Carpenito, 1997b, pp. 126–127).

Many of the same signs and symptoms are present in both *Fear* and *Anxiety*: increased heart and respiratory rate, dilated pupils, diaphoresis, muscle tension, and fatigue. The following comparisons in Table 2 may be helpful:

Table 2

	Anxiety	**Fear**
Physiologic Manifestations	Stimulation of the parasympathetic nervous system with increased gastrointestinal activity	Sympathetic response only; decreased gastrointestinal activity
Type of Threat	Usually psychologic (e.g., to self-image); vague, nonspecific	Often physical (e.g., to safety); specific, identifiable
Feeling	Vague, uneasy feeling	Feeling of dread, apprehension
Source of Feeling	Unknown by the person; unconscious	Known by the person

Because the level of anxiety influences the nursing activities, indicate in the diagnostic statement whether anxiety is moderate, severe, or panic level. Panic may require collaborative interventions, such as medications. Mild anxiety is not a problem, because it is a normal condition present in all human beings. Diagnose *Anxiety* only for patients who require special nursing interventions. Mild anxiety before surgery is a normal, healthy response.

Mild anxiety: Present in day-to-day living; increases alertness and perceptual fields; motivates learning and growth

Moderate anxiety: Narrows perceptual fields; focus is on immediate concerns, with inattention to other communications and details

Severe anxiety: Very narrow focus on specific detail; all behavior is geared toward getting relief

Panic: The person loses control and feels dread and terror. A state of disorganization causes increased physical activity, distorted perceptions and relationships, and loss of rational thought. Panic can lead to exhaustion and death (Stuart and Sundeen, 1995).

Suggested Alternative Diagnoses

Decisional conflict
Fear
Coping, ineffective

NOC Outcomes

Aggression Control: Self-restraint of assaultive, combative, or destructive behavior toward others

Anxiety Control: Personal actions to eliminate or reduce feelings of apprehension and tension from an unidentifiable source

Coping: Actions to manage stressors that tax an individual's resources

Impulse Control: Ability to self-restrain compulsive or impulsive behaviors

Self-Mutilation Restraint: Ability to refrain from intentional self-inflicted injury (nonlethal)

Social Interaction Skills: An individual's use of effective interaction behaviors

Goals/Evaluation Criteria

Examples Using NOC Language

- *Anxiety* relieved, as evidenced by consistently demonstrating Aggression Control, Anxiety Control, Coping, Impulse Control, Self-Mutilation Restraint, and substantially effective Social Interaction Skills

- Demonstrates **Anxiety Control**, as evidenced by the following indicators (specify 1–5: never, rarely, sometimes, often, or consistently demonstrated):

    Plans coping strategies for stressful situations
    Maintains role performance
    Reports absence of sensory perceptual disorders

Reports absence of physical manifestations of anxiety
Behavioral manifestations of anxiety absent

Other Examples

Patient will:

- Continue necessary activities even though anxiety persists
- Demonstrate ability to focus on new knowledge and skills
- Identify symptoms that are indicators of own anxiety
- Not demonstrate aggressive behaviors
- Communicate needs and negative feelings appropriately

NIC Interventions

Anger Control Assistance: Facilitation of the expression of anger in an adaptive nonviolent manner

Anticipatory Guidance: Preparation of patient for an anticipated developmental or situational crisis

Anxiety Reduction: Minimizing apprehension, dread, foreboding, or uneasiness related to an unidentified source of anticipated danger

Behavior Management: Self-Harm: Assisting the patient to decrease or eliminate self-mutilating or self-abusive behaviors

Behavior Modification: Social Skills: Assisting the patient to develop or improve interpersonal social skills

Complex Relationship Building: Establishing a therapeutic relationship with a patient who has difficulty interacting with others

Coping Enhancement: Assisting a patient to adapt to perceived stressors, changes, or threats which interfere with meeting life demands and roles

Impulse Control Training: Assisting the patient to mediate impulsive behavior through application of problem-solving strategies to social and interpersonal situations

Nursing Activities

Assessments

- Assess and document patient's level of anxiety q _____
- Explore with patient techniques that have, and have not, reduced anxiety in the past.
- *(NIC) Anxiety Reduction:* Determine patient's decision-making ability

Patient/Family Teaching

- Develop teaching plan with realistic goals, including need for repetition, encouragement, and praise of the tasks learned

- *(NIC) Anxiety Reduction:*
  Provide factual information concerning diagnosis, treatment, and prognosis
  Instruct patient on the use of relaxation techniques
  Explain all procedures, including sensations likely to be experienced during the procedure

Collaborative Activities

- *(NIC) Anxiety Reduction:* Administer medications to reduce anxiety, as appropriate

Other

- Encourage patient to verbalize thoughts and feelings to externalize anxiety
- Help patient to focus on the present situation as a means of identifying coping mechanisms needed to reduce anxiety
- Provide diversion through television, radio, games, and occupational therapies to reduce anxiety and expand focus
- Provide positive reinforcement when patient is able to continue ADLs and other activities despite anxiety
- Reassure patient by touch and empathetic verbal and nonverbal exchanges, encourage patient to express anger and irritation, and allow patient to cry
- Reduce excessive stimulation by providing a quiet environment, limited contact with others if necessary, and limited use of caffeine and other stimulants
- Suggest alternative therapies for reducing anxiety that are acceptable to patient
- *(NIC) Anxiety Reduction:*
  Use a calm, reassuring approach
  Clearly state expectations for patient's behavior
  Stay with patient [e.g., during procedures] to promote safety and reduce fear
  Administer back rub/neck rub, as appropriate
  Keep treatment equipment out of sight
  Help patient identify situations that precipitate anxiety
  Encourage parents to stay with child, as appropriate

ANXIETY, DEATH
(00147) (1998)

Definition: Apprehension, worry, or fear related to death or dying

Defining Characteristics

Subjective
Anticipated pain related to dying

Concern about meeting one's creator or feeling doubtful about the existence of a god or higher being

Concerns of overworking the caregiver as terminal illness incapacitates self

Deep sadness

Denial of one's own mortality or impending death

Fear of delayed demise

Fear of developing a terminal illness

Fear of leaving family alone after death

Fear of loss of physical or mental abilities when dying

Fear of premature death because it prevents the accomplishment of important life goals

Fear of the process of dying

Negative death images or unpleasant thoughts about any event related to death or dying

Powerlessness over issues related to dying

Total loss of control over any aspect of one's own death

Worrying about being the cause of others' grief and suffering

Worrying about the impact of one's own death on significant others

Related Factors
To be developed

Suggestions for Use
Always use the most specific label. If a dying patient's anxiety is related to death or dying, use *Death anxiety;* if not, use the broader label, *Anxiety*.

Suggested Alternative Diagnoses
Anxiety

Sorrow, chronic

Spiritual distress

NOC Outcomes

Acceptance: Health Status: Reconciliation to health circumstances

Anxiety Control: Personal actions to eliminate or reduce feelings of apprehension and tension from an unidentifiable source

Depression Level: Severity of melancholic mood and loss of interest in life events

Dignified Dying: Maintaining personal control and comfort with the approaching end of life

Fear Control: Personal actions to eliminate or reduce disabling feelings of alarm aroused by an identifiable source

Health Beliefs: Perceived Threat: Personal conviction that a health problem is serious and has potential negative consequences for lifestyle

Hope: Presence of internal state of optimism that is personally satisfying and life-supporting

Goals/Evaluation Criteria

Examples Using NOC Language

- *Anxiety* relieved, as evidenced by consistently demonstrating Anxiety Control, Depression Level, Dignified Dying, Fear Control, Health Beliefs: Perceived Threat, and Hope.
- Demonstrates **Anxiety Control**, as evidenced by the following indicators (specify 1–5: never, rarely, sometimes, often, or consistently demonstrated):
    Reports absence of sensory perceptual disorders
    Reports absence of physical manifestations of anxiety
    Behavioral manifestations of anxiety absent
- Demonstrates **Dignified Dying**, as evidenced by the following indicators (specify 1–5: not at all, to a slight extent, to a moderate extent, to a great extent or to a very great extent):
    Expresses readiness for death
    Resolves important issues and concerns
    Reconciles previous relationships
    Exchanges affection with others
    Disengages gradually from significant others
    Verbalizes comfort
    Expresses pain relief
    Expresses symptom control

Other Examples

Patient will:
- Maintain psychologic comfort during the process of dying

- Verbalize feelings (e.g., anger, sorrow, or loss) and thoughts with staff and/or significant others
- Identify areas of personal control
- Express positive feelings about relationships with significant others
- Accept limitations and seek help as needed

NIC Interventions

Anxiety Reduction: Minimizing apprehension, dread, foreboding, or uneasiness related to an unidentified source of anticipated danger

Coping Enhancement: Assisting a patient to adapt to perceived stressors, changes, or threats which interfere with meeting life demands and roles

Dying Care: Promotion of physical comfort and psychological peace in the final phase of life

Emotional Support: Provision of reassurance, acceptance, and encouragement during times of stress

Hope Instillation: Facilitation of the development of a positive outlook in a given situation

Spiritual Support: Assisting the patient to feel balance and connection with a greater power

Nursing Activities

Assessments

- Monitor for signs and symptoms of anxiety (e.g., vital signs, appetite, sleep patterns, concentration level)
- Assess support provided by significant others
- Monitor for expressions of hopelessness or powerlessness (e.g., "I can't")
- Determine sources of anxiety (e.g., fear of pain, body malfunction, humiliation, abandonment, nonbeing, negative impact on survivors)

Patient/Family Teaching

- Provide information about the patient's illness and prognosis
- Provide honest and direct answers to the patient's questions about the dying process

Collaborative Activities

- Refer to home care or hospice care, as appropriate
- Arrange access to clergy or spiritual advisors as patient wishes
- Connect patient and family with appropriate support groups

Other

- Support spiritual needs without imposing own beliefs on patient
- Use therapeutic communication skills to build trusting relationship and facilitate expression of patient needs
- Listen attentively
- Offer support for difficult feelings without offering false reassurance or too much advice
- Encourage patient to express feelings with significant others
- Help patient to identify areas of personal control; offer choices and options to the extent of the patient's ability
- Spend time with patient to deter fear of being alone
- Assist patient to reminisce and review personal life positively
- Identify and support the patient's usual coping strategies
- Provide for physical comfort and security

ASPIRATION, RISK FOR
(00039) (1988)

Definition: At risk for entry of gastrointestinal secretions, oropharyngeal secretions, solids or fluids into tracheobronchial passages

Risk Factors
Objective
Decreased gastrointestinal motility
Delayed gastric emptying [e.g., secondary to ileus or intestinal obstruction]
Depressed cough and gag reflexes
Facial, oral, and neck surgery or trauma
Gastrointestinal tubes
Hindered elevation of upper body
Impaired swallowing
Incomplete lower esophageal sphincter
Increased gastric residual
Increased intragastric pressure
Medication administration
Presence of tracheostomy or endotracheal tube
Reduced level of consciousness [e.g., secondary to anesthesia, head injury, cerebrovascular accident, seizures]
Tube feedings
Wired jaws

Suggestions for Use

Always use the most specific label for which the patient has the necessary defining characteristics. Do not use *Risk for injury* if the patient has the defining characteristics or risk factors for *Risk for aspiration.*

Suggested Alternative Diagnoses

Airway clearance, ineffective
Injury, risk for
Self-care deficit: feeding
Swallowing, impaired

NOC Outcomes

Aspiration Control: Personal actions to prevent the passage of fluid and solid particles into the lung
Cognitive Ability: Ability to execute complex mental processes
Immobility Consequences: Physiological: Compromise in physiologic functioning due to impaired physical mobility
Neurological Status: Extent to which the peripheral and central nervous systems receive, process, and respond to internal and external stimuli
Respiratory Status: Ventilation: Movement of air in and out of the lungs
Swallowing Status: Extent of safe passage of fluids and/or solids from the mouth to the stomach

Goals/Evaluation Criteria

Examples Using NOC Language

- Will not aspirate, as evidenced by Aspiration Control; uncompromised Cognitive Ability, Neurological Status, Swallowing Status, and Respiratory Status: Ventilation; and no Physiological Immobility Consequences
- Will demonstrate **Cognitive Ability**, as evidenced by the following indicators (specify 1–5: extremely, substantially, moderately, mildly, or not compromised):
  Attentiveness, concentration, and orientation
  Information processing
  Immediate, recent, and remote memory
- Demonstrates **Aspiration Control**, as evidenced by the following indicators (specify 1–5: never, rarely, sometimes, often or consistently demonstrated):
  Avoids risk factors

Positions self upright for eating and drinking

Maintains appropriate consistency of liquids and foods

Selects foods according to swallowing ability

Other Examples

Patient will:

- Demonstrate improved swallowing
- Tolerate oral intake and secretions without aspiration
- Tolerate enteral feedings without aspiration
- Have clear lung sounds and patent airway
- Maintain adequate muscle strength and tone

NIC Interventions

Airway Management: Facilitation of patency of air passages

Aspiration Precautions: Prevention or minimization of risk factors in the patient at risk for aspiration

Respiratory Monitoring: Collection and analysis of patient data to ensure airway patency and adequate gas exchange

Swallowing Therapy: Facilitating swallowing and preventing complications of impaired swallowing

Vomiting Management: Prevention and alleviation of vomiting

Nursing Activities

Assessments

- Check gastric residual prior to feeding and giving medications
- Monitor for signs of aspiration during feedings: coughing, choking, drooling
- Verify placement of enteral tube prior to feeding and giving medications
- Evaluate family's comfort level with feeding, suctioning, positioning, and so forth
- *(NIC) Aspiration Precautions:*

  Monitor level of consciousness, cough reflex, gag reflex, and swallowing ability

  Monitor pulmonary status [e.g., before and after feeding and before and after giving medication]

Patient/Family Teaching

- Instruct family in feeding and swallowing techniques
- Instruct family in use of suction for removal of secretions
- Review with patient and family signs and symptoms of aspiration and preventive measures

- Help family to create an emergency plan in case patient aspirates at home

Collaborative Activities

- Report any change in color of lung secretions that resembles food or feeding intake
- Request occupational therapy consultation
- *(NIC) Aspiration Precautions:* Suggest speech pathology consult as appropriate

Other

- Allow patient time to swallow
- Have a suction catheter available at the bedside and suction during meals, as needed
- Involve the family during patient's ingestion of food and meals
- Provide support and reassurance
- Place the patient in semi- or high-Fowler position when eating, if possible
- Place patients who are unable to sit upright on their sides and elevate the head of the bed as much as possible during and after feedings
- Provide positive reinforcement for attempts to swallow independently
- Use a syringe, if necessary, when feeding the patient
- Vary consistency of foods to identify those foods more easily tolerated
- *(NIC) Aspiration Precautions:*
  Keep head of bed elevated 30 to 45 min after feeding
  Cut food into small pieces
  Feed in small amounts
  Avoid liquids or use thickening agent
  Place dye in NG [nasogastric] feeding
  Break or crush pills before administration
  Request medication in elixir form
- For children:
  Choose age-appropriate toys with no small, removable parts; do not give balloons to small children
  Avoid foods such as nuts, gum, grapes, and small candy
  Teach parents not to prop bottle

ATTACHMENT, PARENT/INFANT/CHILD, RISK FOR IMPAIRED (00058) (1994)

Definition: Disruption of the interactive process between parent and significant other and child or infant that fosters the development of a protective and nurturing reciprocal relationship.

Risk Factors

Anxiety associated with the parent role

Ill infant or child who is unable to effectively initiate parental contact due to altered behavioral organization

Inability of parents to meet personal needs

Lack of privacy

Physical barriers

Premature infant

Separation

Substance abuse

Suggestions for Use

Use this diagnosis when parent(s) are at risk for attachment problems. If actual signs of delayed attachment are observed, use *Risk for impaired parenting related to Impaired parent/infant/child attachment.*

Suggested Alternative Diagnoses

Parenting, impaired

Parenting, risk for impaired

NOC Outcomes

Child Development: 2, 4, 6, and 12 Months and 2, 3, 4, and 5 Years: Milestones of physical, cognitive, and psychosocial progression by 2, 4, 6, and 12 months; and 2, 3, 4, and 5 years of age. [NOTE: NOC has separate outcomes and indicators for each age.]

Family Environment: Internal: Social climate as characterized by family member relationships and goals

Parent–Infant Attachment: Behaviors that demonstrate an enduring affectionate bond between a parent and infant

Parenting: Provision of an environment that promotes optimum growth and development of dependent children

Role Performance: Congruence of an individual's role behavior with role expectations

Substance Addiction Consequences: Compromise in health status and social functioning due to substance addiction

Goals/Evaluation Criteria

Examples Using NOC Language

- Demonstrate **Parent–Infant Attachment**, as evidenced by the following indicators (specify 1–5: never, rarely, sometimes, often, or consistently demonstrated):

  Parent will:

  Practice healthy behaviors during pregnancy

  Assign specific attributes to fetus

  Prepare for infant prior to birth

  Hold, touch, stroke, pat, kiss, and smile at infant

  Talk to infant

  Use en face position and eye contact

  Play with infant

  Respond to infant cues

  Console and soothe infant

  Keep infant dry, clean, and warm

  Infant will:

  Look at parent(s)

  Respond to parent(s)' cues

- Demonstrate **Parenting**, as evidenced by the following indicators (specify 1–5: not, slightly, moderately, substantially, or totally adequate):

  Stimulate child's cognitive and social development

  Facilitate the child's emotional and spiritual growth

  Demonstrate a loving relationship with child

  Verbalize positive attributes of child

NIC Interventions

Attachment Promotion: Facilitation of the development of the parent–infant relationship

Developmental Enhancement: Child: Facilitating or teaching parents and caregivers to facilitate the optimal gross motor, fine motor, language, cognitive, social and emotional growth of preschool and school-aged children

Environmental Management: Attachment Process: Manipulation of the patient's surroundings to facilitate the development of the parent–infant relationship

Parent Education: Infant: Instruction on nurturing and physical care needed during the first year of life

Parenting Promotion: Providing parenting information, support, and coordination of comprehensive services to high-risk families

Role Enhancement: Assisting a patient, significant other, and family to improve relationships by clarifying and supplementing specific role behaviors

Nursing Activities

Assessments

- Assess parent's learning needs
- Identify parent's readiness to learn about infant care
- Assess parent's ability to recognize infant's physiologic needs (e.g., hunger cues)
- *(NIC) Attachment Promotion:*
  Ascertain before birth whether parent(s) has names picked out for both sexes
  Discuss parent's reaction to pregnancy

Patient/Family Teaching

- Teach/demonstrate care of newborn (e.g., feeding, bathing)
- Teach parent(s) about child development
- Assist parents in interpreting infant/child's cues and changing needs (e.g., nonverbal cues, crying, and vocalizations)
- Teach quieting techniques and support parent's ability to relieve child's distress
- *(NIC) Attachment Promotion:*
  Inform parent(s) of care being given to newborn
  Explain equipment used to monitor infant in nursery
  Demonstrate ways to touch infant confined to Isolette
  Share information gained from initial physical assessment of newborn with parent(s)
  Discuss infant behavioral characteristics with parent(s)

Other

Prenatal Period

- *(NIC) Attachment Promotion:*
  Provide parent(s) the opportunity to hear fetal heart tones as soon as possible
  Provide parent(s) the opportunity to see the ultrasound image of the fetus
  Encourage parent(s) to attend prenatal or parenting classes

Intrapartum Period

- *(NIC) Attachment Promotion:*

  Encourage father–significant other to participate in labor and delivery

  Place infant on mother's body immediately after birth

  Provide opportunity for parent(s) to see, hold, and examine newborn immediately after birth

  Provide family privacy during initial interaction with newborn

- *(NIC) Environmental Management: Attachment Process:*

  Limit number of people in delivery room

  Provide comfortable chair for father or significant other

  Maintain low level of stimuli in patient and family environment

Neonatal Period

- *(NIC) Attachment Promotion:*

  Assist parent(s) to participate in infant care

  Reinforce caregiver role behaviors

  Reinforce normal aspects of infant with defect

  Encourage parent(s) to bring personal items, such as toy or picture, to be put in Isolette or at bedside of infant

  Inform parent(s) of care being given to infant in another hospital

  Discuss infant behavioral characteristics with parent(s)

  Point out infant cues that show responsiveness to parent(s)

  Keep infant with parent(s) after birth, when possible

  Encourage parents to massage infant

  Encourage parent(s) to touch and speak to newborn

- *(NIC) Environmental Management: Attachment Process:*

  Permit father or significant other to sleep in room with mother

  Reduce interruptions by hospital personnel

BODY IMAGE, DISTURBED
(00118) (1973, 1998)

Definition: Confusion in mental picture of one's physical self

Defining Characteristics

Either (A) or (B) must be present to justify the diagnosis of *Disturbed Body Image*. The remaining defining characteristics may be used to validate the presence of (A) or (B).

(A) Verbal response to actual or perceived change in structure or function

(B) Nonverbal response to actual or perceived change in structure or function

Subjective

Depersonalization of [body] part or loss by impersonal pronouns

Emphasis on remaining strengths and heightened achievement

Fear of rejection or of reaction by others

Focus on past strength, function, or appearance

Negative feelings about body (e.g., feelings of helplessness, hopelessness, or powerlessness)

Personalization of body part or loss by name

Preoccupation with change or loss

Refusal to verify actual change

Verbalization of change in lifestyle

Objective

Actual change in [body] structure or function

Change in ability to estimate spatial relationship of body to environment

Change in social involvement

Hiding or overexposing body part (intentional or unintentional)

Missing body part

Not looking at body part

Not touching body part

Showing reluctance to touch or look at affected body part

Trauma to nonfunctioning body part

Related Factors

Biophysical [e.g., chronic illness, congenital defects, pregnancy]

Cognitive/perceptual [e.g., chronic pain]

Cultural or spiritual

Developmental changes

Illness

Psychosocial [e.g., eating disorders]

[Situational crisis (specify)]

Trauma or injury

Treatments [e.g., surgery, chemotherapy, radiation]

Suggestions for Use

This label is related to *Low self-esteem*, but is specific to negative feelings about one's body or body parts. Although *Disturbed body image* is often caused by loss of a body part or actual body changes, the changes in body structure or function can be perceived rather than actual. Patients on prolonged bed rest or who are dependent on machines (e.g., dialysis equipment, respirators) may experience distortion of body image. Eating disorders are often related to *Disturbed body image*.

Suggested Alternative Diagnoses

Nutrition: less than body requirements, imbalanced
Nutrition: more than body requirements, imbalanced
Self-esteem, chronic, or situational low

NOC Outcomes

Body Image: Positive perception of own appearance and body functions

Child Development: 2 Years: Milestones of physical, cognitive, and psychosocial progression by 2 years of age. **NOTE:** NOC also suggests Child Development outcomes for 3, 4, and 5 years; middle childhood (6–11 years); and adolescence (12–17 years), all having the same definition

Distorted Thought Control: Self-restraint of disruption in perception, thought processes, and thought content

Grief Resolution: Adjustment to actual or impending loss

Psychosocial Adjustment: Life Change: Psychosocial adaptation of an individual to a life change

Self-Esteem: Personal judgment of self-worth

Goals/Evaluation Criteria

Examples Using NOC Language

- *Disturbed body image* alleviated as demonstrated by positive Body Image, no delay in Child Development, consistently demonstrated Distorted Thought Control, Grief Resolution (to a great extent), substantial Psychosocial Adjustment: Life Change, and positive Self-Esteem
- Demonstrates **Body Image**, as evidenced by the following indicators (specify 1–5: never, rarely, sometimes, often, or consistently positive):
    Congruence between body reality, body ideal, and body presentation
    Satisfaction with body appearance and function
    Willingness to touch affected body part

Other Examples

Patient will:

- Identify personal strengths
- Acknowledge impact of situation on existing personal relationships and lifestyle
- Acknowledge the actual change in body appearance
- Describe actual change in body function
- Express willingness to use suggested resources after discharge
- Maintain close social interaction and personal relationships

NIC Interventions

Anticipatory Guidance: Preparation of patient for an anticipated developmental or situational crisis

Body Image Enhancement: Improving a patient's conscious and unconscious perceptions and attitudes toward his body

Coping Enhancement: Assisting a patient to adapt to perceived stressors, changes, or threats which interfere with meeting life demands and roles

Developmental Enhancement: Adolescent: Facilitating optimal physical, cognitive, social, and emotional growth of individuals during the transition from childhood to adulthood

Developmental Enhancement: Child: Facilitating or teaching parents–caregivers to facilitate the optimal gross motor, fine motor, language, cognitive, social and emotional growth of preschool and school-aged children

Grief Work Facilitation: Assistance with the resolution of a significant loss

Parent Education: Adolescent: Assisting parents to understand and help their adolescent children

Parent Education: Childrearing Family: Assisting parents to understand and promote the physical, psychological, and social growth and development of their toddler, preschool, or school-aged child or children

Risk Identification: Analysis of potential risk factors, determination of health risks, and prioritization of risk reduction strategies for an individual or group

Self-Esteem Enhancement: Assisting a patient to increase his personal judgment of self-worth

Nursing Activities

Assessments

- Assess and document patient's verbal and nonverbal responses to his body

- *(NIC) Body Image Enhancement:*

   Determine how child responds to parents' reactions, as appropriate

   Determine patient's body image expectations based on developmental stage

   Determine whether perceived dislike for certain physical characteristics creates a dysfunctional social paralysis for teenagers and other high-risk groups

   Determine whether a recent physical change has been incorporated into patient's body image

   Identify the significance of the patient's culture, religion, race, gender, and age on body image

   Monitor frequency of statements of self-criticism

Patient/Family Teaching

- *(NIC) Body Image Enhancement:* Teach parents the importance of their responses to the child's body changes and future adjustment, as appropriate

Collaborative Activities

- Refer to social services department for planning care with patient and family
- Offer to make initial phone call to appropriate community resources for patient and family

Other

- Actively listen to patient and family and acknowledge reality of concerns about treatments, progress, and prognosis
- Encourage patient and family to air feelings and to grieve
- Assist patient and family to identify coping mechanisms and personal strengths and acknowledge limitations
- Provide care in a nonjudgmental manner, maintaining the patient's privacy and dignity
- Encourage patient to:

   Maintain usual daily grooming routine

   Verbalize concerns about close personal relationships

   Verbalize consequences of physical and emotional changes that have influenced self-concept

- *(NIC) Body Image Enhancement:*

   Identify means of reducing the impact of any disfigurement through clothing, wigs, or cosmetics, as appropriate.

   Facilitate contact with individuals with similar changes in body image

Use self-picture drawing as a mechanism for evaluating a child's body image perceptions

Instruct children about the functions of the various body parts, as appropriate

Use self-disclosure exercises with groups of teenagers or others distraught over normal physical attributes

---

BODY TEMPERATURE: IMBALANCED, RISK FOR (00005) (1986, 2000)

Definition: At risk for failure to maintain body temperature within normal range

Risk Factors

Objective

Altered metabolic rate

Dehydration

Exposure to cold and cool or warm and hot environments

Extremes of age

Extremes of weight

Illness or trauma affecting temperature regulation

[Immaturity of newborn's temperature-regulating system]

[Inability to perspire]

Inactivity

Inappropriate clothing for environmental temperature

[Low birth weight (neonate)]

Medications causing vasoconstriction or vasodilation

Sedation

Vigorous activity

Suggestions for Use

If the patient is at risk for both *Hypothermia* and *Hyperthermia*, then *Risk for imbalanced body temperature* is the appropriate diagnosis. If the patient is at risk for only an elevation in temperature, use *Risk for hyperthermia*; if at risk for only decreased body temperature, use *Risk for hypothermia*.

Suggested Alternative Diagnoses

Hyperthermia

Hypothermia

Thermoregulation, ineffective

NOC Outcomes

Hydration: Amount of water in the intra- and extracellular compartments of the body

Immune Status: Adequacy of natural and acquired appropriately targeted resistance to internal and external antigens

Infection Status: Presence and extent of infection

Thermoregulation: Balance among heat production, heat gain, and heat loss

Thermoregulation: Neonate: Balance among heat production, heat gain, and heat loss during the neonatal period

Goals/Evaluation Criteria

Examples Using NOC Language

- Exhibits **Hydration**, as evidenced by the following indicators (specify 1–5: extremely, substantially, moderately, mildly, or not compromised):
    Skin hydration
    Neonate: no lethargy
    Moist mucous membranes
    Sunken eyes not present
    Perspiration ability
- Exhibits **Thermoregulation**, as evidenced by the following indicators (specify 1–5: extremely, substantially, moderately, mildly, or not compromised)
    Skin temperature IER
    Body temperature IER
    Reported thermal comfort

Other Examples

Patient will:
- Describe adaptive measures to minimize fluctuations in body temperature
- Report early signs and symptoms of hypo- or hyperthermia
- Maintain body temperature within normal range

NIC Interventions

Newborn Care: Management of neonate during the transition to extrauterine life and subsequent period of stabilization

Temperature Regulation: Attaining or maintaining body temperature within a normal range

Temperature Regulation: Intraoperative: Attaining or maintaining desired intraoperative body temperature

Vital Signs Monitoring: Collection and analysis of cardiovascular, respiratory, and body temperature data to determine and prevent complications

Nursing Activities

Assessments

- Evaluate home environment for factors that may alter body temperature
- Assess for early signs and symptoms of hypo- and hyperthermia
- *(NIC) Temperature Regulation:*

    Monitor temperature at least every 2 hr, as appropriate

    Monitor for and report signs and symptoms of hypo- and hyperthermia

    Monitor newborn's temperature until stabilized

    Wrap infant immediately after birth to prevent heat loss

Patient/Family Teaching

- Instruct patient and family in measures to minimize temperature fluctuations:

    #### *For Hyperthermia*

    Drink adequate fluids

    Limit activity on hot days

    Lose weight, if obese

    Maintain stable environmental temperature

    Remove excess clothing

    #### *For Hypothermia*

    Bathe in warm room, away from drafts

    Increase activity

    Limit alcohol intake

    Maintain adequate nourishment

    Maintain stable environmental temperature

    Wear adequate clothing

- Instruct patient and family to recognize and report early signs and symptoms of hypo- and hyperthermia:

    For Hyperthermia: Dry skin, headache, increased pulse, increased temperature, irritability, temperature above 37.8 °C or 100 °F, weakness

    For Hypothermia: Apathy; cold, hard abdomen that feels like marble; disorientation and confusion, drowsiness, hypertension, hypoglycemia, impaired ability to think; reduced pulse and respirations, skin hard and cold to touch, temperature of less than 95 °F

Collaborative Activities

- Report to physician if adequate hydration cannot be maintained
- *(NIC) Temperature Regulation:* Administer antipyretic medication, as appropriate

Other

- Dry and swaddle infant (or place on skin-to-skin contact with mother) immediately after birth to prevent heat loss by evaporation
- *(NIC) Temperature Regulation:* Adjust environmental temperature to patient needs.

BOWEL INCONTINENCE
(00014) (1975, 1998)

Definition: Change in normal bowel habits characterized by involuntary passage of stool.

Defining Characteristics

Subjective

Inability to recognize urge to defecate

Recognizes rectal fullness but reports inability to expel formed stool

Self-report of inability to feel rectal fullness

Objective

Constant dribbling of soft stool

Fecal odor

Fecal staining of clothing and/or bedding

Inability to delay defecation

Inattention to urge to defecate

Red perianal skin

Urgency

Related Factors

Abnormally high abdominal or intestinal pressure

Chronic diarrhea

Colorectal lesions

Dietary habits

Environmental factors (e.g., inaccessible bathroom)

General decline in muscle tone

Immobility

Impaction
Impaired cognition
Impaired reservoir capacity
Incomplete emptying of bowel
Laxative abuse
Loss of rectal sphincter control
Lower motor nerve damage
Medications
Rectal sphincter abnormality
Self-care deficit—toileting
Stress
Upper motor nerve damage

Suggestions for Use

(1) Differentiate between this label and *Diarrhea*. (2) *Self-care deficit: toileting* may be the cause of *Bowel incontinence*. However, there seems to be no advantage to writing a diagnosis of *Bowel incontinence related to Toileting self-care deficit*. A diagnosis such as *Toileting self-care deficit related to inability to ambulate to toilet or commode* provides more specific information about the self-care deficit and thus more guidance for nursing interventions to alleviate the problem.

Suggested Alternative Diagnoses

Diarrhea
Management of therapeutic regimen: individual, ineffective
Self-care deficit: toileting

NOC Outcomes

Bowel Continence: Control of passage of stool from the bowel
Bowel Elimination: Ability of the gastrointestinal tract to form and evacuate stool effectively
Tissue Integrity: Skin and Mucous Membranes: Structural intactness and normal physiological function of skin and mucous membranes

Goals/Evaluation Criteria

Examples Using NOC Language

- Patient will exhibit **Bowel Continence**, as evidenced by the following indicators (specify 1–5: never, rarely, sometimes, often, or consistently demonstrated):

    Maintains control of passage of stool

Consistently identifies urge to defecate

Consistently responds to urge in timely manner

Manages bowel appliance independently

Reaches toilet facility independently before defecating

Other Examples

Patient will:

- Have progressively fewer incontinent episodes
- Be free of skin irritation to perianal area

NIC Interventions

Bowel Incontinence Care: Promotion of bowel continence and maintenance of perianal skin integrity

Bowel Incontinence Care: Encopresis: Promotion of bowel continence in children

Bowel Management: Establishment and maintenance of a regular pattern of bowel elimination

Bowel Training: Assisting the patient to train the bowel to evacuate at specific intervals

Perineal Care: Maintenance of perineal skin integrity and relief of perineal discomfort

Nursing Activities

Assessments

- Assess condition of perianal skin after each episode of incontinence
- Document frequency of incontinent episodes
- Assess for symptoms of encopresis
- Obtain toilet training history of child, including duration of encopresis and treatment efforts
- *(NIC) Bowel Incontinence Care:*

  Determine physical or psychologic cause of fecal incontinence

  Monitor diet and fluid requirements

  Monitor for adequate bowel evacuation

  Determine goals of bowel management program with patient and family

Patient/Family Teaching

- Instruct patient and family about physiology of normal defecation
- For encopresis: Caution parents not to create feelings of anxiety, guilt, or inadequacy about toileting; teach parents ways to reward desired toileting behaviors

- *(NIC) Bowel Incontinence Care:*

  Instruct patient and family to record fecal output, as appropriate

  Discuss procedures and expected outcomes with patient

  Explain etiology of problem and rationale for actions

Collaborative Activities

- Obtain order from physician to institute bowel-training program (program may include bulk-forming laxative; rectal suppository q day; digital stimulation; and scheduled use of bedpan, commode, or bathroom)
- Refer for family therapy (e.g., for incontinence with emotional etiology)

Other

- Provide care in an accepting, nonjudgmental manner
- Provide bedpan or assist to commode q _____
- Provide privacy for defecation
- Establish a regular time for defecation
- Provide foods high in bulk and ample fluids
- Reinforce that the goal of therapy is to help the child with encopresis learn new bowel habits while avoiding excessive involvement of the parent with daily aspects of bowel function and diet
- *(NIC) Bowel Incontinence Care:*

  Wash perianal area with soap and water and dry it thoroughly after each stool

  Use powder and creams on perianal area with caution

  Keep bed and clothing clean

  Implement bowel-training program, as appropriate

  Place on incontinent pads, as needed

  Provide protective pants, as needed

BREASTFEEDING, EFFECTIVE
(00106) (1990)

Definition: Mother–infant dyad and family exhibit adequate proficiency and satisfaction with breastfeeding process.

Defining Characteristics

Subjective

Contentment of infant after feeding

Maternal verbalization of satisfaction with the breastfeeding process

Objective

Ability of mother to position infant at breast to promote a successful latch-on response

Adequate infant elimination patterns for age

Appropriate infant weight pattern for age

Eagerness of infant to nurse

Effective mother–infant communication patterns [e.g., infant cues, maternal interpretation or response]

Regular and sustained suckling and swallowing at breast

Signs and symptoms of oxytocin release [letdown or milk ejection reflex]

Related Factors

Basic breastfeeding knowledge

Infant gestational age greater than 34 weeks

Maternal confidence

Normal breast structure

Normal infant oral structure

Supportive source

Suggestions for Use

This is a wellness diagnosis; therefore it is not necessary to write it with an etiology (related factors). It represents a clinical judgment that breastfeeding is progressing satisfactorily and that there are no risk factors for *Ineffective breastfeeding*. During the first few days after childbirth, the nursing focus is to prevent or eliminate risk factors that might cause *Ineffective breastfeeding*. It is probably too soon, during that time, to conclude that there are no problems or risk factors, so a better choice might be *Risk for ineffective breastfeeding*.

Suggested Alternative Diagnoses

Ineffective breastfeeding, risk for

NOC Outcomes

Breastfeeding Establishment: Infant: Proper attachment of an infant to and sucking from the mother's breast for nourishment during the first 2–3 weeks

Breastfeeding Establishment: Maternal: Maternal establishment of proper attachment of an infant to and sucking from the breast for nourishment during the first 2–3 weeks

Breastfeeding Maintenance: Continued nourishment of an infant through breastfeeding

Breastfeeding Weaning: Process leading to the eventual discontinuation of breastfeeding

Goals/Evaluation Criteria

Examples Using NOC Language

See Ineffective Breastfeeding, pp. 53–54.

Other Examples

- Mother and infant will establish and maintain breastfeeding for as long as desired
- Infant will demonstrate correct:

  Alignment and areolar grasp

  Latching on technique and tongue placement

  Suck and audible swallow
- Mother will:

  Recognize early hunger cues

  State satisfaction with breastfeeding

  Experience no nipple tenderness

  Verbalize knowledge of signs of decreased milk supply

  Explain how to safely collect and store breast milk

NIC Interventions

Breastfeeding Assistance: Preparing a new mother to breastfeed her infant

Lactation Counseling: Use of an interactive helping process to assist in maintenance of successful breastfeeding

Lactation Suppression: Facilitating the cessation of milk production and minimizing breast engorgement after giving birth

Nursing Activities

Early Postpartum

Assessments

- Observe for correct breastfeeding technique
- *(NIC) Breastfeeding Assistance:*

  Monitor infant's ability to suck

  Monitor infant's ability to grasp the nipple correctly (i.e., latch-on skills)

  Monitor skin integrity of nipples

  Monitor letdown reflex

Patient/Family Teaching

- Discuss breastfeeding schedule, usually a "demand" time every 1½–3 hr
- Instruct mother in usual breastfeeding norms (e.g., increased frequency of nursing in first weeks of life, baby's elimination patterns, uterine contractions during nursing)
- Provide anticipatory guidance for potential problems such as maternal fatigue; breast engorgement; sore, cracked nipples; multiple births
- Discuss ways to enhance milk supply:
    Drink plenty of fluids
    Get enough rest (e.g., between feedings)
    Nurse frequently
    Use alternate breast at start of each feeding
- *(NIC) Breastfeeding Assistance:*
    Assist parents in identifying infant arousal cues as opportunities to practice breastfeeding
    Encourage mother not to restrict infant sucking time
    Inform mother of pump options available if needed to maintain lactation
    Encourage use of comfortable, cotton, supportive nursing bra
    Provide written materials to reinforce instructions at home

Collaborative Activities

- Make referrals to appropriate community resources, such as La Leche League, other nursing mothers, lactation consultant

Other

- Promote maternal confidence by providing positive feedback
- Provide opportunity to breast-feed within 1–2 hr after birth

Home Care

Assessments

- Assess breastfeeding technique within first 5–7 days after birth
- Confirm infant's elimination pattern
- Explore mother's breastfeeding plans, for example, duration, return to work, introduction of solid foods, weaning; provide anticipatory guidance

Patient/Family Teaching

- Discuss mother's need to check with physician prior to taking any medication while breastfeeding

- Provide instruction regarding breast engorgement, cracked/sore nipples, manual expression, infant appetite spurts, supplemental feedings

Collaborative Activities

- Encourage mother to enlist or request available resources for assistance (e.g., family, public health nurse, pediatrician, La Leche League, Nursing Mothers' Council)

Other

- Discuss impact of breastfeeding on family dynamics
- Discuss setting priorities that delegate meal preparation, increase mother's rest, and minimize care of the house
- Promote maternal confidence by providing encouragement, praise, and reassurance

BREASTFEEDING, INEFFECTIVE
(00104) (1988)

Definition: Dissatisfaction or difficulty a mother, infant, or child experiences with the breastfeeding process.

Defining Characteristics

Subjective

Perceived inadequate milk supply

Unsatisfactory breastfeeding process [as stated by mother]

Objective

Actual inadequate milk supply

Arching and crying at the breast

Fussiness and crying within the first hour after breastfeeding

Inability of infant to latch-on to maternal breast correctly

Insufficient emptying of each breast per feeding

Insufficient opportunity for suckling at the breast

No observable signs of oxytocin release

Nonsustained suckling at the breast

Observable signs of inadequate infant intake

Persistence of sore nipples beyond the first week of breastfeeding

Resistance to latching on

Unresponsiveness to other comfort measures

Related Factors

Inadequate sucking reflex in infant
Infant anomaly
Infant receiving supplemental feedings with artificial nipple
Interruption in breastfeeding
Knowledge deficit
Maternal anxiety or ambivalence
Maternal breast anomaly
Nonsupportive partner or family
Prematurity
Previous breast surgery
Previous history of breastfeeding failure

Suggestions for Use

This diagnosis focuses on the mother's satisfaction with the breastfeeding process and includes an actual or perceived inadequate milk supply. The comparisons in Table 3 may be helpful in determining a diagnosis.

Table 3

Diagnosis	Cues (Defining Characteristics)
Ineffective breastfeeding	Dissatisfaction with feeding process
Ineffective infant feeding pattern	Inability of infant to suck or poorly coordinated suck and swallow response
Interrupted breastfeeding	Mother wishes to maintain lactation but unable to put baby to breast for some feedings (e.g., illness or working)

Suggested Alternative Diagnoses

Breastfeeding, interrupted
Infant feeding pattern, ineffective

NOC Outcomes

Breastfeeding Establishment: Infant: Proper attachment of an infant to and sucking from the mother's breast for nourishment during the first 2–3 weeks

Breastfeeding Establishment: Maternal: Maternal establishment of proper attachment of an infant to and sucking from the breast for nourishment during the first 2–3 weeks

Breastfeeding Maintenance: Continued nourishment of an infant through breastfeeding

Breastfeeding Weaning: Process leading to the eventual discontinuation of breastfeeding

Knowledge: Breastfeeding: Extent of understanding conveyed about lactation and nourishment of infant through breastfeeding

Goals/Evaluation Criteria

Examples Using NOC Language

- Mother and infant will experience *Effective breastfeeding* as demonstrated by Knowledge: Breastfeeding; Breastfeeding Establishment: Infant/Maternal; Breastfeeding Maintenance; and Breastfeeding Weaning
- Infant will demonstrate **Breastfeeding Establishment: Infant**, as evidenced by the following indicators (specify 1–5: not, slightly, moderately, substantially, or totally adequate):

  Proper alignment and latch-on

  Proper areolar grasp and compression

  Correct suck and tongue placement

  Audible swallow

  Minimum eight feedings per day (on demand)

  Age-appropriate weight gain

  Infant contentment after feeding

Other Examples

Mother will:

- Maintain effective breastfeeding for as long as desired
- Describe increasing confidence with breastfeeding
- Recognize early hunger cues
- Indicate satisfaction with breastfeeding
- Not experience nipple tenderness
- Recognize signs of decreased milk supply

NIC Interventions

Breastfeeding Assistance: Preparing a new mother to breast-feed her infant

Lactation Counseling: Use of an interactive helping process to assist in maintenance of successful breastfeeding

Lactation Suppression: Facilitating the cessation of milk production and minimizing breast engorgement after giving birth

Nursing Activities

Assessments

- Assess infant's ability to latch-on and suck effectively
- *(NIC) Lactation Counseling:*
  Evaluate newborn suck and swallow pattern
  Determine mother's desire and motivation to breast-feed
  Evaluate mother's understanding of infant's feeding cues (e.g., rooting, sucking, and alertness)
  Monitor maternal skill with latching infant onto the nipple
  Monitor skin integrity of nipples
  Evaluate understanding of plugged milk ducts and mastitis
  Monitor ability to correctly relieve breast congestion

Patient/Family Teaching

- Instruct mother in breastfeeding techniques that increase her skill in feeding infant; consider relaxation techniques, comfortable positioning, stimulation of rooting reflex, establishment of infant alert state before attempting to feed, stimulation of infant to continue to feed, and alternation of breasts
- Instruct mother in breast-pumping techniques to maintain milk supply during interruptions or delays in infant sucking reflex
- Instruct mother in need for adequate rest and intake of fluids
- *(NIC) Lactation Counseling:*
  Provide information about advantages and disadvantages of breastfeeding
  Discuss alternative methods of feeding
  Correct misconceptions, misinformation, and inaccuracies about breastfeeding
  Demonstrate suck training, as appropriate
  Instruct about infant stool and urination patterns, as appropriate
  Recommend nipple care, as needed
  Instruct on signs of problems to report to health care practitioner
  Discuss signs of readiness to wean

Collaborative Activities

- Refer to appropriate community resources, such as La Leche League and the public health department

Other

- Have mother express enough milk to relieve engorgement, allowing nipples to evert

- Increase number of nursings on demand for a crying, wakeful infant
- Increase number of scheduled nursings for the sleepy infant of low birth weight
- Offer food and fluids to mother during day and evening prior to breastfeeding times
- Provide privacy for mother and infant
- Recognize *time-out* behaviors in premature infant
- Schedule rest periods, as needed
- Reinforce successful behaviors
- *(NIC) Lactation Counseling:*
  Provide support of mother's decisions
  Encourage continued lactation on return to work or school

BREASTFEEDING, INTERRUPTED
(00105) (1992)

Definition: Break in the continuity of the breastfeeding process as a result of inability or inadvisability to put baby to breast for feeding.

Defining Characteristics

Subjective
Maternal desire to maintain lactation and provide (or eventually provide) her breast milk for her infant's nutritional needs

Objective
Infant does not receive nourishment at the breast for some or all of feedings

Lack of knowledge regarding expression and storage of breast milk

Separation of mother and infant

Related Factors

Abrupt weaning of infant

Contraindications to breastfeeding

[Engorgement]

Maternal employment [obligations outside the home]

Maternal medications that are contraindicated for the infant

Maternal or infant illness

Prematurity

[Sore or cracked nipples]

Suggestions for Use

Because this diagnosis represents a situation rather than a response, there is little the nurse can do to correct the interruption (e.g., the need for the mother to work). Therefore, this label might function best as an etiology (e.g., *Risk for ineffective breastfeeding related to Interrupted breastfeeding secondary to mother's employment*). Also see Suggestions for Use for Ineffective Breastfeeding, on p. 53.

Suggested Alternative Diagnoses

Breastfeeding, ineffective
Infant feeding pattern, ineffective

NOC Outcomes

Breastfeeding Maintenance: Continued nourishment of an infant through breastfeeding
Knowledge: Breastfeeding: Extent of understanding conveyed about lactation and nourishment of infant through breastfeeding
Parent–Infant Attachment: Behaviors which demonstrate an enduring affectionate bond between a parent and infant

Goals/Evaluation Criteria

Examples Using NOC Language

- Mother and baby will not experience *Interrupted breastfeeding*, as evidenced by substantial Breastfeeding Knowledge, Maintenance of Breastfeeding, and consistently demonstrated Parent–Infant Attachment.
- Mother and baby will demonstrate **Breastfeeding Maintenance**, as evidenced by the following indicators (specify 1–5: not, slightly, moderately, substantially, or totally adequate):
    Infant growth and development in normal range
    Recognition of signs of decreased milk supply
    Mother's continuation of lactation on return to work or school
    Mother's ability to safely collect and store breast milk, if desired
    Care provider's ability to safely thaw, warm, and feed stored breast milk

Other Examples

- Mother and infant will maintain effective breastfeeding for as long as desired

Mother will:

- Choose and demonstrate preferred technique for expression of milk

- Describe safe storage techniques for expressed milk

Baby will:

- Receive mother's milk
- Gain _____ g/day or _____ g/week

NIC Interventions

Attachment Promotion: Facilitation of the development of the parent–infant relationship

Bottle Feeding: Preparation and administration of fluids to an infant via a bottle

Emotional Support: Provision of reassurance, acceptance, and encouragement during times of stress

Environmental Management: Attachment Process: Manipulation of the patient's surroundings to facilitate the development of the parent–infant relationship

Kangaroo Care: Promoting closeness between parent and physiologically stable preterm infant by preparing the parent and providing the environment for skin-to-skin contact

Lactation Counseling: Use of an interactive helping process to assist in maintenance of successful breastfeeding

Lactation Suppression: Facilitating the cessation of milk production and minimizing breast engorgement after giving birth

Nursing Activities

Assessments

- Assess family's ability to support lactation and breastfeeding plan and cope with lifestyle changes
- Assess mother's desire and motivation to continue breastfeeding
- Confirm readiness for transition to breast after interruption (e.g., infant's stability when outside the Isolette; infant's coordination of sucking, swallowing, and breathing; mother's willingness to try)
- Consider a feeding flow sheet to facilitate assessment: Document infant's state, oxygen needs, positioning, time at breast, total nursing time, daily weight, stool pattern
- *(NIC) Bottle Feeding:*

  Determine water source used to dilute concentrated or powdered formula

  Determine fluoride content of water used to dilute concentrated or powdered formula and refer for fluoride supplementation, if indicated

  Monitor infant weight, as appropriate

Patient/Family Teaching

- Assist working mother to maintain lactation by including the following teaching:

    Provide information about lactation and breast milk expression (with manual and electric pump), collection, and storage

    Display and demonstrate variety of breast pumps, providing information about costs, effectiveness, and availability of each

    Educate infant caretaker on topics such as storage and thawing of breast milk and avoidance of bottle feedings in the 2 hr prior to mother's return home

    Provide information to enhance milk volume on topics such as adequate rest, regular expression of milk, and increase in mother's intake of fluid, especially toward the end of the work week

- *(NIC) Bottle Feeding:* Caution parent or caregiver about using microwave oven to warm formula

Other

- Assist mother in setting realistic goals for herself
- Encourage continued feeding of breast milk on return to work or school
- Assist mother and premature infant with transition to breast:

    Encourage skin-to-skin contact for mother and infant, using cover blanket over infant to maintain body temperature

    Help infant open mouth wider

    Position baby with one hand supporting head, leaving the other hand free to manipulate breast; ear, shoulder, and hips of infant should be aligned so that mother's nipples do not become sore

    Provide privacy

- Assist working mother to maintain lactation and effective breastfeeding:

    A few days before mother's return to work, introduce baby to bottle in different situations: someone other than mother presents bottle, mother is not present, baby is hungry, in a different place than usual for breastfeeding

    Develop schedule for expression and storage of milk at work

    Establish support network to ensure that mother has help with day-to-day lactation and breastfeeding problems as they occur

    Provide anticipatory guidance for potential problems (e.g., engorgement, pain, leaking, diminished milk production, feelings of disappointment and anger, depression, guilt, inadequacy)

Allow infant, once latched on, to nurse until sucking and swallowing stop; switch baby to other breast and repeat until suck or swallow stops, then switch back. Time at breast will be longer than at bottle, but not to the point of infant's exhaustion.

- If abrupt weaning is necessary, assist mother to:

  Introduce bottle feeding

  Manage breast discomfort

  Verbalize feelings about sudden change in plans

BREATHING PATTERN, INEFFECTIVE
(00032) (1980, 1996, 1998)

Definition: Inspiration or expiration that does not provide adequate ventilation.

Defining Characteristics

Subjective

Dyspnea

Shortness of breath

Objective

Altered chest excursion

Assumption of three-point position

Decreased inspiratory–expiratory pressure

Decreased minute ventilation

Decreased vital capacity

Depth of breathing (adults V_T 500 ml at rest, infants 6–8 ml/kg)

Increased anterior–posterior diameter

Nasal flaring

Orthopnea

Prolonged expiration phases

Pursed-lip breathing

Respiratory rate (adults ages 14 or older < 11–24 [breaths per minute], infants 25–60, ages 1–4 < 20–30, ages 5–14 < 15–25)

Timing ratio

Use of accessory muscles to breathe

Related Factors

Anxiety

Body position

Bony deformity
Chest wall deformity
Decreased energy and fatigue
Hyperventilation
Hypoventilation syndrome
Musculoskeletal impairment
Neurological immaturity
Neuromuscular dysfunction
Obesity
Pain
Perception and cognitive impairment
Respiratory muscle fatigue
Spinal cord injury

Suggestions for Use

Do not use this label if the condition cannot be treated by independent nursing actions. Consider, too, that *Ineffective breathing pattern* may be a symptom of another more useful diagnosis, such as *Anxiety*; or it may be the etiology of another diagnosis, such as *Activity intolerance*. Differentiate carefully among this and the suggested alternative diagnoses. Also see Suggestions for Use for Airway Clearance, Ineffective, pp. 16–17.

Suggested Alternative Diagnoses

Activity intolerance
Airway clearance, ineffective
Gas exchange, impaired

NOC Outcomes

Respiratory Status: Airway Patency: Extent to which the tracheobronchial passages remain open
Respiratory Status: Ventilation: Movement of air in and out of the
lungs
Vital Signs Status: Temperature, pulse, respiration, and blood
pressure within expected range for the individual

Goals/Evaluation Criteria

Examples Using NOC Language

• Demonstrates effective breathing patterns, as evidenced by
uncompromised Respiratory Status: Ventilation; Respiratory
Status: Airway Patency; and Vital Signs Status

- Demonstrates uncompromised **Respiratory Status: Ventilation**, as evidenced by the following indicators (specify 1–5: extremely, substantially, moderately, mildly, or not compromised):

    Depth of inspiration and ease of breathing

    Chest expansion symmetric

    Accessory muscle use not present

    Adventitious breath sounds not present

    Shortness of breath not present

Other Examples

Patient will:

- Demonstrate optimal breathing while on mechanical ventilator
- Have respiratory rate and rhythm within normal limits
- Have pulmonary function within normal limits for patient
- Request breathing assistance when needed
- Be able to describe plan for care at home

NIC Interventions

Airway Management: Facilitation of patency of air passages

Airway Suctioning: Removal of airway secretions by inserting a suction catheter into the patient's oral airway or trachea

Respiratory Monitoring: Collection and analysis of patient data to ensure airway patency and adequate gas exchange

Ventilation Assistance: Promotion of an optimal spontaneous breathing pattern that maximizes oxygen and carbon dioxide exchange in the lungs

Vital Signs Monitoring: Collection and analysis of cardiovascular, respiratory, and body temperature data to determine and prevent complications

Nursing Activities

Assessments

- Monitor for pallor and cyanosis
- Monitor effect of medications on respiratory status
- Determine location and extent of crepitus over rib cage
- Assess need for airway insertion
- Observe and document bilateral chest expansion of patient on ventilator
- *(NIC) Respiratory Monitoring:*

    Monitor rate, rhythm, depth, and effort of respirations

    Note chest movement, watching for symmetry, use of accessory muscles, and supraclavicular and intercostal muscle retractions

Monitor for noisy respirations, such as crowing or snoring

Monitor breathing patterns: bradypnea; tachypnea; hyperventilation; Kussmaul respirations; Cheyne-Stokes respirations; and apneustic, Biot, and ataxic patterns

Note location of trachea

Auscultate breath sounds, noting areas of decreased/absent ventilation and presence of adventitious sounds

Monitor for increased restlessness, anxiety, and air hunger

Note changes in SaO_2, SvO_2, end-tidal CO_2, and arterial blood gas (ABG) values, as appropriate

Patient/Family Teaching

- Inform patient and family about relaxation techniques to improve breathing pattern; specify techniques
- Discuss the plan for care at home, including medications, supportive equipment, signs and symptoms of reportable complications, community resources
- Teach how to cough effectively
- Inform patient and family that smoking is prohibited in room
- Instruct patient and family that they should notify the nurse at onset of ineffective breathing pattern

Collaborative Activities

- Confer with respiratory therapist to ensure adequate functioning of mechanical ventilator
- Report changes in sensorium, breath sounds, respiratory pattern, ABGs, sputum, and so forth, as needed or per protocols
- Administer medications (e.g., bronchodilators) per order or protocols
- Administer ultrasonic nebulizer treatments and humidified air or oxygen per order or agency protocols
- Give pain medications to allow optimal respiratory pattern, specify schedule

Other

- Correlate and document all assessment data (e.g., patient sensorium, breath sounds, respiratory pattern, ABGs, sputum, effect of medications)
- Help patient to use incentive spirometer, as needed
- Reassure patient during periods of respiratory distress
- Encourage slow abdominal breathing during periods of respiratory distress
- Suction as needed to remove secretions
- Have patient turn, cough, and deep breathe q _____

- Inform patient before beginning intended procedures, to lower anxiety and increase sense of control
- Maintain low-flow oxygen by nasal cannula, mask, hood, or tent, specify flow rate.
- Position patient for optimal breathing, specify position.
- Synchronize patient's breathing pattern with ventilator rate

---

CARDIAC OUTPUT, DECREASED
(00029) (1975, 1996, 2000)

Definition: Inadequate blood pumped by the heart to meet the metabolic demands of the body.

Defining Characteristics

Altered Heart Rate and Rhythm
Arrhythmias (tachycardia, bradycardia)
EKG changes
Palpitations

Altered Preload
Edema
Fatigue
Increased or decreased central venous pressure (CVP)
Increased or decreased pulmonary artery wedge pressure (PAWP)
Jugular vein distention
Murmurs
Weight gain

Altered Afterload
Cold and clammy skin
Decreased peripheral pulses
Increased or decreased pulmonary vascular resistance (PVR)
Increased or decreased systemic vascular resistance (SVR)
Oliguria
Prolonged capillary refill
Shortness of breath or dyspnea
Skin color changes
Variations in blood pressure readings

Altered Contractility
Crackles
Cough
Orthopnea or paroxysmal nocturnal dyspnea
Cardiac output < 4 L/min

Cardiac index < 2.5 L/min

Decreased ejection fraction, stroke volume index (SVI), left ventricular stroke work index (LVSWI)

S_3 or S_4 sounds

Behavioral/Emotional

Anxiety

Restlessness

Related Factors

Altered heart rate or rhythm

Altered Stroke Volume

Altered preload

Altered afterload

Altered contractility

Non-NANDA International related factors:

Cardiac anomaly (specify)

Drug toxicity

Dysfunctional electrical conduction

Hypovolemia

Increased ventricular workload

Ventricular damage

Ventricular ischemia

Ventricular restriction

Suggestions for Use

This label does not suggest independent nursing actions. The nurse can neither conclusively diagnose nor definitively treat this problem. For patients with physiologic decreased cardiac output, you may find it more useful to use a label that represents a human response to this pathophysiology (e.g., *Activity intolerance related to Decreased cardiac output*). If the patient is at risk for developing complications, write them as collaborative problems (e.g., Potential Complication of myocardial infarction: Cardiogenic shock).

Suggested Alternative Diagnoses

Activity intolerance

Self-care deficit

NOC Outcomes

Cardiac Pump Effectiveness: Extent to which blood is ejected from the left ventricle per minute to support systemic perfusion pressure

Circulation Status: Extent to which blood flows unobstructed, unidirectionally, and at an appropriate pressure through large vessels of the systemic and pulmonary circuits

Tissue Perfusion: Abdominal Organs: Extent to which blood flows through the small vessels of the abdominal viscera and maintains organ function

Tissue Perfusion: Peripheral: Extent to which blood flows through the small vessels of the extremities and maintains tissue function

Vital Signs Status: Temperature, pulse, respiration, and blood pressure within expected range for the individual

Goals/Evaluation Criteria

Examples Using NOC Language

- Demonstrates satisfactory cardiac output, as evidenced by Vital Signs Status, Cardiac Pump Effectiveness, Circulation Status, Tissue Perfusion (Abdominal Organs), and Tissue Perfusion (Peripheral)
- Demonstrates **Circulation Status**, as evidenced by the following indicators (specify 1–5: extremely, substantially, moderately, mildly, or not compromised):
    Systolic, diastolic, and mean blood pressure (BP) IER
    Heart rate IER
    Central venous pressure and pulmonary wedge pressure IER
    Orthostatic hypotension not present
    Blood gases IER
    Adventitious breath sounds not present
    Neck vein distention not present
    Peripheral edema not present
    Ascites not present
    Peripheral pulses strong and symmetric
    Cognitive status IER

Other Examples

Patient will:
- Have cardiac index and ejection fraction within normal limits
- Have urine output, urine specific gravity, blood urea nitrogen (BUN), and plasma creatinine within normal limits
- Have normal skin color
- Demonstrate increasing tolerance for physical activity
- Describe the required diet, medications, activity, and limitations
- Identify reportable signs and symptoms of worsening condition

NIC Interventions

Cardiac Care: Limitation of complications resulting from an imbalance between myocardial oxygen supply and demand for a patient with symptoms of impaired cardiac function

Cardiac Care, Acute: Limitation of complications for a patient recently experiencing an episode of an imbalance between myocardial oxygen supply and demand resulting in impaired cardiac function

Circulatory Care: Arterial Insufficiency: Promotion of arterial circulation

Circulatory Care: Mechanical Assist Device: Temporary support of the circulation through the use of mechanical devices or pumps

Circulatory Care: Venous Insufficiency: Promotion of venous circulation

Embolus Care: Peripheral: Limitation of complications for a patient experiencing, or at risk for, occlusion of peripheral circulation

Hemodynamic Regulation: Optimization of heart rate, preload, afterload, and contractility

Intravenous (IV) Therapy: Administration and monitoring of intravenous (IV) fluids and medications

Shock Management: Cardiac: Promotion of adequate tissue perfusion for a patient with severely compromised pumping function of the heart

Vital Signs Monitoring: Collection and analysis of cardiovascular, respiratory, and body temperature data to determine and prevent complications

Nursing Activities

Assessments

- Assess and document BP, presence of cyanosis, respiratory status, and mental status
- Monitor for signs of fluid overload (e.g., dependent edema, weight gain)
- Assess patient's activity tolerance by noting onset of shortness of breath, pain, palpitations, or dizziness
- Evaluate patient's responses to oxygen therapy
- *(NIC) Hemodynamic Regulation:*
  Monitor pacemaker functioning, if appropriate
  Monitor peripheral pulses, capillary refill, and temperature and color of extremities
  Monitor intake and output, urine output, and patient weight, as appropriate

Monitor systemic and pulmonary vascular resistance, as appropriate

Auscultate lung sounds for crackles or other adventitious sounds

Monitor and document heart rate, rhythm, and pulses

Patient/Family Teaching

- Explain purpose of administering oxygen per nasal cannula or mask
- Instruct regarding maintenance of accurate intake and output
- Teach use, dose, frequency, and side effects of medications
- Teach to report and describe palpitations and pain onset, duration, precipitating factors, site, quality, and intensity
- Instruct patient and family in plan for care at home, including activity limitations, diet restrictions, and use of therapeutic equipment
- Provide information on stress-reduction techniques such as biofeedback, progressive muscle relaxation, meditation, and exercise

Collaborative Activities

- Confer with physician regarding parameters for administering or withholding BP medications
- Administer and titrate antiarrhythmic, inotropic, nitroglycerin, and vasodilator medications to maintain contractility, preload, and afterload per medical order or protocols
- Administer anticoagulants to prevent peripheral thrombus formation, per order or protocol
- Promote afterload reduction (e.g., with intraaortic balloon pumping) per medical order or protocol

Other

- Change patient's position to flat or Trendelenburg when BP is in a range lower than normal for patient
- For sudden, severe, or prolonged hypotension, establish IV access for administration of IV fluids or medications to raise BP
- Correlate effects of laboratory values, oxygen, medications, activity, anxiety, and pain on the dysrhythmia
- Do not take rectal temperatures
- Turn patient every 2 hr or maintain other appropriate or required activity to decrease peripheral circulation stasis
- *(NIC) Hemodynamic Regulation:*
  Minimize or eliminate environmental stressors
  Insert urinary catheter, if appropriate

CAREGIVER ROLE STRAIN
(00061) (1992, 1998, 2000)

Definition: Difficulty in performing family caregiver role.

Defining Characteristics

Caregiving Activities

Apprehension about care receiver's care if caregiver becomes ill or dies

Apprehension about possible institutionalization of care receiver

Apprehension about the future regarding care receiver's health and the caregiver's ability to provide care

Difficulty performing or completing required tasks

Dysfunctional change in caregiving activities

Preoccupation with care routine

Caregiver Health Status

Physical

Cardiovascular disease

Diabetes

Fatigue

Gastrointestinal upset (e.g., mild stomach cramps, vomiting, diarrhea, recurrent gastric ulcer episodes)

Headaches

Hypertension

Rash

Weight change

Emotional

Anger

Disturbed sleep

Feeling depressed

Frustration

Impaired individual coping

Impatience

Increased emotional lability

Increased nervousness

Lack of time to meet personal needs

Somatization

Stress

Socioeconomic

Changes in leisure activities

Low work productivity

Refuses career advancement

Withdraws from social life

Caregiver–Care Receiver Relationship

Difficulty watching care receiver go through the illness

Grief or uncertainty regarding changed relationship with care receiver

Family Processes

Concerns about family members

Family conflict

Related Factors/Risk Factors

Care Receiver Health Status

Addiction or codependency

Illness chronicity

Illness severity

Increasing care needs and dependency

Instability of care receiver's health

Problem behaviors

Psychological or cognitive problems

Unpredictability of illness course

Caregiving Activities

24-hr care responsibilities

Amount of activities

Complexity of activities

Discharge of family members to home with significant care needs

Ongoing changes in activities

Unpredictability of care situation

Years of caregiving

Caregiver Health Status

Addiction or codependency

Inability to fulfill one's own or other's expectations

Marginal coping patterns

Physical problems

Psychological or cognitive problems

Unrealistic expectations of self

Socioeconomic

Alienation from family, friends, and coworkers

Competing role commitments

Insufficient recreation

Isolation from others

Caregiver–Care Receiver Relationship

History of poor relationship

Mental status of elder inhibiting conversation

Presence of abuse or violence

Unrealistic expectations of caregiver by care receiver

Family Processes

History of family dysfunction

History of marginal family coping

Resources

Assistance and support (formal and informal)

Caregiver is not developmentally ready for caregiver role

Emotional strength

Inadequate community resources (e.g., respite services, recreational resources)

Inadequate equipment for providing care

Inadequate physical environment for providing care (e.g., housing, temperature, safety)

Inadequate transportation

Inexperience with caregiving

Insufficient finances

Insufficient time

Lack of caregiver privacy

Lack of knowledge about or difficulty accessing community resources

Lack of support

Physical energy

Suggestions for Use

Caregiver role strain focuses on the burden of the individual caregiver who has had to assume the care of a family member. The family diagnoses (*Family coping and Interrupted family processes*) focus on the family system and the manner in which family functioning has been altered by a stressor. The stressor in those diagnoses is not necessarily the need to care for a family member.

Suggested Alternative Diagnoses

Coping: family, compromised

Coping: family, disabled

Family processes, interrupted

Management of therapeutic regimen: families, ineffective

NOC Outcomes

Caregiver Emotional Health: Feelings, attitudes, and emotions of a family care provider while caring for a family member or significant other over an extended period of time

Caregiver Home Care Readiness: Preparedness to assume responsibility for the health care of a family member or significant other in the home

Caregiver Lifestyle Disruption: Disturbances in the lifestyle of a family member due to caregiving

Caregiver–Patient Relationship: Positive interactions and connections between the caregiver and care recipient

Caregiver Performance: Direct Care: Provision by family care provider of appropriate personal and health care for a family member or significant other

Caregiver Performance: Indirect Care: Arrangement and oversight of appropriate care for a family member or significant other

Caregiver Physical Health: Physical well-being of a family care provider while caring for a family member or significant other over an extended period of time

Caregiver Stressors: The extent of biopsychosocial pressure on a family care provider caring for a family member or significant other over an extended period of time

Caregiver Well-Being: Primary care provider's satisfaction with health and life circumstances

Caregiving Endurance Potential: Factors that promote family care provider continuance over an extended period of time

Role Performance: Congruence of an individual's role behavior with role expectations

Goals/Evaluation Criteria

Examples Using NOC Language

- Experiences relief from *Caregiver role strain*, as demonstrated by adequacy of Caregiver Emotional Health, Caregiver Home Care Readiness, Caregiver–Patient Relationship, Caregiver Performance: Direct and Indirect Care, Caregiver Physical Health, Caregiver Well-Being, Caregiving Endurance Potential, and Role Performance; minimal Caregiver Lifestyle Disruption and Caregiver Stressors

- Demonstrates **Caregiver Emotional Health**, as evidenced by the following indicators (specify 1–5: extremely, substantially, moderately, mildly, or not compromised):

Free of anger, resentfulness, guilt, depression, frustration, perceived burden, and ambivalence concerning situation

Satisfaction with life

Sense of control and self-esteem

Perceived spiritual well-being

Other Examples

Caregiver will:

- Verbalize knowledge of treatment regimen and procedures, follow-up care, and emergency care
- Verbalize knowledge of how to obtain and operate needed equipment
- Express willingness to assume caregiving role
- Ensure provision of appropriate level of care
- Balance competing family and personal needs
- Identify and use personal strengths, social supports, and community resources

NIC Interventions

Caregiver Support: Provision of the necessary information, advocacy, and support to facilitate primary patient care by someone other than a health care professional

Coping Enhancement: Assisting a patient to adapt to perceived stressors, changes, or threats which interfere with meeting life demands and roles

Parenting Promotion: Providing parenting information, support and coordination of comprehensive services to high-risk families

Respite Care: Provision of short-term care to provide relief for family caregiver

Role Enhancement: Assisting a patient, significant other, and family to improve relationships by clarifying and supplementing specific role behaviors

Teaching: Individual: Planning, implementation, and evaluation of a teaching program designed to address a patient's particular needs

Nursing Activities

Assessments

- Assess care receiver for signs of emotional or physical neglect or abuse
- Assess caregiver for signs of increasing role strain (e.g., depression, anxiety, increased use or abuse of alcohol or drugs, frustration, helplessness, sleeplessness, lowered morale, physical or emotional exhaustion, and personal health problems)

- *(NIC) Caregiver Support:*
  Determine caregiver's level of knowledge
  Determine caregiver's acceptance of role
  Monitor family interaction problems related to care of patient

Patient/Family Teaching

- Acknowledge and teach that the work of the caregiver is both physical and mental and includes (Bowers, 1987):
  Anticipatory caregiving (making decisions based on possible future needs of care receiver, e.g., place of residence)
  Instrumental caregiving (direct, hands-on care)
  Preventive caregiving (taking action to prevent illness, injury, or complications, e.g., altering the physical environment, preparing meals)
  Protective caregiving (protecting care receiver from threats to self-image, identity, and change in relationship with caregiver)
  Supervisory caregiving (arranging for and monitoring care, e.g., making appointments, arranging transportation)
- Facilitate coping and adjustment by teaching caregiver and care receiver how to (Chilman, Nunnally & Cox, 1988):
  Deal with pain, incapacitation, and illness-related symptoms
  Deal with hospital environment and disease-related treatments and procedures
  Establish and maintain workable relationships with the health care team
- *(NIC) Caregiver Support:*
  Teach caregiver stress management techniques
  Educate caregiver about the grieving process

Collaborative Activities

- Refer as needed for counseling and support during times of stress or crisis
- Refer for necessary assistance with preventive, supervisory, and instrumental caregiving (e.g., Visiting Nurse Association, respite care, hospice care, day treatment, secondary caregivers)
- Report to authorities signs of care receiver physical or emotional neglect or abuse

Other

- Arrange for parent(s) of chronically ill child to receive training in areas of child development and education and compliance-related behavior problems

- Assist caregiver to identify problems or concerns with caregiving (e.g., lack of knowledge, skill, and emotional readiness for caregiving; lack of social support; financial burden; disruptive behavior; increasing need for physical care)
- Develop a plan of care with caregiver that identifies coping mechanisms, personal strengths, social supports, and acknowledged limitations. Consider including the following:

  Assistance with household tasks

  Family therapy

  Self-help and mutual support groups for information, advocacy, and emotional support
- Explore with caregiver the possibility of institutional care (now or in the future) and feelings associated with institutionalization
- Explore with caregiver–care receiver past and current closeness, shared activities, and confiding in one another as indications of emotional investment and commitment to the caregiver role
- Facilitate family's adjustment to illness of family member by assisting them to (Chilman, Nunnally & Cox, 1988):

  Develop flexibility regarding future goals

  Grieve for the loss of pre-illness family identity

  Maintain a sense of mastery over their lives

  Move toward acceptance of changes

  Pull together during short-term crisis
- *(NIC) Caregiver Support:*

  Accept expressions of negative emotion

  Act for caregiver if overburdening becomes apparent

CAREGIVER ROLE STRAIN, RISK FOR
(00062) (1992)

Definition: Caregiver is vulnerable for felt difficulty in performing the family caregiver role.

Risk Factors

Objective

Addiction or codependency

Care receiver exhibits deviant, bizarre behavior

Caregiver health impairment

Caregiver is female

Caregiver is not developmentally ready for caregiver role (e.g., a young adult needing to provide care for middle-aged care receiver)

Caregiver is spouse

Caregiver's competing role commitments

Complexity and amount of caregiving tasks

Developmental delay or retardation of the care receiver or caregiver

Discharge of family member with significant home care needs

Duration of caregiving required

Family–caregiver isolation

Illness severity of the care receiver

Inadequate physical environment for providing care (e.g., housing, transportation, community services, equipment)

Inexperience with caregiving

Lack of respite and recreation for caregiver

Marginal caregiver's coping patterns

Marginal family adaptation or dysfunction prior to the caregiving situation

Past history of poor relationship between caregiver and care receiver

Premature birth or congenital defect

Presence of abuse or violence

Presence of situational stressors which normally affect families (e.g., significant loss, disaster, or crisis; economic vulnerability; major life events)

Psychological or cognitive problems in care receiver

Unpredictable illness course or instability in the care receiver's health

Suggestions for Use

See Caregiver Role Strain, p. 71.

Suggested Alternative Diagnoses

Coping: family, compromised

Coping: family, disabled

Family processes, interrupted

Management of therapeutic regimen: families, ineffective

NOC Outcomes

See Caregiver Role Strain, p. 72.

Family Coping: Family actions to manage stressors that tax family resources

Family Functioning: Ability of the family to meet the needs of its members through developmental transitions

Knowledge: Energy Conservation: Extent of understanding conveyed about energy conservation techniques

Knowledge: Health Behaviors: Extent of understanding conveyed about the promotion and protection of health

Knowledge: Health Resources: Extent of understanding conveyed about health care resources

Rest: Extent and pattern of diminished activity for mental and physical rejuvenation

Risk Control: Actions to eliminate or reduce actual, personal, and modifiable health threats

Risk Detection: Actions taken to identify personal health threats

Goals/Evaluation Criteria

See Caregiver Role Strain, pp. 72–73.

NIC Interventions

Caregiver Support: Provision of the necessary information, advocacy, and support to facilitate primary patient care by someone other than a health care professional

Coping Enhancement: Assisting a patient to adapt to perceived stressors, changes, or threats which interfere with meeting life demands and roles

Emotional Support: Provision of reassurance, acceptance, and encouragement during times of stress

Energy management: Regulating energy use to treat or prevent fatigue and optimize function

Family Involvement Promotion: Facilitating family participation in the emotional and physical care of the patient

Health Screening: Detecting health risks or problems by means of history, examination, and other procedures

Parent Education: Childrearing Family: Assisting parents to understand and promote the physical, psychological, and social growth and development of their toddler, preschool, or school-aged child or children

Parent Education: Infant: Instruction on nurturing and physical care needed during the first year of life

Parenting Promotion: Providing parenting information, support, and coordination of comprehensive services to high-risk families

Respite Care: Provision of short-term care to provide relief for family caregiver

Nursing Activities

Assessments

- Assess caregiver's level of knowledge of medical and care regimen
- Determine caregiver's desire for and acceptance of role
- See Assessments for Caregiver Role Strain, on pp. 73–74.

Patient/Family Teaching

- See Patient and Family Teaching for Caregiver Role Strain, on p. 74.

Collaborative Activities

- See Collaborative Activities for Caregiver Role Strain, on p. 74.

Other

- See Other activities for Caregiver Role Strain, on pp. 74–75.

COMMUNICATION, READINESS FOR ENHANCED
(00157) (2002)

Definition: A pattern of exchanging information and ideas with others that is sufficient for meeting one's needs and life's goals and can be strengthened.

Defining Characteristics

Subjective

Expresses satisfaction with ability to share information and ideas with others

Objective

Able to speak or write a language

Expresses thoughts and feelings

Expresses willingness to enhance communication

Forms words, phrases, and language

Uses and interprets nonverbal cues appropriately

Suggestions for Use

Because this is a wellness diagnosis, an etiology (i.e., related factors) is not needed. If situations exist that pose a risk to effective communication, use *Risk for impaired verbal communication*.

Suggested Alternative Diagnoses

Risk for impaired verbal communication

NOC Outcomes

NOC outcomes have not yet been linked to this diagnosis; however, the following may be useful:

Communication Ability: Ability to receive, interpret, and express spoken, written, and nonverbal messages

Communication: Expressive Ability: Ability to express and interpret verbal and nonverbal messages

Communication: Receptive Ability: Ability to receive and interpret verbal and nonverbal messages

Goals/Evaluation Criteria

Examples Using NOC Language:

- Demonstrates **Communication Ability**, as evidenced by the following indicators (specify 1–5: extremely, substantially, moderately, mildly, or not compromised):

  Use of written, spoken, or nonverbal language

  Use of sign language

  Use of pictures and drawings

  Acknowledgment of messages received

  Exchange [of] messages with others

Other Examples

Patient will:

- Report improved ability to communicate verbally
- Report improved nonverbal communication

NIC Interventions

Interventions have not yet been developed for this diagnosis; however, the following may be useful:

Active Listening: Attending closely to and attaching significance to a patient's verbal and nonverbal messages

Assertiveness Training: Assistance with the effective expression of feelings, needs, and ideas while respecting the rights of others

Learning Readiness Enhancement: Improving the ability and willingness to receive information

Nursing Activities

Assessments

- Assess clarity and effectiveness of verbal messages
- Assess for barriers to assertiveness
- Determine areas in which patient wishes to improve his communication (e.g., verbal, nonverbal, written)

Patient/Family Teaching

- Teach the difference between assertiveness and aggressiveness
- Role model assertive behaviors
- Teach strategies for assertiveness (e.g., saying no appropriately, beginning and ending conversations, making requests)

Other

- Demonstrate interest in the patient
- Encourage to express both positive and negative ideas and feelings
- Use questions and feedback to improve the clarity of verbal and nonverbal messages
- Give praise for improved communication
- Assist with planning opportunities to practice communication techniques

COMMUNICATION, VERBAL, IMPAIRED
(00051) (1983, 1996, 1998)

Definition: Decreased, delayed, or absent ability to receive, process, transmit, and use a system of symbols (anything that has or transmits meaning).

Defining Characteristics

Objective

Absence of eye contact or difficulty in selective attending

Difficulty expressing thoughts verbally (e.g., aphasia, dysphasia, apraxia, dyslexia)

Difficulty forming words or sentences (e.g., aphonia, dyslalia, dysarthria)

Difficulty in comprehending and maintaining the usual communication pattern

Disorientation in the three spheres of time, space, person

Does not or cannot speak

Dyspnea

Inability or difficulty in use of facial or body expressions

Inappropriate verbalization

Partial or total visual deficit

Slurring

Speaks or verbalizes with difficulty

Stuttering

Unable to speak dominant language
Willful refusal to speak

Related Factors

Absence of significant others
Alteration of central nervous system
Alteration of self-esteem or self-concept
Altered perceptions
Anatomical defect (e.g., cleft palate, alteration of the neuromuscular visual system, auditory system, or phonatory apparatus)
Brain tumor
Cultural difference
Decrease in circulation to brain
Differences related to developmental age
Emotional conditions
Environmental barriers
Lack of information
Physical barrier (e.g., tracheostomy, intubation)
Physiological conditions
Psychological barriers (e.g., psychosis, lack of stimuli)
Side effects of medications
Stress
Weakening of the musculoskeletal system

Suggestions for Use

Use this label for those who want to communicate but who have difficulty doing so. If communication problems are caused by psychiatric illness or coping difficulties, a diagnosis of *Fear* or *Anxiety* may be more appropriate. Note that communication problems may be receptive (i.e., difficulty hearing) as well as expressive (i.e., difficulty speaking).

Suggested Alternative Diagnoses

Anxiety
Coping, defensive
Fear
Self-esteem, chronic or situational low
Sensory perception, disturbed: visual, auditory
Thought processes, disturbed

NOC Outcomes

Communication Ability: Ability to receive, interpret, and express spoken, written, and nonverbal messages

Communication: Expressive Ability: Ability to express and interpret verbal and nonverbal messages

Communication: Receptive Ability: Ability to receive and interpret verbal and nonverbal messages

Goals/Evaluation Criteria

Examples Using NOC Language:

- Demonstrates **Communication Ability**, as evidenced by the following indicators (specify 1–5: extremely, substantially, moderately, mildly, or not compromised):

  Use of written, spoken, or nonverbal language

  Use of sign language

  Use of pictures and drawings

  Acknowledgment of messages received

  Exchange [of] messages with others

Other Examples

  Patient will:

- Communicate needs to staff and family with minimal frustration
- Communicate satisfaction with alternative means of communication

NIC Interventions

Active Listening: Attending closely to and attaching significance to a patient's verbal and nonverbal messages

Communication Enhancement, Hearing Deficit: Assistance in accepting and learning alternate methods for living with diminished hearing

Communication Enhancement, Speech Deficit: Assistance in accepting and learning alternate methods for living with impaired speech

Communication Enhancement: Visual Deficit: Assistance in accepting and learning alternate methods for living with diminished vision

Nursing Activities

Assessments

- Assess and document patient's:

  Primary language

Ability to speak, hear, write, read, and understand

Ability to establish communication with staff and family

Response to touch, spatial distance, culture, and male and female roles that may influence communication

Patient/Family Teaching

- Explain to patient why he cannot speak or understand, as appropriate
- Explain to hearing-impaired patient that sounds will be heard differently with use of a hearing aid
- *(NIC) Communication Enhancement: Speech Deficit:*
  Instruct patient and family on use of speech aids (e.g., tracheal-esophageal prosthesis and artificial larynx)
  Teach esophageal speech, as appropriate.

Collaborative Activities

- Consult with physician regarding need for speech therapy
- Help patient and family to locate resources for hearing aids
- *(NIC) Communication Enhancement: Speech Deficit:*
  Use interpreter, as necessary
  Reinforce need for follow-up with speech pathologist after discharge

Other

- Help patient to locate a telephone for the hearing impaired
- Encourage attendance at group meetings for interpersonal contact, specify group
- Encourage frequent family visits to provide stimulation for communication
- Encourage patient to communicate slowly and to repeat requests
- Give frequent positive reinforcement to patient efforts to communicate
- Encourage self-expression in any manner that provides information to staff and family
- Establish one-to-one contact with patient q _____
- Use flash cards, pad, pencil, gestures, pictures, foreign language vocabulary lists, computer, and so forth, to facilitate optimal two-way communication
- Speak slowly, distinctly, and quietly, facing the patient
- When speaking to a patient with hearing impairment, be sure your mouth is visible; do not smoke, talk with a full mouth, or chew gum
- Obtain hearing-impaired patient's attention by touching

- Give clear and simple directions; avoid overwhelming choices that may add to the patient's confusion, for example, take patient by the arm, saying, "Walk with me now."
- Involve patient and family in developing a communication plan
- Provide care in a relaxed, unhurried, nonjudgmental manner
- Provide continuity in nursing assignment to establish trust and reduce frustration
- Reassure patient that frustration and anger are acceptable and expected
- Use family and significant person or hospital translator, as appropriate; specify name, phone number, and relationship in care plan.
- *(NIC) Communication Enhancement: Speech Deficit:*
  Refrain from shouting at patient with communication disorders
  Carry on one-way conversations, as appropriate
  Listen attentively

CONFUSION, ACUTE
(00128) (1994)

Definition: Abrupt onset of a cluster of global, transient changes and disturbances in attention, cognition, psychomotor activity, level of consciousness, or sleep–wake cycle.

Defining Characteristics

Subjective
Lack of motivation to initiate or follow through with goal-directed or purposeful behavior
Misperceptions

Objective
Fluctuation in cognition
Fluctuation in sleep–wake cycle
Fluctuation in level of consciousness
Fluctuation in psychomotor activity
Increased agitation or restlessness
Hallucinations

Related Factors
Alcohol abuse
Delirium
Dementia

Over 60 years of age [NOTE: This is a NANDA International related factor. It does not imply that only people older than 60 can be confused; nor does it imply that one can assume confusion in older adults. What it means is that conditions causing confusion (e.g., organic brain syndrome, Alzheimer disease) are statistically more common in older than in younger adults.]

Drug abuse

Suggestions for Use

Confusion may be used to describe a variety of cognitive impairments. It may be difficult to determine whether *Confusion* is acute or chronic. Therefore, until careful assessment and analysis have been done, it may be necessary to use the more general non-NANDA International term Confusion. *Acute confusion* develops suddenly. *Chronic confusion* develops over time, and is caused by progressive degenerative changes in the brain. *Disturbed thought processes* are caused by functional or emotional rather than physiologic disorders.

Suggested Alternative Diagnoses

Confusion (non-NANDA International)

Confusion, chronic

Environmental interpretation syndrome, impaired

Thought processes, altered

Tissue perfusion, altered (cerebral)

NOC Outcomes

Cognitive Ability: Ability to execute complex mental processes

Cognitive Orientation: Ability to identify person, place, and time

Distorted Thought Control: Ability to self-restrain disruption in perception, thought processes, and thought content

Information Processing: Ability to acquire, organize, and use information

Memory: Ability to cognitively retrieve and report previously stored information

Neurological Status: Consciousness: Extent to which an individual arouses, orients, and attends to the environment

Safety Behavior: Personal: Individual or caregiver efforts to control behaviors that might cause personal injury

Sleep: Extent and pattern of natural periodic suspension of consciousness during which the body is restored

Goals/Evaluation Criteria

Examples Using NOC Language

- Demonstrates **Cognitive Ability**, as evidenced by the following indicators (specify 1–5: extremely, substantially, moderately, mildly, or not compromised):

    Attentiveness, concentration, and orientation

    Immediate, recent, and remote memory

    Makes appropriate decisions

    Communicates clearly and appropriately for age and ability

Other Examples

Patient will:

- Have decreasing episodes of *Confusion*
- Make lifestyle and behavior changes to alleviate or prevent further episodes of *Confusion*
- Demonstrate decreased restlessness and agitation
- Not respond to hallucinations or delusions
- Demonstrate accurate interpretation of environment
- Organize and process information logically
- Correctly identify common objects and familiar persons
- Read and understand short written statements
- Add and subtract numbers accurately
- Obey verbal instructions and commands
- Retain motor responses to noxious stimuli
- Open eyes to external stimuli
- Be awake at appropriate times
- Have a normal electroencephalogram and electromyogram

NIC Interventions

Cerebral Perfusion Promotion: Promotion of adequate perfusion and limitation of complications for a patient experiencing, or at risk for, inadequate cerebral perfusion

Cognitive Stimulation: Promotion of awareness and comprehension of surroundings by utilization of planned stimuli

Delirium Management: Provision of a safe and therapeutic environment for the patient who is experiencing an acute confusional state

Delusion Management: Promoting the comfort, safety, and reality orientation of a patient experiencing false, fixed beliefs that have little or no basis in reality

Environmental Management: Safety: Monitoring and manipulation of the physical environment to promote safety

Fall Prevention: Instituting special precautions with patient at risk for injury from falling

Hallucination Management: Promoting the safety, comfort, and reality orientation of a patient experiencing hallucinations

Neurologic Monitoring: Collection and analysis of patient data to prevent or minimize neurological complications

Reality Orientation: Promotion of patient's awareness of personal identity, time, and environment

Sleep Enhancement: Facilitation of regular sleep–wake cycles

Nursing Activities

Assessments

- Identify possible causes of delirium (e.g., pain, hypoglycemia, infection, medications)
- Monitor neurologic status
- Monitor emotional status
- Obtain baseline history of mental status and any changes
- Perform complete mental status exam
- *(NIC) Delusion Management:*
  Monitor delusions for presence of content that is self-harmful or violent
  Monitor self-care ability

Patient/Family Teaching

- *(NIC) Delusion Management:*
  Educate family and significant others about ways to deal with patient who is experiencing delusions
  Provide illness teaching to patient and significant others, if delusions are illness-based (e.g., delirium, schizophrenia, or depression)
  Provide medication teaching to patient and significant others

Collaborative Activities

- *(NIC) Delusion Management: Administer prn medications for anxiety or agitation*

Other

- Reassure patient with therapeutic communication frequently
- Use touch, as appropriate
- Avoid use of restraints, if possible
- Encourage family and significant others to stay with patient
- Use nursing measures (e.g., mouth care, positioning) to promote comfort and sleep

- Continue patient's usual rituals, to limit anxiety
- Give choices but limit options if patient becomes frustrated or confused
- Be sure patient wears an identification bracelet
- Orient patient (e.g., to staff, surroundings, and care activities), as needed
- Call the patient by name when beginning an interaction
- Explain routines and procedures slowly, briefly, and in simple terms
- Give patient time to respond when presenting options or new information
- *(NIC) Delusion Management:*

  Focus discussion on the underlying feelings, rather than the content of the delusion ("It appears as if you may be feeling frightened")

  Avoid arguing about false beliefs; state doubt matter-of-factly

  Encourage patient to verbalize delusions to caregivers before acting on them

  Assist with self-care, as needed

  Maintain a safe environment

  Provide for the safety and comfort of patient and others when patient is unable to control behavior (e.g., limit setting, area restriction, physical restraint, or seclusion)

  Decrease excessive environmental stimuli, as needed

  Maintain a consistent daily routine

  Assign consistent caregivers on a daily basis

CONFUSION, CHRONIC
(00129) (1994)

Definition: Irreversible, long-standing, or progressive deterioration of intellect and personality characterized by decreased ability to interpret environmental stimuli [and] decreased capacity for intellectual thought processes, and manifested by disturbances of memory, orientation, and behavior

Defining Characteristics
Subjective
Impaired memory (short-term, long-term)

Objective

Altered interpretation and response to stimuli

Altered personality

Clinical evidence of organic impairment

Impaired socialization

No change in level of consciousness

Progressive or long-standing cognitive impairment

Related Factors

Alzheimer disease

Cerebrovascular accident

Head injury

Korsakoff's psychosis

Multi-infarct dementia

Suggestions for Use

See Suggestions for Use for Confusion, Acute, p. 85. For clients with self-care deficits, be sure to include that diagnostic label in the care plan (e.g., *Total self-care deficit related to Chronic confusion*). It is difficult to distinguish between *Chronic confusion* and *Impaired environmental interpretation syndrome*.

Suggested Alternative Diagnoses

Confusion, acute

Environmental interpretation syndrome, impaired

Memory, impaired

Self-care deficit (specify)

Thought processes, distorted

NOC Outcomes

Cognitive Ability: Ability to execute complex mental processes

Cognitive Orientation: Ability to identify person, place, and time

Concentration: Ability to focus on a specific stimulus

Decision Making: Ability to choose between two or more alternatives

Distorted Thought Control: Self-restraint of disruption in perception, thought processes, and thought content

Identity: Ability to distinguish between self and nonself and to characterize one's essence

Information Processing: Ability to acquire, organize, and use information

Memory: Ability to cognitively retrieve and report previously stored information

Neurological Status: Consciousness: Extent to which an individual arouses, orients, and attends to the environment

Goals/Evaluation Criteria

Examples Using NOC Language

- Maintains or improves Concentration, Decision Making, Distorted Thought Control, Information Processing, and Memory
- Exhibits minimal deterioration in Cognitive Orientation
- Experiences no loss of Identity
- Neurological Status: consciousness not compromised
- Demonstrates **Cognitive Ability**, as evidenced by the following indicators (specify 1–5: extremely, substantially, moderately, mildly, or not compromised):

    Attentiveness, concentration, and orientation

    Immediate, recent, and remote memory

    Makes appropriate decisions

    Communicates clearly and appropriately for age and ability.

Other Examples

Patient will:

- Respond to visual and auditory cues, draw a circle, maintain attention
- Identify relevant information and choose among alternatives
- Interact appropriately with others
- Formulate coherent messages
- Obey simple directions and commands
- Not attend to hallucinations or delusions
- Attend to, perceive, and interpret the environmental stimuli correctly
- Correctly identify objects and people
- Balance activity with rest
- Not be restless or agitated
- Participate to maximum ability in therapeutic milieu or ADLs
- Not be combative
- Be content and less frustrated by environmental stressors

NIC Interventions

Anxiety Reduction: Minimizing apprehension, dread, foreboding, or uneasiness related to an unidentified source of anticipated danger

Cerebral Perfusion Promotion: Promotion of adequate perfusion and limitation of complications for a patient experiencing, or at risk for, inadequate cerebral perfusion

Cognitive Restructuring: Challenging a patient to alter distorted thought patterns and view self and the world more realistically

Cognitive Stimulation: Promotion of awareness and comprehension of surroundings by utilization of planned stimuli

Decision-Making Support: Providing information and support for a patient who is making a decision regarding health care

Delusion Management: Promoting the comfort, safety, and reality orientation of a patient experiencing false, fixed beliefs that have little or no basis in reality

Dementia Management: Provision of a modified environment for the patient who is experiencing a chronic confusional state

Family Involvement Promotion: Facilitating family participation in the emotional and physical care of the patient

Memory Training: Facilitation of memory

Mood Management: Providing for safety and stabilization of a patient who is experiencing dysfunctionally depressed mood or elevated mood

Neurologic Monitoring: Collection and analysis of patient data to prevent or minimize neurological complications

Reality Orientation: Promotion of patient's awareness of personal identity, time, and environment

Nursing Activities

Assessments

- Obtain information about past and present patterns of behavior (e.g., sleep, medication use, elimination, food intake, hygiene, social interaction)
- Assess for signs of depression (e.g., insomnia, flat affect, withdrawal, loss of appetite)
- *(NIC) Dementia Management:*
  Monitor cognitive functioning, using a standardized assessment tool [e.g., the Mini-Mental State Examination]
  Determine physical, social, and psychologic history of patient before the onset of confusion; usual habits and routines
  Monitor nutrition and weight
  Monitor carefully for physiologic causes of increased confusion that may be acute and reversible

Patient/Family Teaching

- Teach patient and significant others about patient's medications
- Explain the effect of the patient's illness on his mood (e.g., depression, premenstrual syndrome)

Collaborative Activities

- Administer mood-stabilizing medications
- Refer to social services department for referral to day care programs, Meals On Wheels, respite care, and so forth.

Other

- If client experiences delusions or hallucinations, refer to Nursing Activities in Confusion, Acute, pp. 87–88.
- In early dementia, when the main symptoms are those of Impaired memory, refer to Nursing Activities for Impaired Memory, pp. 302–303.
- Provide opportunity for physical activity
- Alternate activity with scheduled quiet times and activities (e.g., an hour in a recliner or chair, quiet music) at least twice a day to allow for resolution of anxiety and tension
- Provide appropriate outlets for patient's feelings (e.g., art therapy and physical exercise)
- Assist with reality orientation (e.g., provide clocks, calendars, personal items, seasonal decorations)
- For geriatric patients, promote reminiscence and life review (e.g., ask questions about client's work and family, such as: "Looking back, what was really important to you?")
- Keep environment as quiet as possible (e.g., avoid buzzers, alarms, and overhead paging systems)
- *(NIC) Dementia Management:*

    Include family members in planning, providing, and evaluating care, to the extent desired

    Provide a low-stimulation environment (e.g., quiet, soothing music; nonvivid and simple, familiar patterns in decor; performance expectations that do not exceed cognitive-processing ability; and dining in small groups)

    Identify and remove potential dangers in environment for patient

    Place identification bracelet on patient

    Prepare for interaction with eye contact and touch, as appropriate

    Address the patient distinctly by name when initiating interaction and speak slowly

Introduce self when initiating contact

Give one simple direction at a time [and repeat as necessary (e.g., "follow me," or "sit on the chair," or "put on your slippers")]

Use distraction, rather than confrontation, to manage behavior

Provide patient a general orientation to the season of the year by using appropriate cues (e.g., holiday decorations, seasonal decorations and activities, and access to contained, out-of-doors area)

Label familiar photos with names of the individuals

Limit number of choices patient has to make, so not to cause anxiety

Avoid use of physical restraints

Assist with self-care, as needed, [Specify methods.]

Provide boundaries, such as red or yellow tape on the floor when low-stimulus units are not available

---

CONSTIPATION
(00011) (1975, 1998)

Definition: Decrease in normal frequency of defecation accompanied by difficult or incomplete passage of stool or passage of excessively hard, dry stool.

Defining Characteristics

Subjective
Abdominal pain

Abdominal tenderness with or without palpable muscle resistance

Anorexia

Feeling of rectal fullness or pressure

Generalized fatigue

Headache

Increased abdominal pressure

Indigestion

Nausea

Pain with defecation

Objective
Atypical presentations in older adults (e.g., change in mental status, urinary incontinence, unexplained falls, elevated body temperature)

Bright red blood with stool

Change in abdominal growling (borborygmi)

Change in bowel pattern
Dark or black or tarry stool
Decreased frequency
Decreased volume of stool
Distended abdomen
Dry, hard, formed stools
Hypo- or hyperactive bowel sounds
Oozing liquid stool
Palpable abdominal mass
Palpable rectal mass
Percussed abdominal dullness
Presence of soft pastelike stool in rectum
Severe flatus
Straining with defecation
Unable to pass stool
Vomiting

Related Factors

Functional

Abdominal muscle weakness
Habitual denial and ignoring of urge to defecate
Inadequate toileting (e.g., timeliness, positioning for defecation, privacy)
Insufficient physical activity
Irregular defecation habits
Recent environmental changes

Psychological

Depression
Emotional stress
Mental confusion

Pharmacological

Aluminum-containing antacids
Anticholinergics
Anticonvulsants
Antidepressants
Antilipemic agents
Bismuth salts
Calcium carbonate
Calcium channel blockers
Diuretics
Iron salts
Laxative overdose

Nonsteroidal anti-inflammatory agents
Opiates
Phenothiazides
Sedatives
Sympathomimetics

Mechanical

Electrolyte imbalance
Hemorrhoids
Megacolon (Hirschsprung disease)
Neurological impairment
Obesity
Postsurgical obstruction
Pregnancy
Prostate enlargement
Rectal abscess or ulcer
Rectal anal fissures
Rectal anal stricture
Rectal prolapse
Rectocele
Tumors

Physiological

Change in usual foods and eating patterns
Decreased motility of gastrointestinal tract
Dehydration
Inadequate dentition or oral hygiene
Insufficient fiber intake
Insufficient fluid intake
Poor eating habits

Suggested Alternative Diagnoses

Constipation, perceived
Constipation, risk for

NOC Outcomes

Bowel Elimination: Ability of the gastrointestinal tract to form and evacuate stool effectively

Hydration: Amount of water in the intra- and extracellular compartments of the body

Symptom Control: Personal actions to minimize perceived adverse changes in physical and emotional functioning

Goals/Evaluation Criteria

Examples Using NOC Language

- *Constipation* alleviated, as indicated by **Bowel Elimination** (specify 1–5: extremely, substantially, moderately, mildly, or not compromised):

   Elimination pattern in expected range; stool soft and formed

   Passes stool without aids

   Ingests adequate fluids and fiber

   Exercises adequate amount

Other Examples

Patient will:

- Demonstrate knowledge of bowel regimen necessary to overcome the side effects of medications
- Report the passage of stool with a reduction of pain and straining
- Demonstrate adequate hydration (e.g., good skin turgor, intake of fluids approximately equal to output)

NIC Interventions

Bowel Management: Establishment and maintenance of a regular pattern of bowel elimination

Constipation/Impaction Management: Prevention and alleviation of constipation/impaction

Fluid Management: Promotion of fluid balance and prevention of complications resulting from abnormal or undesired fluid levels

Nursing Activities

Assessments

- Gather baseline data on bowel regimen, activity, medications and patient's usual pattern
- Assess and document:

   Color and consistency of first stool postoperatively

   Frequency, color, and consistency of stool q _____

   Passage of flatus

   Presence of impaction

   Presence or absence of bowel sounds and abdominal distention in all four quadrants

- *(NIC) Constipation/Impaction Management:*

   Monitor for signs and symptoms of bowel rupture or peritonitis

   Identify factors (e.g., medications, bed rest, and diet) that may cause or contribute to constipation

Patient/Family Teaching

- Inform patient of possibility of medication-induced constipation
- Instruct patient in bowel elimination aids that will promote optimal bowel pattern at home
- Teach patient the effects of diet (e.g., fluids and fiber) on elimination
- Instruct patient in consequences of long-term laxative use
- Stress the avoidance of straining during defecation to prevent change in vital signs, dizziness, or bleeding
- *(NIC) Constipation/Impaction Management:*
  Explain etiology of problem and rationale for actions to patient
  Teach patient and family how to keep a food diary

Collaborative Activities

- Consult with dietitian for increase in fiber and fluids in diet
- Request a physician's order for elimination aids, such as dietary bran, stool softeners, enemas, and laxatives
- *(NIC) Constipation/Impaction Management:*
  Consult with physician about a decrease or increase in frequency of bowel sounds
  Consult with physician if signs and symptoms of constipation or impaction persist

Other

- Encourage patient to request pain medication prior to defecation to facilitate painless passage of stool
- Encourage optimal activity to stimulate patient's bowel elimination
- Provide privacy and safety for patient during bowel elimination
- Provide care in an accepting, nonjudgmental manner
- Provide fluids of patient's choice, specify

CONSTIPATION, PERCEIVED
(00012) (1988)

Definition: Self-diagnosis of constipation and abuse of laxatives, enemas, and suppositories to ensure a daily bowel movement

Defining Characteristics

Subjective

Expectation of a daily bowel movement

Expected passage of stool at same time every day

Objective

Overuse of laxatives, enemas, and suppositories [to induce a daily bowel movement]

Related Factors

Cultural and family health beliefs

Faulty appraisal [of normal bowel function]

Impaired thought processes

Suggestions for Use

None

Suggested Alternative Diagnoses

Constipation

Constipation, risk for

NOC Outcomes

Bowel Elimination: Ability of the gastrointestinal tract to form and evacuate stool effectively

Health Beliefs: Personal convictions that influence health behaviors

Health Beliefs: Perceived Threat: Personal conviction that a health problem is serious and has potential negative consequences for lifestyle

Goals/Evaluation Criteria

Examples Using NOC Language

- *Perceived constipation* alleviated, as indicated by Bowel Elimination and Health Beliefs.
- Demonstrates **Bowel Elimination**, as evidenced by the following indicators (specify 1–5: extremely, substantially, moderately, mildly, or not compromised):

    Elimination pattern in expected range

    Passes stool without aids

    Abuse of aids not present

    Ingests adequate fluids and fiber

Other Examples

Patient will:

- Verbalize understanding of need to decrease use of laxatives, enemas, and suppositories
- Describe dietary regimen that will more naturally regulate bowel function

NIC Interventions

Bowel Management: Establishment and maintenance of a regular pattern of bowel elimination

Health Education: Developing and providing instruction and learning experiences to facilitate voluntary adaptation of behavior conducive to health in individuals, families, groups, or communities

Teaching: Individual: Planning, implementation, and evaluation of a teaching program designed to address a patient's particular needs

Values Clarification: Assisting another to clarify his own values in order to facilitate effective decision making

Nursing Activities

Assessments

- Assess patient's expectation of normal bowel function
- Observe, document, and report requests for laxatives, enemas, or suppositories
- *(NIC) Bowel Management:*

  Monitor bowel movements, including frequency, consistency, shape, volume, and color, as appropriate

  Note preexistent bowel problems, bowel routine, and use of laxatives

Patient/Family Teaching

- Instruct patient and family in diet, fluid intake, activity, exercise, and the consequence of overuse of laxatives, enemas, and suppositories

Collaborative Activities

- Initiate a multidisciplinary care conference involving the patient and family to encourage positive behaviors (e.g., change in diet)

Other

- Assist patient to identify realistic use of laxatives, enemas, and suppositories
- Provide positive feedback to patient when behavior change occurs
- *(NIC) Bowel Management:* Encourage decreased gas-forming food intake, as appropriate

CONSTIPATION, RISK FOR
(00015) (1998)

Definition: At risk for a decrease in normal frequency of defecation accompanied by difficult or incomplete passage of excessively hard, dry stool.

Risk Factors

Functional

Abdominal muscle weakness

Habitual denial and ignoring of urge to defecate

Inadequate toileting (e.g., timeliness, positioning for defecation, privacy)

Insufficient physical activity

Irregular defecation habits

Recent environmental changes

Psychological

Depression

Emotional stress

Mental confusion

Physiological

Change in usual foods and eating patterns

Decreased motility of gastrointestinal tract

Dehydration

Inadequate dentition or oral hygiene

Insufficient fiber intake

Insufficient fluid intake

Poor eating habits

Pharmacological

Aluminum-containing antacids

Anticholinergics

Anticonvulsants

Antidepressants

Antilipemic agents

Bismuth salts

Calcium carbonate

Calcium channel blockers

Diuretics

Iron salts

Laxative overuse

Nonsteroidal anti-inflammatory agents

Opiates
Phenothiazines
Sedatives
Sympathomimetics

Mechanical

Electrolyte imbalance
Hemorrhoids
Megacolon (Hirschsprung's disease)
Neurological impairment
Obesity
Postsurgical obstruction
Pregnancy
Prostate enlargement
Rectal abscess or ulcer
Rectal anal fissures
Rectal anal stricture
Rectal prolapse
Rectocele
Tumors

Suggested Alternative Diagnoses

None

NOC Outcomes

Bowel Elimination: Ability of the gastrointestinal tract to form and evacuate stool effectively

Hydration: Amount of water in the intra- and extracellular compartments of the body

Mobility Level: Ability to move purposefully

Nutritional Status: Food and Fluid Intake: Amount of food and fluid taken into the body over a 24-hr period

Self-Care: Toileting: Ability to toilet self

Treatment Behavior: Illness or Injury: Personal actions to palliate or eliminate pathology

Goals/Evaluation Criteria

Examples Using NOC Language

- *Risk for constipation* alleviated, as indicated by status of Bowel Elimination, Hydration, Mobility Level, Nutritional Status: Food and Fluid Intake, Toileting Self-Care, and Treatment Behavior: Illness or Injury

- Demonstrates **Bowel Elimination**, as evidenced by the following indicators (specify 1–5: extremely, substantially, moderately, mildly, or not compromised):

    Elimination pattern in expected range

    Passes stool without aids

    Abuse of aids not present

    Ingests adequate fluids and fiber

Other Examples

The patient will:

- Demonstrate knowledge of bowel regimen necessary to overcome the side effects of medications
- Describe dietary requirements (e.g., fluids and fiber) necessary to maintain usual bowel pattern
- Pass stool of usual consistency and frequency for patient
- Report the passage of stool with no pain or straining

NIC Interventions

Constipation/Impaction Management: Prevention and alleviation of constipation/impaction

Self-Care Assistance: Toileting: Assisting another with elimination

Nursing Activities

Assessments

- Gather baseline data on bowel regimen, activity, and medications
- Assess and document postoperatively:

    Color and consistency of first stool

    Passage of flatus

    Presence or absence of bowel sounds and abdominal distention

Patient/Family Teaching

- Inform patient of possibility of medication-induced constipation
- Explain the effects of fluids and fiber in preventing constipation
- Instruct patient in consequences of long-term laxative use

Collaborative Activities

- Refer to dietitian, as needed, to increase fiber and fluids in diet

Other

- Encourage optimal activity to stimulate bowel elimination
- Provide privacy and safety for patient during bowel elimination
- Provide fluids of patient's choice; specify fluids

COPING: COMMUNITY, INEFFECTIVE
(00077) (1994, 1998)

Definition: Pattern of community activities (for adaptation and problem solving) that is unsatisfactory for meeting the demands or needs of the community.

Defining Characteristics

Subjective

Community does not meet its own expectations

Expressed community powerlessness

Expressed vulnerability

Objective

Deficits in community participation

Excessive community conflicts

High illness rates

Increased social problems (e.g., homicides, vandalism, arson, terrorism, robbery, infanticide, abuse, divorce, unemployment, poverty, militancy, mental illness)

Stressors perceived as excessive

Related Factors

Deficits in community social support services and resources

Inadequate resources for problem solving

Ineffective or nonexistent community systems (e.g., lack of emergency medical system, transportation system, or disaster planning systems)

Natural or man-made disasters

Suggestions for Use

This diagnosis is most useful for community health nurses who focus on the health of groups (e.g., unwed mothers, all the people in a county, patients with diabetes).

Suggested Alternative Diagnoses

Coping: community, readiness for enhanced

Management of therapeutic regimen: community, ineffective

NOC Outcomes

Community Competence: The ability of a community to collectively problem solve to achieve goals

Community Health: Immunity: Resistance of a group to the invasion and spread of an infectious agent

Community Health Status: The general state of well-being of a community or population

Community Risk Control: Chronic Disease: Community actions to reduce the risk of chronic diseases and related complications

Community Risk Control: Communicable Disease: Community actions to eliminate or reduce the spread of infectious agents (bacteria, fungi, parasites, and viruses) that threaten public health

Community Risk Control: Lead Exposure: Community actions to reduce lead exposure and poisoning

Goals/Evaluation Criteria

Examples Using NOC Language

- *Ineffective community coping* alleviated, as indicated by status of Community Competence, Community Health: Immunity, Community Health Status, Community Risk Control: Chronic and Communicable Diseases, and Community Risk Control: Lead Exposure

- Demonstrates **Community Health Status**, as evidenced by the following indicators (specify 1–5: poor, fair, average, good, or excellent):

    Prevalence of health promotion programs

    Prevalence of health protection programs

    Health status of infants, children, adolescents, adults, and elders

    Compliance with environmental health standards

    Morbidity rates

    Crime statistics

    Mortality rates

    Health surveillance data systems in place

Other Examples

The community:

- Develops improved communication among its members
- Implements effective problem-solving strategies
- Develops group cohesiveness
- Expresses the power to manage change and improve community functioning

NIC Interventions

See NIC Interventions for Community Coping: Readiness for Enhanced, on pp. 107–108.

Community Disaster Preparedness: Preparing for an effective response to a large-scale disaster

Health Screening: Detecting health risks or problems by means of history, examination, and other procedures

Nursing Activities

Assessments

- Assess and identify causative or risk factors affecting the community's ability to adapt and cope effectively (e.g., lack of information about available resources)
- Assess the effects of health policies and standards on nursing practice, patient outcomes, and health care costs
- Determine the availability of resources and the extent to which they are being used
- *(NIC) Environmental Management: Community:*
  Initiate screening for health risks from the environment
  Monitor status of known health risks
  Teaching
- Help to identify and mobilize available resources and supports (e.g., emergency aid from the Red Cross)
- Inform policy makers of projected effects of policies on patient welfare
- Inform health care consumers of current and proposed changes in health policies and standards and potential effects on health
- *(NIC) Environmental Management: Community:* Conduct educational programs for targeted risk groups [e.g., teenage pregnancy]

Collaborative Activities

- *(NIC) Environmental Management: Community:*
  Participate in multidisciplinary teams to identify threats to safety in the community
  Coordinate services to at-risk groups and communities
  Work with environmental groups to secure appropriate governmental regulations
  Collaborate in the development of community action programs

Other

- Participate in lobbying for changes in health policies and standards to improve health care
- Arrange opportunities for community members to meet and discuss the situation (e.g., civic organizations, church groups, town meetings)

- Assist community members to become aware of conflicts that prevent them from working together (e.g., anger, mistrust)
- Determine ways of disseminating information to the community (e.g., radio and television reports, flyers, meetings)
- Help write grant proposals to obtain funding for programs needed to improve community coping
- Advocate for the community (e.g., write letters to government agencies and newspapers)
- *(NIC) Environmental Management: Community:* Encourage neighborhoods to become active participants in community safety

---

COPING: COMMUNITY, READINESS FOR ENHANCED (00076) (1994)

Definition: Pattern of community activities for adaptation and problem solving that is satisfactory for meeting the demands or needs of the community but can be improved for management of current and future problems and stressors.

Defining Characteristics

Objective
One or more of the following characteristics:
Active planning by community for predicted stressors
Active problem solving by community when faced with issues
Agreement that community is responsible for stress management
Deficits in one or more characteristics that indicate effective coping
Positive communication among community members
Positive communication between community, aggregates, and the larger community
Programs [available] for recreation and relaxation
Resources sufficient for managing stressors

Related Factors

Community has a sense of power to manage stressors
Resources available for problem solving
Social supports available

Suggestions for Use

This diagnosis can be used for a community that is meeting its basic needs for a clean environment, food, shelter, and safety, and wishes to focus on higher levels of functioning, such as wellness promotion. When external threats (e.g., floods, epidemics) occur in such a community, they pose risk factors; as long as the community continues to adapt, *Risk for ineffective community coping* should be used. If the threat produces defining characteristics (symptoms) in the community, use *Ineffective community coping.*

Suggested Alternative Diagnoses

Coping: community, ineffective
Coping: community, risk for ineffective

NOC Outcomes

See NOC Outcomes for Coping: Community, Ineffective, on pp. 103–104.

Goals/Evaluation Criteria

See Goals/Evaluation Criteria for Coping: Community, Ineffective, on p. 104.

The community:

- Has a plan in place to deal with problems and stressors
- Accesses or develops programs designed to improve the well-being of specific groups within the population (e.g., weight-control programs, retirement-planning programs)
- Continues to enhance present methods of communication and problem solving
- Expresses the power to manage change and improve community functioning

NIC Interventions

Communicable Disease Management: Working with a community to decrease and manage the incidence and prevalence of contagious diseases in a specific population

Community Health Development: Facilitating members of a community to identify a community's health concerns, mobilize resources, and implement solutions

Environmental Management: Community: Monitoring and influencing of the physical, social, cultural, economic, and political conditions that affect the health of groups and communities

Environmental Risk Protection: Preventing and detecting disease and injury in populations at risk from environmental hazards

Health Education: Developing and providing instruction and learning experiences to facilitate voluntary adaptation of behavior conducive to health in individuals, families, groups, or communities

Health Policy Monitoring: Surveillance and influence of government and organization regulations, rules, and standards that affect nursing systems and practices to ensure quality care of patients

Immunization/Vaccination Management: Monitoring immunization status, facilitating access to immunizations, and provision of immunizations to prevent communicable disease

Program Development: Planning, implementing, and evaluating a coordinated set of activities designed to enhance wellness, or to prevent, reduce, or eliminate one or more health problems of a group or community

Nursing Activities

Assessments

- Determine the availability of resources and the extent to which they are being used
- Identify groups that are at high risk for unhealthful behavior
- Identify factors in high-risk groups that may motivate or prevent healthful behavior
- Determine sociocultural and historic context of individual and group health behaviors
- Create and implement processes for regular evaluation of client outcomes during and after completion of program or activities
- Assess the effects of health policies and standards on nursing practice, patient outcomes, and health care costs
- *(NIC) Environmental Management: Community*: Initiate screening for health risks from the environment

Teaching

- Help to identify and mobilize available resources and supports (e.g., funding sources, supplies)
- Select learning strategies based on identified characteristics of target population
- Design processes for informing health care consumers of existing and proposed changes in health policies
- Provide educational materials written at an appropriate level for the target group
- *(NIC) Environmental Management: Community*: Conduct educational programs for targeted risk groups [e.g., teenage pregnancy]

Collaborative Activities

- Help the community obtain funding for wellness programs (e.g., education, smoking prevention)

- *(NIC) Environmental Management: Community:*
  Participate in multidisciplinary teams to identify threats to
    safety in the community
  Collaborate in the development of community-action programs
  Work with environmental groups to secure appropriate govern-
    mental regulations

Other
- Establish a collaborative partnership with the community and
  explain the role of a community health nurse in wellness pro-
  motion
- Lobby or write letters to urge policies that promote health (e.g.,
  health education guaranteed as an employee benefit; insurance
  premium reductions for healthy behaviors and lifestyles)
- Help write grants to obtain funding for wellness programs
- Assist in improving educational levels within the community
- *(NIC) Environmental Management: Community:*
  Promote governmental policy to reduce specified risks
  Encourage neighborhoods to become active participants in
    community safety
  Coordinate services to at-risk groups and communities

COPING, DEFENSIVE
(00071) (1988)

Definition: Repeated projection of falsely positive self-evaluation
  based on a self-protective pattern that defends against underlying perceived threats to positive self-regard

Defining Characteristics
Subjective
Denial of obvious problems and weaknesses
Difficulty in reality-testing perceptions
Projection of blame and responsibility
Rationalizes failures

Objective
Grandiosity
Difficulty in establishing or maintaining relationships
Hostile laughter or ridicule of others
Hypersensitive to slight or criticism
Lack of follow-through or participation in treatment or therapy
Superior attitude toward others

Related Factors

Not yet developed by NANDA International. Non-NANDA International Related Factors include the following:

Physical illness (specify)

Situational crisis (specify)

Psychologic impairment (specify)

Suggestions for Use

This diagnosis is less specific than *Ineffective denial*, which is actually one of many manifestations of *Defensive coping* (see Defining Characteristics, p. 109). Use the more specific diagnosis when attempts to cope involve overuse or misuse of denial.

Suggested Alternative Diagnoses

Adjustment, impaired

Communication, verbal, impaired

Coping, ineffective

Denial, ineffective

Thought processes, disturbed

NOC Outcomes

Acceptance: Health Status: Reconciliation to health circumstances

Child Development: Adolescence (12–17 Years): Milestones of physical, cognitive, and psychosocial progression between 12 and 17 years of age

Coping: Actions to manage stressors that tax an individual's resources

Self-Esteem: Personal judgment of self-worth

Social Interaction Skills: An individual's use of effective interaction behaviors

Goals/Evaluation Criteria

Examples Using NOC Language

- Patient will not use *Defensive coping*, as demonstrated by Acceptance: Health Status, effective Coping, positive Self-Esteem and Social Interaction Skills, or normal Child Development: Adolescence

- **Coping** indicators include the following (specify 1–5: never, rarely, sometimes, often, or consistently demonstrated):

    Modifies lifestyle, as needed

    Seeks information concerning illness and treatment

Seeks professional help, as appropriate

Verbalizes acceptance of situation

Uses effective coping strategies

Other Examples

Patient will:

- Acknowledge specific problems and conflicts that interfere with social interactions and relationships
- Demonstrate decrease in defensiveness
- Express feelings about changes in health
- Express feelings of self-worth
- Reformulate previous concept of health
- Maintain effective interactions with others

NIC Interventions

Behavior Modification: Social Skills: Assisting the patient to develop or improve interpersonal social skills

Complex Relationship Building: Establishing a therapeutic relationship with a patient who has difficulty interacting with others

Coping Enhancement: Assisting a patient to adapt to perceived stressors, changes, or threats which interfere with meeting life demands and roles

Counseling: Use of an interactive helping process focusing on the needs, problems, or feelings of the patient and significant others to enhance or support coping, problem solving, and interpersonal relationships

Emotional Support: Provision of reassurance, acceptance, and encouragement during times of stress

Self-Awareness Enhancement: Assisting a patient to explore and understand his thoughts, feelings, motivations, and behaviors

Self-Esteem Enhancement: Assisting a patient to increase his personal judgment of self-worth

Self-Responsibility Facilitation: Encouraging a patient to assume more responsibility for own behavior

Nursing Activities

Assessments

- Assess degree of defensiveness and denial that interferes with self-assessment

Patient/Family Teaching

- Teach alternative behaviors to obtain positive regard through group therapy, individual therapy, role playing, and role modeling

Collaborative Activities

- Refer to appropriate community resources (e.g., family or marriage counseling, substance-abuse groups)

Other

- Assist patient in recognizing negative coping behaviors
- Identify and discuss the subjects, situations, and people that trigger negative coping behaviors
- Include family in treatment, as needed
- Provide feedback in a supportive environment on how behavior is being perceived by others
- Provide reality testing during times of grandiose behavior, denial of obvious problems, and projected blame and responsibility
- *(NIC) Self-Awareness Enhancement:*
  Assist patient to identify the impact of illness on self-concept
  Verbalize patient's denial of reality, as appropriate
  Assist patient to identify life priorities
  Assist patient to identify positive attributes of self

COPING: FAMILY, COMPROMISED
(00074) (1980, 1996)

Definition: Usually supportive primary person (family member or close friend) provides insufficient, ineffective, or compromised support, comfort, assistance, or encouragement which may be needed by the client to manage or master adaptive tasks related to his or her health challenge.

Defining Characteristics

Subjective

Client expresses or confirms a concern or complaint about significant other's response to his health problem

Significant person describes or confirms an inadequate understanding or knowledge base, which interferes with effective assistive or supportive behaviors

Significant person describes preoccupation with personal reaction (e.g., fear, anticipatory grief, guilt, anxiety) to client's illness, disability, or other situational or developmental crises

Objective

Significant person attempts assistive or supportive behaviors with less-than-satisfactory results

Significant person displays protective behavior disproportionate (too little or too much) to the client's abilities or need for autonomy

Significant person withdraws or enters into limited or temporary personal communication with the client at the time of need

Other Possible Defining Characteristics (Non-NANDA International)

Family displays emotional lability

Family displays rigid role boundaries

Family member interferes with necessary medical and nursing actions

Family members are divisive and form unsupportive coalitions

Family verbal interaction with patient is absent or decreased

Related Factors

Developmental crisis of significant person [specify]

Inadequate or incorrect information or understanding by a primary person

Little support provided by client, in turn, for primary person

Prolonged disease or disability progression that exhausts supportive capacity of significant people

Situational crisis of significant person [specify]

Temporary family disorganization and role changes

Temporary preoccupation by a significant person who is trying to manage emotional conflicts and personal suffering and is unable to perceive or act effectively in regard to client's needs

Suggestions for Use

(1) *Caregiver role strain* focuses on the needs of the caregiving family member, whereas *Family coping: compromised* focuses more on the needs of the patient. (2) The distinctions between this diagnosis and *Interrupted family processes* are not clear. (3) For severe malfunction or for abusive or destructive situations, use *Disabled family coping*, which is distinguished by the following defining characteristics:

Denial of existence or severity of illness of a family member

Despair, rejection

Desertion

Abuse (child, spousal, elder)

Suggested Alternative Diagnoses

Caregiver role strain (actual or risk for)
Family coping, disabled
Family processes, interrupted
Management of therapeutic regimen: families, ineffective
Parental role conflict
Parenting, impaired

NOC Outcomes

Caregiver Emotional Health: Feelings, attitudes, and emotions of a family care provider while caring for a family member or significant other over an extended period of time

Caregiver–Patient Relationship: Positive interactions and connections between the caregiver and care recipient

Caregiver Stressors: The extent of biopsychosocial pressure on a family care provider caring for a family member or significant other over an extended period of time

Family Coping: Family actions to manage stressors that tax family resources

Family Normalization: Ability of the family to develop and maintain routines and management strategies that contribute to optimal functioning when a member has a chronic illness or disability

Goals/Evaluation Criteria

Examples Using NOC Language

- Family will not use *Compromised family coping*, as demonstrated by satisfactory status of Caregiver Emotional Health, Caregiver–Patient Relationship, Family Coping, and Family Normalization; and manageable level of Caregiver Stressors
- **Family Coping** indicators include the following (specify 1–5: never, rarely, sometimes, often, or consistently demonstrated):
    Demonstrates role flexibility
    Manages problems
    Cares for needs of all family members
    Maintains financial stability
    Seeks assistance when appropriate

Other Examples

    Family member(s) will:
- Acknowledge needs of patient
- Begin to demonstrate effective interpersonal skills

- Express increased ability to cope with changes in family structure and dynamics
- Express unresolved feelings
- Participate in developing and implementing a treatment plan
- Use more flexible problem-solving strategies
- Achieves financial stability to care for needs of family members

NIC Interventions

Refer to NIC Interventions for Family Coping, Disabled, on p. 120.

Nursing Activities

Assessments

- Identify level of patient's self-care deficits and dependency on family
- Assess interaction between patient and family; be alert for potential destructive behaviors
- Assess ability and readiness of family members to learn
- Determine extent to which family members wish to be involved with the patient
- Identify the family's expectations of and for the patient
- Identify family structure and roles
- *(NIC) Family Support:*
  Appraise family's emotional reaction to patient's condition
  Identify nature of spiritual support for family

Patient/Family Teaching

- Discuss the common responses to health challenges (e.g., anxiety, dependency, depression)
- Provide information about specific health challenge and necessary coping skills
- Teach the family those skills required for care of patient; specify skills
- Teach, role-model, and reinforce communication skills, which may include active listening, reflection, "I" statements, conflict resolution
- *(NIC) Family Support:*
  Teach the medical and nursing plans of care to family
  Provide necessary knowledge of options to family that will assist them to make decisions about patient care

Collaborative Activities

- Explore available hospital resources and support systems with family

- Request social service consultation to help the family determine posthospitalization needs and identify sources of community support
- Initiate a multidisciplinary patient care conference, involving the patient and family in problem solving and facilitation of communication
- *(NIC) Family Support:*
  Provide spiritual resources for family, as appropriate
  Arrange for ongoing respite care, when indicated and desired
  Provide opportunities for peer group support

Other

- Promote an open, trusting relationship with family
- Encourage patient and family to focus on positive aspects of the patient's situation
- Assist family in identifying behaviors that may be hindering prescribed treatment
- Assist family in realistically identifying the needs of patient and family unit
- Assist family with decision making and problem solving
- Encourage family to identify needed role changes to maintain family integrity
- Encourage family to recognize changes in interpersonal relationships
- Explore impact of conflicting values or coping styles on family relationships
- Encourage family to visit or care for patient whenever possible; provide privacy to facilitate family interactions
- Provide structure to family interaction. Consider content of interaction, length of visiting time, staff support during visit, and which family member(s) will visit, based on patient's treatment plan
- *(NIC) Family Support:*
  Foster realistic hope
  Listen to family concerns, feelings, and questions
  Facilitate communication of concerns and feelings between patient and family or between family members
  Answer all questions of family members or assist them to get answers
  Give care to patient in lieu of family to relieve them or when family is unable to give care
  Provide feedback for family regarding their coping

COPING: FAMILY, DISABLED
(00073) (1980, 1996)

Definition: Behavior of significant person (family member or other primary person) that disables his own capacities and the client's capacities to effectively address tasks essential to either person's adaptation to the health challenge.

Defining Characteristics

Subjective

Depression

Distortion of reality of patient's health problem, including extreme denial about its existence or severity

Objective

Abandonment

Aggression and hostility

Agitation

Carrying on usual routines, disregarding client's needs

Client's development of helplessness, inactive dependence

Decisions and actions by family that are detrimental to economic or social well-being

Desertion

Disregarding needs

Impaired individualization

Impaired restructuring of a meaningful life for self

Intolerance

Neglectful care of client in regard to basic human needs or illness treatment

Neglectful relationships with other family members

Prolonged overconcern for client

Psychosomatic symptoms

Rejection

Taking on illness signs of client

Related Factors

Arbitrary handling of family's resistance to treatment, which tends to solidify defensiveness as it fails to deal adequately with underlying anxiety

Dissonant discrepancy of coping styles for dealing with adaptive tasks by the significant person and client or among significant people

Highly ambivalent family relationships

Significant person with chronically unexpressed feelings of (hostility, anxiety, guilt, despair, and so forth)

Other Possible Defining Characteristics (Non-NANDA International)

Emotionally disturbed family member

Substance-abusing family member

Use of violence to manage conflict

Suggestions for Use

This label is appropriate when there is severe malfunction or for abusive or destructive situations. It represents a more dysfunctional situation than does *Interrupted family processes* or *Compromised family coping.* The diagnostic label *Caregiver role strain* focuses on the needs of the caregiving family member, whereas *Disabled family coping* focuses more on the needs of the patient or the family unit. If there is actual violence in the family, the diagnosis might be *Disabled family coping related to use of violence to manage conflict.* When the abusive behavior is potential rather than actual, the label *Risk for violence* should be used.

Suggested Alternative Diagnoses

Caregiver role strain (actual or risk for)

Coping: family, compromised

Management of therapeutic regimen: families/individual, ineffective

Parenting, impaired

Violence: directed at others, risk for

NOC Outcomes

Aggression Control: Self-restraint of assaultive, combative, or destructive behavior toward others

Caregiver Emotional Health: Feelings, attitudes, and emotions of a family care provider while caring for a family member or significant other over an extended period of time

Caregiver–Patient Relationship: Positive interactions and connections between the caregiver and care recipient

Caregiver Well-Being: Primary care provider's satisfaction with health and life circumstances

Caregiving Endurance Potential: Factors that promote family care provider continuance over an extended period of time

Depression Control: Personal actions to minimize melancholy and maintain interest in life events

Depression Level: Severity of melancholic mood and loss of interest in life events

Family Coping: Family actions to manage stressors that tax family resources

Family Normalization: Ability of the family to develop and maintain routines and management strategies that contribute to optimal functioning when a member has a chronic illness or disability

Neglect Recovery: Healing following the cessation of substandard care

Goals/Evaluation Criteria

Examples Using NOC Language

- Family will not use *Disabled family coping*, as demonstrated by satisfactory status of Caregiver Emotional Health, Caregiver–Patient Relationship, Caregiver Well-Being, Caregiving Endurance Potential, Depression Control, Depression Level, Family Normalization, and Neglect Recovery
- **Family Coping** indicators include the following (specify 1–5: never, rarely, sometimes, often, or consistently demonstrated):
    Demonstrates role flexibility
    Manages problems
    Cares for needs of all family members
    Maintains financial stability
    Seeks assistance when appropriate

Other Examples

Family will:
- Acknowledge needs of family unit
- Acknowledge needs of patient
- Begin to demonstrate effective interpersonal skills
- Demonstrate ability to resolve conflict without violence
- Express unresolved feelings
- Identify and maintain intrafamily sexual boundaries
- Identify conflicting coping styles
- Participate in effective problem solving
- Participate in treatment plan

NIC Interventions

Caregiver Support: Provision of the necessary information, advocacy, and support to facilitate primary patient care by someone other than a health care professional

Coping Enhancement: Assisting a patient to adapt to perceived stressors, changes, or threats which interfere with meeting life demands and roles

Emotional Support: Provision of reassurance, acceptance, and encouragement during times of stress

Family Support: Promotion of family interests and goals

Family Therapy: Assisting family members to move their family toward a more productive way of living

Normalization Promotion: Assisting parents and other family members of children with chronic illnesses or disabilities in providing normal life experiences for their children and families

Respite Care: Provision of short-term care to provide relief for family caregiver

Nursing Activities

Also refer to Nursing Activities in Coping: Family, Compromised, pp. 115–116.

Assessments

- Obtain history of family's pattern of behaviors and interactions and changes that have occurred
- Assess interaction between patient and family, being alert for potential destructive behaviors (e.g., elder abuse, child abuse)
- Determine physical, emotional, and educational resources of family members
- Assess family members' motivation and desire for resolving areas of dissatisfaction or conflict
- *(NIC) Family Support:*
  Determine the psychological burden of prognosis for family
  Identify nature of spiritual support for family

Patient/Family Teaching

- Discuss how violence is a learned behavior and can be transmitted to offspring
- Discuss with family effective ways to demonstrate feelings

Collaborative Activities

- Refer family and individual members to support groups, psychiatric treatment, social services (e.g., chemical-dependence programs, Parents United, Incest Survivors Anonymous, child protective services, battered wives' shelters)
- Report indications of physical or sexual abuse as directed by law to appropriate authorities
- *(NIC) Family Support:*
  Provide spiritual resources for family, as appropriate
  Arrange for ongoing respite care, when indicated and desired

Other

- In family discussions, begin with the least emotionally laden subjects
- Assist family in realistically identifying the needs of patient and family unit
- Assist family in recognizing the problem (e.g., managing conflict with violence, sexual abuse)
- Encourage family participation in all group meetings
- Encourage family to express concerns and to help plan post-hospital care
- Help motivate family to change
- Assist family in finding better ways to handle dysfunctional behavior
- Provide "homework" for family members (e.g., a no-television night or eating some meals together)
- Assist family members in clarifying what they expect and need from each other
- *(NIC) Family Support:*
  Foster realistic hope
  Listen to family concerns, feelings, and questions
  Facilitate communication of concerns and feelings between patient and family or between family members
  Answer all questions of family members or assist them to get answers
  Provide feedback for family regarding their coping
  Give care to patient in lieu of family to relieve them or when family is unable to give care

COPING: FAMILY, READINESS FOR ENHANCED (00075) (1980)

Definition: Effective managing of adaptive tasks by family member involved with the client's health challenge, who now exhibits desire and readiness for enhanced health and growth in regard to self and in relation to the client.

Defining Characteristics

Subjective

Individual expressing interest in making contact on a one-to-one basis or on a mutual-aid group basis with another person who has experienced a similar situation

Objective

Family member attempting to describe growth impact of crisis on his own values, priorities, goals, or relationships

Family member moving in direction of health promoting and enriching lifestyle that supports and monitors maturational processes, audits and negotiates treatment programs, and chooses experiences that optimize wellness

Related Factors

Needs sufficiently gratified and adaptive tasks effectively addressed to enable goals of self-actualization to surface

Suggestions for Use

Use this diagnosis for a normally functioning family that wishes to preserve and improve family integrity during changes brought about by illness or developmental and situational crises. Such a family might wish to have control over outcomes or enhance their quality of life. There is some overlap between this label and the following Suggested Alternative Diagnoses. Pending further research, use *Readiness for enhanced family processes* and *Health-seeking behaviors*.

Suggested Alternative Diagnoses

Health-seeking behaviors
Interrupted family processes
Readiness for enhanced family processes

NOC Outcomes

Caregiver Well-Being: Primary care provider's satisfaction with health and life circumstance

Family Coping: Family actions to manage stressors that tax family resources

Family Normalization: Ability of the family to develop and maintain routines and management strategies that contribute to optimal functioning when a member has a chronic illness or disability

Family Participation in Professional Care: Family involvement in decision making, delivery, and evaluation of care provided by health care personnel

Health Promoting Behavior: Actions to sustain or increase wellness

Health Seeking Behavior: Actions to promote optimal wellness, recovery, and rehabilitation

Participation: Health Care Decisions: Personal involvement in selecting and evaluating health care options

Goals/Evaluation Criteria

(Also refer to Goals/Evaluation Criteria for the diagnoses Interrupted Family Processes and Health Seeking Behaviors, on pp. 185 and 240–241, respectively.)

Family member(s) will:

- Develop a plan for personal growth
- Evaluate and change plan as needed
- Identify and prioritize personal goals
- Implement plan

NIC Interventions

Caregiver Support: Provision of the necessary information, advocacy, and support to facilitate primary patient care by someone other than a health care professional

Decision-Making Support: Providing information and support for a patient who is making a decision regarding health care

Family Involvement Promotion: Facilitating family participation in the emotional and physical care of the patient

Family Support: Promotion of family interests and goals

Health Education: Developing and providing instruction and learning experiences to facilitate voluntary adaptation of behavior conducive to health in individuals, families, groups, or communities

Health System Guidance: Facilitating a patient's location and use of appropriate health services

Normalization Promotion: Assisting parents and other family members of children with chronic illnesses or disabilities in providing normal life experiences for their children and families

Respite Care: Provision of short-term care to provide relief for family caregiver

Self-Modification Assistance: Reinforcement of self-directed change initiated by the patient to achieve personally important goals

Nursing Activities

Assessments

- Assess physical, emotional, and educational resources of the family
- Identify family cultural influences
- Identify any self-care deficits in patient
- Identify family structure and roles
- *(NIC) Family Support:*
  Appraise family's emotional reaction to patient's condition
  Determine the psychological burden of prognosis for family
  Identify nature of spiritual support for family

Patient/Family Teaching

- *(NIC) Family Support:*
  Teach the medical and nursing plans of care to family
  Provide necessary knowledge of options to family that will assist them to make decisions about patient care
  Assist family to acquire necessary knowledge, skills, and equipment to sustain their decision about patient care

Collaborative Activities

- Identify community resources that can be used to enhance the health status of the patient with family members
- *(NIC) Family Support:* Arrange for ongoing respite care, when indicated and desired

Other

- Assist family member(s) in developing a plan for personal growth. Plan may include investigation of employment opportunities, school, support groups, enrichment activities, and exercise
- Provide emotional support and availability to family member(s) during implementation, evaluation, and revision of plan
- Assist family member(s) in identifying and prioritizing personal goals

- Encourage family member(s) to compare initial response to the crisis with current situation and to recognize change
- Provide an opportunity for family member(s) to reflect on impact of patient's illness on family structure and dynamics
- Discuss how strengths and resources can be used to enhance health status of the patient with family members
- *(NIC) Family Support:*
  Assure family that best care possible is being given to patient
  Accept the family's values in a nonjudgmental manner
  Listen to family concerns, feelings, and questions
  Facilitate communication of concerns and feelings between patient and family or between family members
  Answer all questions of family members or assist them to get answers
  Respect and support adaptive coping mechanisms used by family
  Provide feedback for family regarding their coping
  Encourage family decision making in planning long-term patient care affecting family structure and finances
  Advocate for family, as appropriate
  Foster family assertiveness in information seeking, as appropriate

COPING [INDIVIDUAL], READINESS FOR ENHANCED (00158)(2002)

Definition: A pattern of cognitive and behavioral efforts to manage demands that is sufficient for well-being and can be strengthened

Defining Characteristics

Subjective
Acknowledges power
Defines stressors as manageable
Is aware of possible environmental changes

Objective
Seeks knowledge of new strategies
Seeks social support
Uses a broad range of problem-oriented and emotion-oriented strategies
Uses spiritual resources

Suggestions for Use

Because this is a wellness diagnosis, an etiology (e.g., related factors) is not needed. If situations exist that pose a risk to effective coping, use *Risk for ineffective coping*. Use individual, family, or community diagnosis, as appropriate

Suggested Alternative Diagnoses

Coping: community, readiness for enhanced
Coping: family, readiness for enhanced
Coping, risk for ineffective

NOC Outcomes

NOC outcomes have not yet been linked to this diagnosis; however, the following may be useful:

Coping: Actions to manage stressors that tax an individual's resources

Health Promoting Behavior: Actions to sustain or increase wellness

Health Seeking Behavior: Actions to promote optimal wellness, recovery, and rehabilitation

Role Performance: Congruence of an individual's role behavior with role expectations

Goals/Evaluation Criteria

Examples Using NOC Language:

- Demonstrates **Health Promoting Behaviors**, as evidenced by the following indicators (specify 1–5: never, rarely, sometimes, often, or consistently demonstrated):

    Seeks balance among exercise, work, leisure, rest, and nutrition
    Uses effective stress reduction behaviors
    Maintains satisfactory social relationships

Other Examples

Patient will:
- Adapt to developmental changes
- Report improved ability to cope with stressors
- Continue to use effective coping strategies
- Identify new coping strategies that may be effective
- Report psychological comfort

NIC Interventions

Interventions have not yet been developed for this diagnosis; however, the following may be useful:

Coping Enhancement: Assisting a patient to adapt to perceived stressors, changes, or threats which interfere with meeting life demands and roles

Resiliency Promotion: Assisting individuals, families, and communities in development, use, and strengthening of protective factors to be used in coping with environmental and societal stressors

Role Enhancement: Assisting a patient, significant other, and family to improve relationships by clarifying and supplementing specific role behaviors

Self-Awareness Enhancement: Assisting a patient to explore and understand his thoughts, feelings, motivations, and behaviors

Simple Relaxation Therapy: Use of techniques to encourage and elicit relaxation for the purpose of decreasing undesirable signs and symptoms such as pain, muscle tension, or anxiety

Assessments

- Identify the patient's view of own condition and its congruence with the view of health care providers
- Assist to identify usual responses to various situations
- Identify areas in which patient wishes to enhance coping
- Identify which relaxation techniques have been effective in the past
- Evaluate effectiveness of relaxation techniques
- *(NIC) Coping Enhancement:*
  Appraise the impact of the patient's life situation on roles and relationships
  Explore with the patient previous methods of dealing with life problems

Patient/Family Teaching

- Teach details of chosen relaxation technique(s) (e.g., visualization)
- *(NIC) Coping Enhancement:*
  Instruct the patient on the use of relaxation techniques, as needed

Other

- Assist patient in identifying personal strengths
- Promote family communication and relationships

- Encourage to develop family traditions (e.g., observance of holidays and birthdays)
- Encourage to attend religious services
- Assist to identify situations that may create role transition
- Provide opportunity for patient to role play new coping strategies
- Assist to identify life priorities
- *(NIC) Coping Enhancement:*
  Arrange situations that encourage patient's autonomy
  Assist patient in identifying positive responses from others
  Support the use of appropriate defense mechanisms
  Encourage verbalization of feelings, perceptions, and fears
  Assist the patient to clarify misconceptions
  Assist the patient to identify available support systems

COPING, INEFFECTIVE
(00069) (1978, 1998)

Definition: Inability to form a valid appraisal of the stressors, inadequate choices or practiced responses, and inability to use available resources

Defining Characteristics

Subjective
Change in usual communication patterns
Fatigue
Verbalization of inability to cope or to ask for help

Objective
Abuse of chemical agents
Decreased use of social support
Destructive behavior toward self and others
High illness rate
Inability to meet basic needs
Inability to meet role expectations
Inadequate problem solving
Lack of goal-directed behavior and resolution of problems, including inability to attend and difficulty with organizing information
Poor concentration
Risk taking
Sleep disturbance
Use of forms of coping that impede adaptive behavior

Other Possible Defining Characteristics (Non-NANDA International)
Evidence of physical and psychologic abuse
Expression of unrealistic expectations
High rate of accidents
Inappropriate use of defense mechanisms
Verbal manipulation

Related Factors

Disturbance in pattern of appraisal of threat
Disturbance in pattern of tension release
Gender differences in coping strategies
High degree of threat
Inability to conserve adaptive energies
Inadequate level of confidence in ability to cope
Inadequate level of perception of control
Inadequate opportunity to prepare for stressor
Inadequate resources available
Inadequate social support created by characteristics of relationships
Situational or maturational crises
Uncertainty

Suggestions for Use

Many labels represent failure to cope (e.g., *Anxiety, Risk for violence, Hopelessness*). Always use the most specific label that fits the patient's defining characteristics. *Ineffective coping* represents a more chronic or long-term pattern than does *Impaired adjustment*. It is also less specific than the label *Defensive coping*.

Suggested Alternative Diagnoses

Adjustment, impaired
Anxiety
Denial, ineffective
Fear
Grieving, dysfunctional
Post-trauma syndrome
Violence, risk for: self-directed or directed at others

NOC Outcomes

Aggression Control: Self-restraint of assaultive, combative, or destructive behavior toward others

Coping: Actions to manage stressors that tax an individual's resources

Decision Making: Ability to choose between two or more alternatives

Impulse Control: Ability to self-restrain compulsive or impulsive behaviors

Information Processing: Ability to acquire, organize, and use information

Role Performance: Congruence of an individual's role behavior with role expectations

Social Support: Perceived availability and actual provision of reliable assistance from other persons

Goals/Evaluation Criteria

Examples Using NOC Language

- Demonstrates effective **Coping**, as evidenced by the following indicators (specify 1–5: never, rarely, sometimes, often, or consistently demonstrated):

    Identifies effective [and ineffective] coping patterns

    Seeks information concerning illness and treatment

    Employs behaviors to reduce stress

    Identifies and uses multiple coping strategies

    Reports decrease in negative feelings

- Demonstrates **Impulse Control** by consistently maintain[ing] self-control without supervision

- Demonstrates normal **Information Processing** by consistently exhibit[ing] logical thought processes

Other Examples

Patient will:

- Demonstrate interest in diversional activities
- Identify personal strengths that may promote effective coping
- Weigh and choose among alternatives and consequences
- Initiate conversation
- Participate in ADLs
- Participate in decision-making process
- Use verbal and nonverbal expressions applicable to situation
- Verbalize plan for either accepting or changing the situation

NIC Interventions

Anger Control Assistance: Facilitation of the expression of anger in an adaptive, nonviolent manner

Coping Enhancement: Assisting a patient to adapt to perceived stressors, changes, or threats which interfere with meeting life demands and roles

Decision-Making Support: Providing information and support for a patient who is making a decision regarding health care

Environmental Management: Violence Prevention: Monitoring and manipulation of the physical environment to decrease the potential for violent behavior directed toward self, others, or environment

Family Involvement Promotion: Facilitating family participation in the emotional and physical care of the patient

Impulse Control Training: Assisting the patient to mediate impulsive behavior through application of problem-solving strategies to social and interpersonal situations

Learning Facilitation: Promoting the ability to process and comprehend information

Learning Readiness Enhancement: Improving the ability and willingness to receive information

Role Enhancement: Assisting a patient, significant other, or family to improve relationships by clarifying and supplementing specific role behaviors

Support Group: Use of a group environment to provide emotional support and health-related information for members

Support System Enhancement: Facilitation of support to patient by family, friends, and community

Nursing Activities

Assessments

- Monitor for aggressive behaviors
- Identify the patient's view of own condition and its congruence with the view of health care providers
- *(NIC) Coping Enhancement:*

    Appraise patient's adjustment to changes in body image, as indicated

    Appraise the impact of the patient's life situation on roles and relationships

    Evaluate the patient's decision-making ability

    Explore with the patient previous methods of dealing with life problems

    Determine the risk of the patient's inflicting self-harm

Patient/Family Teaching

- *(NIC) Coping Enhancement:*

  Provide factual information concerning diagnosis, treatment, and prognosis

  Instruct the patient on the use of relaxation techniques, as needed

  Provide appropriate social skills training

Collaborative Activities

- Initiate a patient care conference to review patient's coping mechanisms and to establish a plan of care
- Involve hospital resources in provision of emotional support for patient and family
- Serve as a liaison between patient, other health care providers, and community resources (e.g., support groups)

Other

- Assist patient in developing a plan for accepting or changing situation
- Assist patient in identifying personal strengths
- Encourage patient to:

  Be involved in planning care activities

  Initiate conversations with others

  Participate in activity
- Ask family to visit whenever possible
- *(NIC) Coping Enhancement:*

  Encourage patient to identify a realistic description of change in role

  Use a calm, reassuring approach

  Reduce stimuli in the environment that could be misinterpreted as threatening

  Provide an atmosphere of acceptance

  Discourage decision making when the patient is under severe stress

  Foster constructive outlets for anger and hostility

  Explore patient's reasons for self-criticism

  Arrange situations that encourage patient's autonomy

  Assist patient in identifying positive responses from others

  Support the use of appropriate defense mechanisms

  Encourage verbalization of feelings, perceptions, and fears

  Assist the patient to clarify misconceptions

  Assist the patient to identify available support systems

  Appraise and discuss alternative responses to situation

DECISIONAL CONFLICT (SPECIFY)
(00083) (1988)

Definition: Uncertainty about course of action to be taken when choice among competing actions involves risk, loss, or challenge to personal life values

Defining Characteristics
Subjective
Focusing on self

Questioning personal values and beliefs while attempting a decision

Verbalized feeling of distress while attempting a decision

Verbalized uncertainty about choices

Verbalization of undesired consequences of alternative actions being considered

Objective
Delayed decision making

Physical signs of distress or tension (e.g., increased heart rate, increased muscle tension, restlessness)

Vacillation between alternative choices

Related Factors

Lack of experience or interference with decision making

Lack of relevant information

Lack of support system

Multiple or divergent sources of information

Perceived threat to value system

Unclear personal values and beliefs

Suggestions for Use

(1) The role of the nurse is to help clients make logical, informed decisions by providing information and support. The nurse should not try to influence the client to decide in a particular way. (2) Do not assume that clients facing a serious, even life-and-death, decision are conflicted. Such decisions may actually be easy to make in some cases.

Suggested Alternative Diagnoses

Parental role conflict

Management of therapeutic regimen, ineffective

Spiritual distress
Spiritual distress, risk for

NOC Outcomes

Decision Making: Ability to choose between two or more alternatives

Information Processing: Ability to acquire, organize, and use information

Participation: Health Care Decisions: Personal involvement in selecting and evaluating health care options

Goals/Evaluation Criteria

Examples Using NOC Language

- *Decisional conflict* will lessen, as demonstrated by Information Processing abilities and Participation: Health Care Decisions
- **Decision Making** will be demonstrated, as evidenced by the following indicators (specify 1–5: never, rarely, sometimes, often, or consistently demonstrated):

  Identifies relevant information

  Recognizes contradiction with others' desires

  Acknowledges relevant legal implications

  Weighs and chooses among alternatives

  Identifies resources necessary to support each alternative

  Acknowledges social context of the situation

Other Examples

Patient will:
- Evaluate available choices in relation to personal values
- Report a decrease in tension or distress
- Exhibit information processing and logical thought processes
- Uses problem solving to achieve chosen outcomes

NIC Interventions

Decision-Making Support: Providing information and support for a patient who is making a decision regarding health care

Health System Guidance: Facilitating a patient's location and use of appropriate health services

Learning Facilitation: Promoting the ability to process and comprehend information

Mutual Goal Setting: Collaborating with patient to identify and prioritize care goals, then developing a plan for achieving those goals

<u>Nursing Activities</u>

Assessments

- Assess patient's understanding of available choices
- Evaluate patient's level of tension or distress
- *(NIC) Decision-Making Support:* Determine whether there are differences between the patient's view of own condition and the view of health care providers

Patient/Family Teaching

- *(NIC) Decision-Making Support:*
  Inform patient of alternative views of solutions
  Provide information requested by patient

Collaborative Activities

- Use resources (e.g., ethics committee) as appropriate.
- *(NIC) Decision-Making Support:*
  Serve as a liaison between patient and other health care providers
  Refer to support groups, as appropriate
  Refer to legal aid, as appropriate
  Facilitate collaborative decision making

Other

- Assist patient in identifying a course of action and adapt as necessary
- *(NIC) Decision-Making Support:*
  Establish communication with patient early in admission
  Facilitate patient's articulation of goals for care
  Facilitate collaborative decision making
  Help patient identify the advantages and disadvantages of each alternative
  Help patient explain decision to others, as needed
  Serve as a liaison between patient and family
  Serve as a liaison between patient and other health care providers
  Respect patient's right to receive or not to receive information

DENIAL, INEFFECTIVE
(00072) (1988)

Definition: Conscious or unconscious attempt to disavow the knowledge or meaning of an event to reduce anxiety and fear, but leading to the detriment of health

Defining Characteristics

Subjective

Displaces fear of impact of the condition

Does not admit fear of death or invalidism

Displays inappropriate affect

Minimizes symptoms

Unable to admit impact of disease in life pattern

Objective

Delays seeking or refuses health care attention to the detriment of health

Displaces source of symptoms to other organs

Does not perceive personal relevance of symptoms or danger

Makes dismissive gestures or comments when speaking of distressing events

Uses home remedies (self-treatment) to relieve symptoms

Related Factors

To be developed

Suggestions for Use

Some denial in response to illness or other crises may be necessary in order for the client to cope with the situation. Such normal denial is gradually replaced by acceptance or changing of the situation, and it does not interfere with the treatment regimen. *Ineffective denial* should be used for clients whose denial persists or interferes with the treatment regimen. For example, a client newly diagnosed with myocardial infarction may respond with denial and, therefore, fail to make changes in lifestyle needed to prevent further heart damage.

Suggested Alternative Diagnoses

Coping, defensive

Coping, ineffective

Family coping, compromised

Family coping, disabled
Grieving, dysfunctional
Management of therapeutic regimen, ineffective
Noncompliance (specify)
Rape-trauma syndrome: silent reaction

NOC Outcomes

Acceptance: Health Status: Reconciliation to health circumstances

Anxiety Control: Personal actions to eliminate or reduce feelings of apprehension and tension from an unidentifiable source

Fear Control: Personal actions to eliminate or reduce disabling feelings of alarm aroused by an identifiable source

Health Beliefs: Perceived Threat: Personal conviction that a health problem is serious and has potential negative consequences for lifestyle

Symptom Control: Personal actions to minimize perceived adverse changes in physical and emotional functioning

Goals/Evaluation Criteria

Examples Using NOC Language

- Patient will not use *Ineffective denial*, as evidenced by Health Beliefs (Perceived Threat), Anxiety Control, Fear Control, and Symptom Control Behavior
- Patient will demonstrate **Acceptance: Health Status** as indicated by:
    Relinquishment of previous concept of health
    Recognition of reality of health situation
    Pursuit of information
    Coping with health situation
    Health-related decision making

Other Examples

Patient will:
- Acknowledge and recognize significance of symptoms
- Report significant symptoms
- Not demonstrate physical and behavioral manifestations of anxiety
- Acknowledge vulnerability to health problem

NIC Interventions

Anxiety Reduction: Minimizing apprehension, dread, foreboding, or uneasiness related to an unidentified source of anticipated danger

Calming Technique: Reducing anxiety in patient experiencing acute distress

Coping Enhancement: Assisting a patient to adapt to perceived stressors, changes, or threats which interfere with meeting life demands and roles

Counseling: Use of an interactive helping process focusing on the needs, problems, or feelings of the patient and significant others to enhance or support coping, problem solving, and interpersonal relationships

Emotional Support: Provision of reassurance, acceptance, and encouragement during times of stress

Health Education: Developing and providing instruction and learning experiences to facilitate voluntary adaptation of behavior conducive to health in individuals, families, groups, or communities

Security Enhancement: Intensifying a patient's sense of physical and psychological safety

Self-Awareness Enhancement: Assisting a patient to explore and understand his thoughts, feelings, motivations, and behaviors

Self-Modification Assistance: Reinforcement of self-directed change initiated by the patient to achieve personally important goals

Self-Responsibility Facilitation: Encouraging a patient to assume more responsibility for own behavior

Teaching: Disease Process: Assisting the patient to understand information related to a specific disease process

Nursing Activities

Assessments

- Assess understanding of symptoms and illness
- Determine whether patient's perception of his health status is realistic
- *(NIC) Anxiety Reduction:*
  Determine patient's decision-making ability
  Identify when level of anxiety changes

Patient Teaching

- Teach recognition of symptoms and desired patient responses
- *(NIC) Anxiety Reduction:* Provide factual information concerning diagnosis, treatment, and prognosis

Collaborative Activities

- Include patient and family in a multidisciplinary conference to develop a plan of action. Plan may include:

  Arranging for follow-up support after discharge

  Meeting with patients in similar situations to learn new ways to cope and to decrease anxiety and fear

Other

- Establish a therapeutic relationship with patient that will allow exploration of denial
- Use every opportunity to reinforce consequences of patient's actions
- Engage patient in discussion about anxiety, fears, symptoms, and impact of illness
- Identify and reinforce patient strengths
- *(NIC) Anxiety Reduction:*

  Seek to understand the patient's perspective of a stressful situation

  Reinforce behavior, as appropriate

  Encourage verbalization of feelings, perceptions, and fears

  Demonstrate empathy, warmth, and genuineness

  Support the use of appropriate defense mechanisms

  Assist patient to articulate a realistic description of an upcoming event

DENTITION, IMPAIRED
(00048) (1998)

Definition: Disruption in tooth development and eruption patterns or structural integrity of individual teeth

Defining Characteristics

Subjective

Toothache

Objective

Asymmetrical facial expression

Crown or root caries

Erosion of enamel

Excessive calculus

Excessive plaque

Halitosis

Incomplete eruption for age (may be primary or permanent teeth)
Loose teeth
Malocclusion or tooth misalignment
Missing teeth or complete absence
Premature loss of primary teeth
Tooth enamel discoloration
Tooth fracture(s)
Worn-down or abraded teeth

Related Factors

Access or economic barriers to professional care
Barriers to self-care
Bruxism
Chronic use of tobacco, coffee, tea, or red wine
Chronic vomiting
Dietary habits
Excessive intake of fluorides
Excessive use of abrasive cleaning agents
Genetic predisposition
Ineffective oral hygiene
Lack of knowledge regarding dental health
Nutritional deficits
Premature loss of primary teeth
Selected prescription medications
Sensitivity to heat or cold

Suggestions for Use

None

Suggested Alternative Diagnosis

Self-care deficit: bathing and hygiene

NOC Outcomes

Oral Health: Condition of the mouth, teeth, gums, and tongue
Self-Care: Oral Hygiene: Ability to care for own mouth and teeth

Goals/Evaluation Criteria

Examples Using NOC Language

- Patient corrects *Impaired dentition*, as evidenced by Oral Health and Self-Care: Oral Hygiene.
- Patient will demonstrate **Oral Health**, as indicated by:
    Cleanliness of mouth, teeth, gums, tongue, and dentures or dental appliances

Moistness of lips, oral mucosa, and tongue

Breath free of halitosis

Free of bleeding

Other Examples

Patient will:

- Be free from debris and plaque on dental surfaces
- Have firm, well-hydrated, nonbleeding gums of uniform color
- Verbalize feeling of oral cleanliness
- Demonstrate correct brushing and flossing procedures
- Follow sound nutritional practices, such as avoiding sweets between meals
- Have a checkup by a dentist every six months
- Be free from caries, loose teeth, or toothaches
- Parent will take child for first dentist visit by age 2 or 3
- Child will not experience premature loss of primary teeth

NIC Interventions

Oral Health Maintenance: Maintenance and promotion of oral hygiene and dental health for the patient at risk for developing oral or dental lesions

Oral Health Restoration: Promotion of healing for a patient who has an oral mucosal or dental lesion

Nursing Activities

Assessments

- Inspect mouth for loose or missing teeth, color and condition of enamel, number of dental fillings and caries, and tartar at base of teeth
- Observe for halitosis
- Determine client's usual oral hygiene practices
- Assess client's level of knowledge of measures to prevent Impaired dentition (e.g., "How often do you see your dentist?")
- Assess client's access to and resources for dental care
- Assess client's ability to perform oral care (e.g., "Do you have any problems caring for your teeth?")
- Assess client's knowledge of oral hygiene practices and routines (e.g., brushing method)
- Identify risk factors for Impaired dentition (e.g., clients who are seriously ill, confused, depressed)

Collaborative Activities

- Refer to dental hygienist, dentist, or clinic, as needed

Client/Family Teaching

- Teach parents the importance of caring for the child's primary teeth
- Teach parents to help children brush or inspect their mouths after brushing
- Teach brushing and flossing techniques, as needed
- Explain the causes of dental problems, such as tooth decay
- Teach to avoid heavy use of tobacco, tea, coffee, and red wine, to prevent discoloration
- Teach measures to avoid tooth decay:
  Brush after meals and at bedtime
  Ensure adequate intake of calcium, phosphorus, and vitamins A, C, and D
  Avoid sweets between meals; take in moderation with meals
  Eat cleansing foods, such as raw fruits and vegetables
  If water is not fluoridated, take a fluoride supplement daily until at least age 14
  Have a dental checkup every six months
  Floss teeth daily

Other

- Provide oral hygiene for patients with *Self-care deficit* (e.g., thorough brushing and rinsing)
- Help patient establish an oral hygiene schedule after meals and at bedtime. For example:
  Use sulcular technique and soft toothbrush
  Rinse with mouthwash or solution of warm water and salt or baking soda

---

DEVELOPMENT: DELAYED, RISK FOR
(00112) (1998)

Definition: At risk for delay of 25% or more in one or more of the areas of social or self-regulatory behavior or cognitive, language, or gross- or fine-motor skills

Risk Factors

Prenatal
Genetic or endocrine disorders
Illiteracy
Inadequate nutrition

Infections
Lack of, late, or poor prenatal care
Maternal age < 15 or > 35 years
Poverty
Substance abuse
Unplanned or unwanted pregnancy

Individual

Behavior disorders
Brain damage (e.g., hemorrhage in postnatal period, shaken baby, abuse, accident)
Chemotherapy
Chronic illness
Congenital or genetic disorders
Failure to thrive, inadequate nutrition
Foster or adopted child
Hearing impairment or frequent otitis media
Lead poisoning
Natural disaster
Positive drug-screening test
Prematurity
Radiation therapy
Seizures
Substance abuse
Technology-dependent
Vision impairment

Environmental

Poverty
Violence

Caregiver

Abuse
Mental illness
Mental retardation or severe learning disability

Suggestions for Use

(1) This diagnosis is made when one or more risk factors are present and the nursing focus is on preventing developmental delays by eliminating the risk factors. (2) Because development is routinely assessed in nursing care of children, a diagnostic statement is usually not required for that application; such assessment is usually included in pediatric standards of care. (3) This label is not appropriate for a mentally impaired child (e.g., *Risk for delayed development related to Down syndrome*). Instead, diagnose the specific

functional task that the child is unable to perform (e.g., *Feeding self-care deficit, Bowel incontinence*).

Suggested Alternative Diagnoses

Bowel incontinence
Communication, impaired verbal
Coping: family, compromised
Coping: family, disabled
Growth, risk for disproportionate
Growth and development, delayed
Coping, ineffective
Parenting, impaired
Self-care deficit (specify)
Urinary incontinence

NOC Outcomes

Child Development: 12 Months; 2, 3, 4, and 5 Years; Middle Childhood (6–11 Years); Adolescence (12–17 Years): Milestones of physical, cognitive, and psychosocial progression by [specify age]
Growth: A normal increase in body size and weight
Social Interaction Skills: An individual's use of effective interaction behaviors

Goals/Evaluation Criteria

NOTE: This text can only provide examples of developmental milestones. Refer to pediatrics or child development texts for complete discussion of growth and development

• The child will achieve developmental milestones, that is, not experience a delay of 25% or more in one or more of the areas of social or self-regulatory behavior or cognitive, language, or gross- or fine-motor skills. For example:

For a 6-month-old: rolls over, sits with support, grasps and mouths objects

For a 3-year-old: demonstrates autonomy, is toilet trained

NIC Interventions

Behavior Modification: Social Skills: Assisting the patient to develop or improve interpersonal social skills
Developmental Enhancement: Adolescent: Facilitating optimal physical, cognitive, social, and emotional growth of individuals during the transition from childhood to adulthood

Developmental Enhancement: Child: Facilitating or teaching parents and caregivers to facilitate the optimal gross-motor, fine-motor, language, cognitive, social, and emotional growth of preschool and school-aged children

Environmental Management: Safety: Monitoring and manipulation of the physical environment to promote safety

Health Screening: Detecting health risks or problems by means of history, examination, and other procedures

Infant Care: Provision of developmentally appropriate family-centered care to the child under 1 year of age

Parent Education: Adolescent: Assisting parents to understand and help their adolescent children

Parent Education: Infant: Instruction on nurturing and physical care needed during the first year of life

Risk Identification: Genetic: Identification and analysis of potential genetic risk factors in an individual, family, or group

Nursing Activities

NOTE: Because this nursing diagnosis is so broad and nonspecific, it is not possible to list every nursing activity here. Refer to age-specific sections in growth and development texts.

Assessments

- Conduct a thorough health assessment (e.g., child's history, temperament, culture, family environment, developmental screening) to determine functional level
- Determine caretakers' level of knowledge, resources, support system, and coping skills
- Identify parental future expectations for child (e.g., ability to learn, developmental achievements)
- Monitor parent and child interactions (e.g., during feedings)
- Assess prenatally for presence of risk factors (e.g., poverty, substance abuse)
- Assess for postnatal risk factors (e.g., chronic illness, seizures, violence, caregiver mental illness)

Patient/Family Teaching

- Teach parents about normal developmental milestones
- Demonstrate activities that promote development
- Teach ways to provide meaningful stimulation for infants and children
- Teach about age-appropriate behaviors
- Teach about age-appropriate toys and materials

Other

- If risk factors cannot be removed (as in a natural disaster), assist family to find resources and support coping efforts
- Assist patient to achieve next level of development through appropriate mastery of tasks specific to his level (refer to growth and development text)
- Establish a therapeutic and trusting relationship with caretakers
- Provide appropriate play activities, encourage activities with other children
- Communicate with patient at appropriate cognitive level of development
- Provide positive rewards or feedback for attempts at self-expression
- Use consistent, structured behavior modification techniques
- Involve patient in self-care and ADLs as much as possible
- Encourage parents to expect and require responsible behavior in child

DIARRHEA
(00013) (1975, 1988)

Definition: Passage of loose, unformed stools

Defining Characteristics

Subjective
Abdominal pain
Cramping
Urgency

Objective
At least three loose liquid stools per day
Hyperactive bowel sounds

Related Factors

Psychological
High stress levels and anxiety

Situational
Adverse effects of medications
Alcohol abuse
Contaminants
Laxative abuse
Radiation

Toxins
Travel
Tube feedings

Physiological

Infectious processes
Inflammation
Irritation
Malabsorption
Parasites

Suggestions for Use

None

Suggested Alternative Diagnosis

Incontinence, Bowel

NOC Outcomes

Bowel Elimination: Ability of the gastrointestinal tract to form and evacuate stool effectively

Electrolyte and Acid–Base Balance: Balance of electrolytes and nonelectrolytes in the intracellular and extracellular compartments of the body

Fluid Balance: Balance of water in the intra- and extracellular compartments of the body

Hydration: Amount of water in the intra- and extracellular compartments of the body

Symptom Severity: Extent of perceived adverse changes in physical, emotional, and social functioning

Goals/Evaluation Criteria

Examples Using NOC Language

- *Diarrhea* will be controlled or eliminated, as demonstrated by effective Bowel Elimination, Electrolyte and Acid/Base Balance, Fluid Balance, adequate Hydration, and Symptom Severity
- Demonstrates effective **Bowel Elimination**, as evidenced by the following indicators (specify 1–5: extremely, substantially, moderately, mildly, or not compromised):
    Elimination pattern in expected range
    Diarrhea not present
    Stool free of blood and mucus
    Painful cramps not present
    Bloating not present

Other Examples

Patient will:

- Follow dietary requirements to alleviate diarrhea
- Practice hygiene adequate to prevent skin breakdown
- Verbalize understanding of the causes of his diarrhea
- Maintain electrolyte balance within normal limits
- Maintain acid–base balance within normal limits
- Be well hydrated (mucous membranes moist; afebrile; good eyeball turgor; BP, hematocrit, and urine output within normal limits)

NIC Interventions

Bowel Management: Establishment and maintenance of a regular pattern of bowel elimination

Diarrhea Management: Prevention and alleviation of diarrhea

Electrolyte Management: Promotion of electrolyte balance and prevention of complications resulting from abnormal or undesired serum electrolyte levels

Fluid Management: Promotion of fluid balance and prevention of complications resulting from abnormal or undesired fluid levels

Fluid/Electrolyte Management: Regulation and prevention of complications from altered fluid and electrolyte levels

Nursing Activities

Assessments

- Perform guaiac test on stools
- Have patient identify usual bowel pattern
- Monitor laboratory values (electrolytes, CBC), and report abnormalities
- Weigh patient daily
- Assess and document:
    Frequency, color, consistency, and amount (measure) of stool
    Skin turgor and condition of oral mucosa as indicators of dehydration
- *(NIC) Diarrhea Management:*
    Obtain stool for culture and sensitivity, if diarrhea continues
    Evaluate medication profile for gastrointestinal side effects
    Evaluate recorded intake for nutritional content
    Monitor skin in perianal area for irritation and ulceration

Patient/Family Teaching

- Inform patient of possibility of medication-induced diarrhea
- *(NIC) Diarrhea Management:*
    Teach patient appropriate use of antidiarrheal medications

Instruct patient and family members to record color, volume, frequency, and consistency of stools

Instruct patient to notify staff of each episode of diarrhea

Teach patient stress-reduction techniques, as appropriate

Collaborative Activities

- Consult with dietitian for adjustment of diet
- Consult with pediatrician for alternative type of feeding
- *(NIC) Diarrhea Management:* Consult physician if signs and symptoms of diarrhea persist

Other

- Help patient to identify stressors that may contribute to diarrhea
- Provide care in an accepting, nonjudgmental manner
- Provide fluids of patient's choice (specify)
- Provide privacy and safety for patient during bowel elimination
- *(NIC) Diarrhea Management:*

  Perform actions to rest the bowel (e.g., NPO or liquid diet)

  Encourage frequent, small feedings and add bulk gradually

DISUSE SYNDROME, RISK FOR
(00040) (1988)

Definition: At risk for deterioration of body systems as the result of prescribed or unavoidable musculoskeletal inactivity. **NOTE:** Complications from immobility can include pressure ulcer, constipation, stasis of pulmonary secretions, thrombosis, urinary tract infection or retention, decreased strength and endurance, orthostatic hypotension, decreased range of joint motion, disorientation, body image disturbance, and powerlessness.

Risk Factors

Subjective

Severe pain

Objective

Altered level of consciousness

Mechanical immobilization

Paralysis

Prescribed immobilization

Suggestions for Use

This label describes the cluster of potential complications of immobility (e.g., *Risk for constipation, Risk for impaired skin integrity*). It is a syndrome diagnosis under which a number of actual and potential problems are clustered. Therefore, when the risk factor is immobility, it is not necessary to write separate risk diagnoses such as *Risk for impaired skin integrity*. Those more specific labels should be used only if an actual problem develops (e.g., actual *Impaired skin integrity related to immobility*), or if the risk factor is something other than immobility (e.g., *Risk for impaired skin integrity related to malnutrition*). Furthermore, this diagnosis should not be written with an etiology. As a syndrome diagnosis, the etiology (disuse) is contained in the label itself.

Even though the NANDA International terminology is still *Risk for disuse syndrome*, Carpenito (1997b, p. 326) recommends that syndrome diagnoses not be written with "risk for," since they include both actual and risk diagnoses. In that case, the diagnosis *Disuse syndrome* would be used both for clients with the risk factor of immobility and those with the defining characteristics for actual *Disuse syndrome*.

Suggested Alternative Diagnoses

If an actual problem occurs as a result of immobility or if the etiology of a potential problem is something other than immobility, consider using a more restricted physiological nursing diagnosis, such as one of the following:

Actual or Risk for:
Activity intolerance
Body image, disturbed
Breathing pattern, ineffective
Constipation
Physical mobility, impaired
Powerlessness
Sensory perception, disturbed: all (specify)
Sexuality patterns, ineffective
Skin integrity, impaired
Swallowing, impaired
Tissue perfusion, ineffective (peripheral)
Urinary retention
Risk for:
Infection
Injury
Peripheral neurovascular dysfunction

NOC Outcomes

Endurance: Extent that energy enables a person's activity

Immobility Consequences: Physiological: Compromise in physiological functioning due to impaired physical mobility

Immobility Consequences: Psychocognitive: Extent of compromise in psycho-cognitive functioning due to impaired physical mobility

Joint Movement: Active: Range of motion of joints with self-initiated movement

Joint Movement: Passive: Range of motion of joints with assisted movement

Mobility Level: Ability to move purposefully

Muscle Function: Adequacy of muscle contraction needed for movement

Neurological Status: Consciousness: Extent to which an individual arouses, orients, and attends to the environment

Goals/Evaluation Criteria

Examples Using NOC Language

- Risk factors will be controlled and patient will not experience *Disuse syndrome*, as evidenced by outcomes of Endurance, Physiological and Psychocognitive Immobility Consequences, Active and Passive Joint Movement, Mobility Level, Muscle Function, and Neurological Status: Consciousness
- Patient will demonstrate **Immobility Consequences: Physiological**, as evidenced by the following indicators (specify 1–5: severe, substantial, moderate, slight, or none):

  Constipation, stool impaction, hypoactive bowel, or paralytic ileus

  Decreased nutritional status

  Urinary calculi, urinary retention, or urinary tract infection

  Pressure sore(s)

  Decreased muscle strength or decreased muscle tone

  Bone fracture, impaired joint movement, contracted joints or ankylosed joints

  Orthostatic hypotension

  Venous thrombosis

  Decreased cough effectiveness, decreased vital capacity, or pneumonia

Other Examples

Goals of care for this label are broad. They focus on preventing complications of immobility for all body systems. For example, patient will:

- Be oriented to time, place, and person
- Have adequate peripheral circulation
- Maintain optimal respiratory function (e.g., effective cough, no lung congestion, normal vital capacity)
- Maintain satisfactory body image
- Demonstrate concentration and interest in surroundings
- Have laboratory values within normal limits (e.g., oxygen, blood glucose, hemoglobin and hematocrit, and serum electrolyte levels)

NIC Interventions

Activity Therapy: Prescription of and assistance with specific physical, cognitive, social, and spiritual activities to increase the range, frequency, or duration of an individual's (or group's) activity

Cognitive Stimulation: Promotion of awareness and comprehension of surroundings by utilization of planned stimuli

Energy Management: Regulating energy use to treat or prevent fatigue and optimize function

Environmental Management: Manipulation of the patient's surroundings for therapeutic benefit

Exercise Therapy: Ambulation: Promotion and assistance with walking to maintain or restore autonomic and voluntary body functions during treatment and recovery from illness or injury

Exercise Therapy: Balance: Use of specific activities, postures, and movements to maintain, enhance, or restore balance

Exercise Therapy: Joint Mobility: Use of active or passive body movement to maintain or restore joint flexibility

Exercise Therapy: Muscle Control: Use of specific body activity or exercise protocols to enhance or restore controlled body movement

Nursing Activities

NOTE: In addition to the following generic activities, the outcomes and interventions selected for this diagnosis are determined by the affected body system and the degree of disuse. For patient goals and nursing activities specific to each body system, refer to plans for the Suggested Alternative Diagnoses listed on p. 150.

Assessments

- Make all assessments indicated in the preceding Goals/Evaluation Criteria, pp. 151–152.
- *(NIC) Energy Management:*
  Monitor nutritional intake to ensure adequate energy resources
  Monitor patient's oxygen response (e.g., pulse rate, cardiac rhythm, and respiratory rate) to self-care or nursing activities
  Determine what and how much activity is required to build endurance

Patient/Family Teaching

- *(NIC) Energy Management:*
  Assist the patient to understand energy conservation principles (e.g., the requirement for restricted activity or bed rest)
  Teach activity organization and time-management techniques to prevent fatigue
  Instruct patient and significant other to recognize signs and symptoms of fatigue that require reduction in activity

Collaborative Activities

- Consult with physical therapy for ways to improve mobility
- *(NIC) Energy Management:* Consult with dietitian about ways to increase intake of high-energy foods

Other

- Plan and implement a turning schedule
- *(NIC) Energy Management:*
  Avoid care activities during scheduled rest periods
  Encourage verbalization of feelings about limitations
  Use passive and active range-of-motion exercises to relieve muscle tension
  Encourage physical activity (e.g., ambulation or performance of ADL) consistent with patient's energy resources
  Assist patient to sit on side of bed ("dangle") if unable to transfer or walk

DIVERSIONAL ACTIVITY, DEFICIENT
(00097) (1980)

Definition: Decreased stimulation from (or interest or engagement in) recreational or leisure activities

Defining Characteristics

Subjective

Patient's statements regarding: boredom, wish there was something to do, to read, etc.

Objective

Usual hobbies cannot be undertaken in hospital

Other Possible Defining Characteristics (Non-NANDA International)

Anger, hostility

Complaints of inability to initiate or continue with usual activity

Disruptive behavior

Flat affect

Increase in daytime sleep periods

Restlessness

Withdrawn behavior

Related Factors

Environmental lack of diversional activity, as in long-term hospitalization

Frequent, lengthy treatments

Other Possible Related Factors (Non-NANDA International)

Deficit in social skills

Forced inactivity

Impaired perception of reality

Lack of motivation

Prolonged bed rest

Suggestions for Use

Deficient diversional activity must be diagnosed from the patient's point of view because only the patient can determine whether the activities available are adequate to meet his needs.

Suggested Alternative Diagnoses

Adjustment, impaired

Coping, ineffective

Loneliness, risk for

Social interaction, impaired

NOC Outcomes

Leisure Participation: Use of restful or relaxing activities as needed to promote well-being

Play Participation: Use of activities as needed for enjoyment, entertainment, and development by children

Social Involvement: Frequency of an individual's social interactions with persons, groups, or organizations

Goals/Evaluation Criteria

Examples Using NOC Language

- *Deficient diversional activity* will be relieved, as evidenced by Leisure Participation, Play Participation, and Social Involvement
- Demonstrates **Social Involvement**, as evidenced by the following indicators (specify 1–5: none, limited, moderate, substantial, or extensive):

    Interaction with close friends, neighbors, family members, or members of work group(s)

    Participation as member of church, club member, club officer, or volunteer group member

Other Examples

Patient will:

- Demonstrate socially acceptable behaviors during activities
- Verbalize acceptance of limitations that interfere with usual leisure activities
- Identify options for recreation
- Verbalize satisfaction with leisure activities
- Participate in appropriate play
- Demonstrate or verbalize enjoyment of play

NIC Interventions

Recreation Therapy: Purposeful use of recreation to promote relaxation and enhancement of social skills

Self-Responsibility Facilitation: Encouraging a patient to assume more responsibility for own behavior

Socialization Enhancement: Facilitation of another person's ability to interact with others

Therapeutic Play: Purposeful and directive use of toys or other materials to assist children in communicating their perception and knowledge of their world and to help in gaining mastery of their environment

Nursing Activities

Assessments

- Identify patient's interests
- Monitor emotional, physical, and social responses to diversional activity
- *(NIC) Self-Responsibility Facilitation:* Monitor level of responsibility that patient assumes

Collaborative Activities

- Identify resources, such as volunteers and occupational therapists, that could assist patient in recreational and leisure activities

Other

- Introduce and encourage new or alternative leisure-time activities, specify activities
- Introduce patient to other patients who have successfully dealt with similar situations
- Provide appropriate stimuli, such as music, games, puzzles, visitors, and relaxation therapy to vary monotonous routines and stimulate thought
- Provide compatible roommate, if possible
- Help patient to choose recreational activities appropriate to capabilities (e.g., physical, psychologic, and social)
- Supervise recreational activities, as necessary
- Encourage family, friends, and significant persons to visit
- *(NIC) Self-Responsibility Facilitation:*
  Encourage patient to take as much responsibility for own self-care as possible
  Encourage independence but assist patient when unable to perform
  Assist parents in identifying age-appropriate tasks for which child could be responsible, as appropriate
  Provide positive reinforcement for accepting additional responsibility and/or behavior change

DYSREFLEXIA, AUTONOMIC
(00009) (1988)

Definition: Life-threatening, uninhibited sympathetic response of the nervous system to a noxious stimulus after a spinal cord injury at T7 or above

Defining Characteristics
Subjective
Blurred vision

Chest pain

Headache (a diffuse pain in different portions of the head and not confined to any nerve distribution area)

Metallic taste in mouth

Paresthesia

Objective
Bradycardia (pulse rate of < 60 beats per minute, bpm)

Chills

Conjunctival congestion

Diaphoresis above injury

Horner syndrome (contraction of pupil, partial ptosis of eyelid, enophthalmos, and sometimes loss of sweating over affected side of face)

Nasal congestion

Pallor below injury

Paroxysmal hypertension (sudden periodic elevation of BP, where systolic is > 140 and diastolic is > 90 bpm)

Pilomotor reflex (gooseflesh formation when skin is cooled)

Red splotches on skin (above the injury)

Tachycardia (pulse rate > 100 bpm)

Related Factors
Bladder distention

Bowel distention

Lack of patient and caregiver knowledge

Skin irritation [or skin lesion]

Suggestions for Use
Autonomic dysreflexia is a potential problem for the patient with high spinal cord injury. *Autonomic dysreflexia* cannot continue as an actual nursing diagnosis. If independent nursing actions do not

resolve it, medical treatment becomes necessary. As a rule, *Risk for automatic dysreflexia* is a more useful label than actual *Autonomic dysreflexia* because the patient is in a potential state most of the time (Carpenito, 1997b, p. 342). The suggested alternative diagnoses represent noxious stimuli that can trigger a sympathetic response in the patient with spinal cord injury. They may be used as actual problems or as the etiology of *Autonomic dysreflexia* or *Risk for autonomic dysreflexia.*

Suggested Alternative Diagnoses

Constipation [fecal impaction]
Skin integrity, impaired
Urinary retention

NOC Outcomes

Neurological Status: Extent to which the peripheral and central nervous systems receive, process, and respond to internal and external stimuli

Neurological Status: Autonomic: Extent to which the autonomic nervous system coordinates visceral function

Vital Signs Status: Temperature, pulse, respiration, and BP within expected range for the individual

Goals/Evaluation Criteria

Examples Using NOC Language

- Patient will not experience *Autonomic dysreflexia*, as demonstrated by Neurological Status, Neurological Status: Autonomic, and Vital Signs Status within expected range for the individual
- Patients will demonstrate satisfactory **Neurological Status**, as evidenced by the following indicators (specify 1–5: extremely, substantially, moderately, mildly, or not compromised):
    Neurological status: consciousness
    Neurological status: central motor control
    Neurological status: cranial sensory and motor function
    Breathing pattern

Other Examples

Patient will:
- Maintain vital signs in expected range: temperature, apical and radial pulse rates, respiration rate, systolic and diastolic BP
- Demonstrate ability to maintain bowel and bladder routine
- Identify early signs and symptoms of dysreflexia (e.g., headache, blurred vision, paresthesia)

NIC Interventions

Dysreflexia Management: Prevention and elimination of stimuli which cause hyperactive reflexes and inappropriate autonomic responses in a patient with a cervical or high thoracic cord lesion

Vital Signs Monitoring: Collection and analysis of cardiovascular, respiratory, and body temperature data to determine and prevent compliations

Nursing Activities

Assessments

- Assess patient's knowledge of condition, including history of previous episodes, early signs and symptoms, and bowel and bladder regimen
- Assess skin condition at least daily, noting any reddened areas above level of spinal cord injury
- Obtain baseline temperature, BP, and pulse
- *(NIC) Dysreflexia Management:*

  Identify and minimize stimuli that may precipitate dysreflexia: bladder distention, renal calculi, infection, fecal impaction, rectal examination, suppository insertion, skin breakdown, and constrictive clothing or bed linen

  Monitor for signs and symptoms of autonomic dysreflexia: paroxysmal hypertension, bradycardia, tachycardia, diaphoresis above the level of injury, facial flushing, pallor below the level of injury, headache, nasal congestion, engorgement of temporal and neck vessels, conjunctival congestion, chills without fever, pilomotor erection, and chest pain

Patient/Family Teaching

- Ask patient to report any early signs and symptoms of condition that occur
- *(NIC) Dysreflexia Management:* Instruct patient and family about causes, symptoms, treatment, and prevention of dysreflexia

Collaborative Activities

- *(NIC) Dysreflexia Management:* Administer IV antihypertensive agents, as ordered

Other

- If symptoms occur, stop activity and have someone notify physician

- Quickly eliminate noxious stimulus in the following order:

    Bladder: Check catheter for patency, or catheterize patient

    Bowel: If distended, apply anesthetic ointment to rectal area and disimpact. Consider enema or flatus tube

    Body temperature: Maintain normal body temperature

- *(NIC) Dysreflexia Management:* Identify and minimize stimuli that may precipitate dysreflexia: bladder distention, renal calculi, infection, fecal impaction, rectal examination, suppository insertion, skin breakdown, and constrictive clothing or bed linen

- During onset of crisis, carry out management plan according to *(NIC) Dysreflexia Management:*

    Administer IV antihypertensive agents, as ordered

    Stay with patient and monitor status every 3–5 min if hyperreflexia occurs

    Place head of bed in upright position, as appropriate, if hyperreflexia occurs

DYSREFLEXIA: AUTONOMIC, RISK FOR
(00010) (1998, 2000)

Definition: At risk for life-threatening uninhibited response of the sympathetic nervous system, post spinal shock, in an individual with a spinal cord injury or lesion at T6 or above (has been demonstrated in patients with injuries at T7 and T8)

Risk Factors

An injury or lesion at T6 or above AND at least one of the following noxious stimuli:

Cardiac/Pulmonary Problems

Pulmonary emboli

Deep Vein thrombosis

Gastrointestinal Problems

Bowel distention

Constipation

Difficult passage of feces

Enemas

Esophageal reflux

Fecal impaction

Gallstones

Gastric ulcers

Gastrointestinal system pathology

Hemorrhoids

Stimulation (e.g., digital, instrumentation, surgery)
Suppositories

Neurological Problems

Painful or irritating stimuli below the level of injury

Reproductive Problems

Ejaculation
Labor and delivery
Menstruation
Ovarian cyst
Pregnancy
Sexual intercourse

Musculoskeletal-Integumentary Problems

Cutaneous stimulations (e.g., pressure ulcer, ingrown toenail, dressings, burns, rash)
Fractures
Heterotrophic bone
Pressure over bony prominences or genitalia
Range-of-motion exercises
Spasm
Sunburns
Wounds

Situational Problems

Constrictive clothing (e.g., straps, stockings, shoes)
Drug reactions (e.g., decongestants, sympathomimetics, vasoconstrictors, narcotic withdrawal)
Positioning
Surgical procedures

Regulatory Stimuli

Extreme environmental temperatures
Temperature fluctuations

Urological Problems

Bladder distention
Bladder spasm
Calculi
Catheterization
Cystitis
Detrusor sphincter dyssynergia
Epididymitis
Instrumentation or surgery
Urethritis
Urinary tract infection

Suggestions for Use

See Suggestions for Use for Autonomic Dysreflexia on pp. 157–158.

Suggested Alternative Diagnoses

Constipation [fecal impaction]
Skin integrity, impaired
Urinary retention

NOC Outcomes

Bowel Elimination: Ability of the gastrointestinal tract to form and evacuate stool effectively

Comfort Level: Feelings of physical and psychological ease

Infection Status: Presence and extent of infection

Neurological Status: Autonomic: Extent to which the autonomic nervous system coordinates visceral function

Symptom Severity: Extent of perceived adverse changes in physical, emotional, and social functioning

Thermoregulation: Balance among heat production, heat gain, and heat loss

Tissue Integrity: Skin and Mucous Membranes: Structural intactness and normal physiological function of skin and mucous membranes

Treatment Behavior: Illness or Injury: Personal actions to palliate or eliminate pathology

Urinary Elimination: Ability of the urinary system to filter waste, conserve solutes, and to collect and discharge urine in a healthy pattern

Vital Signs Status: Temperature, pulse, respiration, and BP within expected range for the individual

NIC Interventions

Dysreflexia Management: Prevention and elimination of stimuli that cause hyperactive reflexes and inappropriate autonomic responses in a patient with a cervical or high thoracic cord lesion

Neurologic Monitoring: Collection and analysis of patient data to prevent or minimize neurological complications

Vital Signs Monitoring: Collection and analysis of cardiovascular, respiratory, and body temperature data to determine and prevent complications

Nursing Activities

Assessments

See Assessments for Autonomic Dysreflexia, p. 159.

Patient/Family Teaching

See Patient/Family Teaching for Autonomic Dysreflexia, p. 159.

Other

- Quickly eliminate any noxious stimulus in the following order:
    Bladder: Check catheter for patency or catheterize patient
    Bowel: If distended, apply anesthetic ointment to rectal area and disimpact; consider enema or flatus tube
    Body temperature: Maintain normal body temperature

ENERGY FIELD, DISTURBED
(00050) (1994)

Definition: Disruption of the flow of energy surrounding a person's being that results in disharmony of the body, mind, and spirit

Defining Characteristics

Objective

Disruption of the field (vacant, hold, spike, bulge)

Movement (wave, spike, tingling, dense, flowing)

Sounds (tone, words)

Temperature change (warmth, coolness)

Visual changes (image, color)

Related Factors

To be developed

Suggestions for Use

This diagnosis suggests independent but nontraditional nursing interventions, which require specialized instruction and practice. Therefore, it should be used only by nurses who possess such expertise (Krieger 1979; Meehan, 1991).

Suggested Alternative Diagnoses

Anxiety

Pain: acute, chronic

NOC Outcomes

Spiritual Well-Being: Personal expressions of connectedness with self, others, higher power, all life, nature, and the universe that transcend and empower the self

Well-Being: An individual's expressed satisfaction with health status

Goals/Evaluation Criteria

Also refer to Goals/Evaluation Criteria for Anxiety and Acute Pain, on pp. 24–25 and 348–349, respectively.

Examples Using NOC Language

- Demonstrates **Spiritual Well-Being**, as evidenced by the following indicators (specify 1–5: extremely, substantially, moderately, mildly, or not compromised):

    Faith, hope, serenity, love, and forgiveness

    Meaning and purpose in life

Other Examples

Patient will:

- Verbalize relief of symptoms (e.g., pain, anxiety) after treatment
- Demonstrate physical evidence of relaxation (e.g., decrease in BP, pulse and respiration rates, and muscle tension)
- Indicate satisfaction with psychologic, social, spiritual, physiologic, and cognitive functioning
- Demonstrate adequate coping skills

NIC Interventions

Hope Instillation: Facilitation of the development of a positive outlook in a given situation

Self-Awareness Enhancement: Assisting a patient to explore and understand his thoughts, feelings, motivations, and behaviors

Spiritual Growth Facilitation: Facilitation of growth in patient's capacity to identify, connect with, and call upon the source of meaning, purpose, comfort, strength, and hope in his life

Therapeutic Touch: Attuning to the universal healing field, seeking to act as an instrument for healing influence, and using the natural sensitivity of the hands to gently focus and direct the intervention process

Nursing Activities

Prior to administering therapeutic touch

- *(NIC) Therapeutic Touch:*

    Center oneself physically and psychologically to purposefully relax tensions

Sit in a relaxed position with body in alignment and hands in lap

Close eyes and breathe evenly and slowly

Attain a sense of inner equilibrium in preparation for directing physical and psychodynamic energies

Assessment

- Position the patient comfortably before beginning assessment
- *NIC (Therapeutic Touch):*

  Place hands 2 or 3 inches from patient's skin

  Move hands slowly and steadily over patient

  Complete total body assessment, typically working from head to toe, front to back

  Note any sign of temperature change, tingling, pressure, electric shock, or pulsation in your hands

  Note objective signs of patient's experience [during and after treatment]: relaxation, slow respirations, peripheral flush, relief of pain, relief of nausea, and increased peristalsis

Treatment

- Provide privacy for the treatment
- Explain the process of therapeutic touch to the patient, obtain verbal permission, discuss findings with patient
- When working in the head area, or for those who may be sensitive to it (e.g., the mentally ill, the elderly, premature infants), use therapeutic touch gently and only for short periods of time
- Use actual, hands-on touch and massage, as needed
- Provide a rest period for the patient after the treatment
- *(NIC) Therapeutic Touch:*

  "Unruffle the field" around pressure areas by placing hands with palms away from the body and moving hands away in a sweeping gesture

  Direct energies to the patient's areas of imbalances

  Stop [therapeutic touch] when there are no longer bilateral differences in the patient's [energy] field

Patient/Family Teaching

- Teach therapeutic touch to family members
- Teach the patient deep-breathing exercises to aid in relaxation
- Teach the patient to use guided imagery in conjunction with the therapeutic-touch treatment

ENVIRONMENTAL INTERPRETATION SYNDROME, IMPAIRED (00127) (1994)

Definition: Consistent lack of orientation to person, place, time, or circumstances over more than 3 to 6 months, necessitating a protective environment

Defining Characteristics
Subjective
Consistent disorientation in known and unknown environments
Objective
Chronic confusional states
Loss of occupation or social functioning from memory decline
Inability to follow simple directions, instructions
Inability to reason
Inability to concentrate
Slow in responding to questions

Related Factors
Alcoholism
Dementia (e.g., Alzheimer disease, multi-infarct dementia, Pick disease, AIDS [-related] dementia)
Depression
Huntington disease
Parkinson disease

Suggestions for Use
Because this diagnosis and those in the Suggested Alternative Diagnoses overlap, careful analysis of the patient's defining characteristics is needed. This diagnosis is especially difficult to differentiate from *Chronic confusion*. The author prefers to use *Chronic confusion*.

Suggested Alternative Diagnoses
Confusion, acute
Confusion, chronic
Injury, risk for
Memory, impaired
Thought processes, disturbed
Tissue perfusion, ineffective (cerebral)

NOC Outcomes

Cognitive Ability: Ability to execute complex mental processes

Cognitive Orientation: Ability to identify person, place, and time

Concentration: Ability to focus on a specific stimulus

Information Processing: Ability to acquire, organize, and use information

Memory: Ability to cognitively retrieve and report previously stored information

Neurological Status: Consciousness: Extent to which an individual arouses, orients, and attends to the environment

Safety Behavior: Home Physical Environment: Individual or caregiver actions to minimize environmental factors that might cause physical harm or injury in the home

Goals/Evaluation Criteria

Examples Using NOC Language

- Maintains or improves Information Processing, Memory, Cognitive Ability, Cognitive Orientation, and Safety Behavior: Home Physical Environment
- Demonstrates **Neurological Status: Consciousness**, as evidenced by the following indicators (specify 1–5: extremely, substantially, moderately, mildly, or not compromised):

     Opens eyes to external stimuli

     Communication appropriate to situation

     Obeys commands

     Motor responses to noxious stimuli

     Attends to environmental stimuli

Other Examples

Patient will:
- Correctly identify common objects
- Speak coherently
- Identify significant other, place, and day
- Remain free from injury or harm
- Participate to maximum level of independence in ADLs
- Be content and less frustrated by environmental stressors

NIC Interventions

Anxiety Reduction: Minimizing apprehension, dread, foreboding, or uneasiness related to an unidentified source of anticipated danger

Cerebral Perfusion Promotion: Promotion of adequate perfusion and limitation of complications for a patient experiencing, or at risk for, inadequate cerebral perfusion

Cognitive Stimulation: Promotion of awareness and comprehension of surroundings by utilization of planned stimuli

Dementia Management: Provision of a modified environment for the patient who is experiencing a chronic confusional state

Environmental Management: Manipulation of the patient's surroundings for therapeutic benefit

Environmental Management: Safety: Monitoring and manipulation of the physical environment to promote safety

Learning Facilitation: Promoting the ability and willingness to receive information

Memory Training: Facilitation of memory

Neurologic Monitoring: Collection and analysis of patient data to prevent or minimize neurological complications

Reality Orientation: Promotion of patient's awareness of personal identity, time, and environment

Surveillance: Safety: Purposeful and ongoing collection and analysis of information about the patient and the environment for use in promoting and maintaining patient safety

Nursing Activities

Also refer to Nursing Activities for Confusion, Chronic, pp. 91–93. In early dementia, when the main symptoms are those of *Impaired memory*, refer to Nursing Activities for Impaired Memory, pp. 302–303.

Assessments

- Determine patient's self-care abilities
- *(NIC) Dementia Management:*

  Identify usual patterns of behavior for such activities as sleep, medication use, elimination, food intake, and self-care

  Monitor cognitive functioning, using a standardized assessment tool

  Identify safety needs of patient based on level of physical and cognitive function and past history of behavior

Patient/Family Teaching

- Teach family and significant others ways to remove safety hazards from the home

Collaborative Activities

- Refer to social services for referral to day care programs

Other

- Modify physical environment to ensure safety for patient
- Accompany ambulatory patient to activities away from the unit
- Encourage family to bring objects from home
- Promote consistency in caregiver assignment
- Orient patient to person, place, and time
- Limit visitors if patient becomes more agitated or disoriented
- Use a calm, unhurried approach
- *(NIC) Dementia Management:*

  Provide a low-stimulation environment (e.g., quiet, soothing music; nonvivid and simple, familiar patterns in décor; performance expectations that do not exceed cognitive-processing ability; and dining in small groups)

  Provide cues—such as current events, seasons, location, and names—to assist orientation

  Address the patient distinctly by name when initiating interaction and speak slowly

  Give one simple direction at a time

FAILURE TO THRIVE, ADULT
(00101) (1998)

Definition: Progressive functional deterioration of a physical and cognitive nature. The individual's ability to live with multisystem diseases, cope with ensuing problems, and manage his care are remarkably diminished.

Defining Characteristics

Subjective

Altered mood state—expresses feelings of sadness, being low in spirit

Expresses loss of interest in pleasurable outlets, such as food, sex, work, friends, family, hobbies, or entertainment

Verbalizes desire for death

Objective

Anorexia—does not eat meals when offered; states does not have an appetite, not hungry, or "I don't want to eat"

Apathy, as evidenced by lack of observable feeling or emotion in terms of normal ADLs and environment

Cognitive decline—decline in mental processing; as evidenced by problems with responding appropriately to environmental stimuli and demonstration of difficulty in reasoning, decision making, judgment, memory and concentration, decreased perception

Decreased participation in ADLs that the older person once enjoyed

Decreased social skills and social withdrawal—noticeable decrease from usual past behavior in attempts to form or participate in cooperative and interdependent relationships (e.g., decreased verbal communication with staff, family, friends)

Frequent exacerbations of chronic health problems, such as pneumonia or urinary tract infections

Inadequate nutritional intake—eating less than body requirements; consumes minimal to no food at most meals (i.e., consumes less than 75% of normal requirements at each or most meals)

Physical decline—decline in bodily function; evidence of fatigue, dehydration, incontinence of bowel and bladder

Self-care deficit—no longer looks after or takes charge of physical cleanliness or appearance; difficulty performing simple self-care tasks; neglects home environment or financial responsibilities

Weight loss (decreased body mass from baseline weight)—5% unintentional weight loss in one month, 10% unintentional weight loss in 6 months

Related Factors

Apathy

Depression

Fatigue

Suggestions for Use

(1) The list of Related Factors shown previously appears to be incomplete for this diagnosis. Considering the multisystem and multifunctional nature of the Defining Characteristics, there are a large number of factors that would cause them. (2) This diagnosis should be used only when several of the Defining Characteristics are present and when all are caused by the same related factors. Many of the Defining Characteristics are actually other nursing diagnoses (see the following Suggested Alternative Diagnoses), and when the patient has only a few of those problems, care planning may be better guided by those more narrowly focused diagnoses.

Suggested Alternative Diagnoses

Anxiety
Confusion, acute or chronic
Coping, ineffective
Fatigue
Fluid volume, deficient
Grieving, dysfunctional
Home maintenance, impaired
Hopelessness
Incontinence, bowel
Incontinence, urinary
Infection, risk for
Injury, risk for
Loneliness, risk for
Memory, impaired
Nutrition: less than body requirements, imbalanced
Powerlessness
Protection, ineffective
Role performance, ineffective
Self-care deficit (specify)
Self-esteem, chronic or situational low
Sexuality patterns, ineffective
Social interaction, impaired
Spiritual distress
Thought processes, disturbed

NOC Outcomes

Nutritional Status: Extent to which nutrients are available to meet metabolic needs

Physical Aging Status: Physical changes that commonly occur with adult aging

Psychosocial Adjustment: Life Change: Psychosocial adaptation of an individual to a life change

Self-Care: Activities of Daily Living (ADLs): Ability to perform the most basic physical tasks and personal care activities

Will to Live: Desire, determination, and effort to survive

Goals/Evaluation Criteria

NOTE: Some examples are given, but the specific goals for this diagnosis will depend upon which of the defining characteristics are present. For other goals, refer to Defining Characteristics for the preceding Suggested Alternative Diagnoses (e.g., the goals for *Anxiety* and *Confusion*).

Examples Using NOC Language

- *Failure to thrive* alleviated, as demonstrated by satisfactory Nutritional Status, Physical Aging Status, Psychosocial Adjustment: Life change, Self-care: (ADLs), and Will to Live.
- Demonstrates **Will to Live**, as evidenced by the following indicators (specify 1–5: extremely, substantially, moderately, mildly, or not compromised)

    Expression of determination to live

    Expression of optimism

    Seeks information about one's illness and treatment

    Use of strategies to compensate for problems associated with disease

    Use of strategies to lengthen life

Other Examples

The patient will:

- Regain energy needed to cope with problems resulting from multisystem diseases
- Eat diet adequate to provide for body requirements
- Regain lost weight
- Not experience further cognitive decline
- Participate in decision making
- Restore relationships with significant others
- Perform ADLs (e.g., bathing, toileting)

NIC Interventions

Coping Enhancement: Assisting a patient to adapt to perceived stressors, changes, or threats which interfere with meeting life demands and roles

Environmental Management: Manipulation of the patient's surroundings for therapeutic benefit

Home Maintenance Assistance: Helping the patient and family to maintain the home as a clean, safe, and pleasant place to live

Hope Instillation: Facilitation of the development of a positive outlook in a given situation

Mood Management: Providing for safety, stabilization, recovery, and maintenance of a patient who is experiencing dysfunctionally depressed mood or elevated mood

Nutrition Management: Assisting with or providing a balanced dietary intake of foods and fluids

Nutrition Therapy: Administration of food and fluids to support metabolic processes of a patient who is malnourished or at high risk for becoming malnourished

Risk Identification: Analysis of potential risk factors, determination of health risks, and prioritization of risk reduction strategies for an individual or group

Self-Care Assistance: Assisting another to perform ADLs

Spiritual Support: Assisting the patient to feel balance and connection with a greater power

Nursing Activities

Because this diagnosis is so broad, a comprehensive list of nursing activities is not practical. Refer to Nursing Activities for the appropriate Suggested Alternative Diagnoses. For example, if the patient is experiencing anorexia and weight loss, refer to *Imbalanced nutrition: less than body requirements* for nursing activities that improve the patient's nutrition. If the patient is incontinent, refer to *Bowel incontinence* or *Urinary incontinence* for the appropriate nursing activities.

FALLS, RISK FOR
(00155) (2000)

Definition: Increased susceptibility to falling that may cause physical harm

Risk Factors

Adults

Age 65 or over
Female (if elderly)
History of falls
Lives alone
Lower limb prosthesis
Use of assistive devices (e.g., walker, cane)
Wheelchair use

Physiological

Anemia
Arthritis
Decreased strength in lower extremities
Diarrhea
Faintness when turning or extending neck

Foot problems
Gait difficulties
Hearing deficits
Impaired balance
Impaired physical mobility
Neoplasms (i.e., causing fatigue or limited mobility)
Neuropathy
Orthostatic hypotension
Postoperative conditions
Postprandial blood sugar changes
Presence of acute illness
Proprioception problems (e.g., unilateral neglect)
Sleeplessness
Urgency or incontinence
Vascular disease
Visual deficits

Cognitive

Diminished mental status (e.g., confusion, delirium, dementia, impaired reality testing)

Medications

ACE inhibitors
Alcohol use
Antianxiety agents
Antihypertensives
Diuretics
Hypnotics
Narcotics
Tranquilizers
Tricyclic antidepressants

Environment

Cluttered environment
No antislip material in bath or shower
Restraints
Throw or scatter rugs
Unfamiliar, dimly lit room
Weather conditions (e.g., ice)
Wet floors

Children

< 2 years of age
Bed located near window

Lack of automobile restraints (i.e., infant carseats)
Lack of parental supervision
Male gender when < 1 year of age
No gate on stairs
No window guards
Unattended infant on bed, changing table, or sofa

Suggestions for Use

When risk factors specific to falls are present, use this diagnosis instead of the more general *Risk for injury* or *Risk for trauma*. If at risk for accidents in addition to falls, the more general diagnoses may be better.

Suggested Alternative Diagnoses

Injury, risk for
Trauma, risk for

NOC Outcomes

NOC has not yet linked outcomes to this diagnosis. However, the following may be useful:

Knowledge: Child Safety: Extent of understanding conveyed about safely caring for a child

Knowledge: Personal Safety: Extent of understanding conveyed about preventing unintentional injuries

Safety Behavior: Fall Prevention: Individual or caregiver actions to minimize risk factors that might precipitate falls

Safety Behavior: Home Physical Environment: Individual or caregiver actions to minimize environmental factors that might cause physical harm or injury in the home

Safety Behavior: Personal: Individual or caregiver efforts to control behaviors that might cause physical injury

Safety Status: Falls Occurrence: Number of falls in the past week

Safety Status: Physical Injury: Severity of injuries from accidents and trauma

Goals/Evaluation Criteria

Examples using NOC Language

- Will decrease or limit *Risk for falls*, as demonstrated by Knowledge: Child and Personal Safety; Safety Behavior: Fall Prevention, Home Physical Environment, and Personal; and Safety Status: Falls Occurrence and Physical Injury

- Demonstrates **Safety Status: Falls Occurrence**, as evidenced by the following indicators (specify 1–5: over 9, 7–9, 4–6, 1–3, and no falls within the past week)

    Number of falls while standing

    Number of falls while walking

    Number of falls while sitting

    Number of falls while transferring

    Number of falls from bed

    Number of falls climbing steps

    Number of falls descending steps

Other Examples

Patient and family will:

- Provide a safe environment (e.g., eliminate clutter and spills, place handrails, and use rubber shower mats and grab bars)
- Identify risks that increase susceptibility to falls
- Avoid physical injury from falls

NOC Interventions

NOC has not yet linked interventions to this diagnosis; however, the following may be useful:

Environmental Management: Safety: Monitoring and manipulation of the physical environment to promote safety

Fall Prevention: Instituting special precautions with patient at risk for injury from falling

Surveillance: Safety: Purposeful and ongoing collection and analysis of information about the patient and the environment for use in promoting and maintaining patient safety

Teaching: Infant Safety: Instruction on safety during the first year of life

Teaching: Toddler Safety: Instruction on safety during the second and third years of life

Nursing Activities

Assessments

- Identify factors that affect safety needs, for example, changes in mental status, degree of intoxication, fatigue, maturational age, medications, and motor or sensory deficit (e.g., with gait, balance)
- *(NIC) Fall Prevention:*

    Identify characteristics of environment that may increase potential for falls (e.g., slippery floors and open stairways)

    Monitor gait, balance, and fatigue level with ambulation

Patient/Family Teaching

- Instruct patient and family in techniques to prevent injury at home, specify techniques
- Provide educational materials related to strategies and measures to prevent falls
- Provide information on environmental hazards and characteristics (e.g., stairs, windows, gates)
- *(NIC) Fall Prevention:*
  Teach patient how to fall so as to minimize injury
  Educate family members about risk factors that contribute to falls and how they can decrease these risks
  Instruct patient to wear prescription glasses, as appropriate, when out of bed
  Instruct family on importance of handrails for stairs, bathrooms, and walkways

Collaborative Activities

- *(NIC) Fall Prevention:* Collaborate with other health care team members to minimize side effects of medications that contribute to falling (e.g., orthostatic hypotension and unsteady gait)

Other

For adults:
- Reorient patient to reality and immediate environment when necessary
- Assist patient with ambulation, as needed
- Provide assistive devices for walking (e.g., cane, walker)
- Use an alarm to alert caretaker when patient is getting out of bed or leaving room
- If necessary, use physical restraints to limit risk of falling
- Place bell or call light within reach of dependent patient at all times
- Instruct patient to call for assistance with movement, as appropriate
- Remove environmental hazards (e.g., provide adequate lighting)
- Make no unnecessary changes in physical environment (e.g., furniture placement)
- Ensure that patient wears proper shoes (e.g., nonskid soles, secure fasteners)

For children:
- Raise side rails when not present at bedside
- For children old enough to climb over bed rails, use a crib with a net or "bubble top"

- *(NIC) Fall Prevention:*

  Remove objects that provide young child with climbing access to elevated surfaces

  Provide close supervision or restraining device (e.g., infant seat with seat belt) when placing infants or young children on elevated surfaces (e.g., table and highchair)

FAMILY PROCESSES, DYSFUNCTIONAL: ALCOHOLISM (00063) (1994)

Definition: Psychosocial, spiritual, and physiologic functions of the family unit are chronically disorganized, leading to conflict, denial of problems, resistance to change, ineffective problem solving, and a series of self-perpetuating crises.

Defining Characteristics

Feelings

Abandonment	Hopelessness
Anger or suppressed rage	Hostility
Anxiety, tension, distress	Hurt
Being different from other people	Insecurity
	Lack of identity
Being unloved	Lingering resentment
Confused love and pity	Loss
Confusion	Mistrust
Decreased self-esteem and worthlessness	Misunderstood
	Moodiness
Depression	Powerlessness
Dissatisfaction	Rejection
Emotional control by others	Repressed emotions
Emotional isolation and loneliness	Responsibility for alcoholic's behavior
Failure	Shame and embarrassment
Fear	Unhappiness
Frustration	Vulnerability
Guilt	

Roles and Relationships

Altered role function and disruption of family roles

Chronic family problems

Closed communication systems

Deterioration in family relationships and disturbed family dynamics

Disrupted family rituals

Economic problems

Family denial

Family does not demonstrate respect for individuality and autonomy of its members

Family unable to meet security needs of its members

Inconsistent parenting and low perception of parental support

Ineffective spouse communication or marital problems

Intimacy dysfunction

Lack of cohesiveness

Lack of skills necessary for relationships

Neglected obligations

Pattern of rejection

Reduced ability of family members to relate to each other for mutual growth and maturation

Triangulating of family relationships

Behaviors

Agitation

Alcohol abuse

Blaming

Broken promises

Chaos

Contradictory, paradoxical communication

Controlling communication and power struggles

Criticizing

Denial of problems

Dependency

Difficulty having fun

Difficulty with intimate relationships

Diminished physical contact

Disturbances in academic performance in children

Disturbances in concentration

Enabling to maintain drinking

Escalating conflict

Expression of anger inappropriately

Failure to accomplish current or past developmental tasks and difficulty with life cycle transitions

Family special occasions are alcohol centered

Harsh self-judgment

Immaturity

Impaired communication

Inability to adapt to change

Inability to deal with traumatic experiences constructively

Inability to express or accept a wide range of feelings

Inability to meet emotional needs of its members

Inability to meet spiritual needs of its members

Inadequate understanding or knowledge of alcoholism

Ineffective problem-solving skills

Isolation

Lack of dealing with conflict

Lack of reliability

Loss of control of drinking

Lying

Manipulation

Nicotine addiction

Orientation toward tension relief rather than achievement of goals

Rationalization and denial of problems

Refusal to get help, inability to accept and receive help appropriately

Seeking approval and affirmation

Self-blaming

Stress-related physical illnesses

Substance abuse other than alcohol

Unresolved grief

Verbal abuse of spouse or parent

Related Factors

Abuse of alcohol

Addictive personality

Biochemical influences

Family history of alcoholism, resistance to treatment

Genetic predisposition

Inadequate coping skills

Lack of problem-solving skills

Suggestions for Use

(1) Note that, by definition, alcohol abuse by a family member must be the related factor. Alcohol abuse may be secondary to the other listed related factors. The diagnostic statement *Interrupted family processes: alcoholism related to alcohol abuse* would not be useful because the etiology is merely a repetition of the problem (alcoholism). (2) *Compromised/disabled family coping* may be more useful for describing the alcoholic family. (3) *Interrupted family processes* cannot be used because it describes a family that has a history of normal functioning.

Suggested Alternative Diagnoses

Coping: family, compromised

Coping: family, disabled

Violence: self-directed or other-directed, risk for

NOC Outcomes

Family Coping: Family actions to manage stressors that tax family resources

Family Environment: Internal: Social climate as characterized by family member relationships and goals

Family Functioning: Ability of the family to meet the needs of its members through developmental transitions

Family Health Status: Overall health status and social competence of family unit

Role Performance: Congruence of an individual's role behavior with role expectations

Substance Addiction Consequences: Compromise in health status and social functioning due to substance addiction

Goals/Evaluation Criteria

Examples Using NOC Language

- Family will resolve *Dysfunctional family coping: alcoholism*, as demonstrated by satisfactory Family Coping, Internal Family Environment, Family Functioning, Family Health Status, and Role Performance
- Alcoholic family member(s) demonstrate(s) **Substance Addiction Consequences**, as evidenced by the following indicators (specify 1–5: severe, substantial, moderate, slight, or none):
    Sustained decrease in physical activity
    Chronic impaired motor function
    Chronic fatigue
    Chronic impaired cognitive function
    Difficulty in maintaining employment
    Habitual arrests within the last year
    Absenteeism from work or school

Other Examples

Patient and family will:
- Acknowledge that alcoholism is a family illness
- Acknowledge the severity of the threat to the well-being of the family
- Identify destructive behaviors
- Begin to change dysfunctional (e.g., codependent) patterns

NIC Interventions

Coping Enhancement: Assisting a patient to adapt to perceived stressors, changes, or threats which interfere with meeting life demands and roles

Family Integrity Promotion: Promotion of family cohesion and unity

Family Process Maintenance: Minimization of family process disruption effects

Substance Use Treatment: Supportive care of patient and family members with physical and psychosocial problems associated with the use of alcohol or drugs

Nursing Activities

Assessments

- Determine history of drug and alcohol use
- Identify nature of spiritual support for family
- *(NIC) Substance Use Treatment:*
  Identify with patient those factors (e.g., genetic, psychological distress, and stress) which contribute to chemical dependency
  Screen patient at frequent intervals for continued substance use, using urine screens or breath analysis, as appropriate
  Determine whether codependent relationships exist in the family

Patient/Family Teaching

- Provide family members with information about alcoholism or help them to find other sources of information
- *(NIC) Substance Use Treatment:* Instruct patient and family about drugs used to treat specific substance used

Collaborative Activities

- *(NIC) Substance Use Treatment:* Identify support groups in the community for long-time substance abuse treatment

Other

- Recognize and accept that resolution of the alcoholism may not be the goal of care
- Emphasize to family members that they must allow the person to be responsible for his own drinking and behaviors
- Explore with the family the methods they use to control the alcoholic's behaviors (e.g., hiding the alcohol)
- Help family to identify realistic goals for changing family interaction patterns
- Assist family members to focus on changing their responses to the drinking instead of trying to control it
- Facilitate communication among family members
- Give positive feedback for adaptive coping mechanisms used by patient and family

- *(NIC) Substance Use Treatment:*
  Establish a therapeutic relationship with patient [and family]
  Assist patient and family to identify use of denial as a substitute
    for confronting the problem
  Facilitate support by significant others
  Encourage patient to take control over own behavior
  Help family members recognize that chemical dependency is a
    family disease
  Discuss with patient the effect of associations with other users
    during leisure or work time
  Discuss the effect of substance use on relationships with family,
    coworkers, and friends
  Encourage patient to keep a detailed chart of substance use to
    evaluate progress
  Assist patient to learn alternate methods of coping with stress
    or emotional distress

FAMILY PROCESSES, INTERRUPTED
(00060) (1982, 1998)

Definition: Change in family relationships or functioning. [The
NANDA International definition does not necessarily describe a
problem. A clearer definition might be: the state in which a family that normally functions effectively experiences dysfunction.]

Defining Characteristics
Subjective
Changes in satisfaction with family
Objective
Changes in [the following factors]:
  Assigned tasks
  Availability for affective responsiveness and intimacy
  Availability for emotional support
  Communication patterns
  Effectiveness in completing assigned tasks
  Expressions of conflict with or isolation from community
  resources
  Expressions of conflict within family
  Mutual support
  Participation in decision making
  Participation in problem solving

Patterns and rituals
Power alliances
Somatic complaints
Stress-reduction behaviors

Related Factors

Developmental transition or crisis
Family roles shift
Informal or formal interaction with community
Modification in family finances
Modification in family social status
Power shift of family members
Shift in health status of a family member
Situational transitions or crises

Suggestions for Use

This label describes a family that normally functions effectively but is experiencing a stressor that alters its functioning. The stressors causing *Interrupted family processes* tend to be situational or developmental transitions and crises, such as death of a family member, divorce, infidelity, loss of a job, serious illness, or hospitalization of a family member. When the interrupted family processes are specifically focused, a diagnosis such as *Dysfunctional grieving* or *Parental role conflict* may describe the problem more specifically.

This label is different from *Compromised family coping*, in which the family coping problem is caused by a change in the relationship between the family members. The stressor in *Compromised family coping* is withdrawal of support by a significant other, not necessarily an external stressor such as death or divorce (as in *Interrupted family processes*). *Compromised family coping* may involve the patient and only one significant other, whereas *Interrupted family processes* involves the entire family. Likewise, *Caregiver role strain* focus on the individual caregiver rather than the whole family. *Interrupted family processes* describes a family that has the resources for coping effectively with stressors, in contrast with *Disabled family coping*, which describes a family that demonstrates destructive behaviors. If stressors are not effectively resolved, *Interrupted family processes* can progress to *Disabled family coping*. To differentiate among the suggested alternative diagnoses, carefully examine the defining characteristics and related factors of each.

Suggested Alternative Diagnoses

Caregiver role strain (actual and at risk for)
Coping: family, compromised
Coping: family, disabled
Grieving, dysfunctional
Management of therapeutic regimen: families, ineffective
Parental role conflict
Parenting, impaired

NOC Outcomes

Family Coping: Family actions to manage stressors that tax family resources

Family Environment: Internal: Social climate as characterized by family member relationships and goals

Family Functioning: Ability of the family to meet the needs of its members through developmental transitions

Family Health Status: Overall health status and social competence of family unit

Parenting: Provision of an environment that promotes optimum growth and development of dependent children

Goals/Evaluation Criteria

Examples Using NOC Language

- Family does not exhibit *Interrupted family processes*, as demonstrated by satisfactory Family Coping, Internal Family Environment, Family Functioning, Family Health Status, and Parenting

Other Examples

Patient and family will:
- Acknowledge change in family roles
- Identify coping patterns
- Participate in decision-making processes regarding posthospital care
- Function to provide mutual support for each family member

NIC Interventions

Coping Enhancement: Assisting a patient to adapt to perceived stressors, changes, or threats which interfere with meeting life demands and roles

Family Integrity Promotion: Promotion of family cohesion and unity

Family Process Maintenance: Minimization of family process disruption effects

Family Support: Promotion of family values, interests, and goals

Normalization Promotion: Assisting parents and other family members of children with chronic illnesses or disabilities in providing normal life experiences for their children and families

Parent Education: Adolescent: Assisting parents to understand and help their adolescent children

Parent Education: Childrearing Family: Assisting parents to understand and promote the physical, psychological, and social growth and development of their toddler or preschool or school-aged child or children

Parenting Promotion: Providing parenting information, support and coordination of comprehensive services to high-risk families

Nursing Activities

Assessments

- Assess interaction between patient and family, being alert for potential destructive behaviors
- Assess child's limitations, so that accommodations can be made to allow child to participate in usual activities
- *(NIC) Family Integrity Promotion:*
  Determine guilt family may feel
  Determine typical family relationships
  Monitor current family relationships
  Determine disruption in typical family processes
  Identify conflicting priorities among family members

Patient/Family Teaching

- Teach the family those skills (e.g., time management, treatments) required for care of patient
- Teach family the need to work with the school system to ensure access to appropriate educational opportunities for the chronically ill or disabled child

Collaborative Activities

- Explore available hospital and community resources with family
- Initiate a multidisciplinary patient care conference, involving the patient and family in problem solving and facilitation of communication
- Provide continuity of care by maintaining effective communication between staff members through nurse report and care planning

- Refer family to a financial counselor
- Request social service consultation to help the family determine posthospitalization needs and identify sources of community support (e.g., for child care)
- *(NIC) Family Integrity Promotion:* Refer for family therapy, as indicated

Other

- Assist family in identifying behaviors that may be hindering prescribed treatment
- Assist family in identifying personal strengths
- Encourage family to verbalize feelings and concerns
- Encourage family to participate in patient's care and help plan posthospital care
- Provide flexible visiting hours to accommodate family visits
- Preserve family routines and rituals (e.g., providing for private meals together or family decision making)
- Provide positive reinforcement for effective use of coping mechanisms
- Help family to focus on the child rather than on the illness or disability
- Encourage opportunities for normal childhood experiences for the chronically ill or disabled child
- *(NIC) Family Integrity Promotion:*
  Provide for family privacy
  Facilitate open communications among family members
  Counsel family members on additional effective coping skills for their own use
  Assist family with conflict resolution

FAMILY PROCESSES, READINESS FOR ENHANCED (00159) (2002)

Definition: A pattern of family functioning that is sufficient to support the well-being of family members and can be strengthened

Defining Characteristics

Objective

Activities support the safety and growth of family members
Balance exists between autonomy and cohesiveness
Boundaries of family members are maintained
Communication is adequate

Energy level of family supports ADLs

Expresses willingness to enhance family dynamics

Family adapts to change

Family functioning meets physical, social, and psychological needs of family members

Family resilience is evident

Family roles are flexible and appropriate for developmental stages

Relationships are generally positive; interdependent with community; family tasks are accomplished

Respect for family members is evident

Related Factors

This is a wellness diagnosis, so an etiology is not necessary. If risk factors suggest the possibility of developing *Interrupted family processes*, use the diagnosis, *Risk for interrupted family processes*.

Suggestions for Use

This label describes a family that is functioning effectively but wishes to improve its functioning and ability to deal with situational or developmental transitions and crises.

Suggested Alternative Diagnoses

Coping: family, readiness for enhanced

Family processes, risk for interrupted

Parenting, readiness for enhanced

NOC Outcomes

NOC outcomes have not yet been developed for this diagnoses; however, the following may be useful:

Family Environment: Internal: Social climate as characterized by family member relationships and goals

Family Functioning: Ability of the family to meet the needs of its members through developmental transitions

Family Health Status: Overall health status and social competence of family unit

Goals/Evaluation Criteria

Examples Using NOC Language

- Family exhibits *Enhanced Family Processes*, as demonstrated by satisfactory Internal Family Environment, Family Functioning, and Family Health Status

Other Examples

Patient and family will:

- Acknowledge change in family roles
- Identify coping patterns
- Function to provide mutual support for each family member

NIC Interventions

NIC interventions have not yet been linked to this diagnosis; however, the following may be useful:

Family Integrity Promotion: Promotion of family cohesion and unity

Family Process Maintenance: Minimization of family process disruption effects

Family Support: Promotion of family values, interests, and goals

Nursing Activities

Assessments

- Assist family members to identify and anticipate situations that have the potential to disrupt family processes
- Identify family's spiritual supports
- Identify family role changes and their effects of family processes
- *(NIC) Family Integrity Promotion:*
  Determine typical family relationships
  Monitor current family relationships
  Identify conflicting priorities among family members

Patient/Family Teaching

- Teach the family those skills (e.g., time management, treatments) that can enhance family processes
- Provide information about existing social support mechanisms that can be used in stressful situations

Other

- Assist family in identifying personal strengths
- Encourage family to verbalize feelings and concerns
- Encourage family to participate in patient's care and help plan posthospital care
- Provide flexible visiting hours to accommodate family visits
- Preserve family routines and rituals (e.g., providing for private meals together or family decision making)
- Provide positive reinforcement for effective use of coping mechanisms
- *(NIC) Family Integrity Promotion:*
  Provide for family privacy

Facilitate open communications among family members

Counsel family members on additional effective coping skills for their own use

Assist family with conflict resolution [if needed]

FATIGUE
(00093) (1988, 1998)

Definition: An overwhelming, sustained sense of exhaustion and decreased capacity for physical and mental work at usual level

Defining Characteristics

Subjective

Compromised concentration

Compromised libido

Disinterest in surroundings, introspection

Drowsy

Feelings of guilt for not keeping up with responsibilities

Increased physical complaints

Perceived need for additional energy to accomplish routine tasks

Tired

Verbalization of unremitting and overwhelming lack of energy

Objective

Decreased performance

Inability to maintain usual routines

Inability to restore energy even after sleep

Increase in rest requirements

Lack of energy or inability to maintain usual level of physical activity

Lethargic or listless

Related Factors

Psychological

Anxiety

Boring lifestyle

Depression

Stress

Environmental

Humidity

Lights

Noise

Temperature

Situational
Negative life events
Occupation

Physiological
Anemia
Disease states
Increased physical exertion
Malnutrition
Poor physical condition
Pregnancy
Sleep deprivation

Other Possible Related Factors (non-NANDA International)
Altered body chemistry (e.g., caused by medications, drug with-
    drawal, chemotherapy)
Excessive social and role demands
Overwhelming psychologic or emotional demands

Suggestions for Use

Do not use this label to describe temporary tiredness resulting
from lack of sleep. *Fatigue* describes a chronic condition. The
patient's previous energy levels and capabilities cannot immediately
be restored, so the nursing focus is to help the patient find ways to
adapt. Discriminate carefully between *Fatigue* and *Activity intolerance*. The energy deficit in *Fatigue* is overwhelming and may exist
even when the patient has not performed any activities. *Fatigue* may
be the etiology of other nursing diagnoses, such as *Self-care deficit*
and *Impaired home maintenance*. Conversely, other labels, such as
Decreased cardiac output, may be the etiology of *Fatigue*.

Suggested Alternative Diagnoses

Activity intolerance
Cardiac output, decreased
Self-care deficit
Sleep pattern, disturbed

NOC Outcomes

Activity Tolerance: Responses to energy-consuming body move-
    ments involved in required or desired daily activities.
Endurance: Extent that energy enables a person's activity
Energy Conservation: Extent of active management of energy to
    initiate and sustain activity

Nutritional Status: Energy: Extent to which nutrients provide cellular energy

Psychomotor Energy: Ability to maintain ADLs, nutrition, personal safety.

Goals/Evaluation Criteria

Examples Using NOC Language

- The patient will adapt to *Fatigue*, as evidenced by Activity Tolerance, Energy Conservation, Endurance, Nutritional Status: Energy, and Psychomotor Energy.
- The patient will demonstrate **Energy Conservation**, as evidenced by the following indicators (specify 1–5: not at all; to a slight, moderate, great, or very great extent):

    Endurance level adequate for activity

    Maintains adequate nutrition

    Balances activity and rest

    Uses energy conservation techniques

    Adapts lifestyle to energy level

Other Examples

Patient will:

- Maintain usual social interaction
- Identify psychologic and physical factors that may cause *Fatigue*
- Maintain ability to concentrate
- Attend and respond appropriately to visual, auditory, verbal, tactile, and olfactory cues
- Report that energy is restored after rest

NIC Interventions

Activity Therapy: Prescription of and assistance with specific physical, cognitive, social, and spiritual activities to increase the range, frequency, or duration of an individual's (or group's) activity.

Energy Management: Regulating energy use to treat or prevent fatigue and optimize function

Environmental Management: Manipulation of the patient's surroundings for therapeutic benefit

Mood Management: Providing for safety, stabilization, recovery, and maintenance of a patient who is experiencing dysfunctionally depressed mood or elevated mood

Nutrition Management: Assisting with or providing a balanced dietary intake of foods and fluids

Nursing Activities

Assessments

- Determine the effects of *Fatigue* on quality of life
- *(NIC) Energy Management:*

  Monitor patient for evidence of excess physical and emotional fatigue

  Monitor cardiorespiratory response to activity (e.g., tachycardia, other dysrhythmias, dyspnea, diaphoresis, pallor, hemodynamic pressures, and respiratory rate)

  Monitor and record patient's sleep pattern and number of sleep hours

  Monitor location and nature of discomfort or pain during movement and activity

  Determine patient's and significant other's perception of causes of *Fatigue*

  Monitor nutritional intake to ensure adequate energy resources

  Monitor administration and effect of stimulants and depressants

Patient/Family Teaching

- Instruct patient in the relationship of Fatigue to disease process and condition
- *(NIC) Energy Management:*

  Instruct patient and significant other to recognize signs and symptoms of *Fatigue* that require reduction in activity

  Teach activity organization and time-management techniques to prevent *Fatigue*

Collaborative Activities

- Make other practitioners aware of the effects of *Fatigue*
- *(NIC) Energy Management:* Consult with dietitian about ways to increase intake of high-energy foods

Other

- Encourage patient and family to express feelings related to life changes caused by *Fatigue*
- Assist patient in identifying measures that increase concentration; consider initiating tasks after rest periods and prioritizing necessary tasks
- Discuss with patient and family ways to modify home environment to maintain usual activities and to minimize *Fatigue*
- Encourage limited social interaction at times of higher energy

- Encourage patient to:
    Report activities that increase *Fatigue*
    Report onset of pain that may produce *Fatigue* (severity, location, precipitating factors)
- Plan activities with patient and family that minimize *Fatigue*. Plan may include:
    Assist with ADLs, as needed, specify
    Reduce low-priority activities
- *(NIC) Energy Management:*
    Reduce physical discomforts that could interfere with cognitive function and self-monitoring or regulation of activity
    Assist the patient and significant other to establish realistic activity goals
    Provide calming diversional activities (e.g., reading, talking to others) to promote relaxation
    Promote bed rest and activity limitation (e.g., increase number of rest periods)
    Avoid care activities during scheduled rest periods
    Limit environmental stimuli (e.g., light and noise) to facilitate relaxation
    Limit number of and interruptions by visitors, as appropriate

FEAR
(00148) (1980, 1996, 2000)

Definition: Response to perceived threat that is consciously recognized as a danger

Defining Characteristics
Subjective
Report of:
Alarm
Apprehension
Being scared
Decreased self-assurance
Dread
Excitement
Increased tension
Jitteriness
Panic

Terror

Worry

Cognitive

Diminished productivity, learning ability, problem-solving ability

Identifies object of fear

Stimulus believed to be a threat

Behaviors

Avoidance or attack behaviors

Impulsiveness

Increased alertness

Narrowed focus on "it" (i.e., the focus of the fear)

Physiological

Anorexia

Diarrhea

Dry mouth

Fatigue

Increased perspiration

Increased pulse

Increased respiratory rate and shortness of breath

Increased systolic blood pressure

Muscle tightness

Nausea

Pallor

Pupil dilation

Vomiting

Related Factors

Innate releasers (neurotransmitters)

Language barrier

Learned response (e.g., conditioning, modeling from or identification with others)

Natural and innate origin (e.g., sudden noise, height, pain, loss of physical support)

Phobic stimulus

Sensory impairment

Separation from support system in potentially stressful situation (e.g., hospitalization, hospital procedures

Unfamiliarity with environmental experience(s)

Suggestions for Use

See Suggestions for Use for Anxiety, pp. 22–24.

Suggested Alternative Diagnoses

Anxiety

Post-trauma syndrome

Rape-trauma syndrome

NOC Outcomes

Anxiety Control: Personal actions to eliminate or reduce feelings of apprehension and tension from an unidentifiable source

Fear Control: Personal actions to eliminate or reduce disabling feelings of alarm aroused by an identifiable source

Goals/Evaluation Criteria

Examples Using NOC Language

- The patient will exhibit **Fear Control**, as evidenced by the following indicators (specify 1–5: never, rarely, sometimes, often, or consistently demonstrated):

    Seeks information to reduce fear

    Avoids source of fear when possible

    Uses relaxation techniques to reduce fear

    Reports decreased duration of episodes

    Reports increased length of time between episodes

    Maintains control over life

    Maintains role performance and social relationships

    Controls fear response

    Remains productive

NIC Interventions

Anxiety Reduction: Minimizing apprehension, dread, foreboding, or uneasiness related to an unidentified source of anticipated danger

Coping Enhancement: Assisting a patient to adapt to perceived stressors, changes, or threats which interfere with meeting life demands and roles

Security Enhancement: Intensifying a patient's sense of physical and psychologic safety

Nursing Activities

Also refer to Nursing Activities for Anxiety, pp. 25–26.

Assessments

- Assess patient's subjective and objective fear responses
- *(NIC) Coping Enhancement:* Appraise the patient's understanding of the disease process

Patient/Family Teaching

- Explain all tests and treatments to patient and family

Collaborative Activities

- Assess need for social service or psychiatric intervention
- Encourage a patient–physician discussion of the patient's fear
- Initiate a multidisciplinary patient care conference to develop a plan of care

Other

- Provide frequent, positive reinforcement when patient demonstrates behaviors that may reduce or eliminate fear
- Stay with patient during new situations
- Remove the source of the patient's fear whenever possible
- Convey acceptance of the patient's perception of fear to encourage open communication regarding the source of the fear
- Provide continuity of patient care through patient assignment and use of care plan
- Provide frequent verbal and nonverbal reassurances that may assist in reducing the patient's fear state, avoid clichés
- Offer pacifier to infant
- Hold or rock child
- Place a night-light in room
- Encourage parent(s) to spend the night at the hospital with a child
- *(NIC) Coping Enhancement:*

  Appraise and discuss alternative responses to situation

  Use a calm, reassuring approach

  Assist the patient in developing an objective appraisal of the event

  Encourage an attitude of realistic hope as a way of dealing with feelings of helplessness

  Discourage decision making when the patient is under severe stress

  Encourage gradual mastery of the situation

  Introduce the patient to persons (or groups) who have successfully undergone the same experience

  Encourage verbalization of feelings, perceptions, and fears

  Reduce stimuli in the environment that could be misinterpreted as threatening

FLUID BALANCE, READINESS FOR ENHANCED (00160) (2002)

Definition: A pattern of equilibrium between fluid volume and chemical composition of body fluids that is sufficient for meeting physical needs and can be strengthened

Defining Characteristics

Subjective

Expresses willingness to enhance fluid balance

No excessive thirst

Objective

Food and fluid intake adequate for daily needs

Good tissue turgor

Moist mucous membranes

No evidence of edema or dehydration

Stable weight

Straw-colored urine with specific gravity within normal limits

Urine output appropriate for intake

Related Factors

This is a wellness diagnosis, so an etiology is not necessary.

Suggestions for Use

If there are risk factors for fluid imbalance, use *Risk for deficient fluid volume* or *Risk for imbalanced fluid volume*.

Suggested Alternative Diagnoses

Fluid volume, risk for deficient

Fluid volume, risk for imbalanced

Nutrition, readiness for enhanced

Urinary elimination, readiness for enhanced

NOC Outcomes

This is a new diagnosis, so NOC outcome linkages have not been developed; however, the following may be useful:

Electrolyte and Acid–Base Balance: Balance of electrolytes and nonelectrolytes in the intra- and extracellular compartments of the body

Fluid Balance: Balance of water in the intra- and extracellular compartments of the body

Hydration: Amount of water in the intra- and extracellular compartments of the body

Nutritional Status: Food and Fluid Intake: Amount of food and fluid taken into the body over a 24-hr period

Goals/Evaluation Criteria

Also refer to Goals/Evaluation Criteria for Deficient Fluid Volume, pp. 202–203, and Excess Fluid Volume, pp. 208–209.

Examples Using NOC Language

- Demonstrates *Enhanced fluid balance*, as evidenced by Electrolyte and Acid–Base Balance, Fluid Balance, adequate Hydration, and adequate Nutritional Status: Food and Fluid Intake
- **Electrolyte and Acid–Base Balance** will be achieved, as evidenced by the following indicators (specify 1–5: extremely, substantially, moderately, mildly, or not compromised):

    Heart rate and rhythm in expected range

    Respiratory rate and rhythm in expected range

    Serum electrolytes (e.g., sodium, potassium, calcium, magnesium) within normal limits

    Serum and urine pH within normal limits

Other Examples

Patient will:
- Not have urine concentration within normal limits
- Have hemoglobin and hematocrit in normal range
- Not experience abnormal thirst
- Have balanced intake and output over 24 hr
- Exhibit good hydration (moist mucous membranes, ability to perspire)
- Have adequate fluid intake

NIC Interventions

NIC interventions have not yet been linked to this new diagnosis; however, the following may be useful:

Fluid Management: Promotion of fluid balance and prevention of complications resulting from abnormal or undesired fluid levels

Nutrition Management: Assisting with or providing a balanced dietary intake of foods and fluids

Teaching: Individual: Planning, implementation, and evaluation of a teaching program designed to address a patient's particular needs

Urinary Elimination Management: Maintenance of an optimum urinary elimination pattern

Nursing Activities

Also refer to Nursing Activities for Excess Fluid Volume, pp. 209–210.

- Ask to describe color, amount, and frequency of fluid loss
- Identify and anticipate factors that may create fluid imbalances (e.g., strenuous exercise, medications, fever, stress, medical orders)
- *(NIC) Fluid Management:*

  Monitor hydration status (e.g., moist mucous membranes, adequacy of pulses, and orthostatic blood pressure)

Patient/Family Teaching

- Teach to monitor hydration status
- Instruct regarding fluid requirements

Other

- Assist, as needed, to make a plan for ingesting adequate fluids
- *(NIC) Fluid Management:*

  Promote oral intake (e.g., provide oral fluids that are the patient's preference, place in easy reach, provide a straw, and provide fresh water), as appropriate

  Provide fluids, as appropriate

FLUID VOLUME, DEFICIENT
(00027) (1978, 1996)

Definition: Decreased intravascular, interstitial, or intracellular fluid; this refers to dehydration—water loss alone without change in sodium

Defining Characteristics

Subjective

Thirst

Objective

Change in mental state

Decreased skin and tongue turgor

Decreased urine output

Decreased venous filling

Dry skin and mucous membrane

Elevated hematocrit

Increased body temperature

Increased pulse rate, decreased blood pressure, decreased pulse
   volume and pressure
Increased urine concentration
Sudden weight loss (except in third-spacing)
Weakness

Related Factors

Active fluid volume loss
[Excessive continuous consumption of alcohol]
Failure of regulatory mechanisms [as in diabetes insipidus, hyper-
   aldosteronism]
[Inadequate fluid intake secondary to _____]

Suggestions for Use

Use this label for patients experiencing vascular, cellular, or intracellular dehydration. Use the label cautiously, because many fluid
balance problems require nurse–physician collaboration. Do not
use this label routinely, even as a potential problem, for patients
who have a medical order of NPO. Independent nursing treatments
for *Deficient fluid volume* are meant to prevent fluid loss (e.g.,
diaphoresis) and encourage oral fluid intake. For a diagnosis such
as *Risk for deficient fluid volume* related to NPO order, there are no
independent nursing actions to prevent or treat either side of the
diagnostic statement. The treatment of *Deficient fluid volume* related
to NPO status, for example, requires a medical order for IV therapy.

Do not use *Deficient fluid volume* to describe patients who are,
at risk for hemorrhage, or are hemorrhaging or in hypovolemic
shock. These situations usually represent collaborative problems.

   Incorrect: Risk for deficient fluid volume related to postpartum
   hemorrhage
   Correct: Potential complication of childbirth: Postpartum hemorrhage
   Correct: Risk for postpartum hemorrhage related to uterine atony
   The most appropriate use of the *Deficient fluid volume* label is as
a diagnosis (either actual or potential) for patients who are not
drinking sufficient amounts of oral fluids, especially in the presence
of increased fluid loss (e.g., *Diarrhea*, vomiting, burns). Actual
Deficient fluid volume may also be the etiology of other nursing diagnoses, such as *Impaired oral mucous membrane*.

Suggested Alternative Diagnoses

Deficient fluid volume, risk for
Fluid volume imbalance, risk for

Oral mucous membrane, impaired

Tissue perfusion, ineffective (renal)

NOC Outcomes

Electrolyte and Acid–Base Balance: Balance of electrolytes and nonelectrolytes in the intra- and extracellular compartments of the body

Fluid Balance: Balance of water in the intra- and extracellular compartments of the body

Hydration: Amount of water in the intra- and extracellular compartments of the body

Nutritional Status: Food and Fluid Intake: Amount of food and fluid taken into the body over a 24-hr period

Goals/Evaluation Criteria

NOTE: Although some NOC outcomes relate to electrolyte and acid–base balance, the focus of this nursing diagnosis is on fluid volume.

Examples Using NOC Language

- *Fluid volume deficit* will be eliminated, as evidenced by Fluid Balance, Electrolyte and Acid–Base Balance, adequate Hydration, and adequate Nutritional Status: Food and Fluid Intake
- **Electrolyte and Acid–Base Balance** will be achieved, as evidenced by the following indicators (specify 1–5: extremely, substantially, moderately, mildly, or not compromised):

  Heart rate and rhythm in expected range

  Respiratory rate and rhythm in expected range

  Mental alertness and cognitive orientation not compromised

  Serum electrolytes (e.g., sodium, potassium, calcium, magnesium) within normal limits

  Serum and urine pH within normal limits

Other Examples

Patient will:

- Have normally concentrated urine. Specify baseline specific gravity
- Have hemoglobin and hematocrit within normal range for patient
- Have central venous and pulmonary wedge pressures in expected range
- Not experience abnormal thirst
- Have balanced intake and output over 24 hr

- Exhibit good hydration (moist mucous membranes, ability to perspire)
- Have adequate oral or IV fluid intake

NIC Interventions

Electrolyte Management: Promotion of electrolyte balance and prevention of complications resulting from abnormal or undesired serum electrolyte levels

Fluid Management: Promotion of fluid balance and prevention of complications resulting from abnormal or undesired fluid levels

Fluid Monitoring: Collection and analysis of patient data to regulate fluid balance

Fluid/Electrolyte Management: Regulation and prevention of complications from altered fluid and electrolyte levels

Hypovolemia Management: Expansion of intravascular fluid volume in a patient who is volume depleted

Intravenous (IV) Therapy: Administration and monitoring of IV fluids and medications

Nutrition Management: Assisting with or providing a balanced dietary intake of foods and fluids

Nutritional Monitoring: Collection and analysis of patient data to prevent or minimize malnourishment

Shock Management, Volume: Promotion of adequate tissue perfusion for a patient with severely compromised intravascular volume

Nursing Activities

NOTE[1]: Some of these activities are specific for patients who are hemorrhaging. Refer to the preceding Suggestions for Use before including those activities in your plan of care.

NOTE[2]: Although some of the NIC interventions relate to electrolyte and acid–base balance, the focus of this nursing diagnosis is on fluid volume.

Assessments

- Monitor color, amount, and frequency of fluid loss
- Observe especially for loss of fluids high in electrolytes (e.g., diarrhea, wound drainage, nasogastric suction, diaphoresis, ileostomy drainage)
- Monitor for bleeding (e.g., check all secretions for frank or occult blood)

- Identify contributing factors that may aggravate dehydration (e.g., medications, fever, stress, medical orders)
- Review electrolytes, especially sodium, potassium, chloride, and creatinine
- Assess for vertigo or postural hypotension
- Assess orientation to person, place, and time
- *(NIC) Fluid Management:*

  Monitor hydration status (e.g., moist mucous membranes, adequacy of pulses, and orthostatic blood pressure)

  Monitor laboratory results relevant to fluid balance (e.g., hematocrit, BUN, albumin, total protein, serum osmolality, and urine specific gravity levels)

  Weigh daily and monitor trends

  Count or weigh diapers

  Maintain accurate intake and output record

Patient/Family Teaching

- Instruct patient to inform nurse of thirst.

Collaborative Activities

- Report and document output less than _____ ml
- Report and document output more than _____ ml
- Report electrolyte abnormalities
- *(NIC) Fluid Management:*

  Arrange availability of blood products for transfusion, if necessary

  Administer prescribed nasogastric replacement based on output, as appropriate

  Administer IV therapy, as prescribed

Other

- Provide frequent oral hygiene
- Specify amount of fluids to be ingested in 24 hr, quantifying desired intake during the day, evening, and night shifts
- Ensure that patient is well hydrated preoperatively
- Position in Trendelenburg or elevate patient's legs when hypotensive, unless contraindicated
- *(NIC) Fluid Management:*

  Promote oral intake (e.g., provide oral fluids that are the patient's preference, place in easy reach, provide a straw, and provide fresh water), as appropriate

  Insert urinary catheter, if appropriate

  Give fluids, as appropriate

FLUID VOLUME, DEFICIENT, RISK FOR
(00028) (1978)

Definition: At risk for experiencing vascular, cellular, or intracellular dehydration

Risk Factors

Objective

Deviations affecting access to or intake or absorption of fluids (e.g., physical immobility)

Excessive losses through normal routes (e.g., diarrhea)

Extremes of age

Extremes of weight

Factors influencing fluid needs (e.g., hypermetabolic state)

Knowledge deficiency related to fluid volume

Loss of fluid through abnormal routes (e.g., indwelling tubes)

Medications (e.g., diuretics)

Suggestions for Use

Do not use routinely for patients who are NPO. Refer to Suggestions for Use for Deficient Fluid Volume, p. 201.

Suggested Alternative Diagnoses

Deficient fluid volume

Fluid volume imbalance, risk for

NOC Outcomes

Electrolyte and Acid–Base Balance: Balance of electrolytes and nonelectrolytes in the intra- and extracellular compartments of the body

Fluid Balance: Balance of water in the intra- and extracellular compartments of the body

Hydration: Amount of water in the intra- and extracellular compartments of the body

Nutritional Status: Food and Fluid Intake: Amount of food and fluid taken into the body over a 24-hr period

Goals/Evaluation Criteria

Also refer to Goals/Evaluation Criteria for Deficient Fluid Volume, pp. 202–203.

Example Using NOC Language

- *Deficient fluid volume* will be prevented, as evidenced by Fluid Balance, Electrolyte and Acid–Base Balance, adequate Hydration, and adequate Nutritional Status: Food and Fluid Intake

NIC Interventions

Autotransfusion: Collecting and reinfusing blood that has been lost intraoperatively or postoperatively from clean wounds

Electrolyte Management: Promotion of electrolyte balance and prevention of complications resulting from abnormal or undesired serum electrolyte levels (e.g., serum calcium, potassium, magnesium, sodium, and phosphate)

Fluid Management: Promotion of fluid balance and prevention of complications resulting from abnormal or undesired fluid levels

Fluid Monitoring: Collection and analysis of patient data to regulate fluid balance

Fluid/Electrolyte Management: Regulation and prevention of complications from altered fluid or electrolyte levels

Hypovolemia Management: Expansion of intravascular fluid volume in a patient who is volume depleted

Intravenous (IV) Therapy: Administration and monitoring of IV fluids and medications

Shock Management: Volume: Promotion of adequate tissue perfusion for a patient with severely compromised intravascular volume

Nursing Activities

NOTE: Nursing Activities for *Risk for deficient fluid volume* are essentially the same as those for actual *Deficient fluid volume*, listed on pp. 203–204. Refer to Suggestions for Use for *Deficient Fluid Volume*, p. 201, before including those activities in your plan of care.

FLUID VOLUME, EXCESS
(00026) (1982, 1996)

Definition: Increased isotonic fluid retention

Defining Characteristics

Subjective
Anxiety
Dyspnea or shortness of breath
Restlessness

Objective

Abnormal breath sounds (rales or crackles)

Altered electrolytes

Anasarca

Azotemia

Blood pressure changes

Change in mental status

Change in respiratory pattern

Decreased hemoglobin and hematocrit

Edema

Increased central venous pressure

Intake exceeds output

Jugular vein distention

Oliguria

Orthopnea

Pleural effusion

Positive hepatojugular reflex

Pulmonary congestion

Restlessness

S_3 heart sound

Specific gravity changes

Weight gain over short period

Related Factors

Compromised regulatory mechanism

Excess fluid intake

Excess sodium intake

[Increased fluid intake secondary to hyperglycemia, medications, compulsive water drinking, and so forth]

[Insufficient protein secondary to decreased intake or increased losses]

[Renal dysfunction, heart failure, sodium retention, immobility, and so forth]

Suggestions for Use

Do not use this label for conditions that nurses cannot prevent or treat (e.g., do not use *Excess fluid volume* to describe renal failure or pulmonary edema as these are medical diagnoses). The main type of fluid volume excess that nurses can treat independently is peripheral, dependent edema, which can be symptomatically relieved by elevating the patient's affected limbs. Edema (a symptom of *Excess fluid volume*) is an important risk factor for

Impaired skin integrity, which can be addressed by patient teaching and protective measures. If the patient requires medical intervention to resolve the fluid excess, use a collaborative problem such as Potential Complication of renal failure: Generalized edema. *Excess fluid volume* can also be the cause of complications, such as Potential Complication of *Excess fluid volume*: Pulmonary edema.

> *Incorrect: Excess fluid volume* related to decreased cardiac output
> *Correct:* Potential Complication of decreased cardiac output: *Excess fluid volume*
> *Correct:* Potential Complication of heart failure: Pulmonary edema
> *Correct: Risk for impaired skin integrity* related to *Excess fluid volume,* as manifested by generalized edema

Suggested Alternative Diagnoses

Cardiac output, decreased
Fluid volume, imbalanced, risk for
Skin integrity, risk for impaired
Tissue perfusion, ineffective

NOC Outcomes

Electrolyte and Acid–Base Balance: Balance of electrolytes and nonelectrolytes in the intra- and extracellular compartments of the body
Fluid Balance: Balance of water in the intra- and extracellular compartments of the body
Hydration: Amount of water in the intra- and extracellular compartments of the body

Goals/Evaluation Criteria

Examples Using NOC Language

- *Excess fluid volume* will be eliminated, as evidenced by Fluid Balance, Electrolyte and Acid–Base Balance, and indicators of adequate Hydration
- **Fluid Balance** will not be compromised (in excess) as evidenced by the following indicators (specify 1–5: extremely, substantially, moderately, mildly, or not compromised):
    24-hr intake and output balanced
    Adventitious breath sounds not present
    Body weight stable
    Ascites, neck vein distention, and peripheral edema not present
    Urine specific gravity within normal limits

Other Examples

Patient will:

- Verbalize understanding of fluid and dietary restrictions
- Verbalize understanding of prescribed medications
- Maintain vital signs within normal limits for patient
- Not experience shortness of breath
- Have hematocrit within normal limits

NIC Interventions

Fluid Management: Promotion of fluid balance and prevention of complications resulting from abnormal or undesired fluid levels

Fluid Monitoring: Collection and analysis of patient data to regulate fluid balance

Hypervolemia Management: Reduction in extra- or intracellular fluid volume and prevention of complications in a patient who is fluid overloaded

Nursing Activities

Assessments

- Specify location and degree of peripheral, sacral, and periorbital edema on scale from 1+ to 4+
- Assess for pulmonary or cardiovascular complications as indicated by increased respiratory distress, increased pulse rate, increased blood pressure, abnormal heart sounds, or abnormal lung sounds
- Assess edematous extremity or body part for impaired circulation and skin integrity
- Assess effects of medications (e.g., steroids, diuretics, lithium) on edema
- Regularly monitor abdominal or limb girth
- *(NIC) Fluid Management:*

  Weigh daily and monitor trends

  Maintain accurate intake and output record

  Monitor laboratory results relevant to fluid retention (e.g., electrolyte changes, increased specific gravity, increased BUN, decreased hematocrit, and increased urine osmolality levels)

  Monitor for indications of fluid overload or retention (e.g., crackles, elevated CVP or pulmonary capillary wedge pressure, edema, neck vein distention, and ascites), as appropriate

Patient/Family Teaching

- Instruct patient regarding causes and resolutions of edema; dietary restrictions; and use, dosage, and side effects of prescribed medications
- *(NIC) Fluid Management:* Instruct patient on NPO status, as appropriate

Collaborative Activities

- Administer dialysis, if indicated
- *(NIC) Fluid Management:*
  Consult physician if signs and symptoms of fluid volume excess persist or worsen
  Administer diuretics, as appropriate

Other

- Change position q _____
- Elevate extremities to increase venous return
- Maintain and allocate patient's fluid restrictions
- *(NIC) Fluid Management:* Distribute the fluid intake over 24 hr, as appropriate

---

FLUID VOLUME, IMBALANCED, RISK FOR (00025) (1998)

Definition: A risk of a decrease, increase, or rapid shift from one to the other of intravascular, interstitial, or intracellular fluid; this refers to the loss or excess or both of body fluids

Risk Factors

Scheduled for major invasive procedures
(Other risk factors and defining characteristics to be developed)

Suggestions for Use

This diagnosis was submitted by the Association of Operating Room Nurses and may have specific applications for that setting. It appears that it should be used when a patient is at risk for both *Deficient fluid volume* and *Excess fluid volume.*

Suggested Alternative Diagnoses

Fluid volume, deficient, risk for
Fluid volume, excess, risk for

NOC Outcomes

Electrolyte and Acid–Base Balance: Balance of electrolytes and nonelectrolytes in the intra- and extracellular compartments of the body

Fluid Balance: Balance of water in the intra- and extracellular compartments of the body

Hydration: Amount of water in the intra- and extracellular compartments of the body

Goals/Evaluation Criteria

Refer to Goals/Evaluation Criteria for Deficient Fluid Volume, pp. 202–203, and Excess Fluid Volume, pp. 208–209.

NIC Interventions

Autotransfusion: Collecting and reinfusing blood that has been lost intra- or postoperatively from clean wounds

Electrolyte Monitoring: Collection and analysis of patient date to regulate electrolyte balance

Fluid Management: Promotion of fluid balance and prevention of complications resulting from abnormal or undesired fluid levels

Fluid Monitoring: Collection and analysis of patient data to regulate fluid balance

Hypervolemia Management: Reduction in extra- or intracellular fluid volume and prevention of complications in a patient who is fluid overloaded

Intravenous (IV) Therapy: Administration and monitoring of IV fluids and medications

Nursing Activities

Refer to Nursing Activities for Deficient Fluid Volume, pp. 203–204, and Excess Fluid Volume, pp. 209–210.

GAS EXCHANGE, IMPAIRED
(00030) (1980, 1996, 1998)

Definition: Excess or deficit in oxygenation or carbon dioxide elimination at the alveolar–capillary membrane

Defining Characteristics

Subjective

Dyspnea

Headache upon awakening
Visual disturbance

Objective
Abnormal arterial blood gases
Abnormal arterial pH
Abnormal rate, rhythm, depth of breathing
Abnormal skin color (e.g., pale, dusky)
Confusion
Cyanosis (in neonates only)
Decreased carbon dioxide
Diaphoresis
Hypercapnia
Hypercarbia
Hypoxia
Hypoxemia
Irritability
Nasal flaring
Restlessness
Somnolence
Tachycardia

Related Factors

Alveolar–capillary membrane changes
Ventilation-perfusion imbalance

Suggestions for Use

Use this label cautiously. Decreased passage of gases between the alveoli of the lungs and the vascular system can be discovered only by means of a medically prescribed diagnostic test—blood gas analysis. A patient might easily have most of the defining characteristics without actually having impaired alveolar gas exchange. It is better to use a diagnostic statement that describes oxygen-related problems that can be diagnosed and treated independently by nurses (e.g., *Activity intolerance*). If the patient is at risk for *Impaired gas exchange*, write the appropriate collaborative problem (e.g., Potential Complication of thrombophlebitis: Pulmonary embolus). See Suggestions for Use for Ineffective Airway Clearance, on pp. 16–17, Ineffective Breathing Pattern, on p. 61, and Dysfunctional Ventilatory Weaning Response, on p. 613.

Impaired gas exchange may be associated with a number of medical diagnoses. For example, decreased functional lung tissue may be secondary to chronic lung disease, pneumonia, thoracotomy, atelectasis, respiratory distress syndrome, mass, and diaphragmatic hernia. In addition, decreased pulmonary blood supply may occur secondary to pulmonary hypertension, pulmonary embolus, congestive heart failure, respiratory distress syndrome, and anemia.

Suggested Alternative Diagnoses

Activity intolerance
Airway clearance, ineffective
Breathing pattern, ineffective
Dysfunctional ventilatory weaning response (DVWR)
Spontaneous ventilation, impaired

NOC Outcomes

Electrolyte and Acid–Base Balance: Balance of the electrolytes and nonelectrolytes in the intra- and extracellular compartments of the body

Respiratory Status: Gas Exchange: Alveolar exchange of CO_2 or O_2 to maintain arterial blood gas concentrations

Respiratory Status: Ventilation: Movement of air in and out of the lungs

Tissue Perfusion: Pulmonary: Extent to which blood flows through intact pulmonary vasculature with appropriate pressure and volume, perfusing alveoli–capillary unit

Vital Signs Status: Temperature, pulse, respiration, and blood pressure within expected range for the individual

Goals/Evaluation Criteria

Examples Using NOC Language

- *Impaired gas exchange* will be alleviated, as evidenced by uncompromised Respiratory Status: Gas Exchange and Respiratory Status: Ventilation
- **Respiratory Status: Gas Exchange** will not be compromised as evidenced by the following indicators (specify 1–5: extremely, substantially, moderately, mildly, or not compromised):
  Neurologic status in expected range
  Dyspnea at rest and on exertion not present
  Restlessness, cyanosis, and fatigue not present
  PaO_2, $PaCO_2$, arterial pH, and O_2 saturation within normal limits
  End-tidal CO_2 in expected range

- **Respiratory Status: Ventilation** will not be compromised as evidenced by the following indicators (specify 1–5: extremely, substantially, moderately, mildly, or not compromised):

    Respiratory rate in expected range

    Respiratory rhythm in expected range

    Depth of inspiration

    Expulsion of air

    Dyspnea at rest not present

    Auscultated breath sounds in expected range

Other Examples

Patient will:

- Have pulmonary function within normal limits
- Describe plan for care at home
- Not use pursed-lip breathing
- Not experience shortness of breath or orthopnea

NIC Interventions

Acid–Base Management: Promotion of acid–base balance and prevention of complications resulting from acid–base imbalance

Acid–Base Management: Respiratory Acidosis: Promotion of acid–base balance and prevention of complications resulting from serum pCO_2 levels higher than desired

Acid–Base Management: Respiratory Alkalosis: Promotion of acid–base balance and prevention of complications resulting from serum pCO_2 levels lower than desired

Airway Management: Facilitation of patency of air passages

Electrolyte Management: Promotion of electrolyte balance and prevention of complications resulting from abnormal or undesired serum electrolyte levels

Embolus Care: Pulmonary: Limitation of complications for a patient experiencing, or at risk for, occlusion of pulmonary circulation

Hemodynamic Regulation: Optimization of heart rate, preload, afterload, and contractility

Laboratory Data Interpretation: Critical analysis of patient laboratory data in order to assist with clinical decision making

Oxygen Therapy: Administration of oxygen and monitoring of its effectiveness

Respiratory Monitoring: Collection and analysis of patient data to ensure airway patency and adequate gas exchange

Ventilation Assistance: Promotion of an optimal spontaneous breathing pattern that maximizes oxygen and carbon dioxide exchange in the lungs

Vital Signs Monitoring: Collection and analysis of cardiovascular, respiratory, and body temperature data to determine and prevent complications

Nursing Activities

Assessments

- Assess lung sounds; respiratory rate, depth, and effort; and production of sputum as indicators of effective use of supportive equipment
- Monitor O_2 saturation with pulse oximeter
- Monitor blood gas results (e.g., low PaO_2 and elevated $PaCO_2$ levels suggest respiratory deterioration)
- Monitor electrolyte levels
- Monitor mental status (e.g., level of consciousness, restlessness, and confusion)
- Increase frequency of monitoring when patient appears somnolent
- Observe for cyanosis, especially of oral mucous membranes
- *(NIC) Airway Management:*
  Identify patient requiring actual or potential airway insertion
  Auscultate breath sounds, noting areas of decreased or absent ventilation and presence of adventitious sounds
  Monitor respiratory and oxygenation status, as appropriate
- *(NIC) Hemodynamic Regulation:*
  Auscultate heart sounds
  Monitor and document heart rate, rhythm, and pulses
  Monitor for peripheral edema, jugular vein distension, and S_3 and S_4 heart sounds
  Monitor pacemaker functioning, if appropriate

Patient/Family Teaching

- Explain proper use of supportive equipment (oxygen, suction, spirometer, IPPB)
- Instruct patient in breathing and relaxation techniques
- Explain to patient and family the reasons for low-flow oxygen and other treatments
- Inform patient and family that smoking is prohibited
- Instruct patient and family in plan for care at home, for example, medications, activity, supportive equipment, reportable signs and symptoms, and community resources

- *(NIC) Airway Management:*
  Instruct how to cough effectively
  Teach patient how to use prescribed inhalers, as appropriate

Collaborative Activities

- Consult with physician regarding future need for arterial blood gas (ABG) test and use of supportive equipment as indicated by a change in the patient's condition
- Report changes in correlated assessment data (e.g., patient sensorium, breath sounds, respiratory pattern, ABGs, sputum, effect of medications)
- Administer prescribed medications (e.g., sodium bicarbonate) to maintain acid–base balance
- Prepare patient for mechanical ventilation, if necessary
- *(NIC) Airway Management:*
  Administer humidified air or oxygen, as appropriate
  Administer bronchodilators, as appropriate
  Administer aerosol treatments, as appropriate
  Administer ultrasonic nebulizer treatments, as appropriate
  Administer humidified air or oxygen
- *(NIC) Hemodynamic Regulation:* Administer antiarrhythmic medications, as appropriate

Other

- Inform patient before beginning intended procedures, to lower anxiety and increase sense of control
- Reassure patient during periods of respiratory distress or anxiety
- Provide frequent oral hygiene
- Institute measures to reduce oxygen consumption (e.g., control fever and pain, reduce anxiety)
- Institute plan of care for a patient on a ventilator, which may include:
  - Ensuring adequate oxygen delivery by reporting abnormal ABGs, having Ambu bag attached to oxygen source at bedside, and hyperoxygenating prior to suctioning
  - Ensuring effective breathing pattern by assessing for synchronization and possible need for sedation
  - Maintaining patent airway by suctioning patient and keeping an endotracheal tube or replacement at bedside
  - Monitoring for complications (e.g., pneumothorax, unilateral aeration)
  - Verifying correct placement of endotracheal tube

- *(NIC) Airway Management:*
  Position to maximize ventilation potential
  Position to alleviate dyspnea
  Insert oral or nasopharyngeal airway, as appropriate
  Remove secretions by encouraging coughing or suctioning
  Encourage slow, deep breathing; turning; and coughing
  Assist with incentive spirometer, as appropriate
  Perform chest physical therapy, as appropriate
- *(NIC) Hemodynamic Regulation:*
  Elevate the head of the bed, as appropriate
  Place in Trendelenburg position, if appropriate

GRIEVING, ANTICIPATORY
(00136) (1980, 1996)

Definition: Intellectual and emotional responses and behaviors by which individuals, families, and communities work through the process of modifying self-concept based on the perception of potential loss

Defining Characteristics

Subjective
Anger
Denial of potential loss
Denial of the significance of the loss
Expression of distress at potential loss
Guilt

Objective
Alteration in eating habits, sleep patterns, dream patterns
Altered activity level
Altered communication patterns
Altered libido
Bargaining
Difficulty taking on new or different roles
Potential loss of significant object (e.g., people, possessions, job, status, home, ideals, parts and processes of the body)
Resolution of grief prior to the reality of loss
Sorrow

Related Factors

To be developed

Other Related Factors (non-NANDA International)
Impending death of self
Potential loss of body parts or functions
Potential loss of significant person, animal, or possession
Potential loss of social role

Suggestions for Use

Anticipatory grieving may be a normal, not necessarily maladaptive, response. If it requires no intervention, do not include it in the patient care plan. *Anticipatory grieving* occurs before the loss. It shares some defining characteristics with *Dysfunctional grieving*; however, the following symptoms of *Dysfunctional grieving* would rule out a diagnosis of *Anticipatory grieving:*

Exaggerated and prolonged feelings of guilt
Interference with life functioning
Prolonged anger or hostility
Suicidal thoughts

Suggested Alternative Diagnoses

Coping, ineffective
Grieving, dysfunctional
Sorrow, chronic

NOC Outcomes

Coping: Actions to manage stressors that tax an individual's resources

Family Coping: Family actions to manage stressors that tax family resources

Family Environment: Internal: Social climate as characterized by family member relationships and goals

Grief Resolution: Adjustment to actual or impending loss

Psychosocial Adjustment: Life Change: Psychosocial adaptation of an individual to a life change

Goals/Evaluation Criteria

Examples Using NOC Language

- Patient successfully resolves *Anticipatory grieving*, as demonstrated by successful Coping, Grief Resolution, and Psychosocial Adjustment: Life Change

- Patient demonstrates **Coping**, as evidenced by the following indicators (specify 1–5: never, rarely, sometimes, often, or consistently demonstrated):

    Identifies and uses effective coping patterns

    Seeks information concerning illness and treatment

    Uses available social supports

    Seeks professional help, as appropriate

    Reports decrease in physical symptoms of stress and in negative feelings

- Patient demonstrates **Grief Resolution**, as evidenced by the following indicators (specify 1–5: not at all, to a slight extent, to a moderate extent, to a great extent, or to a very great extent):

    Expresses feelings about loss

    Verbalizes reality of loss

    Participates in planning funeral

    Shares loss with significant others

    Progresses through stages of grief

    Maintains grooming and hygiene

    Reports decreased preoccupation with loss

    Reports adequate nutritional intake

    Reports normal sexual desire

Other Examples

Patient and family will:

- Demonstrate ability to make mutual decisions regarding anticipated loss
- Express thoughts, feelings, and spiritual beliefs about loss
- Verbalize fears and concerns about potential loss
- Participate in grief work
- Not experience somatic distress
- Express feelings of productivity, usefulness, empowerment, and optimism

NIC Interventions

Anticipatory Guidance: Preparation of patient for an anticipated developmental or situational crisis

Coping Enhancement: Assisting a patient to adapt to perceived stressors, changes, or threats which interfere with meeting life demands and roles

Family Integrity Promotion: Promotion of family cohesion and unity

Family Support: Promotion of family values, interests, and goals

Grief Work Facilitation: Assistance with the resolution of a significant loss

Grief Work Facilitation: Perinatal Death: Assistance with the resolution of a perinatal loss

Nursing Activities

Assessments

- Assess past experience of patient and family with loss, existing support systems, and current grief work
- Determine cause and length of time since diagnosis of fetal or infant death
- *(NIC) Grief Work Facilitation:* Identify the loss

Patient/Family Teaching

- Teach characteristics of normal and abnormal grieving
- Discuss differences in individual patterns of grieving (e.g., male vs. female)
- Help child to clarify misconceptions about death, dying, or loss
- *(NIC) Grief Work Facilitation:* Instruct in phases of the grieving process, as appropriate
- *(NIC) Anticipatory Guidance:*

  Provide information on realistic expectations related to the patient's behavior

  Suggest books and literature for the patient to read, as appropriate

Collaborative Activities

- Refer to appropriate resources, such as support groups, legal assistance, financial assistance, social services, chaplain, grief counselor, genetic counselor
- *(NIC) Grief Work Facilitation:* Identify sources of community support

Other

- Assist patient and family to verbalize fears and concerns of potential loss, including impact on the family unit
- Help patient and family to share mutual fears, plans, concerns, and hopes with each other
- For perinatal loss, encourage parents to hold infant while and after the baby dies, as appropriate
- *(NIC) Grief Work Facilitation:*

  Assist the patient to identify the nature of the attachment to the lost object or person

  Encourage expression of feelings about the loss

  Encourage identification of greatest fears concerning the loss

Include significant others in discussions and decisions, as appropriate

Use clear words, such as "dead" or "died," rather than euphemisms

Encourage patient to implement cultural, religious, and social customs associated with the loss

Encourage expression of feelings in ways comfortable to the child, such as writing, drawing, or playing

- *(NIC) Anticipatory Guidance:*

Provide the patient with a phone number to call for assistance, if necessary

Schedule follow-up phone calls to evaluate success or reinforcement needs

Rehearse techniques needed to cope with upcoming developmental milestone or situational crisis with the patient, as appropriate

GRIEVING, DYSFUNCTIONAL
(00135) (1980, 1996)

Definition: Extended, unsuccessful use of intellectual and emotional responses by which individuals, families, [and] communities attempt to work through the process of modifying self-concept based upon the perception of loss

Defining Characteristics
Subjective
Alteration in dream patterns
Alteration in libido
Anger
Denial of loss
Expression of guilt
Expression of unresolved issues
Sadness
Objective
Alteration in activity level
Alteration in concentration or pursuit of tasks
Alteration in eating habits
Alteration in sleep patterns
Crying
Developmental regression

Difficulty in expressing loss

Idealization of lost object (e.g., people, possessions, job, status, home, ideals, parts and processes of the body)

Interference with life functioning

Labile affect

Onset or exacerbation of somatic or psychosomatic responses

Prolonged interference with life functioning

Reliving past experiences with little or no reduction (diminishment) of intensity of the grief

Repetitive use of ineffectual behaviors associated with attempts to reinvest in relationships

Verbal expressions of distress at loss

Related Factors

Actual or perceived object loss (object loss is used in the broadest sense). Objects may include people, possessions, a job, status, home, ideals, and parts and processes of the body.

[Chronic illness]

[Terminal illness]

Suggestions for Use

Most of the defining characteristics may also be present in the normal or anticipatory grief process. Grieving is dysfunctional only if it is prolonged (perhaps for more than a year after the loss) or if the symptoms are unusually numerous or severe. *Chronic sorrow* describes the patient's feelings, whereas grieving describes behaviors used in trying to cope with the loss. See Suggestions for Use for Grieving, Anticipatory on p. 218.

Suggested Alternative Diagnoses

Adjustment, impaired

Coping, ineffective

Grieving, anticipatory

Sorrow, chronic

Thought processes, disturbed

NOC Outcomes

Concentration: Ability to focus on a specific stimulus

Coping: Actions to manage stressors that tax an individual's resources

Family Coping: Family actions to manage stressors that tax family resources

Grief Resolution: Adjustment to actual or impending loss

Psychosocial Adjustment: Life Change: Psychosocial adaptation of an individual to a life change

Role Performance: Congruence of an individual's role behavior with role expectations

Goals/Evaluation Criteria

Examples Using NOC Language

- Patient will satisfactorily resolve *Dysfunctional grieving*, as demonstrated by successful Coping, Grief Resolution, and Psychosocial Adjustment: Life Change
- See Goals/Evaluation Criteria for Grieving, Anticipatory on p. 218–219, for indicators for **Coping,** and for Other Examples
- Demonstrates **Role Performance,** as evidenced by the following indicators (specify 1–5: not, slightly, moderately, substantially, or totally adequate):

    Ability to meet role expectations

    Performance of family role behaviors

    Performance of community role behaviors

    Reported comfort with role expectation

Other Examples

Patient will:
- Report adequate intake of food and fluids
- Report adequate social support
- Verbalize grief
- Verbalize meaning of loss

NIC Interventions

Coping Enhancement: Assisting a patient to adapt to perceived stressors, changes, or threats which interfere with meeting life demands and roles

Counseling: Use of an interactive helping process focusing on the needs, problems, or feelings of the patient and significant others to enhance or support coping, problem solving, and interpersonal relationships

Family Integrity Promotion: Promotion of family cohesion and unity

Family Therapy: Assisting family members to move their family toward a more productive way of living

Grief Work Facilitation: Assistance with the resolution of a significant loss

Grief Work Facilitation: Perinatal Death: Assistance with the resolution of a perinatal loss

Nursing Activities

See Nursing Activities for Grieving, Anticipatory on pp. 220–221.

Assessments

- Assess and document the presence and source of patient's grief
- *(NIC) Family Integrity Promotion:*
  Determine typical family relationships
  Monitor current family relationships
  Identify typical family coping mechanisms
  Identify conflicting priorities among family members

Patient/Family Teaching

- Provide patient and family with information about hospital and community resources, such as self-help groups

Collaborative Activities

- Initiate a patient care conference to review patient and family needs related to their stage of the grieving process and to establish a plan of care
- Seek support among peers and others to provide patient care as needed
- *(NIC) Grief Work Facilitation: Perinatal Death:* Notify laboratory or funeral home, as appropriate, for disposition of body

Other

- Acknowledge patient's and family's grief reactions while continuing necessary care activities
- Discuss with patient and family the impact of the loss on the family unit and its functioning
- Avoid confrontation of denial and, at the same time, do not reinforce denial
- Balance any misperceptions with reality
- Encourage independence in performance of self-care, assisting patient only as necessary
- Establish a schedule for contact with patient
- Establish a trusting relationship with patient and family
- Help patient and family to participate actively in decision-making process
- Provide a safe, secure, and private environment to facilitate patient and family grieving process
- Recognize and reinforce the strength of each family member

- *(NIC) Grief Work Facilitation: Perinatal Death:*
  Assist in keeping infant alive until parents arrive
  Baptize the infant, as appropriate
  Discuss plans that have been made (e.g., burial, funeral, and infant name)
  Describe mementos that will be obtained, including footprints, handprints, pictures, caps, gowns, blankets, diapers, and blood pressure cuffs, as appropriate
  Prepare infant for viewing by bathing and dressing, including parents in activities as appropriate
  Encourage family members to view and hold infant for as long as desired
  Focus on normal features of infant, while sensitively discussing anomalies
  Transfer infant to morgue or prepare body to be transported by family to funeral home

---

GROWTH, DISPROPORTIONATE, RISK FOR (00113) (1998)

Definition: At risk for growth above the 97th percentile or below the 3rd percentile for age, crossing two percentile channels; disproportionate growth

Risk Factors

Prenatal

Congenital or genetic disorders
Infection
Maternal nutrition
Multiple gestation
Substance use or abuse
Teratogen exposure

Individual

Anorexia
Caregiver or individual maladaptive feeding behaviors
Chronic illness
Infection
Insatiable appetite
Malnutrition
Organic and inorganic factors

Prematurity
Substance abuse

Environmental

Deprivation
Lead poisoning
Natural disasters
Poverty
Teratogens
Violence

Caregiver

Abuse
Mental illness
Mental retardation
Severe learning disability

Suggestions for Use

There are many conditions, including other nursing diagnoses, that create *Risk for disproportionate growth*, for example, *Ineffective breastfeeding*. The diagnosis of *Risk for disproportionate growth* related to *Ineffective breastfeeding* suggests goals focused on weight gain or loss but gives little guidance for nursing activities to correct the breastfeeding problem; whereas a diagnosis of *Ineffective breastfeeding* related to maternal anxiety or ambivalence provides direction for nursing activities to correct the breastfeeding problem and, indirectly, to correct the *Risk for disproportionate growth*. When possible, use the more specific diagnoses rather than the more general diagnosis *Risk for disproportionate growth*.

Because growth is routinely assessed in nursing care of children, a diagnostic statement is usually not required for that application—such assessment is usually included in pediatric standards of care. Likewise, this label is not appropriate for a child with failure to thrive. That condition may be described better by one of the family functioning diagnoses or by a diagnosis of *Imbalanced nutrition: less than body requirements*.

Suggested Alternative Diagnoses

Breastfeeding, ineffective
Disabled family coping
Growth and development, delayed
Ineffective coping
Infant feeding pattern, ineffective

Nutrition: imbalanced, less than body requirements
Parenting, Impaired
Self-care deficit: feeding

NOC Outcomes

Child Development: 2 Months: Milestones of physical, cognitive, and psychosocial progression by 2 months of age

Child Development: 4 Months: Milestones of physical, cognitive, and psychosocial progression by 4 months of age

Child Development: 6 Months: Milestones of physical, cognitive, and psychosocial progression by 6 months of age

Child Development: 12 Months: Milestones of physical, cognitive, and psychosocial progression by 12 months of age

Child Development: 2 Years: Milestones of physical, cognitive, and psychosocial progression by 2 years of age

Child Development: 3 Years: Milestones of physical, cognitive, and psychosocial progression by 3 years of age

Child Development: 4 Years: Milestones of physical, cognitive, and psychosocial progression by 4 years of age

Child Development: 5 Years: Milestones of physical, cognitive, and psychosocial progression by 5 years of age

Child Development: Middle Childhood (6–11 Years): Milestones of physical, cognitive, and psychosocial progression between 6 and 11 years of age

Child Development: Adolescence (12–17 Years): Milestones of physical, cognitive, and psychosocial progression between 12 and 17 years of age

Growth: A normal increase in body size and weight

Physical Aging Status: Physical changes that commonly occur with adult aging

Physical Maturation: Female: Normal physical changes in the female that occur with the transition from childhood to adulthood

Physical Maturation: Male: Normal physical changes in the male that occur with the transition from childhood to adulthood

Goals/Evaluation Criteria

NOTE: This text can provide only examples of growth norms. Refer to pediatrics or child development texts for complete discussion of growth; or refer to *Nursing Outcomes Classification (NOC) Manual* for complete list of indicators for each age group:

2, 4, 6, and 12 months; 2, 3, 4, and 5 years; middle childhood; and adolescence.

- The child will achieve expected growth norms (e.g., weight, head circumference, bone age, mean body mass), that is, not above the 97th percentile or below the 3rd percentile for age
- Physical maturation will progress normally (e.g., for females: growth spurt between 9.5 and 14.5 years of age, breast development, and onset of menstruation; for males: growth spurt between 10.5 and 16 years of age, voice change, penis enlargement, increased muscle mass)

NIC Interventions

Developmental Care: Structuring the environment and providing care in response to the behavioral cues and states of the preterm infant

Developmental Enhancement: Adolescent: Facilitating optimal physical, cognitive, social, and emotional growth of individuals during the transition from childhood to adulthood

Developmental Enhancement: Child: Facilitating or teaching parents and caregivers to facilitate the optimal gross-motor, fine-motor, language, cognitive, social, and emotional growth of preschool and school-aged children

Health Screening: Detecting health risks or problems by means of history, examination, and other procedures

Infant Care: Provision of developmentally appropriate family-centered care to the child under 1 year of age

Nutrition Management: Assisting with or providing a balanced dietary intake of foods and fluids

Nutrition Therapy: Administration of food and fluids to support metabolic processes of a patient who is malnourished or at high risk for becoming malnourished

Nutritional Monitoring: Collection and analysis of patient data to prevent or minimize malnourishment

Parent Education: Childrearing Family: Assisting parents to understand and promote the physical, psychological, and social growth and development of their toddler, or preschool or school-aged child

Parenting Promotion: Providing parenting information, support, and coordination of comprehensive services to high-risk families

Risk Identification: Analysis of potential risk factors, determination of health risks, and prioritization of risk reduction strategies for an individual or group

Self-Responsibility Facilitation: Encouraging a patient to assume more responsibility for own behavior

Teaching: Infant Nutrition: Instruction on nutrition and feeding practices during the first year of life

Teaching: Toddler Nutrition: Instruction on nutrition and feeding practices during the second and third years of life

Weight Management: Facilitating maintenance of optimal body weight and percentage of body fat

Nursing Activities

NOTE: Because this nursing diagnosis is so broad, not every possible nursing activity can be listed here. Refer to age-specific sections in growth and development texts for full lists of activities.

Assessments

- Assess the caretakers' knowledge, resources, support system, coping skills, and level of commitment to develop a plan of care for eliminating risk factors
- Conduct a thorough health assessment (e.g., child's history, temperament, culture, family environment, developmental screening) to determine risk factors
- Monitor parent and child interactions and communication
- Assess adequacy of nutritional intake (e.g., calories, nutrients)
- Monitor trends in weight loss or gain
- Take skinfold measurements
- Determine food preferences

Patient/Family Teaching

- Teach caregivers about normal growth patterns
- Teach patient and family about nutritional needs

Collaborative Activities

- Act as case manager to insure comprehensive care by coordinating medical, school, rehabilitation, and social services efforts
- Refer to nutritionist for diet teaching and planning

Other

- Assist caretakers to develop a plan of care (for possible care plans and interventions, refer to Nursing Activities for the Suggested Alternative Diagnoses presented on pp. 226–227.)
- Establish a therapeutic and trusting relationship with caretakers.

GROWTH AND DEVELOPMENT, DELAYED (00111) (1986)

Definition: Deviations from age-group norms

Defining Characteristics

Objective

Altered physical growth

Decreased responses

Delay or difficulty in performing skills (e.g., motor, social, or expressive) typical of age group

Flat affect

Inability to perform self-care or self-control activities appropriate for age

Listlessness

Related Factors

Effects of physical disability

Environmental and stimulation deficiencies

Inadequate caretaking

Inconsistent responsiveness

Indifference

Multiple caretakers

Prescribed dependence

Separation from significant others

Other Possible Related Factors (non-NANDA International)

Abuse

Changes in family system

Congenital anomaly

Fetal distress during or after birth or delivery

Inadequate bonding

Inadequate prenatal care

Loss

Maternal acute or chronic disease

Neonatal disease

Poverty

Prematurity

Serious illness/injury

Traumatic separation

Unhealthy maternal lifestyle during pregnancy

Suggestions for Use

Use of this label is not recommended. It is too broad to suggest nursing actions. There are many nursing diagnoses that could be considered *Delayed growth and development* or that could be caused by *Delayed growth and development* (e.g., *Self-care deficit, Urinary incontinence, Impaired verbal communication*, and *Impaired parenting*). When possible, use the more specific labels. If the problem is potential rather than actual, use *Risk for disproportionate growth* or *Risk for delayed development*.

Because growth and development are routinely assessed in nursing care of children, a diagnostic statement is usually not required for that application—such an assessment is usually included in pediatric standards of care. This label is not appropriate for a mentally impaired child (e.g., *Delayed growth and development* related to Down syndrome). Instead, diagnose the specific functional task that the child is unable to perform (e.g., *Feeding self-care deficit*). Likewise, this label is probably not appropriate for a child with failure to thrive. That condition may be described better by one of the family functioning diagnoses or by a diagnosis of *Imbalanced nutrition: less than body requirements*. *Delayed growth and development* is most appropriately used for a child who is having difficulty achieving age-specific developmental tasks and growth norms.

Suggested Alternative Diagnoses

Bowel incontinence
Breastfeeding, ineffective
Communication, impaired verbal
Coping: family, compromised
Coping: family, disabled
Coping , ineffective
Incontinence, urinary
Infant feeding pattern, ineffective
Nutrition: imbalanced, less than body requirements
Parenting, impaired
Self-care deficit (specify)

NOC Outcomes

Refer to NOC Outcomes for the preceding nursing diagnosis, *Risk for disproportionate growth*, on p. 227.

Goals/Evaluation Criteria

Examples Using NOC Language

- Normal progression of **Physical Aging Status**, as evidenced by the following indicators (specify 1–5: extreme, substantial, moderate, mild, or no deviation from expected range):

    Mean body mass, bone density, basal metabolic rate, skin elasticity, and muscle strength

    Cardiac output, vital capacity, and BP

    Hearing, visual, olfactory, and taste acuity

Other Examples

This section can only provide examples. Refer to *Nursing Outcomes Classification (NOC)* manual or pediatrics text for complete list of indicators for each age group: 2, 4, 6, and 12 months; 2, 3, 4, and 5 years; middle childhood; and adolescence.

- The child will achieve expected growth norms (e.g., weight, head circumference, bone age, mean body mass), that is, not above the 97th percentile or below the 3rd percentile for age
- The child will achieve milestones of physical, cognitive, and psychosocial progression (specify age of achievement), with no delay from expected range
- Examples of indicators of normal child development for a 6-month-old child are as follows: rolls over, sits with support, grasps and mouths objects
- Physical maturation will progress normally (e.g., for females: growth spurt between 9.5 and 14.5 years of age, breast development, and onset of menstruation; for males: growth spurt between 10.5 and 16 years of age, voice change, penis enlargement, increased muscle mass)
- The patient will achieve the highest level of wellness, independence, and growth and development possible given patient's illness or disability status

NIC Interventions

Refer to NIC Interventions for the nursing diagnosis *Risk for Disproportionate Growth*, on pp. 228–229.

Nursing Activities

NOTE: Because this nursing diagnosis is so broad and nonspecific, not every possible nursing activity can be listed here. Refer to the *Nursing Interventions Classification (NIC)* manual and to age-specific sections in growth and development texts for full lists of activities

Assessments

- Assess the caretakers' knowledge, resources, support systems, coping skills, and level of commitment to develop a plan of care
- Conduct a thorough health assessment (e.g., child's history, temperament, culture, family environment, developmental screening) to determine functional level
- Identify potential related physical problems (e.g., dehydration, falls, upper respiratory infection, skin breakdown), and initiate plans to prevent them
- Monitor parent and child interactions and communication
- Assess adequacy of nutritional intake (e.g., calories, nutrients)
- Monitor trends in weight loss or gain
- Take skinfold measurements
- Determine food preferences
- *(NIC) Self-Responsibility Facilitation:* Monitor level of responsibility that patient assumes

Patient/Family Teaching

- *(NIC) Developmental Enhancement:*
  Teach caregivers about normal developmental milestones and associated behaviors
  Demonstrate activities that promote development to caregivers

Collaborative Activities

- Act as case manager to ensure comprehensive care by coordinating medical, nutritional, school, rehabilitation, and social services
- *(NIC) Developmental Enhancement:* Refer caregivers to support group, as appropriate

Other

- Assist caretakers to develop a plan of care (for possible care plans and interventions, refer to Family Coping: Ineffective, Compromised, on pp. 115–116, and Family Coping: Ineffective, Disabled on pp. 120–121)
- Assist patient in achieving next level of growth and development through appropriate mastery of tasks specific to his level
- Create an environment where ADLs can be performed with maximum independence
- Establish a therapeutic and trusting relationship with caretakers
- Help the family develop a strategy to integrate the patient as an accepted member of the family and community

- *(NIC) Developmental Enhancement:*
  Provide activities that encourage interaction among children
  Encourage child to express self through positive rewards or feedback for attempts
  Offer age-appropriate toys or materials
  Be consistent and structured with behavior management or modification strategies
- *(NIC) Self-Responsibility Facilitation:*
  Encourage patient to take as much responsibility for own self-care as possible
  Encourage parents to clearly communicate and follow through on expectations for responsible behavior in child, as appropriate

HEALTH MAINTENANCE, INEFFECTIVE
(00099) (1982)

Definition: Inability to identify, manage, or seek out help to maintain health

Defining Characteristics
Subjective
Expressed interest in improving health behaviors
Objective
Demonstrated lack of adaptive behaviors to internal and external environmental changes
Demonstrated lack of knowledge regarding basic health practices
History of lack of health-seeking behavior
Reported or observed lack of equipment, financial, or other resources
Reported or observed impairment of personal support system
Reported or observed inability to take responsibility for meeting basic health practices in any or all functional pattern areas

Other Defining Characteristics (non-NANDA International)
History of untreated, chronic symptoms of disease process
Limited use of health care agencies and personnel
Limited use of preventive health measures
Need to adhere to cultural and religious beliefs

Related Factors
Disabling spiritual distress
Dysfunctional grieving

Ineffective family coping

Ineffective individual coping

Lack of ability to make deliberate and thoughtful judgments

Lack of material resources

Lack of or significant alteration in communication skills (e.g., written, verbal, or gestural)

Perceptual and cognitive impairment (complete and partial lack of gross- and fine-motor skills)

Unachieved developmental tasks

Other Related Factors (non-NANDA International)

Cultural beliefs

Lack of social supports

Motor impairment

Religious beliefs

Suggestions for Use

Use this diagnosis for patients who wish to change an unhealthy lifestyle or who lack knowledge of their disease or condition. Do not use it to describe patients who are not motivated to change or learn. Health-seeking behaviors is a wellness diagnosis to be used for clients with a generally healthy lifestyle who are seeking to attain a higher level of wellness (e.g., a client who wishes information about BP screening).

Suggested Alternative Diagnoses

Adjustment, impaired

Coping, ineffective

Denial, ineffective

Health-seeking behaviors

Knowledge, deficient

Management of therapeutic regimen: family and individual, ineffective

Noncompliance (specify)

NOC Outcomes

Health Beliefs: Perceived Resources: Personal conviction that one has adequate means to carry out a health behavior

Health-Promoting Behavior: Actions to sustain or increase wellness

Health-Seeking Behavior: Actions to promote optimal wellness, recovery, and rehabilitation

Knowledge: Health Behaviors: Extent of understanding conveyed about the promotion and protection of health

Knowledge: Health Promotion: Extent of understanding of information needed to obtain and maintain optimal health

Knowledge: Health Resources: Extent of understanding conveyed about health care resources

Knowledge: Treatment Regimen: Extent of understanding conveyed about a specific treatment regimen

Participation: Health Care Decisions: Personal involvement in selecting and evaluating health care options

Psychosocial Adjustment: Life Change: Psychosocial adaptation of an individual to a life change

Risk Detection: Actions taken to identify personal health threats

Self-Direction of Care: Directing others to assist with or perform physical tasks, personal care, and activities needed to function in the home or the community

Social Support: Perceived availability and actual provision of reliable assistance from other persons

Treatment Behavior: Illness or Injury: Personal actions to palliate or eliminate pathology

Goals/Evaluation Criteria

Examples Using NOC Language

- Will demonstrate **Participation: Health Care Decisions**, as evidenced by the following indicators (specify 1–5: never, rarely, sometimes, often, or consistently demonstrated):

    Demonstrates self-direction in decision making

    Seeks information

    Identifies barriers and available supports for achieving desired outcomes

    Seeks services to meet desired outcomes

Other Examples

Patient will:

- Develop and follow strategies to maximize health
- Acknowledge adverse effects of health beliefs
- Demonstrate awareness that healthy behavior requires some effort, and confidence in ability to manage it
- Follow recommended treatment regimens
- Identify potential health risks created by lifestyle
- Verbalize and demonstrate knowledge of preventive health measures (e.g., performs self-examinations, participates in health screenings)

NIC Interventions

Decision-Making Support: Providing information and support for a patient who is making a decision regarding health care

Family Involvement Promotion: Facilitating family participation in the emotional and physical care of the patient

Health Education: Developing and providing instruction and learning experiences to facilitate voluntary adaptation of behavior conducive to health in individuals, families, groups, or communities

Health Screening: Detecting health risks or problems by means of history, examination, and other procedures

Health System Guidance: Facilitating a patient's location and use of appropriate health services

Risk Identification: Analysis of potential risk factors, determination of health risks, and prioritization of risk reduction strategies for an individual or group

Risk Identification: Childbearing Family: Identification of an individual or family likely to experience difficulties in parenting and prioritization of strategies to prevent parenting problems

Self-Modification Assistance: Reinforcement of self-directed change initiated by the patient to achieve personally important goals

Self-Responsibility Facilitation: Encouraging a patient to assume more responsibility for own behavior

Support Group: Use of a group environment to provide emotional support and health-related information for members

Support System Enhancement: Facilitation of support to patient by family, friends, and community

Teaching: Disease Process: Assisting the patient to understand information related to a specific disease process

Teaching: Individual: Planning, implementation, and evaluation of a teaching program designed to address a patient's particular needs

Teaching: Procedure/Treatment: Preparing a patient to understand and mentally prepare for a prescribed procedure or treatment

Nursing Activities

Assessments

- Identify beliefs and knowledge deficits that interfere with health maintenance

- Assess availability and adequacy of support system
- *(NIC) Self-Modification Assistance:*

  Appraise the patient's reasons for wanting to change

  Appraise the patient's knowledge and skill level in relationship to the desired change

Patient/Family Teaching

- *(NIC) Health System Guidance:*

  Explain the immediate health care system, how it works, and what the patient and family can expect

  Give written instructions for purpose and location of health care activities, as appropriate

  Inform the patient the meaning of signing a consent form

  Inform patient of the cost, time, alternatives, and risks involved in a specific test or procedure

  Provide patient with copy of Patient's Bill of Rights
- *(NIC) Self-Modification Assistance:*

  Explain to the patient the function of cues and triggers in producing behavior

  Instruct the patient on the use of "cue expansion"—increasing the number of cues that prompt a desired behavior

  Instruct the patient on the use of "cue restriction"—decreasing the frequency of cues that elicit an undesirable behavior

Collaborative Activities

- Consult with social services to plan for health maintenance needs on discharge
- *(NIC) Health System Guidance:*

  Inform patient of appropriate community resources and contact persons

  Advise use of second opinion

  Coordinate referrals to relevant health care providers, as appropriate

  Coordinate and schedule time needed by each service to deliver care, as appropriate

  Assist individual to complete forms for assistance, such as housing and financial aid, as needed

Other

- Encourage discussion of preventive health measures specific to patient needs, such as dietary changes, cessation of smoking, stress reduction, and implementation of exercise program

- *(NIC) Health System Guidance:* Encourage the patient and family to ask questions about services and charges
- *(NIC) Self-Modification Assistance:*
  Assist the patient in identifying a specific goal for change
  Explore with the patient potential barriers to change behavior
  Encourage the patient to identify appropriate, meaningful reinforcers and rewards
  Foster moving toward primary reliance on self-reinforcement versus family or nurse for rewards
  Assist the patient in evaluating progress by comparing records of previous behavior with present behavior

---

HEALTH-SEEKING BEHAVIORS (SPECIFY)
(00084) (1988)

Definition: Active seeking by a person in stable health* of ways to alter personal health habits and the environment in order to move toward a higher level of health

Defining Characteristics

Subjective

Expression of concern about current environmental conditions on health status

Expressed desire for increased control of health practice

Expressed desire to seek a higher level of wellness

Stated unfamiliarity with wellness community resources

Objective

Demonstrated or observed lack of knowledge of health-promotion behaviors

Observed desire for increased control of health practice

Observed desire to seek a higher level of wellness

Observed unfamiliarity with wellness community resources

Related Factors

Specific to patient (to be developed)

---

*Stable health is defined as achievement of age-appropriate illness-prevention measures; client reports good or excellent health, and signs and symptoms of disease, if present, are controlled.

Suggestions for Use

Use this label for well patients who wish information about disease prevention or health promotion. For patients with an unhealthy lifestyle, consider *Ineffective health maintenance*.

Suggested Alternative Diagnoses

Breastfeeding, effective
Family coping: readiness for enhanced
Health maintenance, ineffective

NOC Outcomes

Adherence Behavior: Self-initiated action taken to promote wellness, recovery, and rehabilitation

Health Beliefs: Personal convictions that influence health behaviors

Health Orientation: Personal view of health and health behaviors as priorities

Health Promoting Behavior: Actions to sustain or increase wellness

Health Seeking Behavior: Actions to promote optimal wellness, recovery, and rehabilitation

Knowledge: Health Promotion: Extent of understanding conveyed about the promotion and protection of health

Knowledge: Health Resources: Extent of understanding conveyed about health care resources

Well-Being: An individual's expressed satisfaction with health status

Goals/Evaluation Criteria

Examples Using NOC Language

- Demonstrates *Health seeking behaviors*, as evidenced by Adherence Behavior, Health Beliefs, Health Orientation, Health-Promoting Behavior, Health-Seeking Behavior, Knowledge: Health Promotion, Knowledge: Health Resources, and Well-Being
- Demonstrates **Adherence Behavior**, as evidenced by the following indicators (specify 1–5: never, rarely, sometimes, often, or consistently demonstrated):
    Seeks health-related information from a variety of sources
    Describes strategies to eliminate unhealthy behavior
    Reports using strategies to maximize health
    Performs self-screening and self-monitoring
    Uses health services congruent with need

- Demonstrates **Health Orientation**, as evidenced by the following indicators (specify 1–5: very weak, weak, moderate, strong, or very strong):

  Focus on wellness

  Focus on disease prevention and management

  Focus on adjustment to life situations

  Expectation that individual is responsible for choices

  Perception that health behavior is relevant to self

  Perception that health is a high priority in making lifestyle choices

Other Examples

Patient will:

- Recognize and act on the need to alter personal health habits
- Strive to balance exercise, work, leisure, and rest
- Maintain a healthy diet
- Avoid risky behaviors (e.g., driving without seat belt)
- Express the desire to seek a higher level of wellness

NIC Interventions

Decision-Making Support: Providing information and support for a patient who is making a decision regarding health care

Health Education: Development and provision of instruction and learning experiences to facilitate voluntary adaptation of behavior conducive to health in individuals, families, groups, or communities

Health System Guidance: Facilitating a patient's location and use of appropriate health services

Risk Identification: Analysis of potential risk factors, determination of health risks, and prioritization of risk reduction strategies for an individual or group

Self-Awareness Enhancement: Assisting a patient to explore and understand his thoughts, feelings, motivations, and behaviors

Self-Modification Assistance: Reinforcement of self-directed change initiated by the patient to achieve personally important goals

Teaching: Individual: Planning, implementation, and evaluation of a teaching program designed to address a patient's particular needs

Values Clarification: Assisting another to clarify his own values in order to facilitate effective decision making

Nursing Activities

Assessments

- Assess patient's motivation to change
- *(NIC) Health Education:*

    Determine personal context and sociocultural history of individual, family, or community health behavior

    Determine current health knowledge and lifestyle behaviors of individual, family, or target group

Patient/Family Teaching

- *(NIC) Health Education:*

    Target high-risk groups and age ranges that would benefit most from health education

    Prioritize identified learner needs based on client preference, skills of nurse, resources available, and likelihood of successful goal attainment

    Avoid use of fear or scare techniques as strategy to motivate people to change health or lifestyle behaviors

    Teach strategies that can be used to resist unhealthful behavior or risk taking, rather than give advice to avoid or change behavior

    Use group presentations to provide support and lessen threat to learners experiencing similar problems or concerns, as appropriate

- *(NIC) Health System Guidance:*

    Explain the immediate health care system, how it works, and what the patient and family can expect

    Instruct patient on what type of services to expect from each type of health care provider (e.g., nurse specialists, registered dietitians, etc.)

    Inform the patient of accreditation and state health department requirements for judging the quality of a facility

    Advise the use of second opinion

    Provide patient with copy of Patient's Bill of Rights

    Give written instructions for purpose and location of health care activities, as appropriate

Collaborative Activities

- Consult with community services as a primary step toward health promotion for patient and family. Involve patient and family in consultation
- *(NIC) Health System Guidance:* Coordinate referrals to relevant health care providers, as appropriate

Other

- Discuss with patient and family personal health habits and determine which behaviors may be changed to achieve optimal health (e.g., through diet, smoking cessation, stress reduction, exercise program)
- Assist patient to recognize potential barriers to changing behaviors
- Stress the importance of self-monitoring when attempting behavior change
- Assist patient to identify extrinsic and intrinsic rewards that can serve as motivators for behavior change
- Help the patient to recognize small successes
- *(NIC) Health Education:* Plan long-term follow-up to reinforce health behavior or lifestyle adaptations
- *(NIC) Health System Guidance:*
  Encourage the patient and family to ask questions about services and charges

  Assist individual to complete forms for assistance, such as housing and financial aid, as needed

  Identify and facilitate transportation needs for obtaining health care services

  Provide follow-up contact with patient, as appropriate

HOME MAINTENANCE, IMPAIRED
(00098) (1980)

Definition: Inability to independently maintain a safe, growth-promoting immediate environment

Defining Characteristics

Subjective
Household members describe outstanding debts or financial crises
Household members express difficulty in maintaining their home in a comfortable fashion
Household members request assistance with home maintenance

Objective
Accumulation of dirt, food wastes, or hygienic wastes
Disorderly surroundings
Inappropriate household temperature
Lack of necessary equipment or aids
Offensive odors
Overtaxed (e.g., exhausted, anxious) family members

Presence of vermin or rodents
Repeated hygienic disorders, infestations, or infections
Unwashed or unavailable cooking equipment, clothes, linen

Related Factors

Impaired cognitive or emotional functioning
Inadequate support system
Individual and family member disease or injury
Insufficient family organization or planning
Insufficient finances
Lack of knowledge
Lack of role modeling
Unfamiliarity with neighborhood resources

Other Related Factors (non-NANDA International)
Developmental disability
Home environment obstacles

Suggestions for Use

This diagnosis emphasizes inability to manage the home environment (e.g., laundry, cleaning, and cooking. If the difficulty is with managing medications or treatments, use *Ineffective management of therapeutic regimen*. If it is primarily a difficulty in managing self-care, such as bathing and dressing, use *Self-care deficit (specify)*. Differentiate also between this label and *Caregiver role strain*.

Suggested Alternative Diagnoses

Caregiver role strain
Family coping, compromised
Injury, risk for (trauma, falls)
Management of therapeutic regimen: family or individual, ineffective
Self-care deficit (specify)

NOC Outcomes

Family Functioning: Ability of the family to meet the needs of its members through developmental transitions
Parenting: Provision of an environment that promotes optimum growth and development of dependent children
Parenting: Social Safety: Parental actions to avoid social relationships that might cause harm or injury
Role Performance: Congruence of an individual's role behavior with role expectations

Self-Care: Instrumental Activities of Daily Living (IADLs): Ability to perform activities needed to function in the home or community

Goals/Evaluation Criteria

Examples Using NOC Language

- *Impaired home maintenance* will be eliminated or moderated, as demonstrated by Family Functioning, Parenting, Parenting: Social Safety, Role Performance, and Self-Care: IADLs
- **Role Performance** will be demonstrated, as evidenced by the following indicators (specify 1–5: not, slightly, moderately, substantially, or totally adequate):

  Ability to meet role expectations

  Performance of family role behaviors
- **Family Functioning** will be demonstrated, as evidenced by the following indicators (specify 1–5: never, rarely, sometimes, often, or consistently demonstrated):

  Cares for dependent family members

  Regulates behavior of members

  Members perform expected roles

  Obtains adequate resources to meet needs of family members

  Members support and help one another

Other Examples

Patient and family/household member will:
- Follow specific plan for home maintenance
- Identify options to overcome financial constraints
- Verbalize awareness of constraints on home situation due to illness of family member
- Verbalize knowledge of available resources
- Perform home maintenance tasks (e.g., shopping, meal preparation, laundry, yard work, housework)
- Drive car (e.g., for shopping)
- Remove environmental hazards from the home
- Provide for the physical needs of dependents in the home
- Provide supervision for children (e.g., of playmates, day care workers)

NIC Interventions

Family Integrity Promotion: Promotion of family cohesion and unity

Family Integrity Promotion: Childbearing Family: Facilitation of the growth of individuals or families who are adding an infant to the family unit

Home Maintenance Assistance: Helping the patient and family to maintain the home as a clean, safe, and pleasant place to live

Parent Education: Adolescent: Assisting parents to understand and help their adolescent children

Parent Education: Childrearing Family: Assisting parents to understand and promote the physical, psychological, and social growth and development of their toddler or preschool or school-aged child or children

Risk Identification: Childbearing Family: Identification of an individual or family likely to experience difficulties in parenting and prioritization of strategies to prevent parenting problems

Role Enhancement: Assisting a patient, significant other, or family to improve relationships by clarifying and supplementing specific role behaviors

Nursing Activities

Assessments

- *(NIC) Home Maintenance Assistance:* Determine patient's home maintenance requirements

Patient/Family Teaching

- Provide written material regarding home maintenance
- *(NIC) Home Maintenance Assistance:* Provide information on how to make home environment safe and clean
- *(NIC) Parent Education: Childrearing Family:*

  Teach importance of balanced diet, three meals a day, and nutritious snacks

  Give parents a variety of strategies to use in managing child's behavior

  Review safety issues with parents, such as children meeting strangers and water and bicycle safety

  Provide parents with readings and other materials that will be helpful in performing parenting role

  Help parents identify evaluation criteria for day care and school settings

Collaborative Activities

- Assess and document need for postdischarge follow-through with public health nurse
- Contact discharge planner or social worker to establish realistic plan for home maintenance

- *(NIC) Home Maintenance Assistance:*
  Provide information on respite care, as needed
  Offer homemaker services, as appropriate

Other

- Accept and support without judgment the realities of the home situation
- Help patient and family/household member identify obstacles and hazards in home that may impede home maintenance
- Help patient and family/household member identify strengths in family unit, as well as support systems that will assist in home maintenance
- Initiate discussion with patient and family about health status of all family members, as illness of other family members may affect home maintenance management
- *(NIC) Home Maintenance Assistance:*
  Involve patient and family in deciding home maintenance requirements
  Suggest necessary structural alterations to make home accessible
  Suggest services for pest control, as needed
  Suggest services for home repair, as needed
  Discuss cost of needed maintenance and available resources
- *(NIC) Parent Education: Childrearing Family:*
  Facilitate parents' discussion of methods of discipline available, selection, and results obtained
  Encourage parents to try different childrearing strategies, as appropriate
  Role play childrearing techniques and communication skills

HOPELESSNESS
(00124) (1986)

Definition: A subjective state in which an individual sees limited or no alternatives or personal choices available and is unable to mobilize energy on own behalf

Defining Characteristics

Subjective
Verbal cues (e.g., despondent content, "I can't," sighing)

Objective
Closing eyes
Decreased appetite

Decreased affect
Decreased response to stimuli
Decreased verbalization
Increased or decreased sleep
Lack of initiative
Lack of involvement in care or passively allowing care
Passivity
Shrugging in response to speaker
Turning away from speaker
Avoiding eye contact (non-NANDA International)

Related Factors

Abandonment
Failing or deteriorating physical condition
Long-term stress
Lost belief in transcendent values or God
Prolonged activity restrictions creating isolation
Lack of social supports (non-NANDA International)

Suggestions for Use

Differentiate between this label and *Powerlessness. Hopelessness* implies that the person believes there is no solution to his problem ("no way out"). In *Powerlessness*, the person may know of a solution to the problem but believes it is beyond his control to achieve the solution. Long-term feelings of *Powerlessness* may lead to *Hopelessness*. Although both diagnoses share some defining characteristics, the following are specific only to *Powerlessness:* irritability, resentment, anger, guilt, and fear of alienation from caregivers. For some patients, *Hopelessness* may be a risk factor for suicide.

Suggested Alternative Diagnoses

Anxiety, death
Coping, ineffective
Failure to thrive, adult
Grieving, dysfunctional (may be an etiology of *Hopelessness*)
Powerlessness
Spiritual distress, actual/risk
Violence: self-directed, risk for

NOC Outcomes

Decision Making: Ability to choose between two or more alternatives

Depression Control: Personal actions to minimize melancholy and maintain interest in life events

Depression Level: Severity of melancholic mood and loss of interest in life events

Hope: Presence of internal state of optimism that is personally satisfying and life supporting

Mood Equilibrium: Appropriate adjustment of prevailing emotional tone in response to circumstances

Quality of Life: An individual's expressed satisfaction with current life circumstances

Goals/Evaluation Criteria

Examples Using NOC Language

- *Hopelessness* will be eliminated, as evidenced by consistent Decision Making, Depression Control, Depression Level, presence of Hope, Mood Equilibrium, and expressed satisfaction with Quality of Life
- **Decision Making** will be demonstrated, as evidenced by the following indicator (specify 1–5: never, rarely, sometimes, often, or consistently demonstrated): Weighs and chooses among alternatives
- **Hope** will be exhibited, as evidenced by the following indicators (specify 1–5: none, limited, moderate, substantial, or extensive):
  Expression of faith, will to live, reasons to live, meaning in life, optimism, and belief in self and others
  Demonstration of a zest for life

Other Examples

Patient will:
- Identify personal strengths
- Initiate behaviors that may reduce feelings of hopelessness
- Report extent and pattern of sleep adequate to produce mental and physical rejuvenation
- Demonstrate appropriate mood and affect
- Maintain appropriate hygiene and grooming
- Demonstrate interest in social and personal relationships
- Show interest in or satisfaction with achieving life goals

NIC Interventions

Decision-Making Support: Providing information and support for a patient who is making a decision regarding health care

Hope Instillation: Facilitation of the development of a positive outlook in a given situation

Mood Management: Providing for safety, stabilization, recovery, and maintenance of a patient who is experiencing dysfunctionally depressed mood or elevated mood

Resiliency Promotion: Assisting individuals, families, and communities in development, use, and strengthening of protective factors to be used in coping with environmental and societal stressors

Self-Modification Assistance: Reinforcement of self-directed change initiated by the patient to achieve personally important goals

Spiritual Growth Facilitation: Facilitation of growth in patient's capacity to identify, connect with, and call upon the source of meaning, purpose, comfort, strength, and hope in his life

Values Clarification: Assisting another to clarify his own values in order to facilitate effective decision-making

Nursing Activities

Assessments

- Assess and document potential for suicide
- Monitor affect and decision-making ability
- Monitor nutrition: intake and body weight
- Assess spiritual needs
- Determine adequacy of relationships and other social supports

Patient/Family Teaching

- Provide information on community resources, such as community agencies, social agencies, self-improvement classes, stress-reduction classes, counseling
- *(NIC) Hope Instillation:* Teach reality recognition by surveying the situation and making contingency plans

Collaborative Activities

- Obtain psychiatric consultation
- *(NIC) Hope Instillation:* Provide patient and family opportunity to be involved with support groups

Other

- Encourage active participation in group activities to provide opportunity for social supports and problem solving
- Explore with patient factors that contribute to feelings of hopelessness
- Provide positive reinforcement for behaviors that demonstrate initiative, such as eye contact, self-disclosure, reduction in amount of sleep time, self-care, increased appetite
- Schedule time with patient to provide opportunity to explore alternative coping measures

- *(NIC) Hope Instillation:*
  Assist patient and family to identify areas of hope in life
  Demonstrate hope by recognizing the patient's intrinsic worth and
    viewing the patient's illness as only one facet of the individual
  Help the patient expand spiritual self
  Employ guided life review or reminiscence, as appropriate
  Avoid masking the truth
  Involve the patient actively in own care
  Encourage therapeutic relationships with significant others

---

HYPERTHERMIA
(00007) (1986)

Definition: A state in which an individual's body temperature is
elevated above his normal range

Defining Characteristics

Objective
Flushed skin
Increase in body temperature above normal range
Increased respiratory rate
Seizures or convulsions
[Skin] warm to touch
Tachycardia

Related Factors

Dehydration
Illness or trauma
Inability or decreased ability to perspire
Inappropriate clothing
Increased metabolic rate
Medication/anesthesia
[Prolonged] exposure to hot environment
Vigorous activity

Suggestions for Use

Nursing activities, such as removal of clothing or a cool sponge
bath, are effective for mild *Hyperthermia*. However, severe *Hyperthermia* is a life-threatening condition requiring both medical and
nursing intervention. An elevated temperature may not be a problem, but merely a symptom of a disease process or infection, and it is

treated by a medication such as acetaminophen or aspirin. Most hyperthermias require no independent nursing treatment.

Suggested Alternative Diagnoses

Body temperature, risk for imbalanced
Hyperthermia, risk for
Thermoregulation, ineffective

NOC Outcomes

Thermoregulation: Balance among heat production, heat gain, and heat loss

Thermoregulation: Neonate: Balance among heat production, heat gain, and heat loss during the neonatal period

Goals/Evaluation Criteria

Examples Using NOC Language

- Patient will demonstrate **Thermoregulation**, as evidenced by the following indicators (specify 1–5: extremely, substantially, moderately, mildly, or not compromised):

    Skin temperature in expected range
    Body temperature within normal limits
    Pulse and respiratory rates in expected range
    Skin color changes not present
    Drowsiness and irritability not present

Other Examples

Patient and family will:
- Demonstrate proper method of taking temperature
- Describe measures to prevent or minimize increase in body temperature
- Report early signs and symptoms of Hyperthermia
Infants will:
- Experience no respiratory distress, restlessness, or lethargy
- Use heat-dissipation posture

NIC Interventions

Fever Treatment: Management of a patient with hyperpyrexia caused by nonenvironmental factors

Malignant Hyperthermia Precautions: Prevention or reduction of a hypermetabolic response to pharmacologic agents used during surgery.

Newborn Care: Management of neonate during the transition to extrauterine life and subsequent period of stabilization

Temperature Regulation: Attaining or maintaining body temperature within a normal range

Temperature Regulation: Intraoperative: Attaining or maintaining desired intraopertive body temperature

Vital Signs Monitoring: Collection and analysis of cardiovascular, respiratory, and body temperature data to determine and prevent complications

Nursing Activities

Also see Nursing Activities for Body Temperature: Imbalanced, Risk for on pp. 44–45.

Assessments

- Monitor for seizure activity
- Monitor hydration (e.g., skin turgor, moist mucous membranes)
- Monitor blood pressure, pulse, and respirations
- *For surgery patients:*
  Obtain personal and family history of malignant hyperthermia, deaths from anesthesia, or postoperative fever
  Monitor for signs of malignant hyperthermia (e.g., fever, tachypnea, arrhythmias, BP changes, mottled skin, rigidity, profuse sweating)
- *(NIC) Temperature Regulation:*
  Monitor temperature at least every 2 hr, as appropriate
  Institute a continuous core temperature monitoring device, as appropriate
  Monitor skin color and temperature

Patient/Family Teaching

- Instruct patient and family in measures for prevention and early recognition of hyperthermia (e.g., heatstroke and heat exhaustion)
- *(NIC) Temperature Regulation:* Teach indications of heat exhaustion and appropriate emergency treatment, as appropriate

Collaborative Activities

- *(NIC) Temperature Regulation:*
  Administer antipyretic medication, as appropriate
  Use cooling mattress and tepid baths to adjust altered body temperature, as appropriate

Other

- Remove excess clothing and cover patient with only a sheet
- Apply cool washcloths (or ice bag covered with a cloth) to axilla, groin, forehead, and nape of neck

- Encourage intake of oral fluids
- Use a circulating fan in patient's room
- Use a cooling blanket
- For malignant hyperthermia:
    Perform emergency care according to protocol
    Keep emergency equipment in operative areas according to protocol

---

HYPOTHERMIA
(00006) (1986, 1988)

Definition: Body temperature below normal range

Defining Characteristics

Objective
Cool skin
Cyanotic nail beds
Hypertension
Pallor
Piloerection
Reduction in body temperature below normal range
Shivering
Slow capillary refill
Cardiac dysrhythmias (non-NANDA International)

Related Factors
Aging
Consumption of alcohol
Damage to hypothalamus
Decreased basal metabolic rate
Evaporation from skin in cool environment
Illness or trauma
Inability or decreased ability to shiver
Inactivity
Inadequate clothing
Medications causing vasodilation
[Prolonged] exposure to cool or cold environment

Other Related Factors (non-NANDA International)
Hypothyroidism
Immaturity of newborn's temperature regulatory system
Loss of subcutaneous fat and malnutrition
Low birth weight

Suggestions for Use

Because severe *Hypothermia* (rectal temperature below 35 °C or 95 °F) may cause complications such as impaired myocardial or respiratory function, such low readings should be reported to the physician. Mild *Hypothermia* (95–97 °F or 35–36 °C) should respond to nursing interventions.

Suggested Alternative Diagnoses

Body temperature, risk for imbalanced
Hypothermia, risk for
Infant behavior, disorganized, risk for
Thermoregulation, ineffective

NOC Outcomes

Thermoregulation: Balance among heat production, heat gain, and heat loss
Thermoregulation: Neonate: Balance among heat production, heat gain, and heat loss during the neonatal period

Goals/Evaluation Criteria

Also see Goals/Evaluation Criteria for Hyperthermia, p. 000 and for Risk for Imbalanced Body Temperature, p. 252.

Examples Using NOC Language

- Demonstrates **Thermoregulation**, as evidenced by the following indicators (specify 1–5: extremely, substantially, moderately, mildly, or not compromised):
     Presence of goose bumps and shivering when cold
     Reported thermal comfort

Other Examples

Patient and family will:
- Describe measures to prevent/minimize decrease in body temperature
- Report early signs and symptoms of hypothermia
- Maintain patient body temperature of at least 97 °F (36 °C)
Infant will:
- Use heat-retaining posture
- Have blood glucose within normal limits
- Not be lethargic

NIC Interventions

Hypothermia Treatment: Rewarming and surveillance of a patient whose core body temperature is below 35 °C

Newborn Care: Management of neonate during the transition to extrauterine life and subsequent period of stabilization

Temperature Regulation: Attaining or maintaining body temperature within a normal range

Temperature Regulation: Intraoperative: Attaining or maintaining desired intraopertive body temperature

Vital Signs Monitoring: Collection and analysis of cardiovascular, respiratory, and body temperature data to determine and prevent complications

Nursing Activities

Also see Nursing Activities for Risk for Imbalanced Body Temperature, pp. 44–45.

Assessments

- Record baseline vital signs
- Place patient on cardiac monitor
- Use a low-range thermometer, if necessary, to obtain accurate temperature
- Assess for symptoms of hypothermia (e.g., skin color changes, shivering, fatigue, weakness, apathy, slurred speech)
- Assess for medical conditions that contribute to hypothermia (e.g., diabetes, myxedema)
- *(NIC) Temperature Regulation:*
  Institute a continuous core temperature monitoring device, as appropriate
  Monitor temperature at least every 2 hr, as appropriate
  Monitor newborn's temperature until stabilized

Patient/Family Teaching

- *(NIC) Temperature Regulation:*
  Teach patient, particularly elderly patients, actions to prevent hypothermia from cold exposure
  Teach indications of hypothermia and appropriate emergency treatment, as appropriate

Collaborative Activities

- For severe hypothermia, assist with core-warming techniques (e.g., hemodialysis, peritoneal dialysis, colonic irrigation)

Other

- Provide warmth, dry clothing, heated blankets, mechanical heating devices, adjusted room temperature, hot-water bottles, submersion in warm water, and warm oral fluids, as tolerated
- Do not give intramuscular (IM) or subcutaneous medications to hypothermic patient
  For intraoperative patient:
- Regulate room temperature to maintain patient's warmth
- Cover patient's head and exposed body parts
- Warm blood before administering
- Cover patient with warm blanket for transport after surgery
- *(NIC) Temperature Regulation:*
  Wrap infant immediately after birth to prevent heat loss
  Apply stockinette cap to prevent heat loss of newborn
  Place newborn in Isolette or under warmer, as needed

IDENTITY: PERSONAL, DISTURBED
(00121) (1978)

Definition: Inability to distinguish between self and nonself

Defining Characteristics

To be developed by NANDA International

Objective (non-NANDA International)
Change in social involvement
Extension of body boundary to incorporate environmental
  objects
Grandiose behavior

Related Factors

To be developed by NANDA International

non-NANDA International
Chronic illness
Chronic pain
Congenital defects
Psychologic impairment (specify)
Situational crisis (specify)

Suggestions for Use

None

Suggested Alternative Diagnoses

Confusion, acute

Confusion, chronic

Self-esteem, chronic low

Self-esteem, situational low

Thought processes, disturbed

NOC Outcomes

Distorted Thought Control: Self-restraint of disruption in perception, thought processes, and thought content

Identity: Ability to distinguish between self and nonself and to characterize one's essence

Self-Mutilation Restraint: Ability to refrain from intentional self-inflicted injury (nonlethal)

Goals/Evaluation Criteria

Examples Using NOC Language

- Demonstrates **Identity**, as evidenced by the following indicators (specify 1–5: never, rarely, sometimes, often, or consistently demonstrated):

    Verbalizes clear sense of personal identity

    Verbalizes affirmations of personal identity

    Exhibits congruent verbal and nonverbal behavior about self

    Differentiates self from environment

    Differentiates self from other human beings

    Establishes personal boundaries

Other Examples

Patient will:

- Express willingness to use suggested resources upon discharge
- Identify personal strengths
- Maintain close personal relationships

NIC Interventions

Behavior Management: Self-Harm: Assisting the patient to decrease or eliminate self-mutilating or self-abusive behaviors

Decision-Making Support: Providing information and support for a patient who is making a decision regarding health care

Delusion Management: Promoting the comfort, safety, and reality orientation of a patient experiencing false, fixed beliefs that have little or no basis in reality

Environmental Management: Violence Prevention: Monitoring and manipulation of the physical environment to decrease the potential for violent behavior directed toward self, others, or environment

Hallucination Management: Promoting the safety, comfort, and reality orientation of a patient experiencing hallucinations

Reality Orientation: Promotion of patient's awareness of personal identity, time, and environment

Self-Esteem Enhancement: Assisting a patient to increase his personal judgment of self-worth

Nursing Activities

Also refer to Nursing Activities for Self-Esteem, Chronic Low, on pp. 442–443 and Self-Esteem, Situational Low, on p. 445–446.

Assessments

- Assess need for assistance from social services department for planning care with patient and family
- *(NIC) Self-Esteem Enhancement:*
  Monitor patient's statements of self-worth
  Determine patient's confidence in own judgment
  Monitor frequency of self-negating verbalizations

Patient/Family Teaching

- *(NIC) Decision-Making Support:* Provide information requested by patient
- *(NIC) Self-Esteem Enhancement:* Instruct parents on the importance of their interest and support in their children's development of a positive self-concept

Collaborative Activities

- Offer to make initial phone call to appropriate community resources for patient and family
- Request psychiatric consultation
- *(NIC) Decision-Making Support:*
  Refer to support groups, as appropriate
  Refer to legal aid, as appropriate

Other

- Encourage patient to verbalize concerns about close personal relationships
- Encourage patient to verbalize consequences of physical and emotional changes that have influenced self-concept
- Encourage patient and family to air feelings and to grieve
- Provide care in a nonjudgmental manner, maintaining the patient's privacy and dignity

- *(NIC) Decision-Making Support:*
  Establish communication with patient early in admission
  Facilitate collaborative decision making
  Serve as a liaison between patient and family
- *(NIC) Self-Esteem Enhancement:*
  Encourage patient to identify strengths
  Provide experiences that increase patient's autonomy, as appropriate
  Refrain from negatively criticizing
  Convey confidence in patient's ability to handle situation
  Encourage the patient to evaluate own behavior

INFANT BEHAVIOR, DISORGANIZED
(00116) (1994, 1998)

Definition: Disintegrated physiological and neurobehavioral responses to the environment

Defining Characteristics

Regulatory Problems

Inability to inhibit
Irritability

State-Organization System

Active–awake (fussy, worried gaze)
Diffuse and unclear sleep
Irritable or panicky crying
Quiet–awake (staring, gaze aversion)
State oscillation

Attention-Interaction System

Abnormal response to sensory stimuli (e.g., difficult to soothe, inability to sustain alert status

Motor System

Altered primitive reflexes
Finger splay, fisting, or hands to face
Hyperextension of arms and legs
Increased, decreased, or limp tone
Jittery, jerky, uncoordinated movement
Tremors, startles, twitches

Physiological

"Time-out" signals (e.g., gaze, grasp, hiccup, cough, sneeze, sigh, slack jaw, open mouth, tongue thrust)

Bradycardia, tachycardia, or arrhythmias

Bradypnea, tachypnea, apnea

Feeding intolerances (aspiration or emesis)

Oximeter desaturation

Pale, cyanotic, mottled, or flushed color

Related Factors

Prenatal

Congenital or genetic disorders

Teratogenic exposure

Postnatal

Feeding intolerance

Invasive and painful procedures

Malnutrition

Oral or motor problems

Pain

Prematurity

Individual

Gestational age

Illness

Immature neurologic system

Postconceptual age

Environmental

Physical environment inappropriateness

Sensory deprivation

Sensory inappropriateness

Sensory overstimulation

Caregiver

Cue knowledge deficit

Cue misreading

Environmental stimulation contribution

Suggestions for Use

This diagnosis is most useful for infants, especially premature infants, in neonatal intensive care units. Immature neurologic development and increased or noxious environmental stimuli create a situation in which the infant must use energy for adaptation rather than for growth and development.

Suggested Alternative Diagnoses

Infant behavior: disorganized, risk for

Growth and development, delayed

Infant behavior: organized, readiness for enhanced
Thermoregulation, ineffective

NOC Outcomes

Child Development: 2 Months, 4 Months, 6 Months, and 12 Months:
Milestones of physical, cognitive, and psychosocial progression
by 2 months, 4 months, 6 months, and 12 months of age. [**NOTE:**
NOC lists these separately for each age group.]

Muscle Function: Adequacy of muscle contraction needed for
movement

Neurologic Status: Extent to which the peripheral and central nervous systems receive, process, and respond to internal and
external stimuli

Preterm Infant Organization: Extrauterine integration of physiological and behavioral function by the infant born 24–37 (term)
weeks' gestation

Sleep: Extent and pattern of natural periodic suspension of consciousness during which the body is restored

Thermoregulation, Neonate: Balance among heat production,
heat gain, and heat loss during the neonatal period

Goals/Evaluation Criteria

Examples Using NOC Language

- **Neurologic Status** is normal, as evidenced by the following indicators (specify 1–5: extremely, substantially, moderately, mildly,
or not compromised):

    Neurologic Status: consciousness, central motor control, cranial sensory or motor function, spinal sensory or motor
    function, and autonomic function

    Breathing pattern

    Rest–sleep pattern

    Seizure activity not present

- **Thermoregulation** is not compromised, as evidenced by the following indicators (specify 1–5: extremely, substantially, moderately, mildly, or not compromised):

    Skin temperature in expected range

    Body temperature within normal limits

    Skin color changes not present

    Pulse and respiratory rates in expected range

    Muscle twitching not present

Other Examples

Infant will:

- Exhibit organized neurobehavioral functioning in all systems
- Not be restless or lethargic
- Utilize nonshivering thermogenesis
- Demonstrate no delay from expected range of development: 2 months (e.g., displays some head control in upright position), 4 months (e.g., controls head well), 6 months (e.g., sits with support), and 12 months (e.g., has precise pincer grasp). **NOTE:** Refer to a child development or pediatrics text for a comprehensive list of developmental milestones for each age.
- Exhibit adequate muscle function (e.g., tone and contraction of muscle; control, steadiness, and speed of muscle movement) Parent/Caregiver will:
- Recognize infant behavioral cues that communicate stress
- Modify the environment in response to infant's behaviors
- Demonstrate appropriate handling techniques to enhance normal development

NIC Interventions

Environmental Management: Manipulation of the patient's surroundings for therapeutic benefit

Neurologic Monitoring: Collection and analysis of patient data to prevent or minimize neurological complications

Newborn Care: Management of neonate during the transition to extrauterine life and subsequent period of stabilization

Positioning: Deliberate placement of the patient or a body part to promote physiological and psychological well-being

Sleep Enhancement: Facilitation of regular sleep–wake cycles

Nursing Activities

Assessments

- Determine whether infant is achieving developmental milestones
- Monitor for signs of stress and maladaptation
- Identify infant's self-regulatory behaviors (e.g., sucking, hand-to-mouth movements)
- Observe for causative external environmental factors (e.g., lights, handling, noise)
- Assess for causative internal factors, such as pain and hunger
- Monitor sleep pattern

Patient/Family Teaching

- Teach parents about infant's needs and abilities
- Demonstrate gentle handling of the baby
- Model appropriate response to infant's behavioral cues
- Instruct parents on normal growth and development

Other

- Use sheepskin, water bed, or other protective mattress or pad for infants who do not tolerate frequent position changes
- Encourage parents to hold infant and participate in care to the extent possible
- Provide a consistent caregiver
- Observe for signs of pain and intervene aggressively to treat pain or remove painful stimuli (e.g., medicate with analgesics before painful procedures)
- Space interventions and handling to allow infant to have uninterrupted sleep for 3–4 hr at a time
- Position infant in correct body alignment
- Provide boundaries (e.g., swaddle, hold close) during all treatments and activities
- *(NIC) Environmental Management:*

  Avoid unnecessary exposure, drafts, overheating, or chilling.

  Control or prevent undesirable or excessive noise, when possible

  Reduce environmental stimuli, as appropriate [e.g., speak in a soft tone at the bedside, limit conversation, open and close incubator slowly and quietly, do not tap on incubator, place rolled blankets near infant's head to absorb sound; cover incubator or warmer during sleep periods]

INFANT BEHAVIOR: DISORGANIZED, RISK FOR (00115) (1994)

Definition: Risk for alteration in integration and modulation of the physiologic and behavioral systems of functioning (i.e., autonomic, motor, state, organizational, self-regulatory, and attention-interaction systems)

Risk Factors

Environmental overstimulation

Invasive or painful procedures

Lack of containment or boundaries

Oral/motor problems

Pain
Prematurity

Suggestions for Use

This diagnosis is most useful for infants, especially premature infants, in neonatal intensive care units. Immature neurologic development and increased or noxious environmental stimuli create the risk for a situation in which the infant must use energy for adaptation rather than for growth and development.

Suggested Alternative Diagnoses

Disorganized infant behavior
Development, risk for delayed
Growth, risk for disproportionate
Growth and development, delayed
Infant behavior: organized, readiness for enhanced
Thermoregulation, ineffective

NOC Outcomes

Child Development: 2 Months, 4 Months, 6 Months, and 12 Months: Milestones of physical, cognitive, and psychosocial progression by 2 months, 4 months, 6 months, and 12 months of age [**NOTE:** NOC lists a separate outcome for each age group.]

Comfort Level: Feelings of physical and psychological ease

Neurologic Status: Extent to which the peripheral and central nervous systems receive, process, and respond to internal and external stimuli

Pain Level: Severity of reported or demonstrated pain

Preterm Infant Organization: Extrauterine integration of physiological and behavioral function by the infant born 24–37 (term) weeks' gestation

Sleep: Extent and pattern of natural periodic suspension of consciousness during which the body is restored

Goals/Evaluation Criteria

Examples Using NOC Language

For Thermoregulation and Neurological Status indicators, refer to Goals/Evaluation Criteria for Disorganized Infant Behavior, p. 262.

- Demonstrates **Pain Level**, as evidenced by the following indicators (specify 1–5: severe, substantial, moderate, slight, or none):
    Oral or facial expressions of pain
    Protective body positions

Restlessness or muscle tension

Change in heart rate or blood pressure

Other Examples

Refer to Goals/Evaluation Criteria for Infant Behavior, Disorganized, pp 262–263.

Infant will:

- Receive sufficient and restful sleep

NIC Interventions

Environmental Management: Manipulation of the patient's surroundings for therapeutic benefit

Health Screening: Detecting health risks or problems by means of history, examination, and other procedures

Infant Care: Provision of developmentally appropriate family-centered care to the child under 1 year of age

Newborn Monitoring: Measurement and interpretation of physiologic status of the neonate the first 24 hr after delivery

Parent Education: Infant: Instruction on nurturing and physical care needed during the first year of life

Positioning: Deliberative placement of the patient or a body part to promote physiological and psychological well-being

Risk Identification: Analysis of potential risk factors, determination of health risks, and prioritization of risk reduction strategies for an individual or group

Surveillance: Purposeful and ongoing acquisition, interpretation, and synthesis of patient data for clinical decision making

Nursing Activities

Refer to Nursing Activities for Infant Behavior, Disorganized, pp. 263–264.

The following assessments should be performed the first 24 hr after delivery:

- *(NIC) Newborn Monitoring:*

Temperature, until stabilized

Respiratory rate and breathing pattern

For respiratory distress, hypoglycemia, and anomalies, if mother has diabetes

Newborn's color

For signs of hyperbilirubinemia

Infant's ability to suck

Newborn's first feeding

Newborn's weight

Newborn's first voiding and bowel movement
Umbilical cord
Male newborn's response to circumcision

INFANT BEHAVIOR: ORGANIZED, READINESS FOR ENHANCED
(00117) (1994)

Definition: A pattern of modulation of the physiologic and behavioral systems of functioning of an infant (i.e., autonomic, motor,
state, organizational, self-regulatory, and attentional-interactional
systems) that is satisfactory but that can be improved, resulting in
higher levels of integration in response to environmental stimuli

Defining Characteristics
Objective
Definite sleep–wake states
Response to visual and auditory stimuli
Stable physiologic measures
Use of some self-regulatory behaviors

Related Factors
Pain
Prematurity

Suggestions for Use
Because this is a wellness diagnosis, related factors are not needed in
the diagnostic statement.

Suggested Alternative Diagnoses
Family coping, readiness for enhanced
Infant behavior, disorganized, risk for

NOC Outcomes
Child Development: 2 Months, 4 Months, 6 Months, and 12 Months:
Milestones of physical, cognitive, and psychosocial progression
by 2 months, 4 months, 6 months, and 12 months of age [**NOTE:**
NOC lists a separate outcome for each age group.]
Neurological Status: Extent to which the peripheral and central
nervous systems receive, process, and respond to internal and
external stimuli

Sleep: Extent and pattern of natural periodic suspension of consciousness during which the body is restored

Thermoregulation: Balance among heat production, heat gain, and heat loss

Thermoregulation: Neonate: Balance among heat production, heat gain, and heat loss during the neonatal period

Goals/Evaluation Criteria

Examples Using NOC Language

For Neurological Status indicators, see Examples Using NOC Language for Infant Behavior, Disorganized, on p. 265.

- Demonstrates no delay from expected range of **Child Development (2, 4, 6, and 12 months)** [NOTE: Refer to pediatrics or child development text or NOC manual for specific examples of normal growth and development in each age group.]
- Demonstrates **Thermoregulation**, as evidenced by the following indicators (specify 1–5: extremely, substantially, moderately, mildly, or not compromised):

  Body temperature within normal limits

  Respiratory distress [not present]

  Restlessness or lethargy [not present]

  Skin color changes

  Nonshivering thermogenesis

  Use of heat-retention or heat-dissipation posture

  Weaning from crib to Isolette

  Blood glucose within normal limits

Other Examples

Infant will:

- Exhibit normal neurobehavioral functioning in all systems
- Demonstrate no maladaptive or abnormal compensatory behaviors
- Have normal pattern, amount, and quality of sleep
- Be wakeful at appropriate times

NIC Interventions

Developmental Care: Structuring the environment and providing care in response to behavioral cues and states of the preterm infant

Environmental Management: Attachment Process: Manipulation of the patient's surroundings to facilitate the development of the parent–infant relationship

Health Screening: Detecting health risks or problems by means of history, examination, and other procedures

Infant Care: Provision of developmentally appropriate family-centered care to the child under 1 year of age

Pain Management: Alleviation of pain or a reduction in pain to a level of comfort that is acceptable to the patient

Sleep Enhancement: Facilitation of regular sleep–wake cycles

Nursing Activities

Assessments

- Monitor infant's pattern and amount of sleep
- Assess ability to regulate all physical and behavioral systems (e.g., cardiac, respiratory, sleep–wake states, reciprocal interactions, self-regulatory)

Patient/Family Teaching

- Teach family measures to promote sleep (e.g., comforting behaviors, lifestyle changes, consistent schedules)
- Review the developmental needs of infants (e.g., stimulation, sleep requirements)
- Help parents to identify the infant's signs of overstimulation and stress
- Role model and teach parents to provide age-appropriate auditory, visual, tactile, vestibular, and gustatory stimulation daily, some examples are the following:

    Auditory: Classical music; high-pitched, melodic speaking
    Visual: Face-to-face positioning with eye contact; mobiles and toys in black, white, and red contrasting colors
    Tactile: Skin-to-skin contact; massage; firm, gentle touch
    Vestibular: Rocking
    Gustatory: Pacifier, sucking fingers (non-nutritive sucking)

- Explain that developmental stimulation should occur when infant is alert
- Teach parents to provide developmental stimulation frequently and for short periods rather than long periods
- Role model and teach parents to use gentle touch; a soft, melodic tone of voice; and mutual gazing
- Teach parents to respond to all of the infant's vocalizations

Collaborative Activities

- Schedule medications and treatments to support infant's sleep pattern

- *(NIC) Environmental Management: Attachment Process:* Develop policies that permit presence of significant others as much as desired

Other

- Adjust environment (e.g., light, noise, temperature, mattress, and bed) to promote sleep
- Maintain infant's usual bedtime routines, (e.g., rocking, pacifier)
- Use massage, positioning, and touch to relax infant and promote sleep
- Schedule treatments to minimize interference with infant's sleep (allow cycle of at least 90 min)
- Support the infant's self-regulatory behaviors (e.g., hand-to-mouth movements, sucking on fingers, limb flexion) for coping with environmental stimuli
- *(NIC) Environmental Management: Attachment Process:*
  Limit number of people in delivery room
  Place infant bassinet at head of mother's bed
  Maintain warm body temperature of newborn
  Provide comfortable chair for father or significant other
  Provide sufficiently long tubing to allow freedom of movement, as appropriate
  Maintain consistency of staff assignment over time
  Maintain low level of stimuli in patient and family environment
  Explain options and then let family choose hospital environment and visitation plan that best meets their needs
  Permit father or significant other to sleep in room with mother
  Reduce interruptions by hospital personnel

INFANT FEEDING PATTERN, INEFFECTIVE (00107) (1992)

Definition: Impaired ability to suck or coordinate the suck and swallow response

Defining Characteristics

Objective
Inability to coordinate sucking, swallowing, and breathing
Inability to initiate or sustain an effective suck

Related Factors

Anatomical abnormalities
Neurologic impairment or delay
Oral hypersensitivity
Prematurity
Prolonged NPO

Suggestions for Use

This label describes a baby with sucking or swallowing difficulties. It focuses on the nutritional needs of the infant. The goal of nursing activities is to prevent weight loss or promote weight gain. Use the defining characteristics in Table 3 on p. 53 to discriminate among this label and the suggested alternative diagnoses.

Suggested Alternative Diagnoses

Breastfeeding, ineffective
Breastfeeding, interrupted
Growth, disproportionate, risk for
Nutrition, imbalanced: less than body requirements

NOC Outcomes

Breastfeeding Establishment: Infant: Proper attachment of an infant to and sucking from the mother's breast for nourishment during the first 2–3 weeks

Breastfeeding Maintenance: Continued nourishment of an infant through breastfeeding

Muscle Function: Adequacy of muscle contraction needed for movement

Nutritional Status: Food and Fluid Intake: Amount of food and fluid taken into the body over a 24-hr period

Swallowing Status: Extent of safe passage of fluids or solids from the mouth to the stomach

Swallowing Status: Esophageal Phase: Adequacy of the passage of fluids or solids from the pharynx to the stomach

Swallowing Status: Oral Phase: Adequacy of preparation, containment, and posterior movement of fluids or solids in the mouth for swallowing

Swallowing Status: Pharyngeal Phase: Adequacy of the passage of fluids or solids from the mouth to the esophagus

Goals/Evaluation Criteria

Examples Using NOC Language

- Demonstrates **Breastfeeding Establishment: Infant**, as evidenced by the following indicators (specify 1–5: not, slightly, moderately, substantially, or totally adequate):

  Proper alignment and latch-on response

  Proper areolar grasp and compression

  Correct suck and tongue placement

  Audible swallow

  Six or more urinations per day (after infant is 2–3 days of age)

- Demonstrates **Breastfeeding Maintenance**, as evidenced by the following indicators (specify 1–5: not, slightly, moderately, substantially, or totally adequate):

  Infant's growth and development is in normal range

  Mother's freedom from breast tenderness

Other Examples

- Infant coordinates suck and swallow with respirations while maintaining heart rate and color
- Oral food and fluid intake are adequate

NIC Interventions

Breastfeeding Assistance: Preparing a new mother to breast-feed her infant

Enteral Tube Feeding: Delivering nutrients and water through a gastrointestinal tube

Lactation Counseling: Use of an interactive helping process to assist in maintenance of successful breastfeeding

Nonnutritive Sucking: Provision of sucking opportunities for infant

Swallowing Therapy: Facilitating swallowing and preventing complications of impaired swallowing

Tube Care: Umbilical Line: Management of a newborn with an umbilical catheter

Nursing Activities

Assessments

- Assess infant's readiness for nipple feeding:

  Coordination of sucking, swallowing, and breathing (34 weeks)

  Presence of gag reflex (32 weeks)

  Presence of mature sucking reflex (32–34 weeks)

  Presence of rooting reflex (28–36 weeks)

- Assess daily whether the infant is ready to advance. Consider a feeding flow sheet to facilitate assessment; document infant's state, oxygen needs, preferred nipple, position, formula type and temperature, amount of feeding taken in first 10 min, total feeding, total feeding time, daily weight, and stool pattern
- At each feeding, assess infant's nipple feeding skills by evaluating if infant:

  Actively initiates swallow in coordination with suck

  Actively sucks liquid from bottle

  Completes feeding in acceptable time

  Coordinates sucking, swallowing, and breathing

  Loses minimal liquid from mouth
- At each feeding, assess respiratory function and behavioral state and monitor infant for problems such as regurgitation, abdominal distention, and increased residuals
- If infant must be tube-fed:

  Monitor for proper placement of the tube (e.g., check for gastric residual or follow appropriate protocol)

  Monitor for presence of bowel sounds
- *(NIC) Lactation Counseling:*

  Determine knowledge base about breastfeeding

  Determine mother's desire and motivation to breast-feed

  Evaluate mother's understanding of infant's feeding cues (e.g., rooting, sucking, and alertness)

  Monitor maternal skill with latching infant to the nipple

Patient/Family Teaching

- Teach the following to increase success with nipple feeding:

  Avoid techniques that interrupt infant's learning by allowing passive flow of liquid without infant's active participation (e.g., jiggling bottle, moving nipple up and down, moving nipple in and out of infant's mouth, moving infant's jaw up and down)

  Burp the infant frequently

  Choose the most appropriate nipple (consider size, shape, firmness, size of hole)

  Consider varying formula (e.g., by thickness, taste, temperature)

  Calming the infant prior to feeding; during feeding, remove nipple at first sign of respiratory or state changes

  Feed the premature infant when fully alert and eager

  Overfill bottle above amount of scheduled feeding to make sucking easier and to minimize sucking of air

    Position the infant in a semiupright position with head slightly forward and chin tilting down

    Provide consistent caregivers to better read infant's cues and facilitate infant learning; involve mother at earliest opportunity

    Remain relaxed and patient during feeding, allow brief rest periods, pace the infant to complete feeding in appropriate time (too quickly may compromise safety, too slowly may increase fatigue and calorie expenditure)

    Use facilitation techniques (e.g., prior to feeding, increase oral sensitivity by stroking the infant's lips, cheeks, and tongue; during feeding, place your fingers on each cheek and under the jaw midway between the chin and throat to provide inward and forward support of the cheeks and tongue)

- If infant must be tube-fed, inform parents on importance of meeting infant sucking needs
- *(NIC) Lactation Counseling:*

  Demonstrate suck training, as appropriate

  Instruct about infant stool and urination patterns, as appropriate

  Instruct on signs of problems to report to health care practitioner

Collaborative Activities

- Establish support network to ensure that mother has help with day-to-day lactation or breastfeeding problems as they occur
- Refer to a lactation specialist or breastfeeding support group, as needed
- Refer to a physical or occupational therapist any infant who is not progressing with feeding or has structural or oral motor defects
- If infant cannot maintain oral nutrition, provide enteral tube feedings, according to protocol
- Consult with physician or nutritionist regarding type and strength of enteral feeding

Other

- Arrange for home visit within 72 hr of discharge
- Determine most appropriate feeding method (e.g., nipple feeding; intermittent gavage; continuous feeding with nasogastric [NG] tube, jejunal tube, or gastrostomy)
- If infant must be tube-fed:

  Elevate head of the bed or hold infant during feedings

  Offer pacifier to infant during feeding

Talk to infant during feeding

Perform daily skin care around feeding device, keep feeding site dry

Change feeding containers and tubing every 24 hr

INFECTION, RISK FOR
(00004) (1986)

Definition: At increased risk for being invaded by pathogenic organisms

Risk Factors

Chronic disease

Immunosuppression

Inadequate acquired immunity

Inadequate primary defenses (e.g., broken skin, traumatized tissue, decrease in ciliary action, stasis of body fluids, change in pH secretions, altered peristalsis)

Inadequate secondary defenses (e.g., decreased hemoglobin, leukopenia, suppressed inflammatory response)

Insufficient knowledge to avoid exposure to pathogens

Invasive procedures

Malnutrition

Pharmaceutical agents

Rupture of amniotic membranes

Tissue destruction and increased environmental exposure

Trauma

Suggestions for Use

Do not use this label routinely for patients with surgical incisions. For the common surgical population, maintaining routine standards of care will prevent incision infection. Likewise, do not use *Risk for infection* routinely for patients who have an indwelling catheter. Aseptic technique is expected. Everyone is, in a sense, at risk for infection. Therefore, use this nursing diagnosis only for those patients who are at higher than "usual" risk, for example, those with nutritional deficits or compromised immune systems. For patients with actual infection, use a collaborative problem (e.g., Potential Complication: sepsis).

Suggested Alternative Diagnoses

Injury, risk for
Nutrition, imbalanced: less than body requirements
Protection, ineffective
Skin integrity, impaired

NOC Outcomes

Immune Status: Adequacy of natural and acquired appropriately targeted resistance to internal and external antigens

Infection Status: Presence and extent of infection

Knowledge: Infection Control: Extent of understanding conveyed about prevention and control of infection

Risk Control: Sexually Transmitted Diseases (STD): Actions to eliminate or reduce behaviors associated with STD

Risk Detection: Actions taken to identify personal health threats

Wound Healing: Primary Intention: The extent to which cells and tissues have regenerated following intentional closure

Wound Healing: Secondary Intention: The extent to which cells and tissues in an open wound have regenerated

Goals/Evaluation Criteria

Examples Using NOC Language

- Risk factors for infection will be eliminated as evidenced by adequacy of patient's Immune Status, substantial Knowledge: Infection Control, and consistently demonstrated Risk Detection and Risk Control behaviors
- Patient will demonstrate **Risk Control**, as evidenced by the following indicators (specify 1–5: never, rarely, sometimes, often, or consistently demonstrated):

    Obtains appropriate immunizations
    Monitors environmental and personal behavior risk factors
    Avoids exposure to health threats
    Modifies lifestyle to reduce risk

Other Examples

   Patient/family will:
- Be free of signs and symptoms of infection
- Demonstrate adequate personal hygiene
- Indicate gastrointestinal, respiratory, genitourinary, and immune status within normal limits
- Describe factors contributing to infection transmission
- Report signs and symptoms of infection and follow screening and monitoring procedures

NIC Interventions

Circulatory Care: Arterial Insufficiency: Promotion of arterial circulation

Health Screening: Detecting health risks or problems by means of history, examination, and other procedures

Immunization/Vaccination Management: Monitoring immunization status, facilitating access to immunizations, and provision of immunizations to prevent communicable disease

Infection Control: Minimizing the acquisition and transmission of infectious agents

Infection Protection: Prevention and early detection of infection in a patient at risk

Incision Site Care: Cleansing, monitoring, and promotion of healing in a wound that is closed with sutures, clips, or staples

Teaching: Safe Sex: Providing instruction concerning sexual protection during sexual activity

Teaching: Sexuality: Assisting individuals to understand physical and psychosocial dimensions of sexual growth and development

Wound Care: Prevention of wound complications and promotion of wound healing

Nursing Activities

Assessments

- Monitor for signs and symptoms of infection (e.g., temperature, pulse rate, drainage, appearance of wound, secretions, appearance of urine, skin temperature, skin lesions, fatigue, malaise)
- Assess for factors that increase vulnerability to infection (e.g., advanced age, immunocompromise, malnutrition)
- Monitor laboratory values (e.g., CBC, absolute granulocyte count, differential results, cultures, serum protein, and albumin)
- Observe performance of personal hygiene practices to protect against infection

Patient/Family Teaching

- Explain to patient and family why illness or therapy increases the risk for infection
- Instruct in performance of personal hygiene practices to protect against infection
- Teach parents recommended immunization schedule for diphtheria, tetanus, pertussis, polio, measles, mumps, and rubella)
- Explain rationale and benefits for and side effects of immunizations
- Provide patient and family a method for keeping a record of immunizations (e.g., form, diary)

- Teach safe methods of food handling, preparation, or storage
- *(NIC) Infection Control:*
  Instruct patient on appropriate hand-washing techniques
  Instruct visitors to wash hands on entering and leaving the
    patient's room
  Teach patient and family about signs and symptoms of infection
    and when to report them to the health care provider

Collaborative Activities

- Refer patient and family to social services or community
  resources to assist in managing home, hygiene, and nutrition
- Follow agency protocol for reporting suspected infections or
  positive cultures
- Refer to social services for help in paying for immunizations
  (e.g., insurance coverage and health department clinics)
- *(NIC) Infection Control:* Administer antibiotic therapy, as appropriate

Other

- Help patient and family identify factors in their environment,
  lifestyle, or health practices that increase risk of infection
- Protect patient from cross-contamination by not assigning same
  nurse to another patient with an infection and not rooming
  patient with an infected patient
- *(NIC) Infection Control:*
  Clean the environment appropriately after each patient use
  Maintain isolation techniques, as appropriate
  Institute universal precautions
  Limit the number of visitors, as appropriate

INJURY, RISK FOR
(00035) (1978)

Definition: At risk of injury as a result of environmental conditions
  interacting with the individual's adaptive and defensive resources

Risk Factors

Internal

Abnormal blood profile (e.g., leukocytosis or leukopenia)
Altered clotting factors
Biochemical or regulatory function (e.g., sensory dysfunction)
Decreased hemoglobin

Developmental age (physiological, psychosocial)
Effector dysfunction
Immune or autoimmune disorder
Integrative dysfunction
Malnutrition
Physical (e.g., broken skin, altered mobility)
Psychologic (affective orientation)
Sickle cells
Thalassemia
Thrombocytopenia
Tissue hypoxia

External

Biological
Immunization level of community
Microorganisms

Chemical
Drugs (e.g., pharmaceutical agents, alcohol, caffeine, nicotine, preservatives, cosmetics, and dyes)
Nutrients (e.g., vitamins, food types)
Poisons
Pollutants

Physical
Design, structure, and arrangement of community, building, or equipment
Mode of transport or transportation
People or provider (nosocomial agents; staffing patterns; cognitive, affective, and psychomotor patterns)

Suggestions for Use

This is a broad label that includes internal risk factors such as altered clotting factors and decreased hemoglobin. It is important to identify only those patients who are at unusually high risk for this problem. Everyone has at least some risk for accidents and injury, but the label should be used only for those who require nursing intervention to prevent injury. **NOTE:** It may be useful to use the label *Disturbed sensory perception* as an etiology for *Risk for injury*.

Several diagnoses describe injury more specifically: *Latex allergy response; Risk for latex allergy response;* and *Risk for suffocation, poisoning, trauma, aspiration,* and *disuse syndrome.* When possible, use these more specific labels instead of *Risk for injury* because they provide clearer direction for nursing care. They need no further specification except for *Risk for trauma,* which includes wounds, burns, and fractures, as well as many other risk factors.

Some nurses use the label *Risk for injury* to describe the potential for such conditions as malignant hyperthermia. It is also sometimes used as a general description for the potential for fetal distress that exists during labor. Those conditions are more usefully described as collaborative problems; however, for nurses who do not use collaborative problems, this text includes goals and nursing interventions for those situations.

Suggested Alternative Diagnoses

Aspiration, risk for
Disturbed sensory perception (visual, auditory, kinesthetic, gustatory, tactile, olfactory)
Home maintenance, impaired
Infection, risk for
Latex allergy response
Latex allergy response, risk for
Poisoning, risk for
Protection, ineffective
Suffocation, risk for
Thought processes, disturbed
Trauma, risk for
Violence: self-directed, risk for

NOC Outcomes

Fetal Status: Intrapartum: Conditions and behaviors indicative of fetal well-being from onset of labor to delivery

Immune Status: Adequacy of natural and acquired appropriately targeted resistance to internal and external antigens

Maternal Status: Intrapartum: Conditions and behaviors indicative of maternal well-being from onset of labor to delivery

Parenting: Social Safety: Parental actions to avoid social relationships that might cause harm or injury

Risk Control: Actions to eliminate or reduce actual, personal, and modifiable health threats

Safety Behavior: Home Physical Environment: Individual or caregiver actions to minimize environmental factors that might cause physical harm or injury in the home

Safety Behavior: Personal: Individual or caregiver efforts to control behaviors that might cause physical injury

Safety Status: Falls Occurrence: Number of falls in the past week

Safety Status: Physical Injury: Severity of injuries from accidents and trauma

Goals/Evaluation Criteria

Examples Using NOC Language

- *Risk for injury* will be decreased, as evidenced by Parenting: Social Safety and Safety Behavior: Fall Prevention.
- **Risk Control** will be demonstrated, as evidenced by the following indicators (specify 1–5: never, rarely, sometimes, often, or consistently demonstrated):

    Monitors environmental and personal behavior risk factors

    Develops and follows selected risk control strategies

    Modifies lifestyle to reduce risk

Other Examples

Patient and family will:

- Provide a safe environment (e.g., eliminate clutter and spills, place handrails, and use rubber shower mats and grab bars)
- Identify risks that increase susceptibility to injury
- Avoid physical injury

Parents will:

- Recognize risk of and monitor for abuse
- Screen playmates, caregivers, and other social contacts
- Recognize signs of gang membership and other high-risk social behaviors

NIC Interventions

Allergy Management: Identification, treatment, and prevention of allergic responses to food, medications, insect bites, contrast material, blood, or other substances

Behavior Modification: Promotion of a behavior change

Electronic Fetal Monitoring: Intrapartum: Electronic evaluation of fetal heart-rate response to uterine contractions during intrapartal care

Environmental Management: Safety: Monitoring and manipulation of the physical environment to promote safety

Fall Prevention: Instituting special precautions with patient at risk for injury from falling

Health Education: Developing and providing instruction and learning experiences to facilitate voluntary adaptation of behavior conducive to health in individuals, families, groups, or communities

Health Screening: Detecting health risks or problems by means of history, examination, and other procedures

Immunization/Vaccination Management: Monitoring immunization status, facilitating access to immunizations, and provision of immunizations to prevent communicable disease

Intrapartal Care: High-Risk Delivery: Assisting vaginal birth of multiple or malpositioned fetuses

Labor Induction: Initiation or augmentation of labor by mechanical or pharmacological methods

Latex Precautions: Reducing the risk of a systemic reaction to latex [**NOTE:** Although this is listed as a priority intervention, no nursing activities will be listed for it. If the patient requires Latex Precautions, use a diagnosis of *Risk for* or *actual Latex allergy response* rather than *Risk for injury.*]

Malignant Hyperthermia Precautions: Prevention or reduction of a hypermetabolic response to pharmacologic agents used during surgery. [**NOTE:** Although NIC lists this as a priority intervention, no nursing activities are provided for it here. If the patient requires Malignant Hyperthermia Precautions, use a nursing diagnosis of *Risk for hyperthermia* instead of *Risk for injury.*]

Parent Education: Adolescent: Assisting parents to understand and help their adolescent children

Parent Education: Childrearing Family: Assisting parents to understand and promote the physical, psychological, and social growth and development of their toddler or preschool or school-aged child or children

Patient Contracting: Negotiating an agreement with a patient that reinforces a specific behavior change

Risk Identification: Analysis of potential risk factors, determination of health risks, and prioritization of risk reduction strategies for an individual or group

Risk Identification: Childbearing Family: Identification of an individual or family likely to experience difficulties in parenting and prioritization of strategies to prevent parenting problems

Self Modification Assistance: Reinforcement of self-directed change initiated by the patient to achieve personally important goals

Surveillance: Safety: Purposeful and ongoing collection and analysis of information about the patient and the environment for use in promoting and maintaining patient safety

Nursing Activities

Because this diagnostic label is so broad, nursing activities vary greatly depending on the problem etiology. It is not possible to anticipate every possible nursing activity that might be used for this diagnosis.

Assessments

- Identify factors that affect safety needs, for example, changes in mental status, degree of intoxication, fatigue, maturational age, medications, and motor or sensory deficit (e.g., with gait, balance)
- Identify environmental factors that create risk for falls (e.g., slippery floors, throw rugs, open stairways, windows, swimming pools)
- Check patient for presence of constrictive clothing, cuts, burns, or bruises
- *(NIC) Electronic Fetal Monitoring: Intrapartum:*

    Institute electronic fetal monitoring during intrapartal care, according to agency protocols

    Review obstetrical history for pertinent information that may influence induction, such as gestational age and length of prior labor and such contraindications as complete placenta previa, classical uterine incision, and pelvic structural deformities

Patient/Family Teaching

- Instruct patient and family in techniques to prevent injury at home, specify techniques
- Instruct patient to use caution in use of heat-therapy devices
- Provide educational materials related to strategies and measures to prevent injury
- Provide information on environmental hazards and characteristics (e.g., stairs, windows, cupboard locks, swimming pools, streets, gates)
- *(NIC) Electronic Fetal Monitoring: Intrapartum:*

    Instruct woman and support person(s) about the reason for electronic monitoring, as well as information to be obtained

    Discuss appearance of rhythm strip with mother and support person

Collaborative Activities

- Refer to educational classes in the community
- *(NIC) Electronic Fetal Monitoring: Intrapartum:*

    Keep physician informed of pertinent changes in the fetal heart rate, interventions for nonreassuring patterns, subsequent fetal response, labor progress, and maternal response to labor

    Assist with procedures to induce labor, if indicated, according to agency protocols and procedures

Other

For adults:

- Reorient patient to reality and immediate environment when necessary
- Assist patient with ambulation, as needed
- Provide assistive devices for walking (e.g., cane, walker)
- Use heating devices with caution to prevent burns in patients with sensory deficit
- Use an alarm to alert caretaker when patient is getting out of bed or leaving room
- If necessary, use physical restraints to limit risk of falling
- Place bell or call light within reach of dependent patient at all times
- Instruct patient to call for assistance with movement, as appropriate
- Remove environmental hazards (e.g., provide adequate lighting)
- Make no unnecessary changes in physical environment (e.g., furniture placement)
- Ensure that patient wears proper shoes (e.g., nonskid soles, secure fasteners)

    For children:

- Raise side rails when not present at bedside
- For children old enough to climb over bed rails, use a crib with a net or bubble top
- *(NIC) Electronic Fetal Monitoring: Intrapartum:* Calibrate equipment, as appropriate, for internal monitoring with a spiral electrode and/or intrauterine pressure catheter

KNOWLEDGE, DEFICIENT (SPECIFY)
(00126) (1980)

Definition: Absence or deficiency of cognitive information related to specific topic

Defining Characteristics
Subjective
Verbalization of the problem
Objective
Inaccurate follow-through of instruction
Inaccurate performance on tests
Inappropriate or exaggerated behaviors (e.g., hysteria, hostility, agitation, or apathy)

Related Factors
Cognitive limitation
Information misinterpretation
Lack of exposure
Lack of interest in learning
Lack of recall
Unfamiliarity with information resources

Suggestions for Use
Deficient knowledge is not recommended as a problem label for the following reasons:
- *Deficient knowledge* is not truly a human response. "Response" suggests a behavior or action; *Deficient knowledge* is simply a state of being.
- *Deficient knowledge* does not necessarily describe a health state.
- *Deficient knowledge* does not necessarily describe a problem. Nursing diagnoses should reflect altered functioning; but *Deficient knowledge* simply means the person lacks some knowledge, not that his functioning is changed as a result of that lack of knowledge.

Deficient knowledge can contribute to a number of problem responses, including *Anxiety, Impaired parenting, Self-care deficit,* or *Ineffective coping.* Therefore, it may be used effectively as the etiology of a nursing diagnosis (e.g., *Risk for injury [trauma]* related to lack of knowledge of proper application of seat belts when pregnant or *Anxiety related to lack of knowledge of procedures involved in bone marrow aspiration*).

If *Deficient knowledge* is used as the problem part of a nursing diagnosis, one goal must be "Patient will acquire knowledge about . . . ." This causes the nurse to focus on giving information rather than focusing on the behaviors caused by the patient's lack of knowledge, reinforcing the belief that giving information will change behavior and solve problems. On the other hand, when *Deficient knowledge* is used as an etiology, it focuses attention on behaviors that indicate self-doubt, decisional conflict, anxiety, and so forth. Note the difference in nursing care suggested by the following diagnostic statements:

Deficient knowledge (bone marrow aspiration) related to lack of prior experience

Anxiety related to Deficient knowledge (bone marrow aspiration)

Patient teaching is an important intervention for most patients and for all nursing diagnoses (e.g., *Constipation, Ineffective breastfeeding*). Therefore, it is not necessary, or even desirable, to have a *Deficient knowledge* diagnosis on every patient's care plan. Nurses should include teaching as one of the nursing interventions for all the other diagnoses that they make.

Some patients, such as a newly diagnosed diabetic, require a great deal of teaching in order to acquire necessary self-care skills. Such special teaching plans should be a part of the routine care on standardized care plans for these patients and should not require an individualized nursing diagnosis. However, if the agency does not have a standardized plan or protocol, it will be necessary to write an individualized teaching plan. Even then, *Deficient knowledge* should be used as the etiology of a response, for example, *Risk for ineffective health maintenance (diabetes management) related to Deficient knowledge (medication, diet, exercise, and skin care) secondary to new diagnosis.*

If used at all, *Deficient knowledge* should describe conditions in which the patient needs new or additional knowledge. It should not be used for problems involving the patient's ability to learn (e.g., *Deficient knowledge related to severe anxiety about outcome of surgery*). Rakel and Bulechek (1990) propose a diagnosis of *Situational learning disability: Impaired ability to learn* or *Situational learning disability: Lack of motivation to learn* for such conditions. However, these are not yet NANDA International labels.

At least two studies have shown that *Deficient knowledge* is one of the diagnoses most frequently used (misused) by nurses (Gordon, 1985; Lambert & Jones, 1989). This may be due in part to premature diagnosing: It is easy to recognize a knowledge deficit, label it as a problem, and not look beyond that to the human response to the lack of knowledge. Misuse of this diagnosis also occurs because of the mistaken belief that information giving effectively changes human behavior.

Suggested Alternative Diagnoses

Adjustment, impaired

Coping [individual], ineffective

Denial, ineffective

Health maintenance, ineffective

Home maintenance, impaired

Management of therapeutic regimen: community/family/individual, ineffective

Noncompliance (specify)

NOC Outcomes

Knowledge: [specify]: Extent of understanding conveyed about, [e.g.,] Breastfeeding.

[**NOTE:** NOC has 26 Knowledge outcomes: Breastfeeding, Child Safety, Conception Prevention, Diabetes Management, Diet, Disease Process, Energy Conservation, Fertility Promotion, Health Behaviors, Health Promotion, Health Resources, Illness Care, Infant Care, Infection Control, Labor and Delivery, Maternal–Child Health, Medication, Personal Safety, Postpartum, Preconception, Pregnancy, Prescribed Activity, Sexual Functioning, Substance Use Control, Treatment Procedure(s), and Treatment Regimen. Conceivably, any subject or outcome could be placed after the NOC Knowledge outcome.]

Goals/Evaluation Criteria

Examples Using NOC Language

- Demonstrates **Knowledge: Diet**, as evidenced by the following indicators (specify 1–5: none, limited, moderate, substantial, or extensive):

    Description of recommended diet

    Explanation of rationale for recommended diet

    Selection of foods recommended in diet

    Development of strategies to change dietary habits

    Performance of self-monitoring activities

Other Examples

Patient and family will:

- Identify need for additional information regarding prescribed treatment (e.g., diet information about)
- Demonstrate ability to _____ (specify skill or behavior)

NIC Interventions

Breastfeeding Assistance: Preparing a new mother to breastfeed her infant

Childbirth Preparation: Providing information and support to facilitate childbirth and to enhance the ability of an individual to develop and perform the role of parent

Family Planning: Contraception: Facilitation of pregnancy prevention by providing information about the physiology of reproduction and methods to control conception

Family Planning: Infertility: Facilitation of pregnancy prevention by providing information about the physiology of reproduction and methods to control conception

Fertility Preservation: Providing information, counseling, and treatment that facilitate reproductive health and the ability to conceive

Health Education: Developing and providing instruction and learning experiences to facilitate voluntary adaptation of behavior conducive to health in individuals, families, groups, or communities

Health System Guidance: Facilitating a patient's location and use of appropriate health services

Infection Protection: Prevention and early detection of infection in a patient at risk

Lactation Counseling: Use of an interactive helping process to assist in maintenance of successful breastfeeding

Parent Education: Adolescent: Assisting parents to understand and help their adolescent children

Parent Education: Childrearing Family: Assisting parents to understand and promote the physical, psychological, and social growth and development of their toddler or preschool or school-aged child or children

Parent Education: Infant: Instruction on nurturing and physical care needed during the first year of life

Preconception Counseling: Screening and providing information and support to individuals of childbearing age before pregnancy to promote health and reduce risks

Preparatory Sensory Information: Describing in concrete and objective terms the typical sensory experiences and events associated with an upcoming stressful health care procedure or treatment

Reproductive Technology Management: Assisting a patient through the steps of complex infertility treatment

Risk Identification: Analysis of potential risk factors, determination of health risks, and prioritization of risk reduction strategies for an individual or group

Substance Use Prevention: Prevention of an alcoholic or drug use lifestyle

Teaching, Disease Process: Assisting the patient to understand information related to a specific disease process

Teaching, Individual: Planning, implementation and evaluation of a teaching program designed to address a patient's particular needs

Teaching: Infant Nutrition: Instruction on nutrition and feeding practices during the first year of life

Teaching: Infant Safety: Instruction on safety during first year of life

Teaching: Preoperative: Assisting a patient to understand and mentally prepare for surgery and the postoperative recovery period

Teaching: Prescribed Activity/Exercise: Preparing a patient to achieve or maintain a prescribed level of activity

Teaching: Prescribed Diet: Preparing a patient to correctly follow a prescribed diet

Teaching: Prescribed Medication: Preparing a patient to safely take prescribed medications and monitor their effects

Teaching: Procedure/Treatment: Preparing a patient to understand and mentally prepare for a prescribed procedure or treatment

Teaching: Psychomotor Skill: Preparing a patient to perform a psychomotor skill

Teaching: Safe Sex: Providing instruction concerning sexual protection during sexual activity

Teaching: Sexuality: Assisting individuals to understand physical and psychosocial dimensions of sexual growth and development

Teaching: Toddler Nutrition: Instruction on nutrition and feeding practices during the second and third years of life

Teaching: Toddler Safety: Instruction on safety during the second and third years of life

Nursing Activities

NOTE: Because *Deficient knowledge* is such a broad label, this text provides only general activities. Refer to the NIC manual for nursing activities associated with a specific intervention, such as Teaching Safe Sex or Teaching Psychomotor Skill.

Assessments

- Check for accurate feedback to ensure that patient understands prescribed treatment and other relevant information
- *(NIC) Teaching: Individual:*
  Determine patient's learning needs

  Appraise the patient's current level of knowledge and understanding of content [e.g., knowledge of prescribed procedure or treatment]

  Determine the patient's ability to learn specific information (e.g., developmental level, physiologic status, orientation, pain, fatigue, unfulfilled basic needs, emotional state, and adaptation to illness)

  Determine the patient's motivation to learn specific information (i.e., health beliefs, past noncompliance, bad experiences with health care and learning, and conflicting goals)

  Appraise the patient's learning style

Patient/Family Teaching

- Provide teaching at patient's level of understanding, repeating information as necessary
- Use multiple teaching approaches, return demonstrations, and verbal and written feedback.
- *(NIC) Teaching: Individual:*
  Establish rapport

  Establish teacher credibility, as appropriate

  Set mutual, realistic learning goals with the patient

  Provide an environment conducive to learning

  Select appropriate teaching methods and strategies

  Select appropriate educational materials

  Reinforce behavior, as appropriate

  Provide time for the patient to ask questions and discuss concerns

  Document on the permanent medical record the content presented, the written materials provided, and the patient's understanding of the information or patient behaviors that indicate learning

  Include the family and significant others, as appropriate

Collaborative Activities

- Provide information on community resources that will help the patient maintain his treatment regimen
- Develop a coordinated multidisciplinary teaching plan, specify plan
- Plan with patient and physician adjustment in treatment to facilitate patient's ability to follow prescribed treatment

Other

- Interact with patient in a nonjudgmental manner to facilitate learning

---

KNOWLEDGE (SPECIFY), READINESS FOR ENHANCED (00161) (2002)

Definition: The presence of acquisition of cognitive information related to a specific topic is sufficient for meeting health-related goals and can be strengthened

Defining Characteristics

Subjective

Explains knowledge of the topic

Expresses an interest in learning

Objective

Behaviors congruent with expressed knowledge

Describes previous experiences pertaining to the topic

Related Factors

This is a wellness diagnosis, so no etiology is needed.

Suggestions for Use

See discussion in this section of the diagnosis, *Deficient knowledge*. When possible, use a more specific diagnosis, such as one of the Suggested Alternative Diagnoses.

Suggested Alternative Diagnoses

Management of therapeutic regimen, readiness for enhanced

Nutrition, readiness for enhanced

Parenting, readiness for enhanced

Sleep, readiness for enhanced

Urinary elimination, readiness for enhanced

NOC Outcomes

NOC outcomes have not yet been linked to this new diagnosis; however, the following may be useful:

Knowledge: [specify]: Extent of understanding conveyed about, [e.g.,] Breastfeeding.

[**NOTE:** NOC has 26 Knowledge outcomes: Breastfeeding, Child Safety, Conception Prevention, Diabetes Management, Diet,

Disease Process, Energy Conservation, Fertility Promotion, Health Behaviors, Health Promotion, Health Resources, Illness Care, Infant Care, Infection Control, Labor and Delivery, Maternal–Child Health, Medication, Personal Safety, Postpartum, Preconception, Pregnancy, Prescribed Activity, Sexual Functioning, Substance Use Control, Treatment Procedure(s), and Treatment Regimen. Conceivably, any subject or outcome could be placed after the NOC Knowledge outcome.]

Goals/Evaluation Criteria

Other Examples

Patient and family will:
- Identify need for additional information regarding health-promoting behaviors or prescribed treatment (e.g., diet information about)
- Demonstrate ability to _____ (specify skill or behavior)

NIC Interventions

NIC interventions have not yet been linked to this new diagnosis. Refer to NIC Interventions for *Deficient Knowledge*, on pp. 288–289. Conceivably, many NIC interventions would apply, depending on the patient's situation.

Nursing Activities

NOTE: Refer to Nursing Activities, for *Deficient knowledge*, on pp. 289–291. Because *Deficient knowledge* is such a broad label, this text provides only general activities.

LATEX ALLERGY RESPONSE
(00041) (1998)

Definition: An allergic response to natural latex rubber products

Defining Characteristics

Type I Reactions: Immediate (< 1 hr), can be life threatening
  Skin and Mucous Membranes: Contact urticaria progressing to generalized symptoms; edema of the lips, tongue, uvula, or throat
  Respiratory: Shortness of breath, tightness in chest, wheezing, bronchospasm leading to respiratory arrest
  Cardiovascular: Hypotension, syncope, cardiac arrest

May also include:

Orofacial characteristics: Edema of sclera or eyelids; erythema or itching of the eyes; tearing of the eyes; nasal congestion, itching, or erythema; rhinorrhea; facial erythema; facial itching; oral itching

Gastrointestinal symptoms: Abdominal pain, nausea

Generalized symptoms: Flushing, general discomfort, generalized edema, increasing complaint of total body warmth, restlessness

Type IV Reactions: Delayed onset (hours), eczema, irritation, reaction to additives causes discomfort (e.g., thirams, carbamates), redness

Irritant Reactions: Blisters, chapped or cracked skin, erythema

Related Factors

No immune mechanism response

Suggestions for Use

For situations that frequently cause sensitization allergy to latex, see Risk Factors for Latex Allergy Response, Risk for on pp. 295–296. For both diagnoses, nursing care would focus on avoiding exposure to latex. When an actual allergic reaction occurs, the dermatitis must be treated medically and the nursing diagnoses of *Impaired skin integrity* and *Risk for infection* may be used.

Suggested Alternative Diagnoses

Infection, risk for
Latex allergy response, risk for
Skin integrity, impaired

NOC Outcomes

Immune Hypersensitivity Control: Extent to which inappropriate immune responses are suppressed

Symptom Severity: Extent of perceived adverse changes in physical, emotional, and social functioning

Tissue Integrity: Skin and Mucous Membranes: Structural intactness and normal physiological function of skin and mucous membranes

Goals/Evaluation Criteria

Examples Using NOC Language

- Demonstrates **Symptom Severity**, as evidenced by the following indicators (specify 1–5: severe, substantial, moderate, slight, or none)

    Symptom intensity, frequency, and persistence

Associated fear and anxiety

Impaired role performance

The patient will:

- Regain skin integrity, as evidenced by good hydration; reduced inflammation, scaling, and flaking; decreased inflammation; and verbalizations of reduced itching
- Experience restful sleep
- Not experience respiratory complications (e.g., asthma)
- Exhibit a positive self-concept, as evidenced by expressed feelings of self-worth and satisfaction with interpersonal interactions
- Not experience recurrence of the allergic response to latex

NIC Interventions

Allergy Management: Identification, treatment, and prevention of allergic responses to food, medications, insect bites, contrast material, blood, or other substances

Latex Precautions: Reducing the risk of a systemic reaction to latex

Nursing Activities

Assessments

- Identify source(s) of latex to which the patient was (or might be) exposed
- Assess skin for signs of healing (e.g., decreased redness, flaking, and scaling)
- Assess comfort level
- Assess sleep–rest pattern
- Observe for signs of *Disturbed body image* or *Social isolation*
- Observe for development of asthmatic response (e.g., wheezing, dyspnea)
- *(NIC) Latex Precautions*:

  Monitor latex-free environment

  Monitor patient for signs and symptoms of a systemic reaction

Patient/Family Teaching

- Explain the relationship between skin dryness, the symptom of itching, and the prescribed therapy (i.e., hydration)
- Explain that scratching will only produce more itching
- Suggest that the client wear loose-fitting, open-weave, cotton clothing and avoid rough or tightly woven fabrics

- Explain that keeping the home and work environments at a constant temperature (68–75 °F) and humidity (about 50%) will help decrease itching
- Advise against self-treating with leftover medication at home
- Explain that the skin lesions are not contagious (unless they are infected)
- Teach to bathe daily for 15–20 min and apply emollient or prescribed medication within 4 min after the bath
- Teach to use warm, not hot, water for bathing
- *(NIC) Latex Precautions:*
  Instruct patient and family about latex content in products and substitution with nonlatex products, as appropriate; wearing a medical alert tag; and notifying care providers
  Instruct patient and family about signs of a reaction
  Instruct patient and family about emergency treatment
  Instruct visitors about latex-free environment

Collaborative Activities

- *(NIC) Latex Precautions:* Report information to physician, pharmacist, and other care providers, as indicated

Other

- Encourage client to maintain existing social activities
- Provide alternatives for supplies and equipment containing latex (e.g., condoms, balloons, gloves, urinary or IV catheters)
- *(NIC) Latex Precautions:*
  Place allergy band on patient
  Post sign indicating latex precautions
  Survey environment and remove latex products

LATEX ALLERGY RESPONSE, RISK FOR
(00042) (1998)

Definition: At risk for allergic response to natural latex rubber products

Risk Factors

Allergies to bananas, avocados, tropical fruits, kiwis, and chestnuts
Allergies to poinsettia plants
Conditions needing continuous or intermittent catheterization
History of allergies and asthma
History of reactions to latex (e.g., balloons, condoms, gloves)

Multiple surgical procedures, especially from infancy (e.g., spina bifida)

Professions with daily exposure to latex (e.g., medicine, nursing, dentistry)

Suggestions for Use

This label may be more useful than actual Latex allergy response. See Suggestions for Use on p. 293.

Suggested Alternative Diagnoses

Body image, disturbed
Infection, risk for
Skin integrity, impaired

NOC Outcomes

Immune Hypersensitivity Control: Extent to which inappropriate responses are suppressed

Goals/Evaluation Criteria

The patient will:
- Not experience allergic reaction to latex (e.g., no skin lesions or symptoms)
- Identify and avoid environmental sources of latex

NIC Interventions

Latex Precautions: Reducing the risk of a systemic reaction to latex

Nursing Activities

Also see Nursing Activities for Latex Allergy Response, on pp. 294–295.

Assessments

- Identify source(s) of latex to which the patient is (or may be) exposed both at work and at home
- Assess patient and family knowledge of sources of latex
- Assess knowledge of sensitization and allergic reactions
- *(NIC) Latex Precautions:*
    Question patient or appropriate other about history of neural tube defect (e.g., spina bifida) or congenital urological condition (e.g., exstrophy of the bladder)
    Question patient or appropriate other about history of systemic reactions to natural rubber latex (e.g., facial or scleral edema, tearing eyes, urticaria, rhinitis, and wheezing)

Patient/Family Teaching

- Teach information about sensitization and allergic reactions, as needed
- Advise against self-treating if allergic reaction is suspected
- *(NIC) Latex Precautions:* Instruct patient and family about risk factors for developing a latex allergy

Collaborative Activities

- Help develop agency and organizational policies to decrease worker exposure to latex products
- *(NIC) Latex Precautions:* Refer patient to allergist for allergy testing, as appropriate

Other

- For clients with risk factors (e.g., allergy to bananas, history of asthma), provide alternatives (or sources for alternatives) for supplies and equipment containing latex (e.g., condoms, balloons, gloves, urinary catheters, IV catheters)

LONELINESS, RISK FOR
(00054) (1994)

Definition: At risk for experiencing vague dysphoria

Risk Factors

Affectional deprivation [e.g., death of a spouse]
Cathectic deprivation [e.g., no one to talk to]
Physical isolation [e.g., isolation because of infectious disease]
Social isolation [e.g., shunning by peer group]

Suggestions for Use

Discriminate between this diagnosis and *Social isolation*. *Social isolation* is objective (perceived by others); *Loneliness* is subjective (an inner feeling state). *Social isolation* may be the risk factor or etiology of *Loneliness*. *Loneliness* better describes the feeling response brought about solitude that is not desired by the person. For *Loneliness* that is brought about by physical disability or disfigurement, see *Disturbed body image*.

Suggested Alternative Diagnoses

Body image, disturbed
Grieving, dysfunctional

Relocation stress syndrome
Social interaction, impaired
Social isolation

NOC Outcomes

Loneliness: The extent of emotional, social, or existential isolation response

Social Involvement: Frequency of an individual's social interactions with persons, groups, or organizations

Goals/Evaluation Criteria

Examples Using NOC Language

- Demonstrates resolution of *Loneliness*, as evidenced by Grief Resolution, Social Interaction Skills, and Social Support
- Demonstrates **Social Involvement**, as evidenced by the following indicators (specify 1–5: none, limited, moderate, substantial, or extensive):

    Interaction with close friends, neighbors, family members, or members of work group(s)

    Participation as a member of a church, club, or volunteer group

    Participation in leisure activities

Other Examples

Patient will:

- Use time alone in a positive way when socialization is not possible
- Identify reasons for feelings of loneliness
- Describe a plan for increasing meaningful relationships
- Use effective interpersonal communication skills (e.g., self-disclosure, cooperation, sensitivity, assertiveness, consideration, genuineness, trust, and compromise), specify skills most relevant to patient
- Verbalize adequacy of social supports (e.g., assistance provided by others)
- Indicate willingness to ask others for help
- Effectively accomplish grief work (e.g., express feelings, verbalize acceptance of loss)

NIC Interventions

Family Integrity Promotion: Promotion of family cohesion and unity

Socialization Enhancement: Facilitation of another person's ability to interact with others

Spiritual Support: Assisting the patient to feel balance and connection with a greater power

Visitation Facilitation: Promoting beneficial visits by family and friends

Nursing Activities

Assessments

- Assess the patient's perceived and actual support systems
- Determine risk factors for loneliness (e.g., lack of energy needed for social interaction, poor communication skills)
- Compare client's desire for visitation and social interaction to actual visitation and social interaction
- Monitor patient's response to visits from family and friends
- *(NIC) Family Integrity Promotion:*
  Determine typical family relationships
  Monitor current family relationships

Patient/Family Teaching

- Teach social skills, as needed (e.g., role model self-disclosure)
- Teach patient to monitor own behaviors that contribute to social isolation

Collaborative Activities

- Refer patient to group or program for increased understanding and practice of communication and interaction skills
- *(NIC) Family Integrity Promotion:*
  Refer family to support group of other families dealing with similar problems
  Refer for family therapy, as indicated

Other

- Encourage patient to talk about feelings of loneliness
- Assist patient to discover new interests
- Role-play communication skills and techniques with patient
- Help patient identify strengths and limitations in communicating
- Give positive feedback when patient uses effective social interaction skills
- Help patient to recognize available social supports
- Encourage patient to reach out to others who have similar interests
- Facilitate family visitation
- *(NIC) Family Integrity Promotion:*
  Assist family to maintain positive relationships

Provide for care of patient by family members, as appropriate

Encourage patient to develop closeness in one existing relationship

---

MEMORY, IMPAIRED
(00131) (1994)

Definition: Inability to remember or recall bits of information or behavioral skills. [**NOTE:** *Impaired memory* may be attributed to pathophysiologic or situational causes that are either temporary or permanent.]

Defining Characteristics

Forgets to perform a behavior at a scheduled time

Inability to determine if a behavior was performed

Inability to learn or retain new skills or information

Inability to perform a previously learned skill

Inability to recall factual information

Inability to recall recent or past events

Observed or reported experiences of forgetting

Related Factors

Acute or chronic hypoxia

Anemia

Decreased cardiac output

[Depression]

Excessive environmental disturbances

Fluid and electrolyte imbalance

Neurologic disturbances

Suggestions for Use

Use this diagnosis only if it is possible for the patient's memory to improve. If the impairment is permanent, consider using it as an etiology of another diagnosis, for example, *Self-care deficit* or *Risk for injury*. *Impaired memory* is also a defining characteristic for some other diagnoses, such as *Chronic confusion* and *Disturbed thought processes*, in which other symptoms are also present.

Suggested Alternative Diagnoses

Confusion, chronic

Environmental interpretation syndrome, impaired

Thought processes, disturbed

Tissue perfusion, ineffective (cerebral)

NOC Outcomes

Cognitive Orientation: Ability to identify person, place, and time

Memory: Ability to cognitively retrieve and report previously stored information

Neurologic Status: Consciousness: Extent to which an individual arouses, orients, and attends to the environment

Goals/Evaluation Criteria

Examples Using NOC language

- Demonstrates unimpaired **Memory** and **Child Development: 12 months . . . Adolescence**
- Demonstrates **Cognitive Orientation**, as evidenced by the following indicators (specify 1–5: never, rarely, sometimes, often, or consistently demonstrated): Identifies significant other; current place; and correct day, month, year, and season
- Demonstrates **Neurologic Status: Consciousness**, as evidenced by the following indicators (specify 1–5: extremely, substantially, moderately, mildly, or not compromised):
  Opens eyes to external stimuli
  Obeys commands
  Attends to environmental stimuli

Other Examples

Patient will:
- Use techniques to help improve memory
- Accurately recall immediate, recent, and remote information
- Verbalize being better able to remember

NIC Interventions

Cerebral Perfusion Promotion: Promotion of adequate perfusion and limitation of complications for a patient experiencing, or at risk for, inadequate cerebral perfusion

Memory Training: Facilitation of memory

Neurologic Monitoring: Collection and analysis of patient data to prevent or minimize neurological complications

Reality Orientation: Promotion of patient's awareness of personal identity, time, and environment

<u>Nursing Activities</u>

Assessments

- Assess for depression, anxiety, and increased stressors that may be contributing to memory loss
- Assess neurologic function to determine whether patient has memory loss only or also has problems, such as dementia, which need to be referred for further treatment
- Assess extent and nature of memory loss (e.g., immediate, recent, or remote events; gradual or sudden loss)
- Determine history and present pattern of alcohol use
- Determine which medications or street drugs the client is taking that might affect memory (e.g., marijuana)
- *(NIC) Memory Training:* Monitor patient's behavior during therapy

Patient/Family Teaching

- Explain to the older patient that short-term memory loss frequently occurs with aging
- *(NIC) Memory Training:* Structure the teaching methods according to patient's organization of information

Collaborative Activities

- Refer patients with sudden memory loss to physician
- *(NIC) Memory Training:* Refer to occupational therapy, as appropriate

Other

- Label items (e.g., the bathroom door, the sink, the refrigerator) to increase recall
- Do not rearrange furniture in the room or the patient's home
- Help the patient to relax in order to improve concentration
- *(NIC) Memory Training:*

  Discuss with patient and family any practical memory problems experienced

  Stimulate memory by repeating patient's last expressed thought, as appropriate

  Reminisce about past experiences with patient, as appropriate

  Implement appropriate memory techniques, such as visual imagery, mnemonic devices, memory games, memory cues, association techniques, making lists, using computers, or using name tags, or rehearsing information

  Assist in associated-learning tasks, such as practice learning and recalling verbal and pictorial information presented, as appropriate

Provide for orientation training, such as patient rehearsing personal information and dates, as appropriate

Provide opportunity for concentration, such as a game matching pairs of cards, as appropriate

Provide opportunity to use memory for recent events, such as questioning patient about a recent outing

Provide for picture recognition memory, as appropriate

Encourage patient to participate in group memory training programs, as appropriate

MOBILITY: BED, IMPAIRED
(00091) (1998)

Definition: Limitation of independent movement from one bed position to another [specify level]

Defining Characteristics

Impaired ability to do the following:

Move from supine to long-sitting or long-sitting to supine

Move from supine to prone or prone to supine

Move from supine to sitting or sitting to supine

Turn side to side

"Scoot" or reposition self in bed

Related Factors

To be developed

Suggestions for Use

1. When the patient's bed mobility cannot be improved, this label should be used as a related or risk factor for other nursing diagnoses, such as *Risk for impaired skin integrity.*

2. Specify level of mobility, the same as you would for *Impaired physical mobility* and *Impaired wheelchair mobility:*

Level 0: Is completely independent

Level 1: Requires use of equipment or device

Level 2: Requires help from another person for assistance, supervision, or teaching

Level 3: Requires help from another person and equipment/ device

Level 4: Is dependent; does not participate in activity

3. See Suggestions for Use for Mobility: Physical, Impaired on p. 307.

Suggested Alternative Diagnoses

Disuse syndrome, risk for
Injury, risk for
Mobility: physical, impaired
Skin integrity, risk for impaired

NOC Outcomes

Body Positioning: Self-Initiated: Ability to change own body positions

Cognitive Ability: Ability to execute complex mental processes

Immobility Consequences: Physiological: Extent of compromise in physiological functioning due to impaired physical mobility

Joint Movement: Active: Range of motion of joints with self-initiated movement

Mobility Level: Ability to move purposefully

Muscle Function: Adequacy of muscle contraction needed for movement

Neurological Status: Extent to which the peripheral and central nervous systems receive, process, and respond to internal and external stimuli

Goals/Evaluation Criteria

Examples Using NOC Language

- Achieves *Bed mobility*, as evidenced by Self-Initiated Body Positioning, Active Joint Movement, and satisfactory Mobility Level, Muscle Function, and Neurological Status
- Demonstrates **Mobility Level**, as evidenced by the following indicators (specify 1–5: is dependent [does not participate], requires assistive person and device, requires assistive person, is independent with assistive device, or is completely independent):
    Body positioning performance
    Muscle and joint movement

Other Examples

The patient will:
- Perform full range-of-motion of all joints
- Turn self in bed or state realistic level of assistance needed
- Demonstrate correct use of assistive devices (e.g., trapeze)
- Request repositioning assistance, as needed

NIC Interventions

Bed Rest Care: Promotion of comfort and safety and prevention of complications for a patient unable to get out of bed

Body Mechanics Promotion: Facilitating the use of posture and movement in daily activities to prevent fatigue and musculoskeletal strain or injury

Exercise Promotion: Strength Training: Facilitating regular resistive muscle training to maintain or increase muscle strength

Exercise Promotion: Stretching: Facilitation of systematic slow-stretch-hold muscle exercises to induce relaxation, to prepare muscles and joints for more vigorous exercise, or to increase or maintain body flexibility

Exercise Therapy: Muscle Control: Use of specific activity or exercise protocols to enhance or restore controlled body movement

Positioning: Deliberative placement of the patient or a body part to promote physiological and psychological well-being

Positioning: Neurologic: Achievement of optimal, appropriate body alignment for the patient experiencing or at risk for spinal cord injury or vertebrae irritability

Self-Care Assistance: Assisting another to perform ADL

Teaching: Prescribed Activity/Exercise: Preparing a patient to achieve or maintain a prescribed level of activity

Nursing Activities

Assessments

- Perform ongoing assessment of patient's mobility
- Assess level of consciousness
- Assess muscle strength and joint mobility (range of motion)
- Assess need for assistance from home health agency or other organization
- Assess need for durable medical equipment

Patient/Family Teaching

- Instruct in active and passive range-of-motion exercises to improve muscle strength and endurance
- Instruct in turning techniques and correct body alignment

Collaborative Activities

- Use occupational and physical therapists as resources in developing plan to maintain and increase bed mobility

Other

- Position call light or button within easy reach
- Provide assistive devices (e.g., trapeze)
- Provide positive reinforcement during activities
- Implement pain control measures before beginning exercises or physical therapy
- Ensure care plan includes number of personnel needed to turn patient

---

MOBILITY: PHYSICAL, IMPAIRED
(00085) (1973, 1998)

Definition: Limitation in independent, purposeful physical movement of the body or of one or more extremities [specify level]:

Level 0: Is completely independent

Level 1: Requires use of equipment or device

Level 2: Requires help from another person for assistance, supervision, or teaching

Level 3: Requires help from another person and equipment or device

Level 4: Is dependent; does not participate in activity

Defining Characteristics

Objective

Decreased reaction time

Difficulty turning

Engages in substitutions for movement (e.g., increased attention to other's activity, controlling behavior, focus on pre-illness or disability activity)

Gait changes (e.g., decreased walk, speed, difficulty initiating gait, small steps, shuffles feet, exaggerated lateral postural sway)

Limited ability to perform fine-motor skills

Limited ability to perform gross-motor skills

Limited range of motion

Movement-induced shortness of breath

Movement-induced tremor

Postural instability during performance of routine ADLs

Slowed movement

Uncoordinated or jerky movements

Related Factors

Altered cellular metabolism

Body mass index above 75th age-appropriate percentile

Cognitive impairment

Cultural beliefs regarding age-appropriate activity

Decreased muscle strength, control, or mass

Depressive mood state or anxiety

Developmental delay

Discomfort

Intolerance to activity and decreased strength and endurance

Joint stiffness or contractures

Lack of knowledge regarding value of physical activity

Lack of physical or social environmental supports

Limited cardiovascular endurance

Loss of integrity of bone structures

Medications

Musculoskeletal impairment

Neuromuscular impairment

Pain

Prescribed movement restrictions

Reluctant to initiate movement

Sedentary lifestyle, disuse, or deconditioning

Selective or generalized malnutrition

Sensoriperceptual impairments

Suggestions for Use

Use *Impaired physical mobility* to describe individuals with limited ability for independent physical movement, such as decreased ability to move arms or legs or generalized muscle weakness, or when nursing interventions will focus on restoring mobility and function or preventing further deterioration. For example, an appropriate diagnosis would be *Impaired physical mobility related to ineffective management of Chronic pain secondary to rheumatoid arthritis.*

Do not use this label to describe temporary immobility that cannot be changed by the nurse (e.g., traction, prescribed bedrest) or permanent paralysis. In these and many other instances, Impaired physical mobility can be used effectively as the etiology of a problem. An example of this would be *Impaired tissue integrity (pressure ulcer) related to Impaired physical mobility +4*. When appropriate, use more specific labels, such as *Impaired bed mobility*, *Impaired transfer ability*, *Impaired wheelchair mobility*, or *Impaired walking*.

Suggested Alternative Diagnoses

Disuse syndrome, risk for
Injury, risk for
Mobility: bed, impaired
Mobility: wheelchair, impaired
Self-care deficit
Transfer ability, impaired
Walking, Impaired

NOC Outcomes

Ambulation: Walking: Ability to walk from place to place
Ambulation: Wheelchair: Ability to move from place to place in a wheelchair
Body Positioning: Self-Initiated: Ability to change own body positions
Joint Movement: Active: Range of motion of joints with self-initiated movement
Mobility Level: Ability to move purposefully
Sensory Function: Proprioception: Extent to which the position and movement of the head and body are sensed
Transfer Performance: Ability to change body locations

Goals/Evaluation Criteria

Examples Using NOC Language

- Demonstrates **Mobility Level**, as evidenced by the following indicators (specify 1–5: is dependent [does not participate], requires assistive person and device, requires assistive person, is independent with assistive device, or is completely independent):
  Balance performance
  Body positioning performance
  Muscle and joint movement
  Transfer performance
  Ambulation: walking
  Ambulation: wheelchair

Other Examples

  Patient will:
- Demonstrate correct use of assistive devices with supervision
- Request assistance with mobilization activities, as needed
- Perform ADLs independently with assistive devices (specify activity and device)

- Bear weight
- Walk with effective gait for _____ (specify distance)
- Transfer to and from chair or wheelchair
- Maneuver wheelchair effectively

NIC Interventions

Exercise Promotion: Strength Training: Facilitating regular resistive muscle training to maintain or increase muscle strength

Exercise Therapy: Ambulation: Promotion and assistance with walking to maintain or restore autonomic and voluntary body functions during treatment and recovery from illness or injury

Exercise Therapy: Balance: Use of specific activities, postures, and movements to maintain, enhance, or restore balance

Exercise Therapy, Ambulation: Promotion and assistance with walking to maintain or restore autonomic and voluntary body functions during treatment and recovery from illness or injury

Exercise Therapy, Joint Mobility: Use of active or passive body movement to maintain or restore joint flexibility

Exercise Therapy: Muscle Control: Use of specific activity or exercise protocols to enhance and restore controlled body movement

Positioning: Deliberative placement of the patient or a body part to promote physiological or psychological well-being

Positioning: Wheelchair: Achievement of optimal, appropriate body alignment for the patient experiencing or at risk for spinal cord injury or vertebrae irritability

Nursing Activities

Assessment is an ongoing process to determine the performance level of the patient's Impaired mobility

Level 1 Nursing Activities

- Assess need for home health assistance and need for durable medical equipment
- Teach patient about and monitor use of mobility devices (e.g., cane, walker, crutches, or wheelchair)
- Instruct and assist him with transfer process (e.g., bed to chair)
- Refer to physical therapist for an exercise program
- Provide positive reinforcement during activities
- Assist patient to use supportive, nonskid footwear for walking
- *(NIC) Positioning:*
  Instruct the patient how to use good posture and good body mechanics while performing any activity
  Monitor traction devices for proper setup

Level 2 Nursing Activities

- Assess patient's learning needs
- Assess need for assistance from home health agency and need for durable medical equipment
- Instruct and encourage patient in active or passive range-of-motion exercises to maintain or develop muscle strength and endurance
- Instruct and encourage patient to use a trapeze or weights to enhance and maintain strength of upper extremities.
- Teach techniques for safe transfer and ambulation.
- Instruct patient regarding weight-bearing status
- Instruct patient regarding correct body alignment
- Use occupational and physical therapists as a resource in developing a plan for maintaining or increasing mobility
- Provide positive reinforcement during activities
- Supervise all mobilization attempts and assist patient, as necessary
- Use a gait belt when assisting with transfer or ambulation

Levels 3 and 4 Nursing Activities

- Determine patient motivation level for maintaining or restoring mobility of joints and muscles
- Use occupational and physical therapists as resource in planning patient care activities
- Encourage patient and family to view limitations realistically
- Provide positive reinforcement during activities
- Administer analgesics before beginning exercises
- Develop a plan specifying the following:
  - Type of assistive device
  - Positioning of patient in bed or chair
  - Ways to transfer and turn patient
  - Number of personnel needed to mobilize patient
  - Necessary elimination equipment (e.g., bedpan, urinal, fracture pan)
  - Schedule of activities
- *(NIC) Positioning:*
  - Monitor traction devices for proper setup
  - Place on an appropriate therapeutic mattress or bed
  - Position patient in proper body alignment
  - Place in the designated therapeutic position (e.g., avoid placing the amputation stump in the flexion position; elevate the affected body part, as appropriate; immobilize or support the affected body part, as appropriate)

Turn the immobilized patient at least every 2 hr, according to a specific schedule

Place bed-positioning switch and call light within easy reach

Encourage active range-of-motion exercises

MOBILITY: WHEELCHAIR, IMPAIRED
(00089) (1998)

Definition: Limitation of independent operation of wheelchair within environment [specify level]

Defining Characteristics

Impaired ability to operate manual or power wheelchair on an incline or decline

Impaired ability to operate manual or power wheelchair on even or uneven surface

Impaired ability to operate wheelchair on curbs

Related Factors

To be developed

Suggestions for Use

Specify levels of independence, which are the same as the options for *Impaired physical mobility* and *Impaired bed mobility*:

Level 0: Is completely independent

Level 1: Requires use of equipment or device

Level 2: Requires help from another person for assistance, supervision, or teaching

Level 3: Requires help from another person and equipment and device

Level 4: Is dependent; does not participate in activity

See Suggestions for Use for Mobility: Physical, impaired on p. 307.

Suggested Alternative Diagnoses

Injury, risk for

Mobility: physical, impaired

Skin integrity, risk for impaired

Transfer ability, impaired

NOC Outcomes

Ambulation: Wheelchair: Ability to move from place to place in a wheelchair

Balance: Ability to maintain body equilibrium

Mobility Level: Ability to move purposefully

Muscle Function: Adequacy of muscle contraction needed for movement

Self-Care: Activities of Daily Living (ADL): Ability to perform the most basic physical tasks and personal care activities

Goals/Evaluation Criteria

Examples Using NOC Language

For each indicator in this set of goals, specify the following parameters: is dependent (does not participate), requires assistive person and device, requires assistive person, is independent with assistive device, or is completely independent

- Patient will demonstrate **Ambulation: Wheelchair**, as evidenced by the following indicators:

    Transfers to and from wheelchair

    Propels wheelchair safely

    Maneuvers curbs, doorways, and ramps

- Demonstrates **Mobility Level**, as evidenced by the following indicators: balance performance, muscle movement, joint movement, body positioning performance, and transfer performance

Other Examples

Patient will:

- Request assistance with mobilization activities, as needed
- Perform ADLs independently with or without assistive devices (specify activity and device)
- Demonstrate moderate active movement of all joints or specify affected joints

NIC Interventions

Exercise Promotion: Strength Training: Facilitating regular resistive muscle training to maintain or increase muscle strength

Exercise Therapy: Balance: Use of specific activities, postures, and movements to maintain, enhance, or restore balance

Exercise Therapy: Joint Mobility: Use of active or passive body movement to maintain or restore joint flexibility

Exercise Therapy: Muscle Control: Use of specific activity or exercise protocols to enhance or restore controlled body movement

Positioning: Wheelchair: Placement of a patient in a properly selected wheelchair to enhance comfort, promote skin integrity, and foster independence

Nursing Activities

Assessments

- Assess patient's learning needs regarding use of wheelchair
- Assess need for assistance from home health agency and need for special modifications to wheelchair (e.g., motor)
- Assess joint mobility and muscle strength
- Assess cognitive abilities
- Determine patient's motivation level for using wheelchair
- *(NIC) Positioning: Wheelchair:*
  Check patient's position in the wheelchair while patient sits on selected pad and wears proper footwear
  Monitor for patient's inability to maintain correct posture in wheelchair

Patient/Family Teaching

- *(NIC) Positioning: Wheelchair:*
  Instruct patient on exercises to increase upper body strength, as appropriate
  Teach how to operate wheelchair, as appropriate

Collaborative Activities

- Collaborate with physical and occupational therapists, as needed (e.g., to be certain that wheelchair size and type is appropriate for patient)

Other

- Provide positive reinforcement during activities
- Supervise attempts to operate wheelchair on curbs and inclines
- Encourage patient and family to view limitations realistically
- *(NIC) Positioning: Wheelchair:*
  Check that foot rests have at least 2 inches of clearance from the floor
  Ensure that wheelchair allows at least 2–3 inches of clearance from the back of knee to front of sling seat
  Provide modifications or appliances to wheelchair to correct for patient problems or muscle weakness

NAUSEA
(00134) (1998, 2002)

Definition: A subjective unpleasant, wavelike sensation in the back of the throat, epigastrium, or throughout the abdomen that may lead to the urge or need to vomit

Defining Characteristics

Subjective
Aversion toward food

Gagging sensation

Increased salivation

Increased swallowing

Reports of "nausea" or "sick to stomach"

Sour taste in mouth

<u>Non-NANDA International Symptoms:</u> May be accompanied by pallor, cold and clammy skin, tachycardia, gastric stasis: Diarrhea usually precedes vomiting, but may be experienced after vomiting or when vomiting does not occur.

Related Factors

Treatment Related
Gastric irritation: pharmaceutical agents (e.g., aspirin, nonsteroidal anti-inflammatory drugs [NSAIDs], steroids, antibiotics), alcohol, iron, and blood

Gastric distention: Delayed gastric emptying caused by pharmaceutical agents (e.g., narcotics administration) and anesthesia agents

Pharmaceutical agents (e.g., analgesics, antiviral for HIV, aspirin, opioids) and chemotherapeutic agents

Toxins (e.g., radiotherapy)

Biophysical
Biochemical disorders (e.g., uremia, diabetic ketoacidosis, pregnancy)

Cardiac pain

Cancer of stomach or intra-abdominal tumors (e.g., pelvic or colorectal cancers)

Esophageal or pancreatic disease

Gastric distention due to delayed gastric emptying; pyloric intestinal obstruction; genitourinary and biliary distention; upper bowel stasis; external compression of the stomach, liver, spleen, or other organs; enlargement that slows stomach functioning (squashed stomach syndrome); excess food intake

Gastric irritation due to pharyngeal and peritoneal inflammation

Liver or splenetic capsule stretch

Local tumors such as acoustic neuroma, primary or secondary brain tumors, bone metastases at base of skull

Motion sickness, Meniere's disease, or labyrinthitis

Physical factors such as increased intracranial pressure and meningitis

Toxins (e.g., tumor-produced peptides) and abnormal metabolites due to cancer

Situational

Psychological factors such as pain, fear, anxiety, noxious odors, taste, or unpleasant visual stimulation

Suggestions for Use

This label is appropriate for short-term episodes of nausea and vomiting (e.g., postoperatively). When *Nausea* is severe or prolonged and may compromise adequate nutrition, use *Risk for imbalanced nutrition: less than body requirements related to Nausea.*

Suggested Alternative Diagnoses

Fluid volume, deficient

Nutrition: less than body requirements, risk for imbalanced

NOC Outcomes

Comfort Level: Feelings of physical and psychologic ease

Hydration: Amount of water in the intra- and extracellular compartments of the body

Nutritional Status: Food and Fluid Intake: Amount of food and fluid taken into the body over a 24-hr period

Symptom Severity: Extent of perceived adverse changes in physical, emotional, and social functioning

Goals/Evaluation Criteria

Examples Using NOC Language

- *Nausea* will be relieved, as evidenced by: substantial Comfort Level, uncompromised Hydration Level, substantially adequate Nutritional Status (Food and Fluid Intake), and slight to no Symptom Severity.
- Demonstrates no **Symptom Severity**, as evidenced by the following indicators (specify 1–5: severe, substantial, moderate, slight, or none):

    Symptom intensity

    Symptom frequency

> Symptom persistence
> Associated discomfort
> Associated restlessness
> Impaired role performance
> Compromised life enjoyment
> Lack of appetite

- Demonstrates **Nutritional Status: Food and Fluid Intake**, as evidenced by the following indicators (specify 1–5: not, slightly, moderately, substantially, or totally adequate):

  > Oral food, tubefeeding, or total parenteral nutrition (TPN) intake
  > Oral or IV fluid intake

- Demonstrates **Hydration**, as evidenced by the following indicators (specify 1–5: extremely, substantially, moderately, mildly, or not compromised):

  > Skin hydration
  > Moist mucous membranes
  > Abnormal thirst not present
  > Sunken eyes not present
  > Fever not present
  > Perspiration ability
  > Urine output within normal limits (WNL)
  > BP WNL
  > Hct WNL

Other Examples

The patient will:

- Report relief from nausea
- Identify measures that decrease nausea

NIC Interventions

Fluid Management: Promotion of fluid balance and prevention of complications resulting from abnormal or undesired fluid levels

Fluid Monitoring: Collection and analysis of patient data to regulate fluid balance

Fluid/Electrolyte Management: Regulation and prevention of complications from altered fluid or electrolyte levels

Medication management: Facilitation of safe and effective use of prescription and over-the-counter drugs

Nausea Management: Prevention and alleviation of nausea

Nutritional Monitoring: Collection and analysis of patient data to prevent or minimize malnourishment

Vomiting Management: Prevention and alleviation of vomiting

Nursing Activities

Assessment

- Monitor patient's subjective symptoms of nausea
- Monitor urine color, quantity, and specific gravity
- *(NIC) Nutritional Monitoring:*
  Monitor trends in weight loss and gain
  Monitor for dry, flaky skin with depigmentation
  Monitor skin turgor, as appropriate
  Monitor gums for swelling, sponginess, receding, and increased
    bleeding
  Monitor energy level, malaise, fatigue, and weakness
  Monitor caloric and nutrient intake
- *(NIC) Fluid Management:*
  Maintain accurate intake and output record
  Monitor food and fluid ingested and calculate daily caloric
    intake, as appropriate
  Monitor nutrition status
  Monitor hydration status (e.g., moist mucous membranes, ade-
    quacy of pulses, and orthostatic BP), as appropriate

Patient/Family Teaching

- Teach patient to use voluntary swallowing or deep breathing to
  suppress the vomiting reflex
- Teach to eat slowly
- Teach to restrict fluids 1 hr before, 1 hr after, and during meals
- Instruct to avoid the smell of food preparation at home (e.g., let
  someone else prepare meals, stay out of the kitchen, go for a
  walk during meal preparation)

Collaborative Activities

- Administer prescribed antiemetics
- Consult with physician to provide adequate pain control with
  medications that do not cause nausea for the patient
- *(NIC) Fluid Management:* Administer IV therapy, as prescribed

Other

- Elevate head of bed or place in lateral position to prevent aspiration (for clients with decreased mobility)
- Keep client and bedding clean when vomiting occurs
- Remove odor-producing substances immediately (e.g., bed-
  pans, food)
- Do not schedule pain- or nausea-producing procedures near
  mealtimes

- Provide oral care after vomiting
- Apply cool, damp cloth to patient's wrists, neck, and forehead
- Offer cold foods and other foods with little odor
- *(NIC) Nutritional Monitoring:* Note significant changes in nutritional status and initiate treatments, as appropriate

---

NEUROVASCULAR DYSFUNCTION: PERIPHERAL, RISK FOR (00086) (1992)

Definition: At risk for disruption in circulation, sensation, or motion of an extremity

Risk Factors

Burns

Fractures

Immobilization

Mechanical compression (e.g., tourniquet, cast, brace, dressing, or restraint)

Orthopedic surgery

Trauma

Vascular obstruction

Suggestions for Use

Use this label for situations nurses can prevent by reducing or eliminating causative factors (e.g., *Risk for peripheral neurovascular dysfunction related to compression from restraints*). For situations requiring medical treatment (e.g., thrombophlebitis), use a collaborative problem such as Potential Complication of thrombophlebitis in left leg: *Peripheral neurovascular dysfunction.*

Suggested Alternative Diagnosis

Perioperative positioning injury, risk for

NOC Outcomes

Joint Movement: Active: Range of motion of joints with self-initiated movement

Muscle Function: Adequacy of muscle contraction needed for movement

Neurological Status: Extent to which the peripheral and central nervous systems receive, process, and respond to internal and external stimuli

Neurological Status: Spinal Sensory/Motor Function: Extent to which spinal nerves convey sensory and motor information

Tissue Perfusion: Peripheral: Extent to which blood flows through the small vessels of the extremities and maintains tissue function

Goals/Evaluation Criteria

Examples Using NOC Language

- Demonstrates **Circulation Status**, as evidenced by the following indicators (specify 1–5: extremely, substantially, moderately, mildly, or not compromised):

    Peripheral tissue perfusion not compromised

    Peripheral pulses strong and symmetric

    Peripheral edema not present

- Demonstrates **Neurological Status**, as evidenced by the following indicators (specify 1–5: extremely, substantially, moderately, mildly, or not compromised):

    Neurological status: consciousness, central motor control, autonomic, and cranial and spinal sensory or motor function

- Demonstrates **Tissue Perfusion: Peripheral**, as evidenced by the following indicators (specify 1–5: extremely, substantially, moderately, mildly, or not compromised):

    Brisk capillary refill

    Intact muscle function

    Intact skin

    Warm extremity temperature

    Lack of localized extremity pain

Other Examples

Patient will:

- Recognize signs and symptoms of peripheral neurovascular dysfunction
- Remain free of injury from compression devices or restraints
- Demonstrate optimal healing and adaptation to cast, traction, or dressing
- Have good muscle tone and strong movement of extremities

NIC Interventions

Circulatory Care: Arterial Insufficiency: Promotion of arterial circulation

Circulatory Care: Venous Insufficiency: Promotion of venous circulation

Circulatory Precautions: Protection of a localized area with limited perfusion

Exercise Promotion: Strength Training: Facilitating regular resistive muscle training to maintain or increase muscle strength

Exercise Therapy: Joint Mobility: Use of active or passive body movement to maintain or restore joint flexibility

Exercise Therapy: Muscle Control: Use of specific activity or exercise protocols to enhance or restore controlled body movement

Peripheral Sensation Management: Prevention or minimization of injury or discomfort in the patient with altered sensation

Positioning: Neurologic: Achievement of optimal, appropriate body alignment for the patient experiencing or at risk for spinal cord injury or vertebrae irritability

Nursing Activities

Assessments

- Perform neurovascular assessments every hour for the first 24 hrs following casting, injury, traction, or restraints. Then, if stable, perform the following activities q4h:

  Assess for and report increasing and progressive pain that is present on passive movement and not relieved by narcotics, which may be first sign of compartmental syndrome

  Assess motor function, movement, and strength of the involved peripheral nerve

- *(NIC) Circulatory Care (Arterial and Venous):* Perform a comprehensive appraisal of peripheral circulation (e.g., check peripheral pulses, edema, capillary refill, color, and temperature of extremity)

- *(NIC) Peripheral Sensation Management:*

  Monitor for paresthesia: numbness, tingling, hyperesthesia, and hypoesthesia

  Monitor sharp and dull or hot and cold discrimination

  Monitor fit of bracing devices, prosthesis, shoes, and clothing

  Check shoes, pockets, and clothing for wrinkles or foreign objects

  Monitor for thrombophlebitis and deep vein thrombosis

Patient/Family Teaching

- Teach patient and family routine cast care and measures to prevent complications

- Teach patient and family signs and symptoms of peripheral nerve injury and importance of immediate medical attention

- Teach patient and family to perform passive, assisted, or active range-of-motion exercises
- *(NIC) Circulatory Care (Arterial and Venous):*
  Instruct the patient on proper foot care
  Instruct the patient on the importance of prevention of venous stasis (e.g., not crossing legs, elevating feet without bending knees, and exercise)
- *(NIC) Peripheral Sensation Management:*
  Instruct patient to use timed intervals, rather than presence of discomfort, as a signal to alter position
  Instruct patient or family to use thermometer to test water temperature

Collaborative Activities

- Collaborate with physical therapist in developing and executing an exercise program

Other

- Avoid tight dressings and appliances to prevent ischemia
- Institute immediate treatment if compartmental syndrome is suspected: keep involved extremity at heart level; notify physician; and anticipate removal of anterior cast, occlusive bandages, and surgical intervention
- Recognize that restlessness, fussiness, and crying may be nonverbal cues of physical distress in infants, children, or adults with impaired verbal communication
- Assure that patient's clothing is not restrictive
- Perform passive or assisted range-of-motion exercises
- *(NIC) Circulatory Care (Arterial and Venous):*
  Elevate affected limb 20 degrees or greater above the level of the heart to improve venous return, as appropriate
  Lower extremity to improve arterial circulation, as appropriate
  Maintain adequate hydration to prevent increased blood viscosity. Restrict smoking [arterial insufficiency]
  Change the patient's position at least every 2 hr, as appropriate
- *(NIC) Peripheral Sensation Management:*
  Avoid or carefully monitor use of heat or cold, such as heating pads, hot-water bottles, and ice packs
  Encourage patient to use the unaffected body part to identify location and texture of objects
  Place cradle over affected body parts to keep bed clothes off affected areas
  Encourage patient to wear well-fitting, low-heeled, soft shoes

NONCOMPLIANCE (SPECIFY)
(00079) (1973, 1996, 1998)

Definition: Behavior of person or caregiver that fails to coincide with a health-promoting or therapeutic plan agreed upon by the person (and family, and community) and health care professional. In the presence of an agreed-upon, health-promoting or therapeutic plan, the behavior of the person or caregiver may be fully of partially nonadherent and may lead to clinically ineffective or partially ineffective outcomes.

Defining Characteristics

Objective

Behavior indicative of failure to adhere (by direct observation or by statements of patient or significant others)

Evidence of development of complications

Evidence of exacerbation of symptoms

Failure to keep appointments

Failure to progress

Objective tests (e.g., physiologic measures, detection of physiologic markers)

Related Factors

Health Care Plan

Complexity

Cost

Duration

Intensity

Significant others

Individual Factors

Cultural influences

Health beliefs

Individual's value system

Knowledge and skill relevant to the regimen behavior

Motivational forces

Personal and developmental abilities

Spiritual values

Health System

Access and convenience of care

Client–provider relationships

Communication and teaching skills of the provider

Credibility of provider
Financial flexibility of plan
Individual health coverage
Provider continuity and regular follow-up
Provider reimbursement of teaching and follow-up
Satisfaction with care

Network

Involvement of members in health plan
Perceived beliefs of significant others
Social value regarding plan

Suggestions for Use

Noncompliance describes failure to adhere to a therapeutic recommendation after having made an informed decision to do so
and after expressing an intention to do so. If the patient is
informed and *intends* to follow instructions, then nursing intervention can be directed at finding and removing the factors that keep
him or her from doing so. For example, a patient may state, "My
husband doesn't need to lose weight, and he loves fried food and
pastries. He just won't eat the diet foods, and I really don't have
time to cook one meal for myself and one for the rest of the family."
This client would like to comply with her diet, but situational
factors make it difficult. You could write a nursing diagnosis of
*Noncompliance with low-calorie diet related to inconvenience of
preparing special foods and lack of family support*. That diagnosis
does suggest independent nursing interventions.

Noncompliance should not be used for a patient who makes an
informed decision to not follow a therapeutic recommendation, for
instance, when a patient decides to stop taking a medication with
unpleasant side effects. Nursing intervention might then be
directed at convincing the patient of the value of continuing with
the therapy, but the nurse should balance this approach with
respect for the patient's autonomy when he or she has truly made
an informed decision. Remember that a decision to refuse therapy
can be as rational as a decision to have therapy.

Noncompliance should not be used for patients who are unable
to follow instructions (e.g., weakness, cognitive disability) or who
lack necessary information. If those factors are contributing to
Noncompliance, then it is better to use the diagnosis *Ineffective
health maintenance*.

Some nurses believe that *Noncompliance* is a negative label. When
using this diagnosis, be sure to express the etiology in neutral,

nonjudgmental terms. Geissler (1991) has suggested the term *non-adherence*, although it is not yet a NANDA International label.

Suggested Alternative Diagnoses

Denial, ineffective

Health maintenance, ineffective

Management of therapeutic regimen: family or individual, ineffective

NOC Outcomes

Adherence Behavior: Self-initiated action taken to promote wellness, recovery, and rehabilitation

Caregiver Performance: Direct Care: Provision by family care provider of appropriate personal and health care for a family member or significant other

Caregiver Performance: Indirect Care: Arrangement and oversight of appropriate care for a family member or significant other by family care provider

Compliance Behavior: Actions taken on the basis of professional advice to promote wellness, recovery, and rehabilitation

Symptom Control: Personal actions to minimize perceived adverse changes in physical and emotional functioning

Treatment Behavior: Illness or Injury: Personal actions to palliate or eliminate pathology

Goals/Evaluation Criteria

Examples Using NOC Language

- *Noncompliance* will decrease, as demonstrated by Adherence Behavior, Compliance Behavior, Symptom Control, and Treatment Behavior: Illness or Injury
- Demonstrates **Adherence Behavior**, as evidenced by the following indicators:

    Reports using strategies to eliminate unhealthy behavior and maximize health

    Describes rationale for deviating from a recommended regimen

    Weighs risks and benefits of health behavior

    Uses health services congruent with need

Other Examples

Patient will:
- Not abuse health care providers physically or verbally
- Use pain control measures

- Comply with prescribed medication and treatment regimens
- Keep appointments with health care providers
- Report significant treatment effects and side effects
- Report controlling illness symptoms

NIC Interventions

Energy Management: Regulating energy use to treat or prevent fatigue and optimize function

Health Education: Developing and providing instruction and learning experiences to facilitate voluntary adaptation of behavior conducive to health in individuals, families, groups, or communities

Health System Guidance: Facilitating a patient's location and use of appropriate health services

Mutual Goal Setting: Collaborating with patient to identify and prioritize care goals, then developing a plan for achieving those goals

Nutrition Management: Assisting with or providing a balanced dietary intake of foods and fluids

Patient Contracting: Negotiating an agreement with a patient that reinforces a specific behavior change

Self-Modification Assistance: Reinforcement of self-directed change initiated by the patient to achieve personally important goals

Self-Responsibility Facilitation: Encouraging a patient to assume more responsibility for own behavior

Teaching: Disease Process: Assisting the patient to understand information related to a specific disease process

Teaching: Individual: Planning, implementation, and evaluation of a teaching program designed to address a patient's particular needs

Nursing Activities

Assessments

- Identify probable cause of patient's noncompliant behavior

Patient/Family Teaching

- Help patient and family to understand the need for following the prescribed treatment and the consequences of noncompliance
- *(NIC) Health System Guidance:*
  Inform patient of appropriate community resources and contact persons

Give written instructions for purpose and location of health care activities, as appropriate

Collaborative Activities

- Consult with physician about possible alteration in medical regimen to encourage patient's compliance
- *(NIC) Health System Guidance:*
  Coordinate referrals to relevant health care providers, as appropriate

  Identify and facilitate communication among health care providers and patient and family, as appropriate.

  Coordinate and schedule time needed by each service to deliver care, as appropriate

  Provide follow-up contact with patient, as appropriate

  Assist individual to complete forms for assistance, such as housing and financial aid, as needed

Other

- Encourage the patient to express feelings and concerns about hospitalization and relationship with health care providers
- Provide emotional support to family members to help them maintain a positive relationship with patient
- Give positive reinforcement for compliance to encourage ongoing positive behaviors
- Develop a written contract with the patient, and evaluate compliant behaviors on a continuing basis. Specify contract.
- *(NIC) Self-Modification Assistance:*
  Encourage the patient to examine personal values and beliefs and satisfaction with them

  Explore with the patient potential barriers to change behavior

  Identify with the patient the most effective strategies for behavior change

  Assist the patient in formulating a systematic plan for behavior change [including intrinsic and extrinsic rewards and reinforcers]

  Assist the patient in identifying even small successes

NUTRITION, IMBALANCED: LESS THAN BODY REQUIREMENTS (00002) (1975)

Definition: Intake of nutrients insufficient to meet metabolic needs

Defining Characteristics

The author recommends using this label only if one of the following cues is present:

Body weight 20% or more under ideal for height and frame

Food intake less than metabolic needs, either total calories or specific nutrients (non-NANDA International)

Loss of weight with adequate food intake

Reported inadequate food intake less than the recommended daily allowance (RDA)

Subjective

Abdominal cramping

Abdominal pain with or without pathology

Aversion to eating

Indigestion (non-NANDA International)

Perceived inability to ingest food

Reported altered taste sensation

Reported lack of food

Satiety immediately after ingesting food

Objective

Capillary fragility

Diarrhea or steatorrhea

Evidence of lack of food

Excessive loss of hair

Hyperactive bowel sounds

Lack of information, misinformation

Lack of interest in food

Misconceptions

Pale conjunctival and mucous membranes

Poor muscle tone

Refusal to eat (non-NANDA International)

Sore, inflamed buccal cavity

Weakness of muscles required for swallowing or mastication

Related Factors

Inability to ingest or digest food or absorb nutrients due to biologic, psychologic, or economic factors, including the following:

Chemical dependence (specify)
Chronic illness (specify)
Difficulty in chewing or swallowing
Economic factors
Food intolerance
High metabolic needs
Inadequate sucking reflex in the infant
Lack of basic nutritional knowledge
Limited access to food
Loss of appetite
Nausea and vomiting
Parental neglect
Psychologic impairment (specify)

Suggestions for Use

Use this label for patients who are able to eat but unable to ingest, digest, or absorb nutrients to adequately meet metabolic needs. Inadequate ingestion might occur because of decreased appetite, nausea, poverty, or many other situations. Examples of patients unable to digest food or absorb particular nutrients are those with allergies, diarrhea, lactose intolerance, or poorly fitting dentures.

Do not use this label routinely for persons who are NPO or for those completely unable to ingest food for other reasons (e.g., unconscious patients). Nurses cannot prescribe independent nursing interventions for a diagnosis such as *Imbalanced nutrition: less than body requirements related to NPO*. They cannot give the missing nutrients, and they cannot change the NPO order. Additionally, the patient is often NPO for only a short time before and after surgery; thus, any lack of nutrients is temporary and resolves without nursing intervention. Long-term NPO status is a risk factor for other nursing diagnoses, such as *Risk for impaired oral mucous membrane*, and for collaborative problems such as Potential Complication: Electrolyte imbalance.

The patient might have a total nutritional deficit or perhaps be deficient in only one nutrient. When the deficit is something other than total, it should be specified like the following example: *Imbalanced nutrition: less than body requirements for protein related to lack of knowledge of nutritious foods and limited budget for food.*

Suggested Alternative Diagnoses

Breastfeeding, ineffective
Dentition, impaired

Failure to thrive, adult

Infant feeding pattern, ineffective

Management of therapeutic regimen, ineffective

Nausea

Self-care deficit: feeding

Swallowing, impaired

NOC Outcomes

Nutritional Status: Extent to which nutrients are available to meet metabolic needs

Nutritional Status: Food and Fluid Intake: Amount of food and fluid taken into the body over a 24-hr period

Nutritional Status: Nutrient Intake: Adequacy of nutrients taken into the body

Weight Control: Personal actions resulting in achievement and maintenance of optimum body weight for health

Goals/Evaluation Criteria

Examples Using NOC Language

- Demonstrates **Nutritional Status: Food, Fluid, and Nutrient Intake**, as evidenced by the following indicators (specify 1–5: not, slightly, moderately, substantially, or totally adequate):

    Oral food, tube feeding, or TPN intake

    Oral or IV fluid intake

Other Examples

Patient will:

- Maintain weight at _____ kg or gain _____ kg by _____ (specify date)
- Describe components of nutritionally adequate diet
- Verbalize willingness to follow diet
- Tolerate prescribed diet
- Maintain body mass and weight WNL
- Have laboratory values (e.g., transferrin, albumin, and electrolytes) WNL
- Report adequate energy levels

NIC Interventions

Diet Staging: Instituting required diet restrictions with subsequent progression of diet as tolerated

Eating Disorders Management: Prevention and treatment of severe diet restriction and overexercising or bingeing and purging of food and fluids

Fluid Monitoring: Collection and analysis of patient data to regulate fluid balance

Nutrition Management: Assistance with or provision of a balanced dietary intake of foods and fluids

Nutritional Monitoring: Collection and analysis of patient data to prevent or minimize malnourishment

Weight Gain Assistance: Facilitation of body weight gain

Nursing Activities

General Activities for all Imbalanced Nutrition

Assessments

- Determine patient motivation for changing eating habits
- Monitor laboratory values, especially transferrin, albumin, and electrolytes
- *(NIC) Nutrition Management:*
  Ascertain patient's food preferences
  Determine patient's ability to meet nutritional needs
  Monitor recorded intake for nutritional content and calories
  Weigh patient at appropriate intervals

Patient/Family Teaching

- Teach a method for meal planning
- Teach patient and family foods that are nutritious, yet inexpensive
- *(NIC) Nutrition Management:* Provide appropriate information about nutritional needs and how to meet them

Collaborative Activities

- Confer with dietitian to establish protein requirements for patients with inadequate protein intake or protein losses (e.g., patients with anorexia nervosa, glomerular disease or peritoneal dialysis)
- Confer with physician regarding need for appetite stimulant, supplemental feedings, nutritional tube feedings, or TPN so that adequate caloric intake is maintained
- Refer to physician to determine cause of altered nutrition
- Refer to appropriate community nutritional programs (e.g., Meals on Wheels, food banks) if patient cannot buy or prepare adequate food
- *(NIC) Nutrition Management:* Determine—in collaboration with dietitian, as appropriate—number of calories and type of nutrients needed to meet nutrition requirements [especially for patients with high-energy needs, such as postoperative patients and those with burns, trauma, fever, and wounds].

Other

- Develop meal plan with patient to include schedule of meals, eating environment, patient likes and dislikes, food temperature
- Encourage family members to bring food of patient's preference from home
- Assist patient to write realistic weekly goals for exercise and food intake
- Encourage patient to display food and exercise goals in a prominent location and review them daily
- Offer largest meal during time of day when patient's appetite is greatest
- Create a pleasant environment for meals (e.g., remove unsightly supplies and excretions)
- Avoid invasive procedures before meals
- Feed patient, as needed
- *(NIC) Nutrition Management:*

  Encourage patient to wear properly fitted dentures or acquire dental care

  Provide patient with high-protein, high-calorie, nutritious finger foods and drinks that can be readily consumed, as appropriate

  Teach patient how to keep a food diary, as needed

Difficulty in Chewing and Swallowing

Also refer to Nursing Activities under the preceding General Activities for all Imbalanced Nutrition, on pp. 330–331 and to Nursing Activities for Swallowing, Impaired on pp. 536–537.

Assessments

- Assess and document degree of chewing and swallowing difficulty

Collaborative Activities

- Request occupational therapy consultation

Other

- Reassure patient and provide calm atmosphere during meals
- Have suction catheters available at bedside and suction during meals, as needed
- Place patient in semi-Fowler or high-Fowler position to facilitate swallowing; have patient remain in this position for 30 minutes following meals to prevent aspiration
- Place food on unaffected side of mouth to facilitate swallowing
- When feeding patient, use syringe, if necessary, to facilitate swallowing

- *(NIC) Nutrition Management:* Encourage patient to wear properly fitted dentures or acquire dental care

Nausea/Vomiting

Also refer to Nursing Activities under General Activities for all Impaired Nutrition, on pp. 330–331 and to Nursing Activities for Nausea, on pp. 317–318.

Assessments

- Identify factors precipitating nausea and vomiting
- Document color, amount, and frequency of emesis

Patient/Family Teaching

- Instruct patient in slow, deep breathing and voluntary swallowing to decrease nausea and vomiting

Collaborative Activities

- Administer antiemetics and/or analgesics before eating or on prescribed schedule

Other

- Minimize factors that may precipitate nausea and vomiting, specify factors.
- Offer cool, wet washcloth to be placed on forehead or back of neck
- Offer oral hygiene before meals
- Limit diet to ice chips and clear liquids when symptoms are severe; progress with diet, as appropriate

Loss of Appetite

Also refer to Nursing Activities under General Activities for all Patients with Impaired Nutrition, on pp. 330–331.

Assessments

- Identify factors that may contribute to patient's loss of appetite (e.g., medications, emotional concerns)

Other

- Give positive feedback to patient who shows increased appetite
- Provide foods in accordance with patient's personal, cultural, and religious preferences
- *(NIC) Nutrition Management:*
  Offer snacks (e.g., frequent drinks and fresh fruits or fruit juice), as appropriate
  Provide a variety of high-calorie, nutritious foods from which to select

Eating Disorders

Also refer to Nursing Activities under General Activities for all Impaired Nutrition, on pp. 330–331.

Assessments

- Monitor patient for behaviors associated with weight loss

Collaborative Activities

- Consult dietitian to determine daily caloric intake necessary to attain target weight
- Notify physician if patient refuses to eat
- Work with physician, nutritionist, and patient to set weight and intake goals

Other

- Establish a trusting, supportive relationship with patient
- Communicate expectations for appropriate intake of food and fluid and amount of exercise
- Confine patient's eating to scheduled meals and snacks
- Accompany patient to bathroom after meals or snacks to observe for self-induced vomiting
- Develop behavior modification program specific to patient's needs
- Provide positive reinforcement for weight gain and appropriate eating behaviors, but do not focus interactions on food or eating
- Explore with patient and significant others personal issues (e.g., body image) that contribute to eating behaviors
- Communicate that the patient is responsible for choices about eating and physical activity
- Discuss the benefits of healthy eating behaviors and the consequences of noncompliance

---

NUTRITION, IMBALANCED: MORE THAN BODY REQUIREMENTS (00001) (1975)

Definition: Intake of nutrients that exceeds metabolic needs

Defining Characteristics

The author recommends using this diagnosis only if one or more of the following NANDA International defining characteristics is present:

Triceps skinfold greater than 15 mm in men and 25 mm in women

Weight 20% over ideal for height and frame

Subjective

Reports of little or no exercise

Objective

Concentration of food intake at end of day

Dysfunctional eating pattern, pairing food with other activities

Eating in response to external cues, such as time of day or social situation

Eating in response to internal cues other than hunger (e.g., anxiety, [anger, depression, boredom, stress, loneliness])

Sedentary activity level

Other Possible Defining Characteristics (non-NANDA International)

Rapid transition across growth percentiles in infants or children

Reported or observed higher baseline weight at beginning of each pregnancy

Related Factors

Excessive intake in relation to metabolic need

Other Possible Related Factors (non-NANDA International)

Chemical dependence

Concentrating food intake at end of day

Decreased metabolic requirements (e.g., secondary to prescribed bed rest)

Dysfunctional eating patterns

Eating in response to external cues (e.g., time of day or social situation)

Eating in response to internal cues other than hunger (e.g., anxiety)

Ethnic and cultural norms

Increased appetite

Lack of basic nutritional knowledge

Lack of physical exercise

Medications that stimulate appetite

Use of food as reward or comfort measure

Obesity in one or both parents

Use of solid food as major food source before 5 months of age

Selecting foods that do not meet daily requirements

Substituting sweets for addiction

Suggestions for Use

This diagnosis is most appropriate for patients who are motivated to lose weight (e.g., a woman who has gained weight after pregnancy). For patients who are overweight but not motivated to participate in a weight loss program, consider *Ineffective health maintenance* instead. Note that *Imbalanced nutrition: more than body requirements* focuses attention on nutrition instead of on lifestyle changes necessary for weight loss (e.g., exercise). Eating in response to stressors might be better described as *Ineffective coping*.

Although some of the nursing actions and one of the NIC interventions specify "eating disorders management" as an intervention for this diagnosis, the focus of nursing for a patient who is bingeing and purging is much more complex than excess calorie intake; this diagnosis has limited use in that situation.

Suggested Alternative Diagnoses

Coping, ineffective

Health maintenance, ineffective

Management of therapeutic regimen, ineffective

Nutrition, imbalanced: risk for more than body requirements

NOC Outcomes

Nutritional Status: Food and Fluid Intake: Amount of food and fluid taken into the body over a 24-hr period

Nutritional Status: Nutrient Intake: Adequacy of nutrients taken into the body

Weight Control: Personal actions resulting in achievement and maintenance of optimum body weight for health

Goals/Evaluation Criteria

Examples Using NOC Language

- Demonstrates **Nutritional Status: Food and Fluid Intake**, as evidenced by the following indicator (specify 1–5: not, slightly, moderately, substantially, or totally adequate): oral food and fluid intake [not excessive]

Other Examples

Patient will:

- Acknowledge weight problem
- Verbalize desire to lose weight
- Participate in a structured weight-loss program
- Participate in a regular exercise program

- Approach ideal weight _____ (specify)
- Refrain from binge eating
- Experience adequate, but not excessive, intake of calories, fats, carbohydrates, vitamins, minerals, iron, and calcium

NIC Interventions

Behavior Modification: Promotion of a behavior change

Eating Disorders Management: Prevention and treatment of severe diet restriction and overexercising or bingeing and purging of food and fluids

Nutrition Management: Assisting with or providing a balanced dietary intake of foods and fluids

Nutritional Monitoring: Collection and analysis of patient data to prevent or minimize malnourishment

Weight Reduction Assistance: Facilitating loss of weight and body fat

Nursing Activities

Assessments

- Monitor patient for behaviors associated with weight gain
- *(NIC) Weight Reduction Assistance:*
  Determine patient's desire and motivation to reduce weight or body fat
  Determine current eating patterns by having patients keep a diary of what, when, and where they eat
- *(NIC) Nutrition Management:* Weigh patient at appropriate intervals

Patient/Family Teaching

- *(NIC) Nutrition Management:*
  Provide appropriate information about nutritional needs and how to meet them
  Encourage patient to follow a diet of complex carbohydrates and protein, and avoid simple sugars, fast food, caffeine, soft drinks
- *(NIC) Weight Reduction Assistance:*
  Discuss with patient and family the influence of alcohol consumption on food ingestion
  Instruct on how to read labels when purchasing food, to control amount of fat and calorie density of food obtained
  Teach food selections, in restaurants and social gatherings, that are consistent with planned calorie and nutrient intake
  Instruct on how to calculate percentage of fat in food products

Collaborative Activities

- Confer with dietitian to implement weight-loss program that includes dietary management and energy expenditure
- *(NIC) Nutrition Management:* Determine—in collaboration with dietitian, as appropriate—number of calories and type of nutrients needed to meet nutrition requirements
- *(NIC) Weight Reduction Assistance:* Encourage attendance at support groups for weight loss (e.g., TOPS Club or Weight Watchers)

Other

- Develop a trusting, supportive relationship with patient
- Help patient to identify physical problems that may be related to obesity or eating disorder
- For patient with compulsive eating disorder, establish expectations for appropriate eating behaviors, intake of food and fluid, and amount of exercise
- Explore with patient personal issues that may contribute to overeating
- Communicate that the patient, alone, is responsible for choices about eating and physical activity
- Provide positive reinforcement for weight loss, maintenance of dietary regimen, improved eating behaviors, and exercise
- Focus on the patient's feelings about himself rather than on the obesity
- Discuss with patient emotions or high-risk situations that stimulate eating (e.g., types of foods, social situations, interpersonal stresses, unmet personal expectations, eating in secret or in private)
- *(NIC) Weight Reduction Assistance:*
  Set a weekly goal for weight loss
  Assist patient to identify motivation for eating and internal and external cues associated with eating
  Determine with the patient the amount of weight loss desired
  Assist with adjusting diet to lifestyle and activity level
  Set a realistic plan with the patient to include reduced food intake and increased energy expenditure [plan should specify frequency of meals and snacks and include self-monitoring activities]
  Encourage substitution of undesirable habits with favorable habits
  Plan an exercise program, taking into consideration the patient's limitations
  Encourage use of internal reward systems when goals are accomplished

NUTRITION, IMBALANCED: MORE THAN BODY REQUIREMENTS, RISK FOR
(00003) (1980)

Definition: At risk of experiencing an intake of nutrients that exceeds metabolic needs

Risk Factors

Subjective
Increased appetite

Eating in response to internal cues other than hunger (e.g., anxiety)

Reported use of solid food as major food source before 5 months of age

Objective
Obesity in one or both parents

Concentration of food intake at end of day

Dysfunctional eating patterns

Eating in response to external cues (e.g., time of day or social situation)

Observed use of food as reward or comfort measure

Pairing food with other activities

Rapid transition across growth percentiles in infants or children

Reported or observed higher baseline weight at beginning of each pregnancy

Other Possible Risk Factors (non-NANDA International)
Chemical dependence

Decreased metabolic requirements

Ethnic and cultural norms

Lack of basic nutritional knowledge

Lack of physical exercise

Suggestions for Use
See Suggestions for Use for Nutrition, Imbalanced: More Than Body Requirements p. 335.

Suggested Alternative Diagnoses
Coping, ineffective

Health maintenance, ineffective

Management of therapeutic regimen, ineffective

NOC Outcomes

Nutritional Status: Food and Fluid Intake: Amount of food and fluid taken into the body over a 24-hr period

Weight Control: Personal actions resulting in achievement and maintenance of optimum body weight for health

Goals/Evaluation Criteria

Examples Using NOC Language

- Demonstrates **Nutritional Status: Food and Fluid Intake**, as evidenced by the following indicator (specify 1–5: not, slightly, moderately, substantially, or totally adequate): oral food and fluid intake not excessive

Other Examples

Patient will:
- Acknowledge presence of risk factors
- Participate in a regular exercise program
- Maintain ideal weight _____ (specify)
- Eat a balanced diet

NIC Interventions

Nutrition Management: Assisting with or providing a balanced dietary intake of foods and fluids

Nutritional Monitoring: Collection and analysis of patient data to prevent or minimize malnourishment

Weight Management: Facilitating maintenance of optimal body weight and percentage of body fat

Nursing Activities

Assessments

- Monitor presence of risk factors for weight gain
- *(NIC) Weight Management:*
  Determine patient's ideal body weight
  Determine patient's ideal percentage of body fat
- *(NIC) Nutrition Management:* Weigh patient at appropriate intervals

Patient/Family Teaching

- Provide information regarding available community resources, such as dietary counseling, exercise programs, self-help groups
- *(NIC) Weight Management:*
  Discuss with the patient the relationship between food intake, exercise, weight gain, and weight loss

Discuss with patient the medical conditions that may affect weight

Discuss with patient the habits and customs and cultural and heredity factors that influence weight

Discuss risks associated with being over- and underweight

Assist in developing well-balanced meal plans consistent with level of energy expenditure

Other

- Develop a weight-management plan
- Develop a plan for management of eating to include the following:

  Frequency of meals and snacks

  Diet high in complex carbohydrates and protein

  Avoidance of simple sugars, fast food, caffeine, and soft drinks

  Recognition of high-risk situations (e.g., types of foods, social situations, interpersonal stresses, unmet personal expectations, eating in secret or in private)

- Provide frequent positive reinforcement for good nutrition and exercise

---

NUTRITION, READINESS FOR ENHANCED (00163) (2002)

Definition: A pattern of nutrient intake that is sufficient for meeting metabolic needs and can be strengthened

Defining Characteristics

Subjective

Attitude toward eating and drinking is congruent with health goals

Expresses knowledge of healthy food and fluid choices

Expresses willingness to enhance nutrition

Objective

Consumes adequate food and fluid

Eats regularly

Follows an appropriate standard for intake (e.g., the food pyramid or American Diabetic Association guidelines)

Safe preparation and storage for food and fluids

Related Factors

This is a wellness diagnosis, so an etiology is not necessary.

Suggestions for Use

If risk factors are present, use *Risk for imbalanced nutrition*.

Suggested Alternative Diagnoses

Fluid balance, readiness for enhanced
Knowledge (specify), readiness for enhanced
Management of therapeutic regimen, effective
Nutrition, risk for imbalanced

NOC Outcomes

This is a new diagnosis, so NOC outcome linkages have not yet been developed; however, the following may be useful:

Nutritional Status: Food and Fluid Intake: Amount of food and fluid taken into the body over a 24-hr period

Weight Control: Personal actions resulting in achievement and maintenance of optimum body weight for health

Goals/Evaluation Criteria

Examples Using NOC Language

• Demonstrates **Nutritional Status: Food and Fluid Intake**, as evidenced by the following indicator (specify 1–5: not, slightly, moderately, substantially, or totally adequate): oral food and fluid intake not excessive

Other Examples

Patient will:

• Maintain ideal weight _____ (specify)
• Eat a balanced diet
• Report enhanced nutritional value of foods consumed (e.g., eats more nonprocessed foods, fewer saturated fats)

NIC Interventions

NIC interventions have not yet been linked to this new diagnosis; however, the following may be useful:

Nutrition Management: Assisting with or providing a balanced dietary intake of foods and fluids

Weight Management: Facilitating maintenance of optimal body weight and percentage of body fat

Nursing Activities

Assessments

• Monitor presence of risk factors for weight gain or loss
• Assess plans for improving diet

- *(NIC) Weight Management:*
  Determine patient's ideal body weight
  Determine patient's ideal percentage of body fat
  Teach patient to weigh at appropriate intervals

Patient/Family Teaching

- Provide information regarding available community resources, such as dietary counseling, exercise programs, self-help groups
- *(NIC) Weight Management:*
  Discuss with the patient the relationship between food intake, exercise, weight gain, and weight loss
  Discuss with patient the medical conditions that may affect weight
  Discuss with patient the habits and customs and cultural and heredity factors that influence weight
  Discuss risks associated with being over- and underweight
  Assist in developing well-balanced meal plans consistent with level of energy expenditure

Other

- Provide frequent positive reinforcement for good nutrition

ORAL MUCOUS MEMBRANE, IMPAIRED
(00045) (1982, 1998)

Definition: Disruptions of the lips and soft tissue of the oral cavity

Defining Characteristics

Subjective

Oral pain and discomfort
Self-report of bad taste
Self-report of difficulty eating or swallowing
Self-report of diminished or absent taste

Objective

Bleeding
Coated tongue
Desquamation
Difficult speech
Edema
Enlarged tonsils beyond what is developmentally appropriate
Fissures, cheilitis
Geographic tongue
Gingival hyperplasia

Gingival or mucosal pallor

Gingival recession, pockets deeper than 4 mm

Halitosis

Hyperemia

Macroplasia

Mucosal denudation

Oral lesions or ulcers

Presence of pathogens

Purulent drainage or exudates

Red or bluish masses (e.g., hemangiomas)

Smooth, atrophic, sensitive tongue

Stomatitis

Vesicles, nodules, or papules

White patches or plaques, spongy patches, or white curdlike exudates

Xerostomia (dry mouth)

<u>Other Defining Characteristics (non-NANDA International)</u>

Discomfort with hot or cold foods

Dry mouth

Dry, cracked lips

Lack of or decreased salivation

Related Factors

Aging-related loss of connective, adipose, or bony tissue

Barriers to oral self-care

Barriers to professional care

Chemotherapy

Chemical (e.g., alcohol, tobacco, acidic foods, regular use of inhalers)

Cleft lip or palate

Decreased platelets

Dehydration

Depression

Diminished hormone levels (women)

Immunocompromised

Immunosuppression

Impaired salivation

Ineffective oral hygiene

Infection

Lack of or decreased salivation

Loss of supportive structures

Malnutrition or vitamin deficiency

Mechanical (e.g., ill-fitting dentures, braces, [and ET or NG] tubes)
Medication side effects
Mouth breathing
NPO for more than 24 hr
Pathologic conditions of the oral cavity
Radiation therapy
Stress
Surgery in oral cavity
Trauma (e.g., drugs, noxious agents)

Suggested Alternative Diagnoses

Dentition, impaired
Tissue integrity, impaired

NOC Outcomes

Oral Health: Condition of the mouth, teeth, gums, and tongue
Tissue Integrity: Skin and Mucous Membranes: Structural intactness and normal physiologic function of skin and mucous membranes

Goals/Evaluation Criteria

Examples Using NOC Language

- Demonstrates **Oral Health**, as evidenced by the following indicators (specify 1–5: extremely, substantially, moderately, mildly, or not compromised):
    Cleanliness of mouth, teeth, gums, tongue, dentures, or dental appliances
    Moisture of oral mucosa and tongue
    Color of mucosa membranes [pink]
    Integrity of oral mucosa, tongue, gum[s], and [teeth]
    Breath free of halitosis
- Demonstrates **Tissue Integrity: Skin and Mucous Membranes**, as evidenced by the following indicators (specify 1–5: extremely, substantially, moderately, mildly, or not compromised):
    Tissue lesion free
    Sensation in expected range

Other Examples

Patient will:
- Ingest foods and fluids with increasing comfort
- Perform essential oral hygiene as prescribed and instructed

NIC Interventions

Oral Health Restoration: Promotion of healing for a patient who has an oral mucosa or dental lesion

Nursing Activities

Assessments

- Identify irritating substances such as tobacco, alcohol, food, medications, extremes in food temperature, seasonings
- Assess patient's understanding of and ability to perform oral care
- *(NIC) Oral Health Restoration:*
  Determine the patient's perception of changes in taste, swallowing, quality of voice, and comfort
  Monitor patient every shift for dryness of the oral mucosa
  Monitor for signs and symptoms of glossitis and stomatitis
  Monitor for therapeutic effects of topical anesthetics, oral protective pastes, and topical or systemic analgesics, as appropriate

Patient/Family Teaching

- *(NIC) Oral Health Restoration:*
  Reinforce oral hygiene regimen as part of discharge teaching
  Instruct patient to avoid commercial mouthwashes
  Instruct patient to report signs of infection to physician immediately

Collaborative Activities

- Confer with physician regarding an order for antifungal mouthwash or oral topical anesthetic if fungal infection exists.
- *(NIC) Oral Health Restoration:*
  Consult physician if signs and symptoms of glossitis and stomatitis persist or worsen
  Apply topical anesthetics, oral protective pastes, and topical or systemic analgesics, as needed

Other

- Provide mouth care prior to meals and as needed
- Avoid use of sugared candies and gum
- Clean dentures after each meal
- *(NIC) Oral Health Restoration:*
  Plan small, frequent meals; select soft foods; and serve chilled or room-temperature foods

Assist patient to select soft, bland, and nonacidic foods

Increase mouth care to every 2 hr and twice at night if stomatitis is not controlled

Use a soft toothbrush for removal of dental debris

Encourage frequent rinsing of the mouth with any of the following: sodium bicarbonate solution, warm saline, or hydrogen peroxide solution

Avoid use of lemon-glycerin swabs

Discourage smoking and alcohol consumption

Remove dentures in case of severe stomatitis

PAIN, ACUTE
(00132) (1996)

Definition: Unpleasant sensory and emotional experience arising from actual or potential tissue damage or described in terms of such damage (International Association for the Study of Pain); sudden or slow onset of any intensity from mild to severe with an anticipated or predictable end and a duration of less than 6 months

Defining Characteristics

Subjective
Verbal or coded report

Objective
Antalgic positioning to avoid pain

Autonomic change in muscle tone (may span from listless to rigid)

Autonomic responses (e.g., diaphoresis; blood pressure, respiration, or pulse changes; pupillary dilation)

Changes in appetite and eating

Distraction behavior (e.g., pacing, seeking out other people and/or activities, repetitive activities)

Expressive behavior (e.g., restlessness, moaning, crying, vigilance, irritability, sighing)

Facial mask [of pain]

Guarding or protective behavior

Narrowed focus (e.g., altered time perception, impaired thought processes, reduced interaction with people and environment)

Self-focus

Sleep disturbance (eyes lack luster, beaten look, fixed or scattered movement, grimace)

<u>Other Defining Characteristics (non-NANDA International)</u>
Communication of pain descriptors (e.g., pain, discomfort,
　　nausea, night sweats, muscle cramps, itching skin, numbness,
　　tingling of extremities)
Grimacing
Limited attention span
Pacing
Pallor
Withdrawal

Related Factors

Injury agents (e.g., biologic, chemical, physical, psychologic)

Suggestions for Use

Acute pain can be diagnosed on the patient's report alone because
that is sometimes the only sign of *Acute pain*. None of the other
defining characteristics taken alone would be sufficient to diagnose *Acute pain*. The related factors indicate that a patient can suf-
fer both physical and psychologic *Acute pain*. Qualifier words
should be added to this diagnosis to indicate the severity, location, and nature of the pain. Two examples of appropriate diagnoses are as follows: *Severe, stabbing chest pain related to fractured
ribs,* and *Mild frontal headache related to sinus congestion.*

　　It is important to differentiate between *Acute Pain* and *Chronic
pain* because the nursing focus is different for each. *Acute pain*
(e.g., postoperative incision pain) is usually a collaborative problem managed primarily by administering narcotic analgesics.
There are a few independent nursing interventions for *Acute pain*,
such as teaching the patient to splint the incision while moving,
but these alone would not provide adequate pain relief. The nurse
takes a more active role in teaching patients self-management of
Chronic pain. When pain is acute or caused by a stressor not
amenable to nursing intervention (e.g., surgical incision), it may be
an etiology rather than a problem, for example, *Ineffective airway
clearance related to weak cough secondary to Acute pain from chest
incision.*

　　In differentiating between *Acute pain* and *Chronic pain*, the comparison in Table 4 may be helpful.

Table 4

Defining Characteristics	Pain	Chronic Pain
Duration less than 6 months	X	
Duration longer than 6 months		X
Autonomic responses, such as pallor, increase in vital signs, and diaphoresis	X	
Personality changes		X
Weight Loss		X

Pain can also be the etiology (i.e., related factor) for other nursing diagnoses, such as *Powerlessness related to inability to cope with Acute pain and Self-care deficit: dressing/grooming, related to joint Pain with movement.*

Suggested Alternative Diagnosis

Pain, chronic

NOC Outcomes

Comfort Level: Feelings of physical and psychologic ease

Pain Control: Personal actions to control pain

Pain: Disruptive Effects: Observed or reported disruptive effects of pain on emotions and behavior

Pain Level: Severity of reported or demonstrated pain

Goals/Evaluation Criteria

Examples Using NOC Language

- Demonstrates **Pain: Disruptive Effects**, as evidenced by the following indicators (specify 1–5: severe, substantial, moderate, slight, or none):
    Impaired role performance or interpersonal relationships
    Compromised work, life enjoyment, or sense of control
    Impaired concentration
    Disrupted sleep
    Lack of appetite or difficulty eating
- Demonstrates **Pain Level**, as evidenced by the following indicators (specify 1–5: severe, substantial, moderate, slight, or none):
    Oral or facial expressions of pain
    Protective body positions
    Restlessness or muscle tension
    Change in respiratory rate, heart rate, or blood pressure

Other Examples

Patient will:

- Demonstrate individualized relaxation techniques that are effective for achieving comfort
- Maintain pain level at _____ or less (on scale of 0–10)
- Report physical and psychologic well-being
- Recognize causal factors and use measures to prevent pain
- Report pain to health care provider
- Use analgesic and nonanalgesic relief measures appropriately

NIC Interventions

Analgesic Administration: Use of pharmacologic agents to reduce or eliminate pain

Conscious Sedation: Administration of sedatives, monitoring of the patient's response, and provision of necessary physiologic support during a diagnostic or therapeutic procedure

Medication Management: Facilitation of safe and effective use of prescription and over-the-counter drugs

Pain Management: Alleviation of pain or a reduction in pain to a level of comfort that is acceptable to the patient

Patient-Controlled Analgesia (PCA) Assistance: Facilitating patient control of analgesic administration and regulation

Nursing Activities

Assessments

- Use self-report as first choice to obtain assessment information
- Ask patient to rate pain or discomfort on a scale of 0–10 (0 = no pain or discomfort, 10 = worst pain)
- Use pain flow sheet to monitor pain relief of analgesics and possible side effects
- Assess the impact of religion, culture, beliefs, and circumstances on patient's pain and responses
- In assessing patient's pain, use words that are consistent with patient's age and developmental level
- *(NIC) Pain Management:*

    Perform a comprehensive assessment of pain to include location, characteristics, onset and duration, frequency, quality, intensity or severity of pain, and precipitating factors

    Observe for nonverbal cues of discomfort, especially in those unable to communicate effectively

Patient/Family Teaching

- Include in discharge instructions the specific medication to be taken, frequency of administration, potential side effects, potential medication interactions, specific precautions when taking the medication (e.g., physical activity limitations, dietary restrictions), and name of person to notify about unrelieved pain
- Instruct patient to inform nurse if pain relief is not achieved
- Inform patient of procedures that may increase pain and offer suggestions for coping
- Correct misconceptions about narcotic or opioid analgesics (e.g., risks of addiction and overdose)
- *(NIC) Pain Management:*

  Provide information about the pain, such as causes of the pain, how long it will last, and anticipated discomforts from procedures

  Use pain-control measures before pain becomes severe

  Teach the use of nonpharmacologic techniques (e.g., biofeedback, transcutaneous electrical nerve stimulation [TENS], hypnosis, relaxation, guided imagery, music therapy, distraction, play therapy, activity therapy, acupressure, hot or cold application, and massage) before, after, and if possible, during painful activities; before pain occurs or increases; and along with other pain-relief measures

Collaborative Activities

- Manage immediate postoperative pain with scheduled opiate (e.g., q4h for 36 hr) or PCA
- *(NIC) Pain Management:* Notify physician if measures are unsuccessful or if current complaint is a significant change from patient's past experience of pain

Other

- Adjust frequency of dosage as indicated by pain assessment and side effects
- Help patient identify comfort measures that have worked in the past, such as distraction, relaxation, or application of heat or cold
- Attend to comfort needs and other activities to assist relaxation, including the following measures:

  Offer position change, back rubs, and relaxation

  Change bed linen, as necessary

  Provide care in an unhurried, supportive manner

  Involve patient in decisions regarding care activities

- Help patient focus on activities rather than on pain and discomfort by providing diversion through television, radio, tapes, and visitors
- Note that the elderly have increased sensitivity to analgesic effects of opiates with higher peak effect and longer duration of pain relief
- Be alert to possible drug-drug and drug-disease interactions in the elderly, who often have multiple illnesses and take multiple medications
- Use a positive approach in order to optimize patient response to analgesics (e.g., "This will help relieve your pain")
- Explore feelings about fear of addiction; to reassure patient, ask: "If you didn't have this pain, would you still want to take this drug?"
- *(NIC) Pain Management:*
  Incorporate the family in the pain relief modality, if possible
  Control environmental factors that may influence the patient's response to discomfort (e.g., room temperature, lighting, and noise)
  Ensure pretreatment analgesia or nonpharmacologic strategies before painful procedures.

PAIN, CHRONIC
(00133) (1986, 1996)

Definition: An unpleasant sensory and emotional experience arising from actual or potential tissue damage or described in terms of such damage (International Association for the Study of Pain); sudden or slow onset of any intensity from mild to severe, constant or recurring, without an anticipated or predictable end and a duration of greater than 6 months

Defining Characteristics

Verbal or coded report or observed evidence of the following:
Depression
Facial mask
Guarding behavior
Irritability
Protective behavior
Restlessness
Self-focusing

Subjective

Fatigue

Fear of reinjury

Objective

Atrophy of involved muscle group

Altered ability to continue previous activities

Anorexia

Changes in sleep pattern

Reduced interaction with people

Sympathetic mediated responses (e.g., temperature, cold, changes of body position, hypersensitivity)

Weight changes

Related Factors

Chronic physical-psychosocial disability (e.g., metastatic cancer, neurologic injury, arthritis)

Suggestions for Use

See Suggestions for Use for Acute Pain on pp. 347–348.

Suggested Alternative Diagnosis

Acute Pain

NOC Outcomes

Comfort Level: Feelings of physical and psychologic ease

Depression Control: Personal actions to minimize melancholy and maintain interest in life events

Depression Level: Severity of melancholic mood and loss of interest in life events

Pain Control: Personal actions to control pain

Pain: Disruptive Effects: Observed or reported disruptive effects of pain on emotions and behavior

Pain Level: Severity of reported or demonstrated pain

Pain: Psychological Response: Cognitive and emotional responses to physical pain

Goals/Evaluation Criteria

Examples Using NOC Language

- Demonstrates **Pain: Disruptive Effects**, as evidenced by the following indicators (specify 1–5: severe, substantial, moderate, slight, or none):

    Impaired role performance or interpersonal relationships

Compromised work, life enjoyment, or sense of control

Impaired concentration

Disrupted sleep

Lack of appetite or difficulty eating

- Demonstrates **Pain Level**, as evidenced by the following indicators (specify 1–5: severe, substantial, moderate, slight, or none):

No oral or facial expressions of pain

No protective body positions

No restlessness or muscle tension

No appetite loss

Frequency of pain and length of pain episodes reported as moderate or slight

Other Examples

- Verbalizes knowledge of alternative measures for pain relief
- Patient's level of pain is maintained at _____ or less (on scale of 0–10)
- Reports physical and psychologic well-being
- Recognizes factors that increase pain and takes preventive measures
- Appropriately uses analgesic and nonanalgesic relief measures

NIC Interventions

Analgesic Administration: Use of pharmacologic agents to reduce or eliminate pain

Behavior Modification: Promotion of a behavior change

Cognitive Restructuring: Challenging a patient to alter distorted thought patterns and view self and the world more realistically

Coping Enhancement: Assisting a patient to adapt to perceived stressors, changes, or threats which interfere with meeting life demands and roles

Medication Management: Facilitation of safe and effective use of prescription and over-the-counter drugs

Mood Management: Providing for safety, stabilization, recovery, and maintenance of a patient who is experiencing dysfunctionally depressed mood or elevated mood

Pain Management: Alleviation of pain or a reduction in pain to a level of comfort that is acceptable to the patient

Patient Contracting: Negotiating an agreement with a patient that reinforces a specific behavior change

Patient-Controlled Analgesia (PCA) Assistance: Facilitation of patient control of analgesic administration and regulation

Nursing Activities

Also refer to Nursing Activities for Acute Pain on pp. 349–351.

Assessments

- Assess and document effects of long-term medication use
- *(NIC) Pain Management:*
  Monitor patient satisfaction with pain management at specified intervals
  Determine the impact of the pain experience on quality of life (e.g., sleep, appetite, activity, cognition, mood, relationships, performance of job, and role responsibilities)

Patient/Family Teaching

- Convey to patient that total pain relief may not be achievable

Collaborative Activities

- Initiate a multidisciplinary patient care planning conference
- *(NIC) Pain Management:*
  Consider referrals for patient, family, and significant others to support groups and other resources, as appropriate

Other

- Offer patient pain-relief measures to supplement pain medication (e.g., biofeedback, relaxation techniques, back rub)
- Assist patient in identifying reasonable and acceptable level of pain
- *(NIC) Pain Management:*
  Promote adequate rest and sleep to facilitate pain relief
  Medicate before an activity to increase participation but evaluate the hazard of sedation

---

PARENTING, IMPAIRED
(00056) (1978, 1998)

Definition: Inability of the primary caretaker to create, maintain, or regain an environment that promotes the optimum growth and development of the child

Defining Characteristics

Infant or Child

Objective
Behavioral disorders
Failure to thrive

Frequent accidents

Frequent illness

Incidence of physical and psychologic trauma or abuse

Lack of attachment

Lack of separation anxiety

Poor academic performance

Poor cognitive development

Poor social competence

Runaway

Parental

Subjective

Negative statements about child

Statements of inability to meet child's needs

Verbalization of role inadequacy frustration

Verbalization that cannot control child

Objective

Abandonment

Child abuse

Child neglect

High punitiveness

Inadequate child health maintenance

Inappropriate child-care arrangements

Inappropriate visual, tactile, and auditory stimulation

Inconsistent behavior management

Inconsistent care

Inflexibility to meet needs of child, situation

Insecure or lack of attachment to infant

Little cuddling

Maternal–child interaction deficit

Poor or inappropriate caretaking skills [e.g., involving toilet training, sleep and rest, feeding, discipline]

Poor parent–child interaction

Rejection or hostility to child

Unsafe home environment

Other Defining Characteristics (non-NANDA International)

Child care from multiple caretakers without consideration of needs of infant or child

Compulsive seeking of role approval from others

Growth and development lag

Noncompliance with child's health appointments

Related Factors

Infant or Child

Altered perceptual abilities

Attention-deficit hyperactivity disorder

Difficult temperament

Handicapping condition or developmental delay

Illness

Lack of goodness of fit (i.e., temperament) with parental expectations

Multiple births

Not gender desired

Premature birth

Prolonged separation from parent

Separation from parent at birth

Unplanned or unwanted child

Knowledge

Inability to recognize and act on infant cues

Lack of cognitive readiness for parenthood

Lack of knowledge about child development

Lack of knowledge about child health maintenance

Lack of knowledge about parenting skills

Limited cognitive functioning

Low educational level or attainment

Poor communication skills

Preference for physical punishment

Unrealistic expectation for self, infant, partner

Physiologic

Physical illness

Psychologic

Depression

Difficult labor or delivery

Disability

High number or closely spaced pregnancies

History of mental illness

History of substance abuse or dependencies

Lack of, or late, prenatal care

Multiple births

Separation from infant or child

Sleep deprivation or disruption

Young age, especially adolescent

Social

Change in family unit
Father of child not involved
Financial difficulties
History of being abused
History of being abusive
Inability to put child's needs before own
Inadequate child-care arrangements
Lack of access to resources
Lack of family cohesiveness
Lack of resources
Lack of social support networks
Lack of transportation
Lack of value of parenthood
Lack of, or poor, parental role model
Legal difficulties
Low self-esteem
Low socioeconomic class
Maladaptive coping strategies
Marital conflict, declining satisfaction
Poor home environments
Poor problem-solving skills
Poverty
Presence of stress (e.g., financial, legal, recent crisis, cultural, move)
Relocations
Role strain or overload
Single parents
Social isolation
Unemployment or job problems
Unplanned or unwanted pregnancy

Suggestions for Use

"Adjustment to parenting in general is a normal maturational process that elicits nursing behaviors of prevention of potential problems and health promotion" (NANDA International, 1999, p. 55). This label represents a less healthy level of functioning than *Parental role conflict*, in which a parent or parents have been functioning satisfactorily but face situational challenges (e.g., divorce, illness) that create role conflict and confusion. Unresolved *Parental role conflict* may progress to *Impaired parenting*.

Suggested Alternative Diagnoses

Caregiver role strain (actual or at risk for)
Coping: family, disabled
Development, risk for delayed
Growth, risk for disproportionate
Family processes, interrupted
Parental role conflict
Parenting, risk for impaired
Role performance, ineffective

NOC Outcomes

Child Development (2, 4, 6, and 12 Months; 2, 3, 4, and 5 Years; 6–11 Years, and 12–17 Years): Milestones of physical, cognitive, and psychosocial progression by_____ age. [**NOTE:** NOC has separate outcomes and indicators for each age.]

Family Coping: Family actions to manage stressors that tax family resources.

Family Environment: Internal: Social climate as characterized by family member relationships and goals

Family Functioning: Ability of the family to meet the needs of its members through developmental transitions

Parent–Infant Attachment: Behaviors that demonstrate an enduring affectionate bond between a parent and infant

Parenting: Provision of an environment that promotes optimum growth

Parenting: Social Safety: Parental actions to avoid social relationships that might cause harm or injury

Role Performance: Congruence of an individual's role behavior with role expectations

Safety Behavior: Home Physical Environment: Individual or caregiver actions to minimize environmental factors that might cause physical harm or injury in the home

Social Support: Perceived availability and actual provision of reliable assistance from other persons

Goals/Evaluation Criteria

Also see Goals/Evaluation Criteria for Delayed Growth and Development, p. 232, and Risk for Impaired Parenting, on p. 369.

Examples Using NOC Language

- Demonstrates **Parent–Infant Attachment**, as evidenced by the following indicators (specify 1–5: never, rarely, sometimes, often, or consistently demonstrated):

    Verbalize positive feelings toward infant

    Touch, stroke, pat, kiss, and smile at infant

    Visit nursery

    Talk to infant

    Use en face position and eye contact

- Demonstrates **Parenting**, as evidenced by the following indicators (specify 1–5: not, slightly, moderately, substantially, or totally adequate):

    Provides for the child's physical needs

    Stimulates cognitive and social development

    Stimulates emotional and spiritual growth

    Demonstrates a loving relationship with child

    Provides regular preventative and episodic health care

- Demonstrates **Role Performance**, as evidenced by the following indicators (specify 1–5: not, slightly, moderately, substantially, or totally adequate):

    Performance of family role behaviors

    Reported comfort with role expectation

- Demonstrates **Safety Behavior: Home Physical Environment**, as evidenced by the following indicators (specify 1–5: not, slightly, moderately, substantially, or totally adequate):

    Smoke detector maintenance

    Disposal of unused medicines

    Storage of firearms to prevent accidents

    Storage of hazardous materials to prevent injury

    Provision of a safe play area

    Use of electrical outlet covers

Other Examples

The parent(s) will:

- Demonstrate constructive discipline
- Identify effective ways to express anger and frustration that are not harmful to child
- Actively participate in counseling and parenting classes
- Identify and use community resources that assist with home care
- Identify people who can provide information and emotional support when needed
- Indicate willingness to ask others for help

The child will:
• Achieve physical, cognitive, and psychosocial milestones at expected times (refer to appropriate age group for specific developmental norms)

NIC Interventions

Abuse Protection Support: Child: Identification of high-risk, dependent child relationships and actions to prevent possible or further infliction of physical, sexual, or emotional harm or neglect of basic necessities of life

Attachment Promotion: Facilitation of the development of the parent–infant relationship

Coping Enhancement: Assisting a patient to adapt to perceived stressors, changes, or threats which interfere with meeting life demands and roles

Developmental Enhancement: Adolescent: Facilitating optimal physical, cognitive, social, and emotional growth of individuals during the transition from childhood to adulthood

Developmental Enhancement: Child: Facilitating or teaching parents and caregivers to facilitate the optimal gross-motor, fine-motor, language, cognitive, social, and emotional growth of preschool and school-aged children

Environmental Management: Attachment Process: Manipulation of the patient's surroundings to facilitate the development of the parent–infant relationship

Environmental Management: Safety: Monitoring and manipulation of the physical environment to promote safety

Family Integrity Promotion: Promotion of family cohesion and unity

Family Integrity Promotion: Childbearing Family: Facilitation of the growth of individuals or families who are adding an infant to the family unit

Family Involvement Promotion: Facilitating family participation in the emotional and physical care of the patient

Family Process Maintenance: Minimization of family process disruption effects

Family Support: Promotion of family values, interests, and goals

Kangaroo Care: Promoting closeness between parent and physiologically stable preterm infant by preparing the parent and providing the environment for skin-to-skin contact

Parent Education: Adolescent: Assisting parents to understand and help their adolescent children

Parent Education: Childrearing Family: Assisting parents to understand and promote the physical, psychological, and social growth and development of their toddler or preschool or school-aged child or children

Parent Education: Infant: Instruction on nurturing and physical care needed during the first year of life

Parenting Promotion: Providing parenting information, support, and coordination of comprehensive services to high-risk families

Risk Identification: Childbearing Family: Identification of an individual or family likely to experience difficulties in parenting and prioritization of strategies to prevent parenting problems

Role Enhancement: Assisting a patient, significant other, or family to improve relationships by clarifying and supplementing specific role behaviors

Support Group: Use of a group environment to provide emotional support and health-related information for members

Support System Enhancement: Facilitation of support to patient by family, friends, and community

Surveillance: Safety: Purposeful and ongoing collection and analysis of information about the patient and the environment for use in promoting and maintaining patient safety

Nursing Activities

Refer to Nursing Activities for Parenting, Risk for Impaired, pp. 370–372.

Collaborative Activities

- Offer to make initial telephone call to appropriate community resources
- *(NIC) Abuse Protection: Child:*

  Refer families to human services and counseling professionals, as needed

  Provide parents with community resource information that includes addresses and phone numbers of agencies that provide respite care, emergency child care, housing assistance, substance abuse treatment, sliding-fee counseling services, food pantries, clothing distribution centers, health care, human services, hot lines, and domestic abuse shelters

  Report suspected abuse or neglect to proper authorities

  Refer parents to Parents Anonymous for group support, as appropriate

Other

- Encourage expression of feelings (e.g., guilt, anger, ambivalence) regarding parenting role
- Help parent identify deficits and alterations in parenting skills

- Provide frequent opportunities for parent–child interaction
- Role model parenting skills
- Help identify realistic expectations of parenting role
- Acknowledge and reinforce parenting strengths and skills
- *(NIC) Family Integrity Promotion:*
   Establish trusting relationship with family members
   Assist family with conflict resolution
   Assist family to resolve feelings of guilt
   Facilitate a tone of togetherness within or among the family
   Facilitate open communications among family members

During Pregnancy

- *(NIC) Attachment Promotion:*
   Discuss parent's reaction to pregnancy
   Provide parent(s) the opportunity to hear fetal heart tones as
      soon as possible
   Discuss parent's reaction to hearing fetal heart tones, viewing
      ultrasound image, etc.
   Assist father or significant other during participation in labor
      and delivery

At Delivery

- *(NIC) Attachment Promotion:*
   Place infant on mother's body immediately after birth
   Provide father opportunity to hold newborn in delivery area
   Provide pain relief for mother
   Provide family privacy during initial interaction with newborn
   Encourage parents to touch and speak to newborn

PARENTING, READINESS FOR ENHANCED (00164) (2002)

Definition: A pattern of providing an environment for children or
   other dependent person(s) that is sufficient to nurture growth
   and development and can be strengthened

Defining Characteristics

Subjective
Children or other dependent person(s) express satisfaction with
   home environment
Expresses willingness to enhance parenting

Objective

Emotional and tacit support of children or dependent person(s) is evident; bonding or attachment evident

Physical and emotional needs of children or dependent person(s) are met

Realistic expectations of children or dependent person(s) exhibited

Related Factors

This is a wellness diagnosis, so an etiology is not needed. If risk factors exist, use *Risk for impaired parenting.*

Suggestions for Use

NANDA International states that, in general, adjustment to parenting is a normal maturational process that calls for nursing interventions to prevent potential problems and promote health. If interventions are not limited to parenting, consider one of the Suggested Alternative Diagnoses.

Suggested Alternative Diagnoses

Coping: family, readiness for enhanced

Family processes, readiness for enhanced

NOC Outcomes

NOC outcomes have not yet been linked to this new diagnosis; however, the following may be useful

Parent–Infant Attachment: Behaviors that demonstrate an enduring affectionate bond between a parent and infant

Parenting: Provision of an environment that promotes optimum growth and development of dependent children

Parenting: Social Safety: Parental actions to avoid social relationships that might cause harm or injury

Role Performance: Congruence of an individual's role behavior with role expectations

Goals/Evaluation Criteria

Also see Goals/Evaluation Criteria for Parenting, Impaired, pp. 359–360.

Examples Using NOC Language

- Demonstrates **Coping**, as evidenced by the following indicators (specify 1–5: never, rarely, sometimes, often, or consistently demonstrated):

    Employs behaviors to reduce stress

    Identifies and uses multiple, effective coping strategies

- Demonstrates **Parenting**, as evidenced by the following indicators (specify 1–5: not, slightly, moderately, substantially, or totally adequate):
    Uses appropriate discipline
    Has realistic expectations of parental role
    Verbalizes positive attributes of child
- Demonstrates **Parent–Infant Attachment** (during pregnancy), as evidenced by the following indicators (specify 1–5: never, rarely, sometimes, often, or consistently demonstrated):
    Practice healthy behaviors
    Assign specific attributes to fetus
    Prepare for infant prior to birth

Other Examples

Parent(s) will:
- Identify own risk factors that may lead to ineffective parenting
- Identify high-risk situations that may lead to ineffective parenting
- Recognize and compensate for physical, cognitive, or psychologic limitations for caregiving
- Verbalize a sense of control over own behaviors and life situation
- Report having positive interpersonal relationships
- Demonstrate constructive discipline
- Identify and use community resources that assist with home care
- Identify people who can provide information and emotional support when needed
- Indicate willingness to ask others for help
The child will:
- Achieve physical, cognitive, and psychosocial milestones at expected times (refer to appropriate age group for specific developmental norms)

NIC Interventions

This is a new diagnosis, so NIC intervention linkages are not yet available; however, the following may be useful:

Attachment Promotion: Facilitation of the development of the parent–infant relationship

Developmental Enhancement: Adolescent: Facilitating optimal physical, cognitive, social, and emotional growth of individuals during the transition from childhood to adulthood

Developmental Enhancement: Child: Facilitating or teaching parents and caregivers to facilitate the optimal gross-motor,

fine-motor, language, cognitive, social, and emotional growth of
preschool and school-aged children

Environmental Management: Attachment Process: Manipulation
of the patient's surroundings to facilitate the development of
the parent–infant relationship

Family Integrity Promotion: Promotion of family cohesion and
unity

Parenting Promotion: Providing parenting information, support,
and coordination of comprehensive services to high-risk families

Role Enhancement: Assisting a patient, significant other, or family
to improve relationships by clarifying and supplementing specific role behaviors

Nursing Activities

Assessment

- Determine whether parents have realistic expectations for child's
  behavior
- *(NIC) Attachment Promotion:*
  Determine parent's knowledge of infant or child basic care needs
    and provide appropriate child-care information, as indicated
- *(NIC) Family Integrity Promotion:*
  Determine typical family relationships
  Monitor current family relationships

Patient/Parent Teaching

- Provide information about child care, as needed
- Teach problem-solving, decision-making, and childrearing skills,
  as needed
- Instruct regarding noncorporal punishment methods for disci-
  plining children
- *(NIC) Attachment Promotion:*
  Demonstrate ways to touch infant confined to Isolette
  Discuss infant behavioral characteristics with parent(s)
  Instruct parent(s) on signs of overstimulation
- *(NIC) Developmental Enhancement: Child:* Teach caregivers about
  normal developmental milestones and associated behaviors

Collaborative Activities

- *(NIC) Attachment Promotion:* Encourage parent(s) to attend prenatal classes

Other

- *(NIC) Attachment Promotion:*

  Encourage father or significant other to participate in labor and delivery

  Provide opportunity for parent(s) to see, hold, and examine newborn immediately after birth

  Share information gained from initial physical assessment of newborn with parent(s)

  Provide family privacy during initial interaction with newborn

  Reinforce attachment behaviors (e.g., eye contact)

  Acknowledge and reinforce parenting strengths and skills

  [For newborns who are premature or ill], explain equipment used to monitor infant in nursery, encourage parent(s) to visit infant in the nursery, place pictures of family in Isolette so infant can "see" the family, take picture of infant to leave with mother before transporting infant to another hospital, and reinforce normal aspects of infant with defect

- *(NIC) Family Integrity Promotion:*

  Be a listener for the family members

  Facilitate a tone of togetherness within/among the family

  Facilitate open communications among family members

PARENTING, RISK FOR IMPAIRED
(00057) (1978, 1998)

Definition: Risk for inability of the primary caretaker to create, maintain, or regain an environment that promotes the optimum growth and development of the child

Risk Factors

Infant or Child

Altered perceptual abilities

Attention-deficit hyperactivity disorder

Difficult temperament

Handicapping condition or developmental delay

Illness

Lack of goodness of fit (i.e., temperament) with parental expectations

Multiple births

Not gender desired

Premature birth

Prolonged separation from parent

Separation from parent at birth
Unplanned or unwanted child

Knowledge

Inability to recognize and act on infant cues
Lack of cognitive readiness for parenthood
Lack of knowledge about child development
Lack of knowledge about child health maintenance
Lack of knowledge about parenting skills
Low cognitive functioning
Low educational level or attainment
Poor communication skills
Preference for physical punishment
Unrealistic expectations of child

Physiologic

Physical illness

Psychologic

Depression
Difficult labor or delivery
Disability
High number or closely spaced children
History of mental illness
History of substance abuse or dependence
Lack of, or late, prenatal care
Multiple births
Separation from infant or child
Sleep deprivation or disruption
Young ages, especially adolescent

Social

Change in family unit
Father of child not involved
Financial difficulties
History of being abused
History of being abusive
Inability to put child's needs before own
Inadequate child-care arrangements
Lack of access to resources
Lack of family cohesiveness
Lack of or poor parental role model
Lack of resources
Lack of social support network
Lack of transportation
Lack of value of parenthood

Legal difficulties
Low self-esteem
Low socioeconomic class
Maladaptive coping strategies
Marital conflict, declining satisfaction
Poor home environment
Poor problem-solving skills
Poverty
Relocation
Role strain or overload
Single parent
Social isolation
Stress
Unemployment or job problems
Unplanned or unwanted pregnancy

Suggestions for Use

NANDA International states that, in general, adjustment to parenting is a normal maturational process that calls for nursing interventions to prevent potential problems and promote health.

Suggested Alternative Diagnoses

Caregiver role strain, risk for
Coping: family, compromised
Coping: family, readiness for enhanced
Family processes, interrupted
Parent/infant/child attachment, risk for impaired
Role conflict, parental
Role performance, ineffective

NOC Outcomes

Caregiver Stressors: The extent of biopsychosocial pressure on a family care provider caring for a family member or significant other over an extended period of time

Coping: Actions to manage stressors that tax an individual's resources

Parent–Infant Attachment: Behaviors that demonstrate an enduring affectionate bond between a parent and infant

Parenting: Provision of an environment that promotes optimum growth and development of dependent children

Parenting: Social Safety: Parental actions to avoid social relationships that might cause harm or injury

Role Performance: Congruence of an individual's role behavior with role expectations

Goals/Evaluation Criteria

Also see Goals/Evaluation Criteria for Parenting, Impaired, pp. 358–360.

Examples Using NOC Language

- Demonstrates **Coping**, as evidenced by the following indicators (specify 1–5: never, rarely, sometimes, often, or consistently demonstrated):

    Employs behaviors to reduce stress

    Identifies and uses multiple, effective coping strategies

- Demonstrates **Parenting**, as evidenced by the following indicators (specify 1–5: not, slightly, moderately, substantially, or totally adequate):

    Uses appropriate discipline

    Has realistic expectations of parental role

    Verbalizes positive attributes of child

- Demonstrates **Parent–Infant Attachment** (during pregnancy), as evidenced by the following indicators (specify 1–5: never, rarely, sometimes, often, or consistently demonstrated):

    Practice healthy behaviors

    Assign specific attributes to fetus

    Prepare for infant prior to birth

Other Examples

Parent(s) will:

- Identify own risk factors that may lead to ineffective parenting
- Identify high-risk situations that may lead to ineffective parenting
- Recognize and compensate for physical, cognitive, or psychologic limitations for caregiving
- Demonstrate recovery from past emotional abuses (e.g., verbalize confidence and self-esteem)
- Seek help for emotional problems/neuroses
- Verbalize a sense of control over own behaviors and life situation
- Report having positive interpersonal relationships

NIC Interventions

Abuse Protection Support: Child: Identification of high-risk, dependent child relationships and actions to prevent possible or further infliction of physical, sexual, or emotional harm or neglect of basic necessities of life

Attachment Promotion: Facilitation of the development of the parent–infant relationship

Developmental Enhancement: Adolescent: Facilitating optimal physical, cognitive, social, and emotional growth of individuals during the transition from childhood to adulthood

Developmental Enhancement: Child: Facilitating or teaching parents and caregivers to facilitate the optimal gross-motor, fine-motor, language, cognitive, social, and emotional growth of preschool and school-aged children

Environmental management: Attachment Process: Manipulation of the patient's surroundings to facilitate the development of the parent–infant relationship

Family Integrity Promotion: Promotion of family cohesion and unity

Normalization Promotion: Assisting parents and other family members of children with chronic illnesses or disabilities in providing normal life experiences for their children and families

Parenting Promotion: Providing parenting information, support and coordination of comprehensive services to high-risk families

Role Enhancement: Assisting a patient, significant other, or family to improve relationships by clarifying and supplementing specific role behaviors

Nursing Activities

Assessment

- Determine whether parents have unrealistic expectations for child's behavior or negative attributions for their child's behavior
- *(NIC) Abuse Protection Support: Child:*

    Identify parents who have had another child removed from the home or have placed previous children with relatives for extended periods

    Identify parents who have a history of substance abuse, depression, or major psychiatric illness

    Identify parents who have a history of domestic violence or a mother who has a history of numerous "accidental" injuries

    Identify crisis situations that may trigger abuse (e.g., poverty, unemployment, divorce, homelessness, and domestic violence)

    Identify infants or children with high-care needs (e.g., prematurity, low birth weight, colic, feeding intolerances, major health problems in the first year of life, developmental disabilities, hyperactivity, and attention-deficit disorders)

- *(NIC) Attachment Promotion:*

  Ascertain before birth whether parent(s) has names picked out for both sexes

  Monitor new parents' reactions to their infant, observing for feelings of disgust, fear, or disappointment in gender

  Determine parent's knowledge of infant or child basic care needs and provide appropriate child-care information, as indicated
- *(NIC) Family Integrity Promotion:*

  Determine typical family relationships

  Monitor current family relationships
- *(NIC) Normalization Promotion:*

  [For a child with a chronic illness] determine the following:

  Accessibility of activity and child's ability to participate in activity

  Need for respite care for parents or other care providers

Patient/Parent Teaching

- *(NIC) Abuse Protection Support: Child:*

  Determine parent's knowledge of infant or child basic care needs and provide appropriate child-care information, as indicated

  Instruct parents on problem-solving, decision-making, and child-rearing and parenting skills or refer parents to programs where these skills can be learned

  Provide parents with information on how to cope with protracted infant crying, emphasizing that they should not shake the baby

  Provide the parents with noncorporal punishment methods for disciplining children
- *(NIC) Attachment Promotion:*

  Demonstrate ways to touch infant confined to Isolette

  Discuss infant behavioral characteristics with parent(s)

  Instruct parent(s) on signs of overstimulation
- *(NIC) Developmental Enhancement: Child:* Teach caregivers about normal developmental milestones and associated behaviors

Collaborative Activities

- Refer to community support and educational programs to assist with development of parenting skills and provide anticipatory guidance
- *(NIC) Abuse Protection Support: Child:*

  Refer at-risk pregnant women and parents of newborns to nurse home visitation services

Provide at-risk families with a public health nurse referral to ensure that the home environment is monitored, that siblings are assessed, and that families receive continued assistance

- *(NIC) Attachment Promotion:* Encourage parent(s) to attend prenatal classes
- *(NIC) Family Integrity Promotion:* Refer for family therapy, as indicated

Other

- *(NIC) Attachment Promotion:*

  Encourage father or significant other to participate in labor and delivery

  Provide opportunity for parent(s) to see, hold, and examine newborn immediately after birth

  Share information gained from initial physical assessment of newborn with parent(s)

  Provide family privacy during initial interaction with newborn

  Reinforce attachment behaviors (e.g., eye contact)

  Acknowledge and reinforce parenting strengths and skills

  [For newborns who are premature or ill], explain equipment used to monitor infant in nursery, encourage parent(s) to visit infant in the nursery, place pictures of family in Isolette so infant can "see" the family, take picture of infant to leave with mother before transporting infant to another hospital, and reinforce normal aspects of infant with defect

- *(NIC) Family Integrity Promotion:*

  Be a listener for the family members

  Facilitate a tone of togetherness within or among the family

  Facilitate open communications among family members

- *(NIC) Normalization Promotion [for ill child]:*

  Encourage parents to have same parenting expectations and techniques for affected child as with other children in family, as appropriate

  Assist family in making changes in home environment that decrease reminders of child's special needs

PERIOPERATIVE POSITIONING INJURY, RISK FOR (00087) (1994)

Definition: At risk for injury as a result of the environmental conditions found in the perioperative setting

Risk Factors

[Advanced age]
Disorientation
Edema
Emaciation
Immobilization, muscle weakness
Obesity
Sensory or perceptual disturbances due to anesthesia

Suggestions for Use

This diagnosis is a specific variation of *Risk for injury*. All surgery patients have at least some risk for *Perioperative positioning injury (PPI)*. For those with no preexisting risk factors, no etiology is needed because the perioperative positioning itself is the etiology. When there are preexisting risk factors (e.g., edema, advanced age, diabetes, arthritis, vascular disease), include them as the etiology (e.g., *Risk for PPI related to generalized edema*). A long surgical procedure also increases the risk for *PPI*. Actual *PPI* may be the etiology of other nursing diagnoses (e.g., *Impaired skin integrity*).

Suggested Alternative Diagnoses

Neurovascular dysfunction: peripheral, risk for
Skin integrity, risk for impaired
Tissue integrity, risk for impaired
Trauma, risk for

NOC Outcomes

Circulation Status: Extent to which blood flows unobstructed, unidirectionally, and at an appropriate pressure through large vessels of the systemic and pulmonary circuits

Neurological Status: Extent to which the peripheral and central nervous systems receive, process, and respond to internal and external stimuli

Respiratory Status: Ventilation: Movement of air in and out of the lungs

Tissue Perfusion: Peripheral: Extent to which blood flows through the small vessels of the extremities and maintains tissue function

Goals/Evaluation Criteria
Examples Using NOC Language
- *PPI* will not occur, as demonstrated by uncompromised Neurological Status, Respiratory Status: Ventilation, Peripheral Tissue Perfusion, and Circulation Status.
- Demonstrates **Neurological Status** (specify 1–5; extremely, substantially, moderately, mildly, or not compromised)
- Demonstrates **Respiratory Status: Ventilation** (specify 1–5; extremely, substantially, moderately, mildly, or not compromised)
- Demonstrates **Tissue Perfusion: Peripheral** (specify 1–5: extremely, substantially, moderately, mildly, or not compromised)
- Demonstrates **Circulation Status**, as evidenced by the following indicators (specify 1–5: extremely, substantially, moderately, mildly, or not compromised):
    Peripheral tissue perfusion
    Peripheral pulses strong and symmetric
    Systolic and diastolic blood pressure in expected range

Other Examples
    Patient will have:
- No skin, tissue, or neuromuscular injury as a result of perioperative positioning
- Brisk capillary refill
- Normal peripheral sensation
- Normal skin color and temperature
- Unimpaired muscle function
- No peripheral edema
- No localized extremity pain

NIC Interventions
Airway Insertion and Stabilization: Insertion or assisting with insertion and stabilization of an artificial airway

Airway Management: Facilitation of patency of air passages

Cerebral Perfusion Promotion: Promotion of adequate perfusion and limitation of complications for a patient experiencing, or at risk for, inadequate cerebral perfusion

Circulatory Care: Arterial Insufficiency: Promotion of arterial circulation

Circulatory Care: Venous Insufficiency: Promotion of venous circulation

Circulatory Precautions: Protection of a localized area with limited perfusion

Embolus Care: Peripheral: Limitation of complications for a patient experiencing, or at risk for, occlusion of peripheral circulation

Positioning: Intraoperative: Moving the patient or body part to promote surgical exposure while reducing the risk of discomfort and complications

Skin Surveillance: Collection and analysis of patient data to maintain skin and mucous membrane integrity

Nursing Activities

Assessments

- Determine preexisting factors (e.g., poor nutrition, diseases) that create risk for PPI
- *(NIC) Positioning: Intraoperative:*
  Determine patient's range of motion and stability of joints
  Check peripheral circulation and neurologic status
  Monitor patient's position intraoperatively
- *(NIC) Skin Surveillance (postoperative period):*
  Observe extremities for color, warmth, swelling, pulses, texture, edema, and ulcerations
  Monitor skin for areas of redness and breakdown
  Monitor skin color and temperature

Patient/Family Teaching

- *(NIC) Skin Surveillance:* Instruct family member or caregiver about signs of skin breakdown, as appropriate.

Collaborative Activities

- *(NIC) Positioning: Intraoperative:* Communicate to postanesthesia nurses any preexisting risk factors or any symptoms observed during the intraoperative period

Other

- Lift patient when positioning; do not slide or pull patient
- Always reposition patient slowly and gently
- Ensure that surgical team members do not lean on the patient
- *(NIC) Positioning: Intraoperative:*
  Use assistive devices [e.g., leg restraint strap] for immobilization
  Use an adequate number of personnel to transfer patient

Support the head and neck during transfer

Protect IV lines, catheters, and breathing circuits

Maintain patient's proper body alignment [refer to agency procedures or a surgical textbook for details of supine, prone, lateral, and lithotomy positions]

Elevate extremities, as appropriate

Apply padding [e.g., to bony prominences] to avoid pressure to superficial nerves

Apply safety strap and arm restraint, as needed

Protect the eyes, as appropriate

POISONING, RISK FOR
(00037) (1980)

Definition: Accentuated risk of accidental exposure to or ingestion of drugs or dangerous products in doses sufficient to cause poisoning

Risk Factors

Internal (Individual)

Cognitive or emotional difficulties

Insufficient finances

Lack of proper precautions

Lack of safety or drug education

Reduced vision

Verbalization of occupational setting without adequate safeguards

External (Environmental)

Availability of illicit drugs potentially contaminated by poisonous additives

Chemical contamination of food and water

Dangerous products placed or stored within the reach of children or confused persons

Flaking, peeling paint or plaster in presence of young children

Large supplies of drugs in house

Medicines stored in unlocked cabinets accessible to children or confused persons

Paint, lacquer, and so forth in poorly ventilated areas or without effective protection

Presence of atmospheric pollutants

Presence of poisonous vegetation

Unprotected contact with heavy metals or chemicals

Suggestions for Use

Use the most specific label for which defining characteristics are present (i.e., if required risk factors are present, use *Risk for poisoning* instead of *Risk for injury*)

Suggested Alternative Diagnoses

Home maintenance, impaired
Injury, risk for
Parenting, impaired
Violence: self-directed, risk for

NOC Outcomes

Medication Response: Therapeutic and adverse effects of prescribed medication

Risk Control: Actions to eliminate or reduce actual, personal, and modifiable health threats

Safety Behavior: Home Physical Environment: Individual or caregiver actions to minimize environmental factors that might cause physical harm or injury in the home

Safety Behavior: Personal: Individual or caregiver efforts to control behaviors that might cause physical injury

Safety Status: Physical Injury: Severity of injuries from accidents and trauma

Goals/Evaluation Criteria

Examples Using NOC Language

- Demonstrates **Risk Control**, as evidenced by the following indicators (specify 1–5: never, rarely, sometimes, often, or consistently demonstrated):

    Monitors personal behavior risk factors
    Monitors environmental risk factors
    Follows selected risk-control strategies

Other Examples

Patient will:
- Develop strategies to prevent poisoning
- Demonstrate understanding of safe use of medication, as indicated by description of proper methods of administration, dosage, storage, and disposal
- Seek information about potential risks

NIC Interventions

Environmental Management, Safety: Monitoring and manipulation of the physical environment to promote safety

Health Education: Developing and providing instruction and learning experiences to facilitate voluntary adaptation of behavior conducive to health in individuals, families, groups, or communities

Surveillance, Safety: Purposeful and ongoing collection and analysis of information about the patient and the environment for use in promoting and maintaining patient safety

Nursing Activities

Assessments

- *(NIC) Environmental Management: Safety:* Monitor the environment for changes in safety status
- *(NIC) Surveillance: Safety:*
  Monitor patient for alterations in physical or cognitive function that might lead to unsafe behavior
  Identify the safety needs of patient based on level of physical and cognitive function and past history of behavior

Patient/Family Teaching

- Provide educational materials related to safety strategies and countermeasures for poisons
- *(NIC) Environmental Management: Safety:*
  Educate high-risk individuals and groups about environmental hazards (e.g., lead and radon)
  Provide patient with emergency phone numbers (e.g., police, local health department, and poison control center)

Collaborative Activities

- Refer to community classes (e.g., cardiopulmonary resuscitation [CPR], first aid)
- *(NIC) Environmental Management: Safety:* Collaborate with other agencies to improve environmental safety (e.g., health department, police, and Environmental Protection Agency [EPA])

Other

- *(NIC) Environmental Management: Safety:*
  Modify the environment to minimize hazards and risk
  Use protective devices (e.g., restraints, side rails, locked doors, fences, and gates) to physically limit mobility or access to harmful situations

- *(NIC) Surveillance: Safety:* Provide appropriate level of supervision and surveillance to monitor patient and to allow for therapeutic actions, as needed

POST-TRAUMA SYNDROME
(00141) (1986, 1998)

Definition: Sustained maladaptive response to a traumatic, overwhelming event

Defining Characteristics

Subjective

Anger or rage
Fear
Flashbacks
Guilt
Headaches
Intrusive thoughts
Numbing
Palpitations
Shame

Objective

Aggression
Alienation
Altered mood states
Anxiety
Avoidance
Compulsive behavior
Denial
Depression
Detachment
Difficulty concentrating
Enuresis (in children)
Exaggerated startle response
Gastric irritability
Grief
Hopelessness
Horror
Hypervigilant
Intrusive dreams
Irritability

Neurosensory irritability
Nightmares
Panic attacks
Psychogenic amnesia
Repression
Substance abuse

Related Factors

Being held prisoner of war or criminal victimization (torture)
Epidemics
Events outside the range of usual human experience
Industrial and motor vehicle accidents
Military combat
Natural or man-made disasters
Physical and psychosocial abuse
Rape
Serious accidents
Serious threat or injury to self or loved ones
Sudden destruction of one's home or community
Tragic occurrence involving multiple deaths
Wars
Witnessing mutilation, violent death, or other horrors

Suggestions for Use

(1) If the related factor is rape, use one of the *Rape-trauma syndrome* diagnoses. (2) Because this is a syndrome diagnosis, the diagnostic statement does not need related factors and the second part of the statement (etiology) is omitted. (3) Other nursing diagnoses (e.g., *Risk for suicide*) may be needed in addition to *Rape-trauma syndrome* in order to focus nursing interventions more specifically.

Suggested Alternative Diagnoses

Coping: family, compromised or disabled
Coping, ineffective
Rape-trauma syndrome: compound reaction
Rape-trauma syndrome: silent reaction
Self-mutilation, risk for
Suicide, risk for
Violence: self-directed, risk for

NOC Outcomes

Abuse Cessation: Evidence that the victim is no longer abused

Abuse Protection: Protection of self or dependent others from abuse

Abuse Recovery: Emotional: Healing of psychologic injuries due to abuse

Abuse Recovery: Financial: Regaining monetary and legal control or benefits following financial exploitation

Abuse Recovery: Physical: Healing of physical injuries due to abuse

Abuse Recovery: Sexual: Healing following sexual abuse or exploitation

Coping: Actions to manage stressors that tax an individual's resources

Fear Control: Personal actions to eliminate or reduce disabling feelings or alarm aroused by an identifiable source

Impulse Control: Ability to self-restrain compulsive or impulsive behaviors

Self-Mutilation Restraint: Ability to refrain from intentional self-inflicted injury (nonlethal)

Goals/Evaluation Criteria

Examples Using NOC Language

- Demonstrates **Abuse Recovery: Sexual**, as evidenced by the following indicators (specify 1–5: none, limited, moderate, substantial, or extensive):

    Details of abuse

    Feelings about the abuse

    Appropriate and inappropriate guilt

    Accurate information about sexual functioning

    Confidence with sexual orientation

    Right to have been protected from abuse

    Hope

- Demonstrates **Abuse Recovery: Emotional**, as evidenced by the following indicators (specify 1–5: none, limited, moderate, substantial, or extensive):

    Demonstrates appropriate affect for situation

    Does not attempt suicide

    Reports feeling less depressed

    Is able to control impulses

    Reports satisfaction with social interactions

Other Examples

Patient will:

- Acknowledge value of counseling
- Identify feelings and situations that lead to impulsive actions
- Control destructive and harmful impulses without supervision
- Seeks help when unable to control impulses
- Report relief from physical symptoms (e.g., headache, gastrointestinal upset)

NIC Interventions

Behavior Management: Self-Harm: Assisting the patient to decrease or eliminate self-mutilating or self-abusive behaviors

Coping Enhancement: Assisting a patient to adapt to perceived stressors, changes, or threats which interfere with meeting life demands and roles

Counseling: Use of an interactive helping process focusing on the needs, problems, or feelings of the patient and significant others to enhance or support coping, problem-solving, and interpersonal relationships

Financial Resource Assistance: Assisting an individual and family to secure and manage finances to meet health care needs

Impulse Control Training: Assisting the patient to mediate impulsive behavior through application of problem-solving strategies to social and interpersonal situations

Rape-Trauma Treatment: Provision of emotional and physical support immediately following a reported rape

Security Enhancement: Intensifying a patient's sense of physical and psychological safety

Support System Enhancement: Facilitation of support to patient by family, friends, and community

Nursing Activities

Also refer to Nursing Activities for Post-Trauma Syndrome, Risk for, pp. 385–386.

Collaborative Activities

- Follow hospital and agency policy regarding legal responsibility for reporting to authorities

Other

- Enhance patient's feeling of safety in the following ways:
    Monitor and hold phone calls at patient's request
    Monitor and limit visitation

Consider private versus semiprivate assignment and choice of roommate

Institute precautions to prevent physical harm to the patient or others

- *(NIC) Counseling:*

Establish a therapeutic relationship based on trust and respect

Demonstrate empathy, warmth, and genuineness

Use techniques of reflection and clarification to facilitate expression of concerns

Encourage expression of feelings in a nondestructive manner

Reveal selected aspects of one's own experiences or personality to foster genuineness and trust, as appropriate

Discourage decision making when the patient is under severe stress

POST-TRAUMA SYNDROME, RISK FOR
(00145) (1998)

Definition: A risk for sustained maladaptive response to a traumatic or overwhelming event

Risk Factors

Diminished ego strength

Displacement from home

Duration of the event

Exaggerated sense of responsibility

Inadequate social support

Nonsupportive environment

Occupation (e.g., police, fire, rescue, corrections, emergency room staff, mental health)

Perception of event

Survivor's role in the event

Suggestions for Use

(1) As a rule, syndrome diagnoses are one-part diagnostic statements, omitting the related factors. However, because this is a "risk for" (potential) diagnosis, it may be helpful to write a two-part statement with the related factors as the etiology (e.g., *Risk for post-trauma syndrome related to inadequate social support to aid in coping with aftermath of surviving a fire in which friends died*). (2) If defining characteristics are present for any of the suggested

alternative diagnoses, the nurse will need to decide whether it is more useful to write an actual diagnosis (e.g., *Social isolation related to unacceptable social values*) or to use the alternative diagnosis as an etiology (e.g., *Risk for post-trauma syndrome related to Social isolation*).

Suggested Alternative Diagnoses

Coping: community, ineffective
Coping: family, compromised or disabled
Coping: ineffective
Family processes, interrupted
Identity: personal, disturbed
Self-esteem, chronic or situational low
Social isolation
Spiritual distress

NOC Outcomes

Abuse Recovery: Emotional: Healing of psychologic injuries due to abuse

Abuse Recovery: Sexual: Healing following sexual abuse or exploitation

Coping: Actions to manage stressors that tax an individual's resources

Depression Control: Personal actions to minimize melancholy and maintain interest in life events

Depression Level: Severity of melancholic mood and loss of interest in life events

Goals/Evaluation Criteria

Examples Using NOC Language

- Recovery from *Post-trauma Syndrome* is indicated by Emotional or Sexual Abuse Recovery (if appropriate); Depression Control; and satisfactory Coping and Depression Level.

Other Examples

- Risk factors will be identified and controlled or eliminated so that *Post-trauma syndrome* does not occur.
  Patient will:
- Display adequate ego strength
- Have adequate social support
- Demonstrate appropriate affect for the situation
- Demonstrate adequate social interaction
- Identify and use effective coping strategies

NIC Interventions

Abuse Protection Support: Identification of high-risk, dependent relationships and actions to prevent further infliction of physical or emotional harm

Coping Enhancement: Assisting a patient to adapt to perceived stressors, changes, or threats which interfere with meeting life demands and roles

Counseling: Use of an interactive helping process focusing on the needs, problems, or feelings of the patient and significant others to enhance or support coping, problem-solving, and interpersonal relationships

Crisis Intervention: Use of a short-term counseling to help the patient cope with a crisis and resume a state of functioning comparable to or better than the precrisis state

Hope Instillation: Facilitation of the development of a positive outlook in a given situation

Mood Management: Providing for safety, stabilization, recovery, and maintenance of a patient who is experiencing dysfunctionally depressed mod or elevated mood

Rape-Trauma Treatment: Provision of emotional and physical support immediately following a reported rape

Support System Enhancement: Facilitation of support to patient by family, friends, and community

Nursing Activities

Assessments

- Assess psychologic response to the trauma
- Assess adequacy and availability of support system and community resources
- Assess family situation

Patient/Family Teaching

- Explain to significant others how they can provide support

Collaborative Activities

- Provide information on or referral to community resources (e.g., rape counselors, clergy, crisis centers, support groups, mental health professionals, social services, Victims' Assistance, Survivors of Trauma)

Other

- Provide opportunity for social supports and problem solving (e.g., participation in social and community activities)

- Encourage patient to verbalize account of the event
- Support the patient needing an invasive medical procedure, which may precipitate flashbacks:

  Explain necessity of procedure

  Premedicate if needed to minimize distress and discomfort

  Stay with patient during procedure

  Encourage patient to discuss feelings after procedure

POWERLESSNESS
(00125) (1982)

Definition: Perception that one's own action will not significantly affect an outcome; a perceived lack of control over a current situation or immediate happening

Defining Characteristics

Severe

Subjective

Verbal expressions of having no control or influence over situation, self-care, or outcome

Objective

Apathy

Depression over physical deterioration that occurs despite patient compliance with regimens

Moderate

Subjective

Anger

Expressions of dissatisfaction and frustration over inability to perform previous tasks or activities

Expression of doubt regarding role performance

Fear of alienation from caregivers

Guilt

Reluctance to express true feelings

Objective

Dependence on others that may result in irritability, resentment, anger, and guilt

Inability to seek information regarding care

No defense of self-care practices when challenged

No monitoring of progress

Nonparticipation in care or decision making when opportunities are provided
Passivity
Resentment

Low

Subjective
Expressions of uncertainty about fluctuating energy levels
Objective
Passivity

Related Factors

Health care environment
Illness-related regimen [e.g., long-term, difficult, complex]
Interpersonal interaction
Lifestyle of helplessness
Chronic or terminal illness (non-NANDA International)
Complications threatening pregnancy (non-NANDA International)

Suggestions for Use

Differentiate between *Powerlessness* and *Hopelessness. Hopelessness* implies that the person believes there is no solution to his problem (i.e., "no way out"). In *Powerlessness,* patients may know of a solution to their problem but believe it is beyond their control to achieve the solution. If *Powerlessness* is prolonged, it can lead to *Hopelessness.* Nurses should be careful to diagnose *Powerlessness* from the patient's perspective and not assume the patient perceives the situation as they would. Cultural and individual differences exist in a person's need to feel in control of a situation (e.g., to be told they have a fatal illness).

Suggested Alternative Diagnoses

Coping, ineffective
Disuse syndrome, risk for
Grieving, dysfunctional
Hopelessness
Rape-trauma syndrome: silent reaction
Self-esteem, chronic low
Spiritual distress

NOC Outcomes

Depression Control: Personal actions to minimize melancholy and maintain interest in life events

Depression Level: Severity of melancholic mood and loss of interest in life events

Family Participation in Professional Care: Family involvement in decision making, delivery, and evaluation of care provided by health care personnel

Health Beliefs: Personal convictions that influence health behaviors

Health Beliefs: Perceived Ability to Perform: Personal conviction that one can carry out a given health behavior

Health Beliefs: Perceived Control: Personal conviction that one can influence a health outcome

Health Beliefs: Perceived Resources: Personal conviction that one has adequate means to carry out a health behavior

Participation: Health Care Decisions: Personal involvement in selecting and evaluating health care options

Goals/Evaluation Criteria

Examples Using NOC Language

- Demonstrates Health Beliefs: Perceived Ability to Perform, Perceived Control, and Perceived Resources (specify 1–5: very weak, weak, moderate, strong, or very strong)
- Demonstrates **Participation: Health Care Decisions**, as evidenced by the following indicators (specify 1–5: never, rarely, sometimes, often, or consistently demonstrated):
    Identifies health outcome priorities
    Uses problem-solving techniques to achieve desired outcomes
    Negotiates for care preferences

Other Examples

Patient will:
- Verbalize any feelings of powerlessness
- Identify actions that are within his control
- Relate absence of barriers to action
- Verbalize ability to perform necessary actions
- Report adequate support from significant others, friends, and neighbors
- Report sufficient time, personal finances, and health insurance
- Report availability of equipment, supplies, services, and transportation

NIC Interventions

Cognitive Restructuring: Challenging a patient to alter distorted thought patterns and view self and the world more realistically

Decision-Making Support: Providing information and support for a patient who is making a decision regarding health care

Family Involvement Promotion: Facilitating family participation in the emotional and physical care of the patient

Health Education: Developing and providing instruction and learning experiences to facilitate voluntary adaptation of behavior conducive to health in individuals, families, groups, or communities

Health System Guidance: Facilitating a patient's location and use of appropriate health services

Mood Management: Providing for safety, stabilization, recovery, and maintenance of a patient who is experiencing dysfunctionally depressed mood or elevated mood

Mutual Goal Setting: Collaborating with patient to identify and prioritize care goals, then developing a plan for achieving those goals

Self-Esteem Enhancement: Assisting a patient to increase his personal judgment of self-worth

Self-Responsibility Facilitation: Encouraging a patient to assume more responsibility for own behavior

Values Clarification: Assisting another to clarify his own values in order to facilitate effective decision making

Nursing Activities

Assessments

- *(NIC) Self-Esteem Enhancement:*
  Determine patient's locus of control
  Determine patient's confidence in own judgment
  Monitor levels of self-esteem over time, as appropriate
- *(NIC) Self-Responsibility Facilitation:*
  Monitor level of responsibility that patient assumes
  Determine whether patient has adequate knowledge about health care condition

Collaborative Activities

- Initiate a multidisciplinary patient care conference to discuss and develop patient care routine

Other

- Help patient to identify factors that may contribute to powerlessness
- Discuss with patient realistic options in care, providing explanations for these options
- Involve patient in decision making about care routine
- Explain to patient the rationale for any change in the plan of care
- *(NIC) Self-Esteem Enhancement:*
  Explore previous achievements of success
  Reinforce the personal strengths that the patient identifies
  Convey confidence in patient's ability to handle situation
- *(NIC) Self-Responsibility Facilitation:*
  Encourage verbalizations of feelings, perceptions, and fears about assuming responsibility
  Encourage independence but assist patient when unable to perform

---

POWERLESSNESS, RISK FOR
(00152) (2000)

Definition: At risk for perceived lack of control over a situation or one's ability to significantly affect an outcome

Risk Factors

Physiological

Acute injury or progressive debilitating disease process (e.g., spinal cord injury, multiple sclerosis)

Aging (e.g., decreased physical strength, decreased mobility)

Chronic or acute illness (hospitalization, intubation, ventilator, suctioning)

Dying

Psychosocial

Absence of integrality (e.g., essence of power)

Decreased self-esteem

Lack of knowledge of illness or health care system

Lifestyle of dependency with inadequate coping patterns

Low or unstable body image

NOC Outcomes

NOC has not yet linked outcomes to this diagnosis; however, the outcomes for actual *Powerlessness,* on p. 388, may be useful.

Goals/Evaluation Criteria

Examples Using NOC Language

Refer to examples for *Powerlessness,* on p. 388.

Other Examples:

Patient will:

- Identify actions that are within his control
- Relate absence of barriers to action
- Verbalize ability to perform necessary actions
- Report adequate support from significant others, friends, and neighbors
- Report sufficient time, personal finances, and health insurance
- Report availability of equipment, supplies, services, and transportation

NIC Interventions

NIC has not yet linked interventions to this diagnosis; however, the interventions for actual *Powerlessness,* on p. 389, may be useful.

Nursing Activities

Refer to Nursing Activities for Powerlessness, on pp. 389–390.

PROTECTION, INEFFECTIVE
(00043) (1990)

Definition: Decrease in the ability to guard self from internal or external threat such as illness or injury

Defining Characteristics

Subjective
Chilling
Dyspnea
Fatigue
Itching
Objective
Altered clotting
Anorexia
Cough
Deficient immunity
Disorientation
Immobility

Impaired healing
Insomnia
Maladaptive stress response
Neurosensory alteration
Perspiring
Pressure ulcers
Restlessness
Weakness

Related Factors

Abnormal blood profiles (e.g., leukopenia, thrombocytopenia, anemia, coagulation)
Alcohol abuse
Diseases (e.g., cancer, immune disorders)
Drug therapies (e.g., antineoplastic, corticosteroid, immune, anticoagulant, thrombolytic)
Extremes of age
Inadequate nutrition
Treatments (e.g., surgery, radiation)
Abuse (non-NANDA International)

Suggestions for Use

(1) When possible, use a more specific label such as *Risk for infection, Impaired skin integrity, Impaired tissue integrity, Altered oral mucous membrane,* or *Fatigue.* (2) *Ineffective protection* should not be used as a "catchall" diagnosis for patients who are immunosuppressed or who have abnormal clotting factors. (3) Although NOC suggests *Abuse Protection* as an outcome, this author does not recommend using *Ineffective protection* to describe child or spousal abuse situations. Instead, consider *Impaired parenting, Compromised/disabled family coping, Risk for violence,* or similar diagnoses. Likewise, although Intrapartum Fetal Monitoring is a NIC priority intervention, the author does not recommend routine use of *Ineffective protection* during labor.

Suggested Alternative Diagnoses

Coping: family, compromised or disabled
Infection, risk for
Injury, risk for
Neurovascular dysfunction: peripheral, risk for
Parenting, impaired

Perioperative positioning injury, risk for
Skin integrity, risk for impaired

NOC Outcomes

Abuse Protection: Protection of self or dependent others from abuse

Coagulation Status: Extent to which blood clots within expected period of time

Endurance: Extent that energy enables a person to sustain activity

Fetal Status: Antepartum: Conditions indicative of fetal physical well-being from conception to the onset of labor

Fetal Status: Intrapartum: Conditions and behaviors indicative of fetal well-being from onset of labor to delivery

Immune Status: Adequacy of natural and acquired appropriately targeted resistance to internal and external antigens

Immunization Behavior: Actions to obtain immunization to prevent a communicable disease

Neurological Status: Consciousness: Extent to which an individual arouses, orients, and attends to the environment

Goals/Evaluation Criteria

Examples Using NOC Language

- Demonstrates **Abuse Protection** (specify 1–5: not, slightly, moderately, substantially, or totally adequate)
- Demonstrates **Immune Status** as evidenced by the following indicators (specify 1–5: extremely, substantially, moderately, mildly, or not compromised):

    Recurrent infections not present

    Chronic fatigue not present

    Immunizations current

    Antibody titers WNL

    Differential WBC values WNL

    T4-cell, T8-cell, and complement levels WNL

Other Examples

Patient will:

- Demonstrate behaviors that decrease risk of injury, infection, or bleeding
- Report early signs and symptoms of injury, infection, or bleeding
- Be free of signs and symptoms of injury, infection, or bleeding
- Verbalize a plan to provide safety for self and children (e.g., obtaining a restraining order)

NIC Interventions

Abuse Protection Support: Identification of high-risk, dependent relationships and actions to prevent further infliction of physical or emotional harm

Abuse Protection Support: Child: Identification of high-risk dependent child relationships and actions to prevent possible or further infliction of physical, sexual, or emotional harm or neglect of basic necessities of life

Abuse Protection Support: Domestic Partner: Identification of high-risk dependent domestic relationships and actions to prevent possible or further infliction of physical, sexual, or emotional harm, or exploitation of partner

Abuse Protection Support: Elder: Identification of high-risk dependent elder relationships and actions to prevent possible or further infliction of physical, sexual, or emotional harm; neglect of basic necessities of life; or exploitation

Allergy Management: Identification, treatment, and prevention of allergic responses to food, medications, insect bites, contrast material, blood, or other substances

Bleeding Precautions: Reduction of stimuli that may induce bleeding or hemorrhage in at-risk patients

Cerebral Perfusion Promotion: Promotion of adequate perfusion and limitation of complications for a patient experiencing, or at risk for, inadequate cerebral perfusion

Electronic Fetal Monitoring: Antepartum: Electronic evaluation of fetal heart rate response to movement, external stimuli, or uterine contractions during antepartal testing

Electronic Fetal Monitoring: Intrapartum: Electronic evaluation of fetal heart rate response to uterine contractions during intrapartal care

Emergency Care: Providing life-saving measures in life-threatening situations

Energy Management: Regulating energy use to treat or prevent fatigue and optimize function

Environmental Management, Violence Prevention: Monitoring and manipulation of the physical environment to decrease the potential for violent behavior directed toward self, others, or environment

Immunization/Vaccination Management: Monitoring immunization status, facilitating access to immunizations, and provision of immunizations to prevent communicable disease

Infection Control: Minimizing the acquisition and transmission of infectious agents

Infection Protection: Prevention and early detection of infection in a patient at risk

Neurologic Monitoring: Collection and analysis of patient data to prevent or minimize neurological complications

Postanesthesia Care: Monitoring and management of the patient who has recently undergone general or regional anesthesia

Risk Identification: Analysis of potential risk factors, determination of health risks, and prioritization of risk reduction strategies for an individual or group

Surgical Precautions: Minimizing the potential for iatrogenic injury to the patient related to a surgical procedure

Surveillance, Safety: Purposeful and ongoing collection and analysis of information about the patient and the environment for use in promoting and maintaining patient safety

Ultrasonography: Limited Obstetric: Performance of ultrasound exams to determine ovarian, uterine, or fetal status

Nursing Activities

Prevention of Infection

See Nursing Activities for Risk for Infection, pp. 277–278.

Prevention of Injury

See Nursing Activities for Risk for Injury, pp. 283–284.

Assessments

- *(NIC) Environmental Management, Violence Prevention:*
  Monitor the safety of items being brought to the environment by visitors

  Remove potential weapons from environment (e.g., sharps and ropelike objects)

  Assign single room to patient with potential for violence toward others

  Lock utility and storage rooms

Prevention of Bleeding

Assessments

- Evaluate extent of patient's bleeding risk

Patient/Family Teaching

- Advise patient to wear medical identification bracelet and to alert dentist or physician

- Instruct patient to avoid trauma (e.g., from contact sports, sharp objects, stiff toothbrush)
- Teach patient signs and symptoms of bleeding and when to report it
- Teach patient first aid for bleeding

Intraoperative and Postoperative Periods

Also refer to Nursing Activities for Perioperative Positioning Injury, Risk for, pp. 375–376.

Assessments

- *(NIC) Postanesthesia Care:*
  Monitor oxygenation
  Ventilate, as appropriate
  Monitor and record vital signs q15 minutes or more often, as appropriate
  Monitor urinary output
  Monitor level of consciousness
- Check surgical site, as appropriate.
- *(NIC) Surgical Precautions:*
  Ensure documentation and communication of any allergies
  Inspect the patient's skin at the site of grounding pad

Collaborative Activities

- *(NIC) Postanesthesia Care:*
  Administer IV medication to control shivering, per agency protocol
  Administer narcotic antagonists, as appropriate, per agency protocol

Other

- *(NIC) Postanesthesia Care:*
  Restrain patient, as appropriate
  Provide warm blankets, as appropriate
- *(NIC) Surgical Precautions:*
  Verify the correct functioning of equipment
  Count sponges, sharps, and instruments before, during, and after surgery, per agency policy
  Inspect the patient's skin for injury after use of electrosurgery

Intrapartum
Assessments

- *(NIC) Electronic Fetal Monitoring: Intrapartum:*
  Verify maternal and fetal heart rates before initiation of electronic fetal monitoring

Palpate [abdomen] to determine contraction intensity with tocotransducer use

Use intermittent or telemetry fetal monitoring, if available, to facilitate maternal ambulation and comfort

Apply internal fetal electrode after rupture of membranes when necessary for evaluation of short-term variability

Apply internal uterine pressure catheter after rupture of membranes when necessary for obtaining pressure data for uterine contractions and resting tone

Patient/Family Teaching

- *(NIC) Electronic Fetal Monitoring:*

Instruct woman and support person(s) about the reason for electronic monitoring, as well as information to be obtained

Discuss appearance of rhythm strip with mother and support person

Collaborative Activities

- *(NIC) Electronic Fetal Monitoring:* Keep physician informed of pertinent changes in the fetal heart rate, interventions for non-reassuring patterns, subsequent fetal response, labor progress, and maternal response to labor

Other

- *(NIC) Electronic Fetal Monitoring:*

Adjust monitors to achieve and maintain clarity of the tracing

Interpret strip when at least a 10-min tracing has been obtained of the fetal heart and uterine activity signals

Remove electronic monitors, as needed for ambulation, after verifying that the tracing is normal (i.e., reassuring)

Calibrate equipment, as appropriate, for internal monitoring with a spiral electrode or intrauterine pressure catheter

Restoration and Growth

Patient/Family Teaching

- Provide information on community resources and support groups

Collaborative Activities

- Consult dietitian for suggestions to improve nutrition
- Confer with social services to identify appropriate referral for counseling

Other

- Explore with patient ways to enhance sleep and rest
- Assist patient in achieving optimum sleep, rest, nutrition, activity, and stress management
- Discuss relaxation techniques with patient/family
- Assist patient and family in identifying and planning an appropriate exercise program

---

RAPE-TRAUMA SYNDROME

(00142) (1980, 1998)

Definition: Sustained maladaptive response to a forced, violent sexual penetration against the victim's will and consent*

Defining Characteristics

Subjective	*Objective*
Anger	Aggression
Anxiety	Agitation
Confusion	Change in relationships
Embarrassment	Denial
Fear	Dependence
Guilt	Depression
Humiliation	Disorganization
Loss of self-esteem	Dissociative disorders
Mood swings	Helplessness
Muscle tension or spasms	Hyperalertness
Nightmares and sleep disturbances	Inability to make decisions
Powerlessness	Paranoia
Self-blame	Phobias
Shame	Physical trauma (e.g., bruising, tissue irritation)
	Revenge
	Sexual dysfunction
	Shock
	Substance abuse
	Suicide attempts
	Vulnerability

*NOTE: This syndrome includes three components: Rape-Trauma, Compound Reaction, and Silent Reaction. Because the defining characteristics are different each appears as a separate diagnosis in the NANDA International taxonomy and in this text.

Related Factors

Rape [patient's biopsychosocial response to event]

Suggestions for Use

Use this diagnosis only if the specific diagnoses of *Rape-trauma syndrome: compound reaction* and *silent reaction* do not apply. This diagnosis does not need an etiology; the etiology, rape, is implied in the label itself.

Suggested Alternative Diagnoses

Rape-trauma syndrome: compound reaction
Rape-trauma syndrome: silent reaction

NOC Outcomes

Abuse Cessation: Evidence that the victim is no longer abused
Abuse Protection: Protection of self or dependent others from abuse
Abuse Recovery: Emotional: Healing of psychological injuries due to abuse
Abuse Recovery: Sexual: Healing following sexual abuse or exploitation
Coping: Actions to manage stressors that tax an individual's resources
Impulse Control: Ability to self-restrain compulsive or impulsive behaviors

Goals/Evaluation Criteria

Examples Using NOC Language

- Demonstrates **Abuse Recovery: Sexual**, as evidenced by the following indicators (specify 1–5: none, limited, moderate, substantial, or extensive):
    Verbalization of details of abuse
    Verbalization of feelings about the abuse
    Verbalization of appropriate and inappropriate guilt
    Verbalization of accurate information about sexual functioning
    Expressions of right to have been protected from abuse
    Expressions of hope
    Expressions of confidence with sexual orientation
    Freedom from sleep disturbances
    Evidence of appropriate same-sex and opposite-sex relationships

- Demonstrates **Coping**, as evidenced by the following indicators (specify 1–5: never, rarely, sometimes, often, or consistently demonstrated):

  Identifies and uses effective coping strategies

  Uses available social support

  Reports decrease in physical symptoms of stress

  Reports decrease in negative feelings

  Expresses feelings of empowerment

Other Examples

Patient will:
- Report cessation of sexual abuse
- Engage in positive interpersonal relationships
- Resolve feelings of depression
- Have appropriate affect for situation
- Obtain treatment for, and resolve, emotional problems and behaviors resulting from the trauma
- Be able to control negative or destructive impulses

NIC Interventions

Abuse Protection Support: Identification of high-risk, dependent relationships and actions to prevent further infliction of physical or emotional harm

Abuse Protection Support: Child: Identification of high-risk dependent child relationships and actions to prevent possible or further infliction of physical, sexual, or emotional harm or neglect of basic necessities of life

Abuse Protection Support: Domestic Partner: Identification of high-risk dependent domestic relationships and actions to prevent possible or further infliction of physical, sexual, or emotional harm, or exploitation of partner

Abuse Protection Support: Elder: Identification of high-risk dependent elder relationships and actions to prevent possible or further infliction of physical, sexual, or emotional harm; neglect of basic necessities of life; or exploitation

Coping Enhancement: Assisting a patient to adapt to perceived stressors, changes, or threats which interfere with meeting life demands and roles

Counseling: Use of an interactive helping process focusing on the needs, problems, or feelings of the patient and significant others to enhance or support coping, problem solving, and interpersonal relationships

Crisis Intervention: Use of short-term counseling to help the patient cope with a crisis and resume a state of functioning comparable to or better than the precrisis state

Rape-Trauma Treatment: Provision of emotional and physical support immediately following a reported rape

Nursing Activities

Assessments

- *(NIC) Crisis Intervention*: Determine whether patient presents safety risk to self or others
- *(NIC) Rape-Trauma Treatment:*

  Document whether patient has showered, douched, or bathed since incident

  Document mental state, physical state (clothing, dirt, and debris), history of incident, evidence of violence, and prior gynecologic history

  Determine presence of cuts, bruises, bleeding, lacerations, or other signs of physical injury

Patient/Family Teaching

- Support and educate significant others; discuss therapeutic response to victim and changes in victim's behaviors that can be anticipated
- *(NIC) Rape-Trauma Treatment:*

  Inform patient of HIV testing, as appropriate

  Give clear, written instructions about medication use, crisis support services, and legal support

  Explain legal proceedings available to patient

Collaborative Activities

- *(NIC) Rape-Trauma Treatment:*

  Refer patient to rape advocacy program

  Offer medication to prevent pregnancy, as appropriate

  Offer prophylactic antibiotic medication against venereal disease

Other

- Approach patient in a nonjudgmental and supportive manner
- Allow adequate time for patient to respond to even simple questions
- Counsel immediate family, spouse, or partner to maintain close relationship with victim, with attention to dispelling feelings of blame (e.g., self or projected)

- Encourage patient and family to verbalize feelings
- *(NIC) Rape-Trauma Treatment:*
  Provide support person to stay with patient
  Use the term "alleged rape" in documentation
  Implement rape protocol (e.g., label and save soiled clothing, vaginal secretions, and vaginal hair combings)
  Implement crisis intervention counseling

RAPE-TRAUMA SYNDROME: COMPOUND REACTION (00143) (1980)

Definition: Forced, violent sexual penetration against the victim's will and consent. The trauma syndrome that develops from this attack or attempted attack includes an acute phase of disorganization of the victim's lifestyle and a long-term process of reorganization of lifestyle*

Defining Characteristics

Subjective
Emotional reaction (e.g., anger, embarrassment, fear of physical violence and death, humiliation, revenge, self-blame in acute phase)

Objective
Change in lifestyle (e.g., changes in residence, dealing with repetitive nightmares and phobias, seeking family support, seeking social network support in long-term phase)

Multiple physical symptoms (e.g., gastrointestinal irritability, genitourinary discomfort, muscle tension, sleep pattern disturbance in acute phase)

Reactivated symptoms of such previous conditions (e.g., physical illness, psychiatric illness in acute phase)

Reliance on aicohol or drugs in acute phase

Other Possible Defining Characteristics (non-NANDA International)
Body image disturbance
Initiating period of celibacy

---

*NOTE: This syndrome includes three components: Rape-Trauma, Compound Reaction, and Silent Reaction. Because the defining characteristics are different each appears as a separate diagnosis in the NANDA International taxonomy and in this text.

Physical trauma (e.g., general soreness, bruises, lesions, trauma to
mouth and rectum)

Promiscuity

Sexual fears

Suicidal or homicidal behavior

Related Factors

To be developed

Patient's biopsychosocial response to rape (non-NANDA International)

Suggestions for Use

When appropriate, use this label instead of the more general
diagnosis of *Rape-trauma syndrome.* This diagnosis does not need
an etiology because the etiology (i.e., rape) is implied by the label
itself.

Suggested Alternative Diagnoses

Rape-trauma syndrome

Rape-trauma syndrome: silent reaction

NOC Outcomes

See NOC Outcomes for Rape-Trauma Syndrome, p. 399.

Self-Mutilation Restraint: Ability to refrain from intentional self-
inflicted injury (nonlethal)

Goals/Evaluation Criteria

Examples Using NOC Language

See Goals/Evaluation Criteria for Rape-Trauma Syndrome, pp.
399–400.

Other Examples

NOTE: In addition to the general goals for Rape-Trauma Syndrome on pp. 399–400, specific goals for this diagnosis depend on
the extent to which the patient's previous psychiatric or medical
conditions are reactivated and what those conditions are. It is not
possible to address here all possibilities that might occur. Some
examples are that the patient will:

- Be kept safe during reactivation of psychiatric or medical conditions
- Actively participate in rape counseling

- Not use alcohol or drugs as a coping mechanism
- Identify the existence of a relationship between his own psychiatric or medical conditions and the rape episode
- Return to previous level of biopsychosocial functioning

NIC Interventions

Also see NIC Interventions for Rape-Trauma Syndrome, on pp. 400–401.

Anger Control Assistance: Facilitation of the expression of anger in an adaptive nonviolent manner

Behavior Management: Self-Harm: Assisting the patient to decrease or eliminate self-mutilating or self-abusive behaviors

Counseling: Use of an interactive helping process focusing on the needs, problems, or feelings of the patient and significant others to enhance or support coping, problem solving, and interpersonal relationships

Crisis Intervention: Use of short-term counseling to help the patient cope with a crisis and resume a state of functioning comparable to or better than the precrisis state

Environmental Management: Violence Prevention: Monitoring and manipulation of the physical environment to decrease the potential for violent behavior directed toward self, others, or environment

Impulse Control Training: Assisting the patient to mediate impulsive behavior through application of problem-solving strategies to social and interpersonal situations

Rape-Trauma Treatment: Provision of emotional and physical support immediately following a reported rape

Nursing Activities

NOTE: Refer to Nursing Activities for Rape-Trauma Syndrome, pp. 401–402. In addition, the following apply:

Assessments

- Assess and document patient's orientation to person, place, time, and situation
- Perform physical assessment based on patient's complaints to determine presenting medical conditions
- Perform psychosocial assessment that focuses on rape
- *(NIC) Counseling:* Determine how family behavior affects patient

Patient/Family Teaching

• Educate significant others regarding psychiatric or medical conditions that reoccur. Discuss therapeutic response to victim and changed behaviors.

Collaborative Activities

• Refer patient and family for medical or psychiatric treatment, as needed

Other

• Establish a plan of care to stabilize medical or psychologic condition to proceed with rape-trauma counseling
• Provide necessary safety precautions indicated by suicide risk assessment
• Support significant others
• *(NIC) Counseling:*
  Establish a therapeutic relationship based on trust and respect
  Provide privacy and ensure confidentiality
  Discourage decision making when the patient is under severe stress

---

RAPE-TRAUMA SYNDROME: SILENT REACTION (00144) (1980)

Definition: Forced, violent sexual penetration against the victim's will and consent. The trauma syndrome that develops from this attack or attempted attack includes an acute phase of disorganization of the victim's lifestyle and a long-term process of reorganization of lifestyle.*

Defining Characteristics

Subjective
Increase in nightmares
Increased anxiety during assessment interview (i.e., blocking of associations, long periods of silence, minor stuttering, physical distress)
No verbalization of the occurrence of rape

---

*NOTE: This syndrome includes three components: Rape-Trauma, Compound Reaction, and Silent Reaction. Because the defining characteristics are different each appears as a separate diagnosis in the NANDA International taxonomy and in this text.

Objective
Abrupt changes in relationships with men
Pronounced changes in sexual behavior
Sudden onset of phobic reactions

Other Possible Defining Characteristics (non-NANDA International)
Avoidance of close relationships
Irritability toward gender of perpetrator
Persistently low self-confidence and self-esteem
Suspiciousness

Related Factors

To be developed

Suggestions for Use

If defining characteristics are present, use this label instead of the more general diagnosis of *Rape-trauma syndrome*. An etiology is not necessary for this diagnosis because the etiology (i.e., rape) is implied in the label itself.

Suggested Alternative Diagnoses

Rape-trauma syndrome
Rape-trauma syndrome: compound reaction

NOC Outcomes

Abuse Protection: Protection of self or dependent others from abuse

Abuse Recovery: Emotional: Healing of psychological injuries due to abuse

Abuse Recovery: Sexual: Healing following sexual abuse or exploitation

Coping: Actions to manage stressors that tax an individual's resources

Impulse Control: Ability to self-restrain compulsive or impulsive behaviors

Self-Mutilation Restraint: Ability to refrain from intentional self-inflicted injury (nonlethal)

Goals/Evaluation Criteria

Examples Using NOC Language

See Goals/Evaluation Criteria for Rape-Trauma Syndrome, pp. 399–400.

Other Examples

NOTE: In addition to the general goals for Rape-Trauma Syndrome on pp. 399–400, specific goals for this diagnosis depend on the extent to which the patient's previous psychiatric or medical conditions are reactivated and what those conditions are. It is not possible to address here all possibilities that might occur. Some examples are that the patient will:

- Acknowledge the rape or attempted rape
- Verbalize details of the rape or attempted rape as a means of catharsis
- Verbalize feelings associated with rape or attempted rape
- Describe a plan that includes safety measures to reduce future risk
- Experience a decrease in stress response symptoms (e.g., nightmares)
- Return to previous level of biopsychosocial functioning, specify level

NIC Interventions

See NIC Interventions for Rape-Trauma Syndrome, pp. 400–401, in addition to the following:

Anger Control Assistance: Facilitation of the expression of anger in an adaptive nonviolent manner

Behavior Management: Self-Harm: Assisting the patient to decrease or eliminate self-mutilating or self-abusive behaviors

Environmental Management: Violence Prevention: Monitoring and manipulation of the physical environment to decrease the potential for violent behavior directed toward self, others, or environment

Impulse Control Training: Assisting the patient to mediate impulsive behavior through application of problem-solving strategies to social and interpersonal situations

Suicide Prevention: Reducing risk of self-inflicted harm with intent to end life

Nursing Activities

Also refer to Nursing Activities for Rape-Trauma Syndrome, pp. 401–402, and for Rape-Trauma Syndrome: Compound Reaction, pp. 404–405.

Other

- Confirm with patient that a traumatic event recently occurred and specifically identify it as "rape"

- Encourage patient to express thoughts, feelings, and behaviors
- Establish therapeutic relationship that will allow exploration of silent reaction
- Assist patient and family to establish support network
- *(NIC) Counseling:* Verbalize the discrepancy between the patient's feelings and behaviors

RELOCATION STRESS SYNDROME
(00114) (1992, 2000)

Definition: Physiological or psychosocial disturbances as a result of transfer from one environment to another

Defining Characteristics

Subjective
Alienation
Aloneness
Anger
Anxiety (e.g., separation)
Fear
Frustration
Loneliness
Loss of identity, self-worth, or self-esteem
Sleep disturbance
Worry

Objective
Dependency
Increased physical symptoms or illness (e.g., GI disturbance, weight change)
Increased verbalization of needs, unwillingness to move, or concern over relocation
Insecurity
Pessimism
Temporary or permanent move
Voluntary or involuntary move
Withdrawal

Related Factors
Decreased physical health status
Feeling of powerlessness
Impaired psychosocial health status

Isolation from family and friends
Lack of adequate support system
Lack of departure counseling
Passive coping
Past, concurrent, and recent losses
Unpredictability of experience

Other (Non-NANDA International) Related Factors
Little or no preparation for the impending move
Losses involved with decision to move
Moderate to high degree of environmental change

Suggestions for Use

Because this is a syndrome diagnosis, no etiology is needed in the diagnostic statement. A syndrome nursing diagnosis represents a group of other nursing diagnoses that are present together. If only one or two of the defining characteristics are present (e.g., anxiety, loneliness), write separate nursing diagnoses for those responses (e.g., *Anxiety*) instead of using *Relocation stress syndrome*.

Suggested Alternative Diagnoses

Anxiety
Confusion, acute
Grieving, dysfunctional
Hopelessness
Loneliness, risk for
Powerlessness
Sleep pattern, disturbed
Sorrow, chronic
Spiritual distress

NOC Outcomes

Anxiety Control: Personal actions to eliminate or reduce feelings of apprehension and tension from an unidentifiable source

Child Adaptation to Hospitalization: Child's adaptive response to hospitalization

Coping: Actions to manage stressors that tax an individual's resources

Depression Control: Personal actions to minimize melancholy and maintain interest in life events

Depression Level: Severity of melancholic mood and loss of interest in life events

Loneliness: The extent of emotional, social, or existential isolation response

Psychosocial Adjustment: Life Change: Psychosocial adaptation of an individual to a life change

Quality of Life: An individual's expressed satisfaction with current life circumstances

Goals/Evaluation Criteria

Examples Using NOC Language

- Demonstrates **Coping**, as evidenced by the following indicators (specify 1–5: never, rarely, sometimes, often, or consistently demonstrated):
    Verbalizes acceptance of situation
    Reports decrease in negative feelings
    Reports decrease in physical symptoms of stress
    Modifies lifestyle, as needed
- Demonstrates **Psychosocial Adjustment: Life Change**, as evidenced by the following indicators (specify 1–5: none, limited, moderate, substantial, or extensive):
    Maintenance of self-esteem
    Expressions of usefulness
    Expressions of adequate social support

Other Examples

Patient will:
- Demonstrate ability to adjust to new environment
- Verbalize satisfaction with new living arrangements
- Express optimism about the present and the future
- Express satisfaction with life achievements
- Participate in diversions (e.g., hobbies)
Child will:
- Adapt to hospitalization (e.g., will not demonstrate agitation, regressive behaviors, anxiety, fear, or anger)
- Respond to play therapy and comfort measures
- Show resolution of separation anxiety

NIC Interventions

Anticipatory Guidance: Preparation of patient for an anticipated developmental or situational crisis

Anxiety Reduction: Minimizing apprehension, dread, foreboding, or uneasiness related to an unidentified source of anticipated danger

Coping Enhancement: Assisting a patient to adapt to perceived stressors, changes, or threats which interfere with meeting life demands and roles

Counseling: Use of an interactive helping process focusing on the needs, problems, or feelings of the patient and significant others to enhance or support coping, problem solving, and interpersonal relationships

Family Involvement Promotion: Facilitating family participation in the emotional and physical care of the patient

Discharge Planning: Preparation for moving a patient from one level of care to another within or outside the current health care agency

Hope Instillation: Facilitation of the development of a positive outlook in a given situation

Mood Management: Providing for safety, stabilization, recovery, and maintenance of a patient who is experiencing dysfunctionally depressed mood or elevated mood

Security Enhancement: Intensifying a patient's sense of physical and psychological safety

Self-Responsibility Facilitation: Encouraging a patient to assume more responsibility for own behavior

Socialization Enhancement: Facilitation of another person's ability to interact with others

Spiritual Support: Assisting the patient to feel balance and connection with a greater power

Values Clarification: Assisting another to clarify his own values in order to facilitate effective decision making

Nursing Activities

Assessments

- Assess patient's orientation, mood (e.g., depressed, angry, anxious), and physiologic status on admission and q _____.
- Identify patient's previous schedules and routines
- Assess readiness for discharge
- (NIC) Coping Enhancement: Appraise patient's needs or desires for social support
- (NIC) Self-Responsibility Facilitation: Monitor level of responsibility that patient assumes

Collaborative Activities

- Maintain consistency in caregivers and care routines as much as possible, consider a case manager

- Utilize other resources to assist in transition to new environment
- Coordinate referrals among health care providers and agencies to effect a smooth transfer or relocation

Other

- Orient patient to new environment as often as needed
- Establish new environment as close to previous environment as possible to maintain consistency in placement of personal belongings, furniture, pictures, and so forth
- To ease the transfer, encourage family to stay with patient, bring familiar objects from home, and provide familiar socialization
- Avoid unplanned or abrupt transfers; also avoid transfers at night or at change of shift
- *(NIC) Coping Enhancement:*

    Assist the patient in developing an objective appraisal of the event

    Use a calm, reassuring approach

    Seek to understand the patient's perspective of a stressful situation

    Discourage decision making when the patient is under severe stress

    Foster constructive outlets for anger and hostility

    Arrange situations that encourage patient's autonomy

    Introduce patient to persons (or groups) who have successfully undergone the same experience

    Encourage verbalization of feelings, perceptions, and fears [about the relocation]

- *(NIC) Hope Instillation:*

    Inform the patient about whether the current situation is a temporary state

    Facilitate the reliving and savoring past achievements and experiences by patient and family

    Create an environment that facilitates patient practicing religion

    Involve the patient actively in own care

- *(NIC) Self-Responsibility Facilitation:*

    Encourage patient to take as much responsibility for own self-care as possible

    Facilitate family support for new level of responsibility sought or attained by patient

RELOCATION STRESS SYNDROME, RISK FOR (00149) (2000)

Definition: At risk for physiologic or psychosocial disturbance following transfer from one environment to another

Risk Factors

Subjective

Feelings of powerlessness

Objective

Decreased psychosocial or physical health status

Lack of adequate support system or group

Lack of predeparture counseling

Moderate mental competence (e.g., alert enough to experience changes)

Moderate to high degree of environmental change (e.g., physical, ethnic, cultural)

Passive coping

Past, current, recent losses

Temporary or permanent moves

Unpredictability of experiences

Voluntary or involuntary move

Suggestions for Use

None

Suggested Alternative Diagnoses

Loneliness, risk for

Powerlessness, risk for

Relocation stress syndrome

NOC Outcomes

See NOC Outcomes for Relocation Stress Syndrome, on pp. 409–410.

Goals/Evaluation Criteria

Examples Using NOC Language

See Examples Using NOC Language for Relocation Stress Syndrome, on p. 410.

Other Examples

See Other Examples for Relocation Stress Syndrome, on p. 410.

NIC Interventions

NIC has not yet linked interventions to this diagnosis; however, the following may be useful:

Anticipatory Guidance: Preparation of patient for an anticipated developmental or situational crisis

Anxiety Reduction: Minimizing apprehension, dread, foreboding, or uneasiness related to an unidentified source of anticipated danger

Coping Enhancement: Assisting a patient to adapt to perceived stressors, changes, or threats which interfere with meeting life demands and roles

Family Involvement Promotion: Facilitating family participation in the emotional and physical care of the patient

Discharge Planning: Preparation for moving a patient from one level of care to another within or outside the current health care agency

Security Enhancement: Intensifying a patient's sense of physical and psychological safety

Socialization Enhancement: Facilitation of another person's ability to interact with others

Spiritual Support: Assisting the patient to feel balance and connection with a greater power

Values Clarification: Assisting another to clarify his own values in order to facilitate effective decision making

Nursing Activities

See Nursing Activities: for Relocation Stress Syndrome, on pp. 411–412.

ROLE CONFLICT, PARENTAL
(00064) (1988)

Definition: Parent experience of role confusion and conflict in response to crisis

Defining Characteristics

Subjective

Expressed concern about perceived loss of control over decisions relating to child

Expressed concern or feelings of inadequacy to provide for child's physical or emotional needs during hospitalization or in the home

Expressed concerns about changes in parental role, family functioning, family communication, family health

Verbalized or demonstrated feelings of guilt, anger, fear, anxiety, or frustrations about effect of child's illness on family process

Objective

Demonstrated disruption in caretaking routines

Reluctance to participate in usual caretaking activities, even with encouragement and support

Related Factors

Change in marital status [e.g., career, roles]

[Financial crisis]

Home care of a child with special needs [e.g., apnea monitoring, postural drainage, hyperalimentation]

Interruptions in family life due to home care regimen [e.g., treatments, caregivers, lack of respite]

Intimidation with invasive or restrictive modality [e.g., isolation, intubation]

Specialized care centers, policies

Separation from child due to chronic illness

Suggestions for Use

Use this label when a situation causes unsatisfactory role performance by previously effective parents

Suggested Alternative Diagnoses

Caregiver role strain (actual or at risk for)

Coping: family, compromised

Family processes, interrupted

Parenting, impaired

Parenting, impaired, risk for

NOC Outcomes

Caregiver Adaptation to Patient Institutionalization: Family caregiver adaptation of role when the care recipient is transferred outside the home

Caregiver Home Care Readiness: Preparedness to assume responsibility for the health care of a family member or significant other in the home

Coping: Actions to manage stressors that tax an individual's resources

Family Environment: Internal: Social climate as characterized by family member relationships and goals

Family Functioning: Ability of the family to meet the needs of its members through developmental transitions

Parenting: Provision of an environment that promotes optimum growth and development of dependent children

Role Performance: Congruence of an individual's role behavior with role expectations

Goals/Evaluation Criteria

Examples Using NOC Language

- *Parental role conflict* will be resolved or alleviated, as evidenced by satisfactory Caregiver Adaptation to Patient Institutionalization, Caregiver Home Care Readiness, Coping, Family Environment: Internal, Family Functioning, Parenting, and Role Performance.
- **Coping** will be demonstrated, as evidenced by the following indicators (specify 1–5: never, rarely, sometimes, often, or consistently demonstrated):

  Uses available social supports

  Uses effective coping strategies

  Seeks professional help, as appropriate

  Seeks information concerning illness and treatment
- **Parenting** will be demonstrated, as evidenced by the following indicators (specify 1–5: not, slightly, moderately, substantially, or totally adequate):

  Provides for the child's physical needs

  Provides for the child's special needs

  Stimulates cognitive and social development

  Stimulates emotional and spiritual growth

  Demonstrates a loving relationship with child
- **Role Performance** will be demonstrated, as evidenced by the following indicators (specify 1–5: not, slightly, moderately, substantially, or totally adequate): performance of family and work role behaviors

Other Examples

The parent or caregiver will:

- Demonstrate ability to modify parenting role in response to crisis
- Express a sense of adequacy in providing for child's needs
- Be available to support child and give consent for treatments
- Develop trust in health care providers
- Express willingness to assume caregiving role
- Demonstrate knowledge of the child's illness, treatment regimen, and emergency care

NIC Interventions

Caregiver Support: Provision of the necessary information, advocacy, and support to facilitate primary patient care by someone other than a health care professional

Coping Enhancement: Assisting a patient to adapt to perceived stressors, changes, or threats which interfere with meeting life demands and roles

Counseling: Use of an interactive helping process focusing on the needs, problems, or feelings of the patient and significant others to enhance or support coping, problem solving, and interpersonal relationships

Crisis Intervention: Use of short-term counseling to help the patient cope with a crisis and resume a state of functioning comparable to or better than the precrisis state

Family Involvement Promotion: Facilitating family participation in the emotional and physical care of the patient

Family Process Maintenance: Minimization of family process disruption effects

Parenting Promotion: Providing parenting information, support, and coordination of comprehensive services to high-risk families

Role Enhancement: Assisting a patient, significant other, and family to improve relationships by clarifying and supplementing specific role behaviors

Nursing Activities

Assessment

- Ask parents to describe how they want to be involved in the care of their hospitalized child
- *(NIC) Family Process Maintenance:*
  Determine typical family processes
  Identify effects of role changes on family processes

Patient/Family Teaching

- Teach new role behaviors created by the crisis situation
- Explain rationale for treatments and encourage questions to minimize misunderstandings and maximize participation
- *(NIC) Family Process Maintenance:* Teach family time management and organization skills when performing patient home care, as needed

Collaborative Activities

- *(NIC) Family Process Maintenance:* Assist family members to use existing support mechanisms

Other

- Confront parents with their ineffective parenting behaviors (during this crisis) and discuss alternatives
- Help parents to identify personal strengths and coping skills that may be useful in resolving the crisis
- Discuss with parent(s) a strategy for meeting personal and family current needs
- Give positive reinforcement for constructive parental actions
- *(NIC) Family Process Maintenance:*

    Keep opportunities for visiting flexible to meet needs of family members and patient

    Provide mechanisms for family members staying at health care agency to communicate with other family members (e.g., telephones, tape recordings, open visiting, photographs, and videotapes)

    Assist family members to facilitate home visits by patient, when appropriate

ROLE PERFORMANCE, INEFFECTIVE
(00055) (1978, 1996, 1998)

Definition: Patterns of behavior and self-expression that do not match the environmental context, norms, and expectations

Defining Characteristics

Subjective

Altered role perceptions

Anxiety or depression

Change in self-perception of role

Inadequate confidence

Inadequate motivation

Powerlessness

Role ambivalence, conflict, confusion, denial, dissatisfaction, overload, or strain

Uncertainty

Objective

Change in capacity to resume role

Change in other's perception of role

Change in usual patterns of responsibility

Discrimination

Domestic violence

Harassment
Inadequate adaptation to change or transition
Inadequate coping
Inadequate external support for role enactment
Inadequate knowledge
Inadequate opportunities for role enactment
Inadequate role competency and skills
Inadequate self-management
Inappropriate developmental expectations
Pessimistic attitude
System conflict

Related Factors

Knowledge

Developmental transitions
Education attainment level
Inadequate role preparation (e.g., role transition, skill, rehearsal, validation)
Lack of knowledge about role
Lack of knowledge about role skills
Lack of opportunity for role rehearsal
Lack of or inadequate role model
Role transition
Unrealistic role expectations

Physiological

Body image alteration
Cognitive deficits
Depression
Fatigue
Health alterations (e.g., physical health, body image, self-esteem, mental health, psychosocial health, cognition, learning style, neurologic health)
Inadequate and inappropriate linkage with health care system
Low self-esteem
Mental illness
Pain
Physical illness
Substance abuse

Social

Domestic violence

Family conflict

Inadequate or inappropriate linkage with health care system

Inadequate role socialization (e.g., role model, expectations, responsibilities)

Inadequate support system

Job schedule demands

Lack of resources

Lack of rewards

Low socioeconomic status

Poverty

Stress and conflict

Young age, developmental level

Suggestions for Use

When applicable, use more specific labels such as *Parental role conflict, Sexual dysfunction,* and *Interrupted family processes.* Some degree of role conflict and disruption is present for everyone. If the patient is having difficulty with role performance, consider using *Ineffective role performance* as the etiology of another diagnosis that describes the impact on functioning (e.g., *Impaired home maintenance related to Ineffective role performance*).

"There is a typology of roles [that applies to this diagnosis]: sociopersonal (e.g., friendship, family, marital, parenting, community), home management, intimacy (e.g., sexuality, relationship building), leisure/exercise/recreation, self-management, socialization (e.g., developmental transitions), community contributor, and religious." (NANDA International, 2003, p. 150).

Suggested Alternative Diagnoses

Caregiver role strain, actual and risk for

Family processes, interrupted

Home maintenance, impaired

Role conflict, parental

Self-esteem, situational low

NOC Outcomes

Caregiver Lifestyle Disruption: Disturbances in the lifestyle of a family member due to caregiving

Coping: Actions to manage stressors that tax an individual's resources

Depression Level: Severity of melancholic mood and loss of interest in life events

Psychomotor Energy: Ability to maintain ADLs, nutrition, personal safety

Psychosocial Adjustment: Life Change: Psychosocial adaptation of an individual to a life change

Role Performance: Congruence of an individual's role behavior with role expectations

Goals/Evaluation Criteria

Examples Using NOC Language

- Demonstrates **Role Performance**, as evidenced by the following indicators (specify 1–5: not, slightly, moderately, substantially, or totally adequate):

    Ability to meet role expectations

    Knowledge of role transition periods

    Performance of family, community, work, intimate, and friendship role behaviors

    Reported strategies for role change(s)

Other Examples

Patient will:

- Acknowledge impact of situation on existing personal relationships, lifestyle, and role performance
- Describe actual change in function
- Express willingness to use resources upon discharge
- Verbalize feelings of productivity and usefulness
- Demonstrate ability to manage finances

NIC Interventions

Anticipatory Guidance: Preparation of patient for an anticipated developmental or situational crisis

Coping Enhancement: Assisting a patient to adapt to perceived stressors, changes, or threats which interfere with meeting life demands and roles

Hope Instillation: Facilitation of the development of a positive outlook in a given situation

Mood Management: Providing for safety, stabilization, recovery, and maintenance of a patient who is experiencing dysfunctionally depressed mood or elevated mood

Role Enhancement: Assisting a patient, significant other, and family to improve relationships by clarifying and supplementing specific role behaviors

Nursing Activities

Assessments

- Assess need for assistance from social services department for planning care with patient and family

Patient/Family Teaching

- *(NIC) Role Enhancement:* Teach new behaviors needed by patient/parent to fulfill a role

Other

- Assist patient in identifying personal strengths
- Actively listen to patient and family and acknowledge reality of concerns
- Encourage patient and family to air feelings and to grieve
- *(NIC) Role Enhancement:*

  Assist patient to identify various roles in life

  Assist patient to identify usual role in family

  Assist patient to identify role insufficiency

  Assist adult children to accept elderly parent's dependency and the role changes involved, as appropriate

  Facilitate discussion of how siblings' roles will change with newborn's arrival, as appropriate

  Facilitate discussion of role adaptations related to children leaving home (i.e., empty-nest syndrome), as appropriate

SELF-CARE DEFICIT—DISCUSSION

Self-care deficit describes a state in which a person experiences impaired ability to perform self-care activities such as bathing, dressing, eating, and toileting. If the person is unable to perform any self-care, the situation is described as *Total self-care deficit.* However, the diagnoses are classified into more specific problems, each with its own defining characteristics; these problems can exist alone or in various combinations, such as *Feeding self-care deficit* and *Feeding and bathing/hygiene self-care deficit.*

Self-care deficits are often caused by *Activity intolerance, Impaired physical mobility, Pain, Anxiety,* or perceptual or cognitive impairment (e.g., *Feeding self-care deficit +2 related to disorientation*). As an etiology, *Self-care deficit* can cause depression, *Fear* of becoming dependent, and *Powerlessness* (e.g., *Fear of becoming totally dependent related to total self-care deficit +2 secondary to residual weakness from CVA*).

Self-care deficit should be used to label only those conditions in which the focus is to support or improve the patient's self-care abilities. Outcome and evaluation criteria for these labels must reflect improved functioning. Therefore, if the diagnosis is used for states not amenable to treatment, there is no hope of achieving the stated outcomes. The focus of nursing interventions in this case is twofold: (1) to increase the patient's ability to perform self-care and (2) to help patients with limitations and perform care the patient cannot do.

SELF-CARE DEFICIT, BATHING/HYGIENE (SPECIFY LEVEL) (00108) (1980, 1998)

Definition: Impaired ability to perform or complete bathing or hygiene activities for oneself

Defining Characteristics

Objective
Inability to [perform the following tasks]:
Dry body
Get bath supplies
Get in and out of bathroom
Obtain or get to water source
Regulate temperature or flow of bathwater
Wash body or body parts

Related Factors

Decreased or lack of motivation
Environmental barriers
Inability to perceive body part or spatial relationship
Musculoskeletal impairment
Neuromuscular impairment
Pain
Perceptual or cognitive impairment
Severe anxiety
Weakness and tiredness

Other Related Factors (non-NANDA International)
Decreased strength and endurance
Depression
Developmental disability
Intolerance to activity

Medically imposed restrictions
Psychologic impairment (specify)

Suggestions for Use

See Self-Care Deficits—Discussion on pp. 422–423.

In order to promote efforts to restore functioning, the patient's functional level must be classified. NANDA International uses the following scale.

0 = Completely independent
1 = Requires use of equipment or device
2 = Requires help from another person for assistance, supervision, or teaching
3 = Requires help from another person and equipment or device
4 = Dependent, does not participate in activity

The following definitions and descriptors in Table 5 may be helpful in determining which number to assign to a patient's functional level:

Table 5

	Totally Dependent (+4)	Moderately Dependent (+3)	Semi-dependent (+2)
Bathing	Patient needs complete bath; cannot assist at all	Nurse supplies all equipment; positions patient; washes back, legs, perineum, and all other parts, as needed; patient can assist	Nurse provides all equipment; positions patient in bed and bathroom. Patient completes bath, except for back and feet
Oral Hygiene	Nurse completes entire procedure	Nurse prepares brush, rinses, mouth, positions patient	Nurse provides equipment; patient does task

Suggested Alternative Diagnoses

Activity intolerance
Physical mobility, impaired
Sensory perception, disturbed
Thought processes, disturbed
Self-care deficit, total

NOC Outcomes

Self-Care: Activities of Daily Living (ADLs): Ability to perform the most basic physical tasks and personal care activities

Self-Care: Bathing: Ability to cleanse own body

Self-Care: Hygiene: Ability to maintain own hygiene

Goals/Evaluation Criteria

Examples Using NOC Language

- Demonstrates **Self-Care: Activities of Daily Living (ADLs)**, as evidenced by the following indicators (specify 1–5: dependent (does not participate), requires assistive person and device, requires assistive person, independent with assistive device, or is completely independent):

    Bathing

    Hygiene

Other Examples

Patient will:

- Accept assistance or total care by caregiver, if needed
- Verbalize satisfactory body cleanliness and oral hygiene
- Maintain mobility needed to get to bathroom and get bath supplies
- Be able to turn on and regulate water temperature and flow
- Wash and dry body
- Perform mouth care
- Apply deodorant

NIC Interventions

Bathing: Cleaning of the body for the purposes of relaxation, cleanliness, and healing

Self-Care Assistance, Bathing/Hygiene: Assisting patient to perform personal hygiene

Nursing Activities

Assessments

- Assess ability to use assistive devices
- Assess oral mucous membranes and body cleanliness daily
- Assess skin condition during bath
- Monitor for changes in functional abilities
- *(NIC) Self-Care Assistance: Bathing/Hygiene:* Monitor cleaning of nails, according to patient's self-care ability

Patient/Family Teaching

- Instruct patient and family in alternative methods for bathing and oral hygiene

Collaborative Activities

- Offer pain medications prior to bathing
- Refer patient and family to social services for home care
- Use occupational and physical therapy as resources in planning patient care activities

Other

- Encourage independence in bathing and oral hygiene, assisting patient only as necessary
- Encourage patient to set own pace during self-care
- Include family in provision of care
- *(NIC) Self-Care Assistance: Bathing/Hygiene:*
  Provide assistance until patient is fully able to assume self-care
  Place towels, soap, deodorant, shaving equipment, and other needed accessories at bedside or in bathroom
  Wash hair, as needed and desired
  Shave patient, as indicated
  Offer hand washing after toileting and before meals

SELF-CARE DEFICIT: DRESSING/ GROOMING (SPECIFY LEVEL)

(00109) (1980, 1998)

Definition: Impaired ability to perform or complete dressing and grooming activities for self

Defining Characteristics

Objective

Impaired ability to:
  Fasten clothing
  Obtain or replace articles of clothing
  Put on or take off necessary items of clothing
Inability to:
  Choose clothing
  Maintain appearance at a satisfactory level

Pick up clothing
Put on clothing on lower body
Put on clothing on upper body
Put on shoes
Put on socks
Remove clothes
Use assistive devices
Use zippers

Related Factors

Decreased or lack of motivation
Discomfort
Environmental barriers
Musculoskeletal impairment
Neuromuscular impairment
Pain
Perceptual or cognitive impairment
Severe anxiety
Weakness or tiredness

Other Related Factors (non-NANDA International)
Depression
Developmental disability
Intolerance to activity
Psychologic impairment (specify)

Suggestions for Use

See Self-Care Deficits—Discussion on pp. 422–423. NANDA International uses the following scale to classify patient's functional level:

0 = Completely independent
1 = Requires use of equipment or device
2 = Requires help from another person for assistance, supervision, or teaching
3 = Requires help from another person and equipment or device
4 = Dependent; does not participate in activity

The following definitions and descriptors in Table 6 may be helpful in determining which number to assign to a patient's functional level:

Table 6

	Totally Dependent (+4)	Moderately Dependent (+3)	Semi-dependent (+2)
Dressing or grooming	Patient needs to be dressed and cannot assist the nurse; nurse combs patient's hair	Nurse combs patient's hair, assists with dressing, buttons and zips clothing, ties shoes	Nurse gathers items for patient; may button, zip or tie clothing. Patient dresses self

Suggested Alternative Diagnoses

Activity intolerance

Fatigue

Physical mobility, impaired

Sensory perception, disturbed

Thought processes, disturbed

Self-care deficit, total

NOC Outcomes

Self-Care: Activities of Daily Living (ADLs): Ability to perform the most basic physical tasks and personal care activities

Self-Care: Dressing: Ability to dress self

Self-Care: Grooming: Ability to maintain kempt appearance

Goals/Evaluation Criteria

Examples Using NOC Language

- Demonstrates **Self-Care: Activities of Daily Living (ADLs)**, as evidenced by the following indicators (specify 1–5: dependent (does not participate), requires assistive person and device, requires assistive person, independent with assistive device, or completely independent):

    Dressing

    Grooming

Other Examples

Patient will:

- Accept care by caregiver
- Express satisfaction with dressing and hair grooming
- Dress and comb hair independently
- Use adaptive devices to facilitate dressing
- Choose clothes and obtain them from closet or drawers

- Zip and button clothing
- Be neatly dressed
- Be able to remove clothing, socks, and shoes
- Have clean, neat hair
- Apply makeup

NIC Interventions

Dressing: Choosing, putting on, and removing clothes for a person who cannot do this for self

Hair Care: Promotion of neat, clean, attractive hair

Self-Care Assistance: Dressing/Grooming: Assisting patient with clothes and makeup

Nursing Activities

Assessments

- Assess ability to use assistive devices
- Monitor energy level and activity tolerance
- Monitor for improved or deteriorating ability to dress and perform hair care
- Monitor for sensory, cognitive, or physical deficits that may make dressing difficult for the patient

Patient/Family Teaching

- Demonstrate use of assistive devices and adaptive activities
- Instruct patient in alternative methods for dressing and hair care, specify methods

Collaborative Activities

- Offer pain medications prior to dressing and grooming
- Refer patient and family to social services for obtaining home health aide, as needed
- Use occupational and physical therapy as resource in planning patient care activities
- *(NIC) Self-Care Assistance: Dressing/Grooming:* Facilitate assistance of a barber or beautician, as necessary

Other

- Encourage independence in dressing and grooming, assisting patient only as necessary
- Accommodate cognitive deficits in the following ways:
  Use nonverbal cues (e.g., give patient one article of clothing at a time, in the order needed)
  Speak slowly and keep directions simple

- Use Velcro fasteners and closures when possible
- Create opportunities for small successes, specify
- Encourage patient to set own pace during dressing and grooming
- Help patient choose clothing that is loose fitting and easy to put on
- Provide for safety by keeping environment uncluttered and well-lighted
- *(NIC) Self-Care Assistance: Dressing/Grooming:*
  Provide patient's clothes in accessible area (e.g., at bedside) [and in the order they will be needed for dressing]
  Facilitate patient's combing hair, as appropriate
  Maintain privacy while the patient is dressing
  Help with laces, buttons, and zippers, as needed
  Use extension equipment [e.g., long-handled shoehorn, button-hook, zipper pull] for pulling on clothing, if appropriate
  Reinforce efforts to dress self

SELF-CARE DEFICIT: FEEDING
(00102) (1980, 1998)

Definition: Impaired ability to perform or complete feeding activities

Defining Characteristics

Objective
Inability to:
  Bring food from a receptacle to the mouth
  Chew food
  Complete a meal
  Get food onto utensil
  Handle utensils
  Ingest food in a socially acceptable manner
  Ingest food safely
  Ingest sufficient food
  Manipulate food in mouth
  Open containers
  Pick up cup or glass
  Prepare food for ingestion
  Swallow food
  Use assistive device

Related Factors

Decreased or lack of motivation

Discomfort

Environmental barriers

Musculoskeletal impairment

Neuromuscular impairment

Pain

Perceptual or cognitive impairment

Severe anxiety

Weakness or tiredness

Other Related Factors (non-NANDA International)

Depression

Developmental disability

Intolerance to activity

Psychologic impairment

Suggestions for Use

Feeding self-care deficit may be the etiology (i.e., related factor) for *Imbalanced nutrition: less than body requirements.* Also see Self-Care Deficits—Discussion on pp. 422–423. NANDA International uses the following scale to classify patient's functional level:

0 = Completely independent

1 = Requires use of equipment or device

2 = Requires help from another person for assistance, supervision, or teaching

3 = Requires help from another person and equipment or device

4 = Dependent, does not participate in activity

The following definitions and descriptors in Table 7 may be helpful in determining which number to assign to a patient's functional level:

Table 7

	Totally Dependent (+4)	Moderately Dependent (+3)	Semi-dependent (+2)
Feeding	Patient needs to be fed totally	Nurse cuts food, opens containers, positions patient, monitors, and encourages eating	Nurse positions patient, gathers supplies, and monitors eating

Suggested Alternative Diagnoses

Activity intolerance

Physical mobility, impaired

Sensory perception, disturbed

Total self-care deficit

NOC Outcomes

Nutritional Status: Extent to which nutrients are available to meet metabolic needs

Nutritional Status: Food and Fluid Intake: Amount of food and fluid taken into the body over a 24-hr period

Self-Care: Activities of Daily Living (ADLs): Ability to perform the most basic physical tasks and personal care activities

Self-Care: Eating: Ability to prepare and ingest food

Swallowing Status: Extent of safe passage of fluids or solids from the mouth to the stomach

Goals/Evaluation Criteria

Examples Using NOC Language

- Demonstrates **Self-Care: Activities of Daily Living (ADLs)**, as evidenced by the following indicator (specify 1–5: dependent (does not participate), requires assistive person and device, requires assistive person, independent with assistive device, or completely independent):

    Feeding

Other Examples

Patient will:

- Accept feeding by caregiver
- Be able to feed self independently (or specify level)
- Express satisfaction with eating and with ability to feed self
- Demonstrate adequate intake of food and fluids
- Use adaptive devices to eat
- Open containers and prepare food

NIC Interventions

Feeding: Providing nutritional intake for patient who is unable to feed self

Nutrition Management: Assisting with or providing a balanced dietary intake of foods and fluids

Nutritional Counseling: Use of an interactive helping process focusing on the need for diet modification

Nutritional Monitoring: Collection and analysis of patient data to prevent or minimize malnourishment

Self-Care Assistance: Feeding: Assisting a person to eat

Swallowing Therapy: Facilitating swallowing and preventing complications of impaired swallowing

Nursing Activities

Assessments

- Assess ability to use assistive devices
- Assess energy level and activity tolerance
- Assess for improved or deteriorating ability to feed self
- Assess for sensory, cognitive, or physical deficits that may make self-feeding difficult
- Assess ability to chew and swallow
- Assess intake for nutritional adequacy

Patient/Family Teaching

- Demonstrate use of assistive devices and adaptive activities
- Instruct patient in alternative methods for eating and drinking, specify method and teaching plan

Collaborative Activities

- Refer patient and family to social services for obtaining home health aide
- Use occupational and physical therapy as resources in planning patient care activities
- *(NIC) Self-Care Assistance: Feeding*: Provide for adequate pain relief before meals, as appropriate

Other

- Accommodate cognitive deficits in the following ways:
    Avoid using sharp eating utensils (e.g., steak knives)
    Check for food in cheeks
    Have meals in quiet environment to limit distraction from task
    Keep verbal communication short and simple
- Serve one food at a time in small amounts
- Acknowledge and reinforce patient's accomplishments
- Encourage independence in eating and drinking, assisting patient only as necessary
- Encourage patient to wear dentures and eyeglasses
- Provide for privacy while eating if patient is embarrassed
- When feeding, allow patient to determine order of foods
- Sit down while feeding; do not hurry

- Serve finger foods (e.g., fruit, bread) to promote independence
- Include parents and family in feeding and meals
- *(NIC) Self-Care Assistance: Feeding:*
  Create a pleasant environment during mealtime (e.g., put bed-
    pans, urinals, and suctioning equipment out of sight)
  Provide for oral hygiene before meals
  Fix food on tray, as necessary, such as cutting meat or peeling
    an egg
  Avoid placing food on a person's blind side
  Provide a drinking straw, as needed or desired
  Provide adaptive devices to facilitate patient's feeding self (e.g.,
    long handles, handle with large circumference, or small strap
    on utensils), as needed
  Provide frequent cuing and close supervision, as appropriate

SELF-CARE DEFICIT: TOILETING
(00110) (1980, 1998)

Definition: Impaired ability to perform or complete own toileting
  activities

Defining Characteristics

Objective
Inability to manipulate clothing for toileting
Unable to carry out proper toilet hygiene
Unable to flush toilet or commode
Unable to get to toilet or commode
Unable to sit on or rise from toilet or commode

Related Factors
Decreased or lack of motivation
Environmental barriers
Impaired mobility status
Impaired transfer ability
Musculoskeletal impairment
Neuromuscular impairment
Pain
Perceptual or cognitive impairment
Severe anxiety
Weakness or tiredness

Other Possible Defining Characteristics (non-NANDA International)

Depression

Developmental disability

Intolerance to activity

Medically imposed restrictions

Psychologic impairment (specify)

Suggestions for Use

Self-care deficit: toileting may be an etiology (i.e., related factor) for *Impaired skin integrity* or *Social isolation*. Also see Self-Care Deficits—Discussion on pp. 422–423. NANDA International uses the following scale to classify functional levels:

0 = Completely independent

1 = Requires use of equipment or device

2 = Requires help from another person for assistance, supervision, or teaching

3 = Requires help from another person and equipment or device

4 = Dependent, does not participate in activity

The following definitions and descriptors in Table 8 may be helpful in determining which number to assign to a patient's functional level:

Table 8

	Totally Dependent (+4)	Moderately Dependent (+3)	Semi-dependent (+2)
Toileting	Patient is incontinent; nurse places patient on bedpan or commode	Nurse provides bedpan, positions patient on or off bedpan, places patient on commode	Patient can walk to bathroom or commode with assistance; nurse helps with clothing

Suggested Alternative Diagnoses

Activity intolerance

Bowel incontinence

Fatigue

Physical mobility, impaired

Sensory perception, disturbed

Thought processes, disturbed

Total self-care deficit
Transfer ability, impaired
Urinary incontinence (functional, stress, total, urge)
Urinary incontinence: urge, risk for

NOC Outcomes

Self-Care: Activities of Daily Living (ADLs): Ability to perform the
most basic physical and personal care activities
Self-Care: Hygiene: Ability to maintain own hygiene
Self-Care: Toileting: Ability to toilet self

Goals/Evaluation Criteria

Examples Using NOC Language

- Demonstrates **Self-Care: Activities of Daily Living (ADLs)**, as
  evidenced by the following indicators (specify 1–5: dependent
  (does not participate), requires assistive person and device,
  requires assistive person, independent with assistive device, or
  completely independent):
    Toileting

Other Examples

Patient will:
- Accept help from caregiver
- Recognize or acknowledge need for help with toileting
- Recognize and respond to urge to urinate and/or defecate
- Be able to get to and from toilet
- Wipe self after toileting

NIC Interventions

Bowel Training: Assisting the patient to train the bowel to evacuate at specific intervals
Environmental Management: Manipulation of the patient's surroundings for therapeutic benefit
Self-Care Assistance: Bathing/Hygiene: Assisting patient to perform personal hygiene
Self-Care Assistance: Toileting: Assisting another with elimination

Nursing Activities

Also see Nursing Activities for Bowel Incontinence on pp. 47–48
and for Urinary Incontinence: Functional, Reflex, Stress, Total, and
Urge on pp. 595–596, 598–599, 601–602, and 603–604.

Assessments

- Assess ability to ambulate independently and safely
- Assess ability to use assistive devices (e.g., walkers, canes)
- Monitor energy level and activity tolerance
- Assess for improved or deteriorating ability to toilet self
- Assess for sensory, cognitive, or physical deficits that may limit self-toileting

Patient/Family Teaching

- Instruct patient and family in transfer and ambulation techniques
- Demonstrate use of assistive equipment and adaptive activities
- *(NIC) Self-Care Assistance: Toileting*: Instruct patient and appropriate others in toileting routine
- *(NIC) Environmental Management:* Provide family and significant other with information about making home environment safe for patient

Collaborative Activities

- Offer pain medications prior to toileting
- Refer patient and family to social services for obtaining home health aide
- Use occupational and physical therapy as resources in planning patient care activities and obtaining necessary equipment

Other

- Specify functional level and assist with toileting or provide basic care, as needed
- Accommodate cognitive deficits (e.g., keep verbal instructions short and simple)
- Allow sufficient time for toileting to avoid fatigue and frustration
- Avoid use of indwelling catheters and condom catheters if possible
- Encourage patient to wear clothes that are easy to manage; assist with clothing, as needed
- Keep bedpan or urinal within patient's reach
- *(NIC) Self-Care Assistance: Toileting:*
  Assist patient to toilet, commode, bedpan, fracture pan, and urinal [specify] at specified intervals
  Facilitate toilet hygiene after completion of elimination
  Flush toilet; cleanse elimination utensil
  Replace patient's clothing after elimination
  Provide privacy during elimination

- *(NIC) Environmental Management:*

  Remove environmental hazards (e.g., loose rugs and small, movable furniture)

  Provide room deodorizers, as needed

  Provide immediate and continuous means to summon nurse and let the patient and family know they will be answered immediately

SELF-CONCEPT, READINESS FOR ENHANCED (00167) (2002)

Definition: A pattern of perceptions or ideas about the self that is sufficient for well-being and can be strengthened

Defining Characteristics

Subjective

Accepts strengths and limitations

Expresses confidence in abilities

Expresses satisfaction with thoughts about self, sense of worthiness, role performance, body image, and personal identity

Expresses willingness to enhance self-concept

Objective

Actions are congruent with expressed feelings and thoughts

Related Factors

This is a wellness diagnosis, so an etiology is not needed.

Suggestions for Use

Self-concept is a broad diagnosis that includes body image, self-esteem, personal identity, and role performance. *Readiness for enhanced self-concept* can be used when there are no risk factors for the more specific problems (e.g., *Chronic or situational low self-esteem, Ineffective role performance*). If risk factors are present, consider a diagnosis such as *Risk for situational low self-esteem*.

Suggested Alternative Diagnoses

Coping (individual), readiness for enhanced

Self-esteem, risk for situational low

NOC Outcomes

Not yet developed, however, the following may be useful:

Body Image: Positive perception of own appearance and body functions

Quality of Life: An individual's expressed satisfaction with current life circumstance

Role Performance: Congruence of an individual's role behavior with role expectations

Self-Esteem: Personal judgment of self-worth

Goals/Evaluation Criteria

Examples Using NOC Language

- Demonstrates **Self-Esteem**, as evidenced by the following indicators (specify 1–5: never, rarely, sometimes, often, or consistently demonstrated):

    Verbalization of self-acceptance

    Acceptance of compliments from others

    Description of success in work, school, or social groups

Other Examples

Patient will:

- Acknowledge personal strengths
- Exhibit realistic self-appraisal
- Express a willingness to enhance self-concept
- Participate in making decisions regarding plan of care
- Practice behaviors that generate self-confidence
- Verbalize positive feelings about body, self, abilities, and role performance

NIC Interventions

NIC interventions have not yet been linked to this new diagnosis; however, the following may be helpful:

Active Listening: Attending closely to and attaching significance to a patient's verbal and nonverbal messages

Body Image Enhancement: Improving a patient's conscious and unconscious perceptions and attitudes toward his body

Self-Awareness Enhancement: Assisting a patient to explore and understand his thoughts, feelings, motivations, and behaviors

Self-Esteem Enhancement: Assisting a patient to increase his personal judgment of self-worth

Nursing Activities

Assessments

- Assess for evidence of positive self-concept (e.g., mood, positive body image, satisfaction with role responsibilities, perception of and satisfaction with self in general)
- *(NIC) Self-Esteem Enhancement:*
  Monitor patient's statements of self-worth
  Determine patient's confidence in own judgment

Patient/Family Teaching

- Teach positive behavioral skills through role play, role modeling, discussion, and so forth
- *(NIC) Self-Esteem Enhancement:* Instruct parents on the importance of their interest and support in their children's development of a positive self-concept

Other

- Help client to anticipate developmental and situational changes that may influence role performance and self-esteem
- *(NIC) Self-Esteem Enhancement:*
  Convey confidence in patient's ability to handle situation(s)
  Encourage patient to accept new challenges
  Reinforce the personal strengths that patient identifies
  Assist patient to identify positive responses from others
  Assist in setting realistic goals to achieve higher self-esteem
  Explore previous achievements of success
  Reward or praise patient's progress toward reaching goals

SELF-ESTEEM, CHRONIC LOW
(00119) (1988, 1996)

Definition: Long-standing, negative self-evaluation or feelings about self or self-capabilities

Defining Characteristics

Subjective

Evaluates self as unable to deal with events (long-standing or chronic)

Expressions of shame and guilt (long-standing or chronic)

Rationalizes away or rejects positive feedback and exaggerates negative feedback about self (long-standing or chronic)

Self-negating verbalization (long-standing or chronic)

Objective

Dependent on others' opinions

Excessively seeks reassurance

Frequent lack of success in work or other life events

Hesitant to try new things and situations (long-standing or chronic)

Indecisive

Lack of eye contact

Nonassertive or passive

Overly conforming

Other Possible Defining Characteristics (non-NANDA International)

Projection of blame or responsibility for problems

Self-destructive behaviors (e.g., alcohol, drug abuse)

Self-neglect

Related Factors

To be developed

Related Factors (non-NANDA International)

Chronic illness

Congenital anomaly

Psychologic impairment (specify)

Repeated unmet expectations

Suggestions for Use

Chronic low self-esteem is different from *Situational low self-esteem* in that the symptoms are long-standing and seem to result from frequent, actual, or perceived lack of success in work or role performance.

Suggested Alternative Diagnoses

Coping, ineffective

Hopelessness

Powerlessness

Self-concept disturbance (non-NANDA International)

Self-esteem, situational low

NOC Outcomes

Depression Level: Personal actions to minimize melancholy and maintain interest in life events

Quality of Life: An individual's expressed satisfaction with current life circumstance

Self-Esteem: Personal judgment of self-worth

Goals/Evaluation Criteria

Examples Using NOC Language

- Demonstrates **Self-Esteem**, as evidenced by the following indicators (specify 1–5: never, rarely, sometimes, often, or consistently demonstrated):

    Verbalization of self-acceptance

    Maintenance of erect posture

    Maintenance of eye contact

    Maintenance of grooming and hygiene

    Acceptance of compliments from others

    Description of success in work, school, or social groups

Other Examples

Patient will:

- Acknowledge personal strengths
- Express a willingness to seek counseling
- Participate in making decisions regarding plan of care
- Practice behaviors that generate self-confidence

NIC Interventions

Hope Instillation: Facilitation of the development of a positive outlook in a given situation

Mood Management: Facilitation of the development of a positive outlook in a given situation

Self-Esteem Enhancement: Assisting a patient to increase his personal judgment of self-worth

Values Clarification: Assisting another to clarify his own values in order to facilitate effective decision making

Nursing Activities

Assessments

- *(NIC) Self-Esteem Enhancement:*

    Monitor patient's statements of self-worth

    Determine patient's confidence in own judgment

    Monitor frequency of self-negating verbalizations

Patient/Family Teaching

- Provide information about the value of counseling and available community resources
- Teach positive behavioral skills through role play, role modeling, discussion, and so forth

- *(NIC) Self-Esteem Enhancement:* Instruct parents on the importance of their interest and support in their children's development of a positive self-concept

Collaborative Activities

- Seek assistance from hospital resources (e.g., social workers, psychiatric clinical specialist, pastoral care services), as needed

Other

- Set limits about negative verbalization (e.g., regarding frequency, content, audience)
- *(NIC) Self-Esteem Enhancement:*
  Reinforce the personal strengths that patient identifies
  Assist patient to identify positive responses from others
  Refrain from teasing
  Assist in setting realistic goals to achieve higher self-esteem
  Assist patient to reexamine negative perceptions of self
  Assist the patient to identify the impact of peer group on feelings of self-worth
  Explore previous achievements of success
  Reward or praise patient's progress toward reaching goals
  Facilitate an environment and activities that will increase self-esteem

SELF-ESTEEM, SITUATIONAL LOW
(00120) (1988, 1996, 2000)

Definition: Development of a negative perception of self-worth in response to a current situation

Defining Characteristics

Subjective

Evaluation of self as unable to deal with situations or events
Expressions of helplessness and uselessness
Self-negating verbalizations
Verbally reports current situational challenge to self-worth

Objective

Indecisive, nonassertive behavior

Related Factors

Behavior inconsistent with values
Developmental changes (specify)

Disturbed body image
Failures and rejections
Functional impairment (specify)
Lack of recognition or rewards
Loss (specify)
Social role changes (specify)

Related Factors (non-NANDA International)
Situational crisis (specify)

Suggestions for Use

Situational low self-esteem can be differentiated from *Chronic low self-esteem* in that the symptoms are episodic. Symptoms occur in a person with previously good self-esteem and are in response to some actual or perceived event or situation. Goals and nursing activities, therefore, may focus on problem solving the situation in addition to building the patient's self-esteem.

Suggested Alternative Diagnoses

Adjustment, impaired
Body image, disturbed
Coping, ineffective
Personal identity, disturbed
Self-esteem, chronic low

NOC Outcomes

Decision Making: Ability to choose between two or more alternatives
Grief Resolution: Adjustment to actual or impending loss
Psychosocial Adjustment: Life Change: Psychosocial adaptation of an individual to a life change
Self-Esteem: Personal judgment of self-worth

Goals/Evaluation Criteria

Examples Using NOC Language

- Demonstrates **Self-Esteem**, as evidenced by the following indicators (specify 1–5: never, rarely, sometimes, often, or consistently demonstrated):
    Verbalization of self-acceptance
    Open communication
    Fulfillment of personally significant roles
    Acceptance of compliments from others

Willingness to confront others

Description of success in work, school, and social groups

- Demonstrates **Decision Making**, as evidenced by the following indicators (specify 1–5: never, rarely, sometimes, often, or consistently demonstrated):

    Identifies alternatives and potential consequences of each

    Identifies resources necessary to support each alternative

    Weighs and chooses among alternatives

Other Examples

Patient will:

- Acknowledge personal strengths
- Practice behaviors that generate self-confidence
- Verbalize episodic change/loss

NIC Interventions

Anticipatory Guidance: Preparation of patient for an anticipated developmental or situational crisis

Coping Enhancement: Assisting a patient to adapt to perceived stressors, changes, or threats which interfere with meeting life demands and roles

Decision-Making Support: Providing information and support for a patient who is making a decision regarding health care

Grief Work Facilitation: Assistance with the resolution of a significant loss

Grief Work Facilitation: Perinatal Death: Assistance with the resolution of a perinatal loss

Self-Esteem Enhancement: Assisting a patient to increase his personal judgment of self-worth

Nursing Activities

Also refer to Nursing Activities for Self-Esteem, Chronic Low on pp. 442–443.

Patient/Family Teaching

- Teach positive behavioral skills through role play, role modeling, discussion, and so forth

Collaborative Activities

- Refer to appropriate community resources
- Seek assistance from hospital resources (social worker, clinical nurse specialist, pastoral care services), as needed

Other

- Explore recent changes with patient that may have influenced low self-esteem
- *(NIC) Self-Esteem Enhancement:*
  Convey confidence in patient's ability to handle situation
  Encourage increased responsibility for self, as appropriate
  Explore reasons for self-criticism or guilt
  Encourage patient to accept new challenges

SELF-ESTEEM, SITUATIONAL LOW, RISK FOR (00153) (2000)

Definition: At risk for developing negative perception of self-worth in response to a current situation (specify)

Risk Factors

Subjective
Disturbed body image
Unrealistic self-expectations

Objective
Behavior inconsistent with values
Decreased power or control over environment
Developmental changes (specify)
Failures and rejections
Functional impairment (specify)
History of abuse, neglect, or abandonment
History of learned helplessness
Lack of recognition or rewards
Physical illness (specify)
Social role changes (specify)

Suggestions for Use

None

Suggested Alternative Diagnoses

Body image, disturbed
Coping, ineffective
Personal identity, disturbed
Self-concept, readiness for enhanced
Self-esteem, situational low

NOC Outcomes

NOC outcomes have not yet been linked to this diagnosis; however, the following may be useful:

Decision Making: Ability to choose between two or more alternatives

Grief Resolution: Adjustment to actual or impending loss

Psychosocial Adjustment: Life Change: Psychosocial adaptation of an individual to a life change

Self-Esteem: Personal judgment of self-worth

Goals/Evaluation Criteria

Refer to Goals/Evaluation Criteria for Self-Esteem: Situational Low, on pp. 444–445.

NIC Interventions

NIC interventions have not yet been linked to this diagnosis; however, the following may be useful:

Anticipatory Guidance: Preparation of patient for an anticipated developmental or situational crisis

Coping Enhancement: Assisting a patient to adapt to perceived stressors, changes, or threats which interfere with meeting life demands and roles

Grief Work Facilitation: Assistance with the resolution of a significant loss

Grief Work Facilitation: Perinatal Death: Assistance with the resolution of a perinatal loss

Self-Esteem Enhancement: Assisting a patient to increase his personal judgment of self-worth

Nursing Activities

Refer to Nursing Activities for Self-Esteem, Situational Low on pp. 445–446.

SELF-MUTILATION
(00151) (2000)

Definition: Deliberate self-injurious behavior causing tissue damage with the intent of causing nonfatal injury to attain relief of tension

Defining Characteristics

Objective

Abrading

Biting

Constricting a body part

Cuts or scratches on body

Hitting

Ingestion or inhalation of harmful substances or objects

Insertion of object(s) into body orifice(s)

Picking at wounds

Self-inflicted burns (e.g., eraser, cigarette)

Severing

Related Factors

Adolescence

Borderline personality disorder

Chaotic or disturbed interpersonal relationships

Character disorder

Childhood illness or surgery

Childhood sexual abuse

Developmentally delayed or autistic individual

Eating disorders

Emotionally disturbed; battered child

Experiences dissociation or depersonalization

Family alcoholism

Family divorce

Family history of self-destructive behaviors

Feelings of depression, rejection, self-hatred, separation anxiety, guilt, depersonalization

Feels threatened with actual or potential loss of significant relationship (e.g., loss of parent or parental relationship)

Foster, group, or institutional care

History of inability to plan solutions or see long-term consequences

History of self-injurious behavior

Impulsivity

Inability to express tension verbally

Inadequate coping

Incarceration

Irresistible urge to cut or damage self

Isolation from peers

Labile behavior (mood swings)

Lack of family confidant

Low or unstable body image

Low or unstable self-esteem

Mounting tension that is intolerable

Needs quick reduction of stress

Peers who self-mutilate

Perfectionism

Poor parent–adolescent communication

Psychotic state (command hallucinations)

Sexual identity crisis

Substance abuse

Use of manipulation to obtain nurturing relationship with others

Violence between parental figures

Suggestions for Use

Use Self-mutilation for a patient who has already inflicted injury on self. Use *Risk for Self-mutilation* when risk factors are present, but the person has not actually exhibited injurious behavior.

Suggested Alternative Diagnoses

Suicide, risk for

NOC Outcomes

NOC outcomes have not yet been linked to this diagnosis; however, the following may be useful:

Anxiety Control: Personal actions to eliminate or reduce feelings of apprehension and tension from an unidentifiable source

Impulse Control: Ability to self-restrain compulsive or impulsive behaviors

Risk Detection: Actions taken to identify personal health threats

Self-Mutilation Restraint: Ability to refrain from intentional self-inflicted injury (nonlethal)

Goals/Evaluation Criteria

See Goals/Evaluation Criteria: for Self-Mutilation, Risk for, on p. 455.

NIC Interventions

NIC interventions have not yet been linked to this diagnosis; however, the following may be useful:

Anger Control Assistance: Facilitation of the expression of anger in an adaptive nonviolent manner

Behavior Management: Self-Harm: Assisting the patient to decrease or eliminate self-mutilating or self-abusive behaviors

Environmental Management, Safety: Monitoring and manipulation of the physical environment to promote safety

Impulse Control Training: Assisting the patient to mediate impulsive behavior through application of problem-solving strategies to social and interpersonal situations

Nursing Activities

For All Patients

Assessments

- Assess self-injury behaviors, including methods used, known triggers, and so forth
- Assess nature and extent of the injuries
- *(NIC) Anger Control Assistance*: Monitor potential for inappropriate aggression and intervene before its expression
- *(NIC) Behavior Management: Self-Harm*: Determine the motive or reason for the behaviors

Collaborative Activities

- Obtain medical orders, as needed, to treat self-inflicted injuries (e.g., cuts, abrasions)

Patient/Family Teaching

- Provide support and education to family regarding patient status and methods of treatment
- *(NIC) Behavior Management: Self-Harm:* Instruct patient in coping strategies (e.g., assertiveness training, impulse control training, and progressive muscle relaxation, as appropriate)

Other

- Provide patient safety, using least restrictive measures (e.g., environmental manipulation, assign roommate, assign patient room close to nursing station, family and visitor restriction, patient within eyesight at all times, patient within arm's length, other interventions specific to patient)
- Accompany patient to activities outside of the unit, as needed
- *(NIC) Behavior Management: Self-Harm:*
  Develop appropriate behavioral expectations and consequences, given the patient's level of cognitive functioning and capacity for self-control

Remove dangerous items from the patient's environment

Use a calm, nonpunitive approach when dealing with self-harmful behaviors

- *(NIC) Anger Control Assistance:*

Use external controls (e.g., physical or manual restraint, time-outs) as needed to calm patient who is expressing anger in a maladaptive manner

Identify consequences of inappropriate expression of anger

Establish basic trust and rapport with patient

Psychotic Patients

Assessments

- Observe for behavioral changes from baseline assessment (e.g., increased withdrawal, agitation)
- Assess patient for morbid preoccupation with suicide, self-mutilation, hopelessness, and worthlessness
- Assess patient with command hallucinations to determine content and source (e.g., ask patient: "Whose voice is it? What did the voice tell you to do? Did the voice tell you to hurt yourself and how? Does the voice have control over you?")
- Monitor intensity of hallucinations and delusions and attempt reality testing q _____
- Determine whether religious, persecutory, or somatic delusions contributed to the self-injury.

Collaborative Activities

- Obtain physician order if intervention is a denial of rights
- *(NIC) Behavior Management: Self-Harm*: Administer medications, as appropriate, to decrease anxiety, stabilize mood, and decrease self-stimulation

Other

- If patient exhibits calmness abruptly following a period of agitation, provide increased safety measures to prevent self-injury
- Assist patient to differentiate internal stimuli from outside world
- Encourage patient to verbalize thoughts and impulses instead of storing up tension
- Search patient and environment for potentially harmful items
- Trim patient's fingernails and toenails to prevent scratching
- Encourage physical activity
- Contract with patient to not injure self

- If patient is unable to make contract or follow directions, stay with patient at all times until either patient reports a decrease in command hallucinations, delusions, or self-mutilation impulses, or until seclusion or restraint is used
- *(NIC) Behavior Management: Self-Harm:*
  Place patient in a more protective environment (e.g., area restriction and seclusion) if self-harmful impulses or behaviors escalate
  Apply, as appropriate, mitts, splints, helmets, or restraints to limit mobility and ability to initiate self-harm
  Assist patient to identify trigger situations and feelings that prompt self-harmful behavior

Personality Disorder Patients

Assessments

- Assess patient's level of impulsivity and frustration tolerance

Patient/Family Teaching

- Teach patient alternative stress-tension-relieving measures (e.g., relaxation techniques; physical exercise; journal writing; self-affirmations; and distracting techniques such as music, television, and conversation)
- Provide family and significant other with guidelines explaining how self-harmful behavior can be managed outside the care environment
- *(NIC) Behavior Management: Self-Harm:* Provide illness teaching to patient and significant others if self-harmful behavior is illness-based (e.g., borderline personality disorder or autism)

Collaborative Activities

- Consider antianxiety or neuroleptic medications according to physician order
- Provide consistent responses to patient by collaborating closely with other health care providers. Review treatment plan frequently to prevent staff splitting and conflict regarding treatment goals.

Other

- Encourage patient to seek out staff and peers instead of using alcohol or drugs
- Establish regular and frequent check-in times with assigned staff
- *(NIC) Behavior Management: Self-Harm:*
  Contract with patient, as appropriate, for "no self-harm"
  Provide predetermined consequences if patient is engaging in self-harmful behaviors

Retarded/Autistic Patients

Assessments

- Assess patient's response to environment to determine if there were stressors that led to self-injury

Patient/Family Teaching

- *(NIC) Behavior Management: Self-Harm:* Provide illness teaching to patient and significant others if self-harmful behavior is illness-based (e.g., borderline personality disorder or autism)

Other

- Alter environmental situations that produce stress that provokes self-injury behaviors
- Remove reinforcement that may induce self-injury behavior (e.g., comforting patient after headbanging, excusing patient from perceived unpleasant tasks
- Develop behavioral plan that will decrease the incidence of self-injury
- Use protective devices to prevent self-injury (e.g., mitts, helmet, jacket restraint, protective clothing)

SELF-MUTILATION, RISK FOR
(00139) (1992, 2000)

Definition: At risk for deliberate self-injurious behavior causing tissue damage with the intent of causing nonfatal injury to attain relief of tension

Risk Factors

Adolescence

Borderline personality disorder

Chaotic or disturbed interpersonal relationships

Character disorder

Childhood illness or surgery

Childhood sexual abuse

Developmentally delayed or autistic individual

Eating disorders

Emotionally disturbed; battered child

Experiences dissociation or depersonalization

Family alcoholism

Family divorce

Family history of self-destructive behaviors

Feelings of depression, rejection, self-hatred, separation anxiety, guilt, depersonalization

Feels threatened with actual or potential loss of significant relationship

Foster, group, or institutional care

History of inability to plan solutions or see long-term consequences

History of self-injurious behavior

Impulsivity

Inability to express tension verbally

Inadequate coping

Incarceration

Irresistible urge to cut or damage self

Isolation from peers

Loss of control over problem-solving situations

Loss of parent or parental relationship

Low or unstable body image

Low or unstable self-esteem

Mounting tension that is intolerable

Needs quick reduction of stress

Peers who self-mutilate

Perfectionism

Psychotic state (command hallucinations)

Sexual identity crisis

Substance abuse

Use of manipulation to obtain nurturing relationship with others

Suggestions for Use

Risk for self-mutilation is a more specific diagnosis than *Risk for self-directed violence*, although the two diagnoses have some of the same defining characteristics (i.e., risk factors). *Risk for self-directed violence* includes actions such as drug and alcohol abuse and high-risk lifestyle (e.g., driving fast), which are not included in *Risk for self-mutilation*.

Suggested Alternative Diagnoses

Self-directed violence, risk for

Self-mutilation

Suicide, risk for

NOC Outcomes

Aggression Control: Self-restraint of assaultive, combative, or destructive behavior toward others. [**NOTE:** This outcome refers to behavior toward others; however, the diagnosis of *Risk for self-mutilation* refers to acts that are harmful to oneself. Therefore, although NOC lists it, I do not recommend Aggression Control as an outcome for self-mutilation.]

Impulse Control: Ability to self-restrain compulsive or impulsive behaviors

Risk Detection: Actions taken to identify personal health threats

Self-Mutilation Restraint: Ability to refrain from intentional self-inflicted injury (nonlethal)

Goals/Evaluation Criteria

Examples Using NOC Language

• Demonstrates **Self-Mutilation Restraint**, as evidenced by the following indicators (specify 1–5: never, rarely, sometimes, often, or consistently demonstrated):

Seeks help when feeling urge to injure self

Upholds contract to not harm self

Refrains from gathering means for self-injury

Maintains self-control without supervision

Other Examples

Patient will:

• Be free from self-injury

• Verbalize reduction or absence of command hallucinations or delusions

• Identify feelings that lead to impulsive actions

• Identify and avoid high-risk environments and situations

NIC Interventions

Anger Control Assistance: Facilitation of the expression of anger in an adaptive nonviolent manner

Behavior Management: Self-Harm: Assisting the patient to decrease or eliminate self-mutilating or self-abusive behaviors

Environmental Management, Safety: Monitoring and manipulation of the physical environment to promote safety

Impulse Control Training: Assisting the patient to mediate impulsive behavior through application of problem-solving strategies to social and interpersonal situations

Nursing Activities

For All Patients

Assessments

- Assess patient for history of self-injury behaviors, including methods used, known triggers, and so forth
- *(NIC) Anger Control Assistance*: Monitor potential for inappropriate aggression and intervene before its expression
- *(NIC) Behavior Management: Self-Harm:* Determine the motive or reason for the behaviors

Patient/Family Teaching

- Provide support and education to family regarding patient status and methods of treatment
- *(NIC) Behavior Management: Self-Harm:* Instruct patient in coping strategies (e.g., assertiveness training, impulse control training, and progressive muscle relaxation, as appropriate)

Other

- Provide patient safety, using least restrictive measures (e.g., environmental manipulation, assign roommate, assign patient room close to nursing station, family and visitor restriction, patient within eyesight at all times, patient within arm's length, other interventions specific to patient)
- Accompany patient to activities outside of the unit, as needed
- *(NIC) Behavior Management: Self-Harm:*
  Develop appropriate behavioral expectations and consequences, given the patient's level of cognitive functioning and capacity for self-control
  Remove dangerous items from the patient's environment
  Use a calm, nonpunitive approach when dealing with self-harmful behaviors
- *(NIC) Anger Control Assistance:*
  Use external controls (e.g., physical or manual restraint, time-outs) as needed to calm patient who is expressing anger in a maladaptive manner
  Identify consequences of inappropriate expression of anger
  Establish basic trust and rapport with patient

Psychotic Patients

Assessments

- Observe for behavioral changes from baseline assessment (e.g., increased withdrawal, agitation)

- Assess patient for morbid preoccupation with suicide, self-mutilation, hopelessness, and worthlessness
- Assess patient with command hallucinations to determine content and source (e.g., ask patient: "Whose voice is it? What is the voice telling you to do? Is the voice telling you to hurt yourself and how? Does the voice have control over you?")
- Monitor intensity of hallucinations or delusions and attempt reality testing q _____
- Assess patient for religious or persecutory delusions that may lead to self-injury
- Assess patient for somatic delusions that may lead to self-injury (e.g., beliefs that part of body is diseased, rotten, or unnecessary)

Collaborative Activities

- Obtain physician order if intervention is a denial of rights
- *(NIC) Behavior Management: Self-Harm*: Administer medications, as appropriate, to decrease anxiety, stabilize mood, and decrease self-stimulation

Other

- If patient exhibits calmness abruptly following a period of agitation, provide increased safety measures to prevent self-injury
- Assist patient to differentiate internal stimuli from outside world
- Encourage patient to verbalize thoughts and impulses instead of storing up tension
- Search patient as needed for potentially harmful items
- Trim patient's fingernails and toenails to prevent scratching
- Encourage physical activity
- Contract with patient to not injure self
- If patient is unable to make contract or follow directions, stay with patient at all times until either patient reports a decrease in command hallucinations, delusions, or self-mutilation impulses, or until seclusion or restraint is used
- *(NIC) Behavior Management: Self-Harm:*

  Place patient in a more protective environment (e.g., area restriction and seclusion) if self-harmful impulses or behaviors escalate

  Apply, as appropriate, mitts, splints, helmets, or restraints to limit mobility and ability to initiate self-harm

  Assist patient to identify trigger situations and feelings that prompt self-harmful behavior

Personality Disorder Patients

Assessments

- Assess patient's level of impulsivity and frustration tolerance

Patient/Family Teaching

- Teach patient alternative stress-tension-relieving measures (e.g., relaxation techniques; physical exercise; journal writing; self-affirmations; and distracting techniques such as music, television, and conversation)
- Provide family and significant other with guidelines explaining how self-harmful behavior can be managed outside the care environment
- *(NIC) Behavior Management: Self-Harm:* Provide illness teaching to patient and significant others if self-harmful behavior is illness-based (e.g., borderline personality disorder or autism)

Collaborative Activities

- Consider antianxiety or neuroleptic medications according to physician order
- Provide consistent responses to patient by collaborating closely with other health care providers. Review treatment plan frequently to prevent staff splitting and conflict regarding treatment goals.

Other

- Encourage patient to seek out staff and peers instead of using alcohol or drugs
- Establish regular and frequent check-in times with assigned staff
- *(NIC) Behavior Management: Self-Harm:*

Contract with patient, as appropriate, for "no self-harm"

Provide predetermined consequences if patient is engaging in self-harmful behaviors

Retarded/Autistic Patients

Assessments

- Assess patient's response to environment to determine if there is a stressor that may lead to self-injury

Patient/Family Teaching

- *(NIC) Behavior Management: Self-Harm:* Provide illness teaching to patient and significant others if self-harmful behavior is illness-based (e.g., borderline personality disorder or autism)

Other

- Alter environmental situations that may produce stress that provokes self-injury behaviors
- Remove reinforcement that may induce self-injury behavior (e.g., comforting patient after headbanging, excusing patient from perceived unpleasant tasks
- Develop behavioral plan that will prevent or decrease incidence of self-injury
- Use protective devices to prevent self-injury (e.g., mitts, helmet, jacket restraint, protective clothing)

SENSORY PERCEPTION, DISTURBED (SPECIFY: VISUAL, AUDITORY, KINESTHETIC, GUSTATORY, TACTILE, OLFACTORY) (00122) (1978, 1980, 1998)

Definition: Change in the amount or patterning of incoming stimuli, accompanied by a diminished, exaggerated, distorted, or impaired response to such stimuli

Defining Characteristics

Subjective

Auditory distortions
Reported change in sensory acuity
Visual distortions

Objective

Altered communication patterns
Change in behavior pattern
Change in problem-solving abilities
Change in usual response to stimuli
Disoriented in time, in place, or with people
Hallucinations
Irritability
Measured change in sensory acuity
Poor concentration
Restlessness

Other Possible Defining Characteristics (non-NANDA International)

Alteration in posture
Altered abstraction

Anxiety

Apathy

Change in muscular tension

Inappropriate responses

Indication of alteration in body image

Related Factors

Altered sensory perception

Altered sensory reception, transmission, or integration

Biochemical imbalance

Biochemical imbalances for sensory distortion (e.g., illusions, hallucinations)

Electrolyte imbalance

Excessive environmental stimuli

Insufficient environmental stimuli

Psychological stress

Suggestions for Use

A diagnosis of *Disturbed sensory perception* represents a change from the individual's usual response to stimuli; the changes in response are not a result of mental or personality disorders. Use this label to describe patients whose perceptions have been influenced by physiologic factors such as pain, sleep deprivation, or immobility or by disease states such as CVA, brain trauma, and increased intracranial pressure (ICP).

Altered cognition and perception can be symptoms of both *Disturbed sensory perception* and *Impaired thought processes*. When a person's ability to interpret stimuli is affected by physical or physiologic factors, use *Disturbed sensory perception*; when the ability to interpret stimuli is affected by mental disorders, use *Impaired thought processes*. To further help differentiate between the two diagnoses, note that the following defining characteristics and related factors may be present in *Impaired thought processes* but not in *Disturbed sensory perception:*

Obsessive thinking

Loss of memory

Impaired judgment

In addition, the following defining characteristics are present in *Disturbed sensory perception,* but not in *Impaired thought processes.*

Visual and auditory distortions

Discoordinated motor activity

Changes in sensory acuity

Disturbed sensory perception may be more useful as the etiology of other problems, for example, the following:

Risk for injury related to Disturbed sensory perception (visual)

Self-care deficit related to Disturbed sensory perception (visual)

Impaired communication related to Disturbed sensory perception (auditory)

Risk for injury related to Disturbed sensory perception (kinesthetic or tactile)

Imbalanced nutrition related to Disturbed sensory perception (olfactory or gustatory)

When *Disturbed sensory perception* exists as a result of immobility, consider using *Risk for disuse syndrome.*

Suggested Alternative Diagnoses

Confusion, acute or chronic

Disuse syndrome, risk for

Environmental interpretation syndrome, impaired

Peripheral neurovascular dysfunction, risk for

Thought processes, disturbed

Unilateral neglect

NOC Outcomes

Auditory

Cognitive Ability: Ability to execute complex mental processes

Cognitive Orientation: Ability to identify person, place, and time

Communication: Receptive Ability: Ability to receive and interpret verbal and nonverbal messages

Distorted Thought Control: Self-restraint of disruption in perception, thought processes, and thought content

Hearing Compensation Behavior: Actions to identify, monitor, and compensate for hearing loss

Gustatory

Cognitive Orientation: Ability to identify person, place, and time

Distorted Thought Control: Self-restraint of disruption in perception, thought processes, and thought content

Nutritional Status: Food and Fluid Intake: Amount of food and fluid taken into the body over a 24-hr period

Sensory Function: Taste and Smell: Extent to which chemicals inhaled or dissolved in saliva are sensed

Kinesthetic

Balance: Ability to maintain body equilibrium

Body-Positioning: Self-Initiated: Ability to change own body positions

Cognitive Orientation: Ability to identify person, place, and time

Distorted Thought Control: Self-restraint of disruption in perception, thought processes, and thought content

Muscle Function: Adequacy of muscle contraction needed for movement

Neurological status: Central Motor Control: Extent to which skeletal muscle activity (body movement) is coordinated by the central nervous system

Sensory Function: Proprioception: Extent to which the position and movement of the head and body are sensed

Olfactory

Cognitive Orientation: Ability to identify person, place, and time

Distorted Thought Control: Self-restraint of disruption in perception, thought processes, and thought content

Nutritional Status: Food & Fluid Intake: Amount of food and fluid taken into the body over a 24-hr period

Sensory Function: Taste & Smell: Extent to which chemicals inhaled or dissolved in saliva are sensed

Tactile

Cognitive Orientation: Ability to identify person, place, and time

Distorted Thought Control: Self-restraint of disruption in perception, thought processes, and thought content

Neurological Status: Spinal Sensory/Motor Function: Extent to which spinal nerves convey sensory and motor information

Sensory Function: Cutaneous: Extent to which stimulation of the skin is sensed in an impaired area

Visual

Body Image: Positive perception of own appearance and body function

Cognitive Orientation: Ability to identify person, place, and time

Distorted Thought Control: Self-restraint of disruption in perception, thought processes, and thought content

Sensory Function: Vision: Extent to which visual images are sensed, with or without assistive devices

Vision Compensation Behavior: Actions to compensate for visual impairment

Goals/Evaluation Criteria

Examples Using NOC Language

- Demonstrates **Anxiety Control**, as evidenced by the following indicators (specify 1–5: never, rarely, sometimes, often, or consistently demonstrated):

  Reports absence of physical and behavioral manifestations of anxiety

  Reports absence of sensory perceptual distortions

- Demonstrates **Body Image**, as evidenced by the following indicators (specify 1–5: never, rarely, sometimes, often, or consistently positive):

  Congruence between body reality, body ideal, and body presentation

- Demonstrates **Cognitive Ability**, as evidenced by the following indicators (specify 1–5: extremely, substantially, moderately, mildly, or not compromised):

  Attentiveness, concentration, and orientation

  Demonstrates immediate, recent, and remote memory

  Makes appropriate decisions

  Communicates clearly and appropriately for age and ability

- Demonstrates **Cognitive Orientation**, as evidenced by the following indicators (specify 1–5: never, rarely, sometimes, often, or consistently demonstrated): Identifies self, significant other, current place, and correct day, month, year, and season

Other Examples

Patient will:

- Interact appropriately with others and with the environment
- Exhibit logical organization of thoughts
- Correctly interpret ideas communicated by others
- Compensate for sensory deficits by maximizing the use of unimpaired senses

NOTE: Consider other outcomes specific to the particular deficit (i.e., visual, auditory, kinesthetic, gustatory, tactile, olfactory)

NIC Interventions

Auditory

Cognitive Stimulation: Promotion of awareness and comprehension of surroundings by utilization of planned stimuli

Communication Enhancement: Hearing Deficit: Assistance in accepting and learning alternate methods for living with diminished hearing

Delusion Management: Promoting the comfort, safety, and reality orientation of a patient experiencing false, fixed beliefs that have little or no basis in reality

Hallucination Management: Promoting the safety, comfort, and reality orientation of a patient experiencing hallucinations

Reality Orientation: Promotion of patient's awareness of personal identity, time, and environment

Gustatory, Olfactory

Cognitive Stimulation: Promotion of awareness and comprehension of surroundings by utilization of planned stimuli

Delusion Management: Promoting the comfort, safety, and reality orientation of a patient experiencing false, fixed beliefs that have little or no basis in reality

Hallucination Management: Promoting the safety, comfort, and reality orientation of a patient experiencing hallucinations

Fluid Monitoring: Collection and analysis of patient data to regulate fluid balance

Nausea Management: Prevention and alleviation of nausea

Nutrition Management: Assisting with or providing a balanced dietary intake of foods and fluids

Reality Orientation: Promotion of patient's awareness of personal identity, time, and environment

Kinesthetic

Body Mechanics Promotion: Facilitating the use of posture and movement in daily activities to prevent fatigue and musculoskeletal strain or injury

Cognitive Stimulation: Promotion of awareness and comprehension of surroundings by utilization of planned stimuli

Delusion Management: Promoting the comfort, safety, and reality orientation of a patient experiencing false, fixed beliefs that have little or no basis in reality

Exercise Promotion: Strength Training: Facilitating regular resistive muscle training to maintain or increase muscle strength

Exercise Therapy: Balance: Use of specific activities, postures, and movements to maintain, enhance, or restore balance

Hallucination Management: Promoting the safety, comfort, and reality orientation of a patient experiencing hallucinations

Neurologic Monitoring: Collection and analysis of patient data to prevent or minimize neurological complications

Reality Orientation: Promotion of patient's awareness of personal identity, time, and environment

Olfactory

Cognitive Stimulation: Promotion of awareness and comprehension of surroundings by utilization of planned stimuli

Delusion Management: Promoting the comfort, safety, and reality orientation of a patient experiencing false, fixed beliefs that have little or no basis in reality

Environmental Management: Manipulation of the patient's surroundings for therapeutic benefit

Hallucination Management: Promoting the safety, comfort, and reality orientation of a patient experiencing hallucinations

Nutrition Management: Assisting with or providing a balanced dietary intake of foods and fluids

Reality Orientation: Promotion of patient's awareness of personal identity, time, and environment

Tactile

Cognitive Stimulation: Promotion of awareness and comprehension of surroundings by utilization of planned stimuli

Delusion Management: Promoting the comfort, safety, and reality orientation of a patient experiencing false, fixed beliefs that have little or no basis in reality

Environmental Management: Safety: Monitoring and manipulation of the physical environment to promote safety

Peripheral Sensation Management: Prevention or minimization of injury or discomfort in the patient with altered sensation

Reality Orientation: Promotion of patient's awareness of personal identity, time, and environment

Surveillance: Safety: Purposeful and ongoing collection and analysis of information about the patient and the environment for use in promoting and maintaining patient safety

Visual

Body Image Enhancement: Improving a patient's conscious and unconscious perceptions and attitudes toward his body

Cognitive Stimulation: Promotion of awareness and comprehension of surroundings by utilization of planned stimuli

Communication Enhancement: Visual Deficit: Assistance in accepting and learning alternate methods for living with diminished vision

Delusion Management: Promoting the comfort, safety, and reality orientation of a patient experiencing false, fixed beliefs that have little or no basis in reality

Environmental Management: Manipulation of the patient's surroundings for therapeutic benefit

Hallucination Management: Promoting the safety, comfort, and reality orientation of a patient experiencing hallucinations

Reality Orientation: Promotion of patient's awareness of personal identity, time, and environment

Self-Esteem Enhancement: Assisting a patient to increase his personal judgment of self-worth

Nursing Activities

NOTE: Choose nursing activities specific to the identified deficit(s) (e.g., visual, auditory, kinesthetic, gustatory, tactile, olfactory).

Assessments

- Monitor and document changes in patient's neurologic status
- Monitor patient's level of consciousness
- Identify factors that contribute to *Disturbed sensory perception*, such as sleep deprivation, chemical dependence, medications, treatments, electrolyte imbalance, and so forth
- *(NIC) Peripheral Sensation Management:*
  Monitor sharp, dull and hot or cold discrimination
  Monitor for paresthesia: numbness, tingling, hyperesthesia, and hypoesthesia
- *(NIC) Surveillance: Safety:*
  Monitor patient for alterations in physical or cognitive function that might lead to unsafe behavior
  Monitor environment for potential safety hazards

Patient/Family Teaching

- *(NIC) Communication Enhancement: Hearing Deficit:* Teach patient that sounds will be experienced differently with the use of a hearing aid
- *(NIC) Peripheral Sensation Management:* Instruct patient or family to examine skin daily for alteration in skin integrity

Collaborative Activities

- Initiate occupational therapy referral, as appropriate

Other

- Ensure access to and use of sensory assistive devices, such as hearing aid and glasses
- Increase number of stimuli to achieve appropriate sensory input (e.g., increase social interaction; schedule contacts; and provide radio, television, and clock with large numbers)

- Reduce number of stimuli to achieve appropriate sensory input (e.g., dim lights, provide a private room, limit visitors, establish rest periods for patient)
- Orient to person, place, time, and situation with each interaction
- Reassure patient and family that sensory or perceptual deficit is temporary, whenever appropriate
- *(NIC) Communication Enhancement: Hearing Deficit:*
  Give one simple direction at a time
  Increase voice volume, as appropriate
  Obtain patient's attention through touch
  Do not cover your mouth, smoke, talk with a full mouth, or chew gum when speaking
  Refrain from shouting at patient with communication disorders
- *(NIC) Communication Enhancement: Visual Deficit:*
  Identify yourself when you enter the patient's space
  Build on patient's remaining vision, as appropriate
  Do not move items in patient's room without informing patient.
- *(NIC) Nutrition Management:*
  Provide patient with high-protein, high-calorie, nutritious finger foods and drinks that can be readily consumed, as appropriate
  Provide food selection
- *(NIC) Peripheral Sensation Management:*
  Avoid or carefully monitor use of heat or cold, such as heating pads, hot-water bottles, and ice packs
  Instruct patient to visually monitor position of body parts, if proprioception is impaired

---

SEXUAL DYSFUNCTION
(00059) (1980)

Definition: Change in sexual function that is viewed as unsatisfying, unrewarding, or inadequate

Defining Characteristics
Subjective
Alteration in achieving sexual satisfaction
Change of interest in self or others
Inability to achieve desired satisfaction
Seeking confirmation of desirability
Verbalization of problem

Objective

Actual or perceived limitations imposed by disease or therapy

Alterations in achieving perceived sex role

Alteration in relationship with significant other

Conflicts involving values

Other Possible Defining Characteristics (non-NANDA International)

Alteration in orgasm or ejaculation

Change in sexual desire

Concern over adequacy in meeting sexual desire of partner

Impotence

Painful coitus

Phobic avoidance of sexual experience

Vaginal dryness

Related Factors

Altered body function or structure (e.g., pregnancy, recent childbirth, drugs, surgery, anomalies, disease process, trauma, radiation)

Biopsychosocial alteration of sexuality

Ineffectual or absent role models

Lack of knowledge

Lack of privacy

Lack of significant other

Misinformation

Medical treatment

Physical abuse

Psychosocial abuse (e.g., harmful relationships)

Values conflict

Vulnerability

Other Possible Related Factors (non-NANDA International)

Body image disturbance

Disturbance in self-esteem

Hormonal changes

Impaired relationship

Pain

Sexual trauma or exploitation

Unrealistic expectations of self and partner

Suggestions for Use

If patient data does not fit the defining characteristics, consider the more general label *Ineffective sexuality patterns*. **NOTE:** *Sexual dysfunction* may be a symptom of other diagnoses, such as *Rape-trauma syndrome*.

Suggested Alternative Diagnoses

Body image, disturbed
Rape-trauma syndrome: silent reaction
Self-esteem, disturbed
Sexuality patterns, ineffective

NOC Outcomes

Abuse Recovery: Sexual: Healing following sexual abuse or exploitation

Child Development: Adolescence (12–17 Years): Milestones of physical, cognitive, and psychosocial progression between 12 and 17 years of age

Physical Aging Status: Physical changes that commonly occur with adult aging

Risk Control: Sexually Transmitted Diseases (STDs): Actions to eliminate or reduce behaviors associated with sexually transmitted disease

Sexual Functioning: Integration of physical, socioemotional, and intellectual aspects of sexual expression

Goals/Evaluation Criteria

Examples Using NOC Language

- Demonstrates **Abuse Recovery: Sexual**, as evidenced by the following indicators (specify 1–5: none, limited, moderate, substantial, or extensive):

    Evidence of appropriate same-sex relationships
    Evidence of appropriate opposite-sex relationships
    Expressions of confidence with gender identity and sexual orientation

- Demonstrates **Child Development: Adolescence (12–17 Years),** as evidenced by the following indicators (specify 1–5: extreme, substantial, moderate, mild, or no delay from expected range):

    Describes sexual development
    Expresses comfort with own sexual identity
    Maintains good peer relationships with same gender

Maintains good peer relationships with opposite gender

Demonstrates capacity for intimacy

Practices responsible sexual behaviors

- Demonstrates **Sexual Functioning**, as evidenced by the following indicators (specify 1–5: never, rarely, sometimes, often, or consistently demonstrated):

Attains sexual arousal

Sustained arousal through orgasm

Expresses ability to be intimate

Expresses acceptance of partner

Expresses willingness to be sexual

Other Examples

Patient and partner will:

- Demonstrate willingness to discuss changes in sexual function
- Request needed information about changes in sexual function
- Verbalize understanding of medically imposed restrictions
- Adapt modes of sexual expression to accommodate age- or illness-related physical changes
- Verbalize ways to avoid STDs

NIC Interventions

Abuse Protection Support: Identification of high-risk, dependent relationships and actions to prevent further infliction of physical or emotional harm

Behavior Modification: Promotion of a behavior change

Coping Enhancement: Assisting a patient to adapt to perceived stressors, changes, or threats which interfere with meeting life demands and roles

Counseling: Use of an interactive helping process focusing on the needs, problems, or feelings of the patient and significant others to enhance or support coping, problem solving, and interpersonal relationships

Infection Protection: Prevention and early detection of infection in a patient at risk

Risk Identification: Analysis of potential risk factors, determination of health risks, and prioritization of risk reduction strategies for an individual or group

Sexual Counseling: Use of an interactive helping process focusing on the need to make adjustments in sexual practice or to enhance coping with a sexual event or disorder

Teaching: Safe Sex: Providing instruction concerning sexual protection during sexual activity

Nursing Activities

Assessments

- Monitor for indicators of resolution of *Sexual dysfunction* (e.g., capacity for intimacy)
- *(NIC) Sexual Counseling:*
  Preface questions about sexuality with a statement that tells the patient that many people experience sexual difficulties
  Determine amount of sexual guilt associated with the patient's perception of the illness

Patient/Family Teaching

- Provide information necessary to enhance sexual function (e.g., anticipatory guidance, educational materials, stress-reduction exercises, sensation-enhancing exercises, prosthetics, implants, focused counseling)
- *(NIC) Sexual Counseling:*
  Discuss the effect of the illness, health situation, and medication on sexuality, as appropriate [e.g., medication side effects; normal aspects of aging; postsurgical adjustments, especially after surgery on sexual organs or ostomy; postmyocardial infarction]
  Discuss the necessary modifications in sexual activity, as appropriate
  Inform patient initially that sexuality is an important part of life and that illness, medications, and stress (or other problems or events the patient is experiencing) often alter sexual functioning
  Provide factual information about sexual myths and misinformation that patient may verbalize
  Instruct the patient only on techniques compatible with values and beliefs

Collaborative Activities

- Encourage continuation of counseling after discharge
- *(NIC) Sexual Counseling:*
  Provide referral or consultation with other members of the health care team, as appropriate
  Refer the patient to a sex therapist, as appropriate

Other

- Encourage verbalization of sexual concerns by utilizing caregivers who have an established rapport with patient and are comfortable discussing patient's sexual concerns, specify caregiver

- Allow time and privacy to address patient's sexual concerns
- Alert patient and partner to possibility of disinterest in, decreased capacity for, or discomfort during sexual activity
- *(NIC) Sexual Counseling:*

    Encourage patient to verbalize fears and to ask questions

    Help patient to express grief and anger about alterations in body functioning and appearance, as appropriate

    Include the spouse or sexual partner in the counseling as much as possible, as appropriate

    Introduce patient to positive role models who have successfully conquered a similar problem, as appropriate

    Provide reassurance and permission to experiment with alternative forms of sexual expression, as appropriate

---

SEXUALITY PATTERNS, INEFFECTIVE
(00065) (1986)

Definition: Expressions of concern regarding own sexuality

Defining Characteristics

Subjective
Reported difficulties, limitations, or changes in sexual behaviors or activities

Related Factors

Conflicts with sexual orientation or variant preferences
Fear of pregnancy or acquiring sexually transmitted disease
Impaired relationship with significant other
Ineffective or absent role models
Knowledge or skill deficit about alternative responses to health-related transitions, altered body function or structure, illness, or medical condition
Lack of privacy
Lack of significant other

Other Possible Related Factors (non-NANDA International)
Body image disturbance
Low self-esteem
Illness or medical treatments

Suggestions for Use

When possible, use a more specific label, such as *Sexual dysfunction*.

Suggested Alternative Diagnoses

Body image, disturbed
Rape-trauma syndrome: silent reaction
Self-esteem, disturbed
Sexual dysfunction

NOC Outcomes

Abuse Recovery: Sexual: Healing following sexual abuse or exploitation

Body Image: Positive perception of own appearance and body function

Child Development: Middle Childhood (6–11 Years): Milestones of physical, cognitive, and psychosocial progression between 6 and 11 years of age

Child Development: Adolescence (12–17 Years): Milestones of physical, cognitive, and psychosocial progression between 12 and 17 years of age

Role Performance: Congruence of an individual's role behavior with role expectations

Self-Esteem: Personal judgment of self-worth

Sexual Identity: Acceptance: Acknowledgement and acceptance of own sexual identity

Goals/Evaluation Criteria

Examples Using NOC Language

- Demonstrates **Abuse Recovery: Sexual** (see Goals/Evaluation Criteria for Sexual Dysfunction, pp. 469–470)
- Demonstrates **Child Development: Adolescence (12–17 Years)** (see Goals/Evaluation Criteria for Sexual Dysfunction, pp. 469–470)
- Demonstrates **Child Development: Middle Childhood (6–11 Years)**, as evidenced by the following indicators (specify 1–5: extreme, substantial, moderate, mild, or no delay from expected range):

    Identifies with same-sex peer group
    Develops close friendships

Other Examples

Patient and partner will:
- Actively participate in counseling
- Request needed information about sexuality
- Acknowledge importance of discussing sexual issues with partner
- Discuss concerns about sexuality
- Express satisfaction with sexuality

NIC Interventions

Body Image Enhancement: Improving a patient's conscious and unconscious perceptions and attitudes toward his body

Coping Enhancement: Assisting a patient to adapt to perceived stressors, changes, or threats which interfere with meeting life demands and roles

Counseling: Use of an interactive helping process focusing on the needs, problems, or feelings of the patient and significant others to enhance or support coping, problem solving, and interpersonal relationships

Developmental Enhancement: Child: Facilitating or teaching parents and caregivers to facilitate the optimal gross-motor, fine-motor, language, cognitive, social, and emotional growth of preschool and school-aged children

Family Planning: Contraception: Facilitation of pregnancy prevention by providing information about the physiology or reproduction and methods to control conception

Parent Education: Adolescent: Assisting parents to understand and help their adolescent children

Parent Education: Childrearing Family: Assisting parents to understand and promote the physical, psychological, and social growth and development of their toddler or preschool or school-aged child or children

Role Enhancement: Assisting a patient, significant other, or family to improve relationships by clarifying and supplementing specific role behaviors

Self-Esteem Enhancement: Assisting a patient to increase his personal judgment of self-worth

Self-Responsibility Facilitation: Encouraging a patient to assume more responsibility for own behavior

Sexual Counseling: Use of an interactive helping process focusing on the need to make adjustments in sexual practice or to enhance coping with a sexual event or disorder

Teaching: Safe Sex: Providing instruction concerning sexual protetion during sexual activity

Nursing Activities

Refer to Nursing Activities for Sexual Dysfunction, pp. 471–472.

SKIN INTEGRITY, IMPAIRED
(00046) (1975, 1998)

Definition: Altered epidermis and dermis

Defining Characteristics
Objective
Disruption of skin surface (epidermis)
Destruction of skin layers (dermis)
Invasion of body structures

Related Factors

External [Environmental]
Chemical substance
Humidity
Hyperthermia
Hypothermia
Mechanical factors (e.g., shearing forces, pressure, restraint)
Medications
Moisture
Physical immobilization
Radiation

Internal [Somatic]
Alterations in turgor (changes in elasticity)
Altered circulation
Altered fluid status
Altered metabolic state
Altered nutritional state (e.g., obesity, emaciation)
Altered pigmentation
Altered sensation
Immunological deficit
Skeletal Prominence

Developmental Factors
Extremes in age

Suggestions for Use

Impaired skin integrity is rather nonspecific. A disruption of the skin surface could be a surgical incision, abrasion, blisters, or decubitus ulcers. When this label is used, the type of disruption should be specified in the problem, not in the etiology. **NOTE:** In the following example, the dermal ulcer is a specific type of *Impaired skin integrity,* not a cause of *Impaired skin integrity:*

> **Correct:** *Impaired skin integrity: dermal ulcer related to complete immobility*
>
> **Incorrect:** *Impaired skin integrity related to dermal ulcer*

When an ulcer is deeper than the epidermis, use *Impaired tissue integrity* instead of *Impaired skin integrity.* Deeper ulcers may require a collaborative approach (i.e., surgical treatment). Do not use *Impaired skin integrity* as a label for a surgical incision, because there are no independent nursing actions to treat this type of "impairment" and the condition is usually self-limiting. The usual nursing care for a surgical incision is to prevent and detect infection; therefore, a diagnosis of *Risk for infection of surgical incision* or the collaborative problem Potential Complication of surgery: Incision infection might be used instead of *Impaired skin integrity.*

Suggested Alternative Diagnoses

Infection, risk for

Skin integrity, risk for impaired

Tissue integrity, impaired

NOC Outcomes

Tissue Integrity: Skin and Mucous Membranes: Structural intactness and normal physiologic function of skin and mucous membranes

Wound Healing: Primary Intention: The extent to which cells and tissues have regenerated following intentional closure

Wound Healing: Secondary Intention: The extent to which cells and tissues in an open wound have regenerated

Goals/Evaluation Criteria

Examples Using NOC Language

- Demonstrates **Tissue Integrity: Skin and Mucous Membranes**, as evidenced by the following indicators (specify 1–5: extremely, substantially, moderately, mildly, or not compromised):

  Tissue temperature, elasticity, hydration, pigmentation, and color in expected range

Tissue lesion-free

Skin intactness

- Demonstrates **Wound Healing: Primary Intention**, as evidenced by the following indicators (specify 1–5: none, slight, moderate, substantial, or complete):

  Skin approximation

  Resolution of drainage from wound or drain

  Resolution of surrounding skin erythema

  Resolution of wound odor

- Demonstrates **Wound Healing: Secondary Intention**, as evidenced by the following indicators (specify 1–5: none, slight, moderate, substantial, or complete):

  Purulent (or other) drainage or wound odor

  Blistered or macerated skin

  Necrosis, sloughing, tunneling, undermining, or sinus tract formation

  Skin and periwound erythema

  Wound size

Other Examples

- Patient and family demonstrate optimal skin or wound care routine

NIC Interventions

Incision Site Care: Cleansing, monitoring, and promotion of healing in a wound that is closed with sutures, clips, or staples

Pressure Management: Minimizing pressure to body parts

Pressure Ulcer Care: Facilitation of healing in pressure ulcers

Skin Surveillance: Collection and analysis of patient data to maintain skin and mucous membrane integrity

Wound Care: Prevention of wound complications and promotion of wound healing

Nursing Activities

Also see Nursing Activities for Skin Integrity, Risk for Impaired pp. 482–484.

Assessments

- Assess functioning of equipment such as pressure-relieving devices, including static-air mattress, low-air loss therapy, air-fluidized therapy, and water bed
- *(NIC) Incision Site Care:* Inspect the incision site for redness, swelling, or signs of dehiscence or evisceration

- *(NIC) Wound Care:*
  Inspect the wound with each dressing change
NOTE: Characteristics of the wound should include the following:
- Location, dimensions, and depth of wound
- Presence and character of exudate, including tenacity, color, and odor
- Presence or absence of granulation or epithelialization
- Presence or absence of necrotic tissue, describe color, odor, amount
- Presence or absence of symptoms of local wound infection (e.g., pain on palpation, edema, pruritus, induration, warmth, foul odor, eschar, exudate)
- Presence or absence of undermining or sinus-tract formation

Patient/Family Teaching

- Instruct in care of surgical incision, including signs and symptoms of infection, ways to keep incision dry during bath, and minimization of stress on the incision
- *(NIC) Skin Surveillance:* Instruct family member and caregiver about signs of skin breakdown, as appropriate
- *(NIC) Wound Care:* Teach patient or family member(s) wound care procedures

Collaborative Activities

- Consult dietitian for foods high in proteins, minerals, calories, and vitamins
- Consult physician regarding implementation of enteral feedings or parenteral nutrition to increase wound healing potential
- Refer to enterostomal therapy nurse for assistance with assessment, staging, treatment, and documentation of wound care or skin breakdown
- *(NIC) Wound Care:* Apply TENS unit for wound healing enhancement, as appropriate

Other

- Evaluate topical dressing and treatment measures, which may include hydrocolloid dressings, hydrophilic dressings, absorbent dressings, and so forth
- Establish a wound or skin care routine, which may include the following:
  Frequently turn and reposition patient
  Keep surrounding tissue free from excess moisture and drainage
  Protect patient from fecal and urinary contamination

Protect patient from other wound and drain-tube excretions into wound

- Clean and dress surgical incision site using the following principles of sterility or medical asepsis, as appropriate:

  Wear disposable gloves (sterile, if needed)

  Clean incision from "clean to dirty," using one swab for each wipe

  Clean around staples or sutures, using sterile cotton-tipped applicator

  Clean around drain last, moving from center outward in a circular motion

  Apply antiseptic ointment, as ordered

  Change dressing at appropriate intervals or leave open to air according to order

- (NIC) Wound Care:

  Remove adhesive tape and debris

  Clean with antibacterial soap, as appropriate

  Place affected area in a whirlpool bath, as appropriate

  Administer IV site, Hickman line, or central venous line site care, as appropriate

  Massage the area around the wound to stimulate circulation

  Administer skin ulcer care, as needed

  Position to avoid placing tension on the wound, as appropriate

---

SKIN INTEGRITY, RISK FOR IMPAIRED
(00047) (1975, 1998)

Definition: At risk for skin being adversely altered [**NOTE**: Risk should be determined by the use of a risk assessment tool (e.g., Braden Scale)].

Risk Factors

External [Environmental]

Chemical substance

Excretions and secretions

Extremes of age

Humidity

Hyperthermia

Hypothermia

Mechanical factors (e.g., shearing forces, pressure, restraint)

Medications

Moisture
Physical immobilization
Radiation

Internal [Somatic]

Alterations in nutritional state (e.g., obesity, emaciation)
Alterations in skin turgor (i.e., changes in elasticity)
Altered circulation
Altered metabolic state
Altered pigmentation
Altered sensation
Developmental factors
Medication
Immunologic [deficit]
Psychogenic
Skeletal prominence

Suggestions for Use

Use this diagnosis for patients who have no symptoms but who are at risk of developing disruption of skin surface or destruction of skin layers if preventive measures are not instituted. The presence of more than one risk factor increases the likelihood of skin damage. When *Risk for impaired skin integrity* occurs as a result of immobility and when other body systems are also at risk for impairment, consider using *Risk for disuse syndrome.*

Suggested Alternative Diagnosis

Disuse syndrome, risk for
Skin integrity, impaired

NOC Outcomes

Dialysis Access Integrity: The extent to which a dialysis access site is functional and free of inflammation

Immobility Consequences: Physiological: Extent of compromise in physiologic functioning due to impaired physical mobility

Nutritional Status: Extent to which nutrients are available to meet metabolic needs

Physical Aging Status: Physical changes that commonly occur with adult aging

Self-Mutilation Restraint: Ability to refrain from intentional self-inflicted injury (nonlethal)

Tissue Integrity: Skin and Mucous Membranes: Structural intactness and normal physiological function of skin and mucous membranes

Tissue Perfusion: Peripheral: Extent to which blood flows through the small vessels of the extremities and maintains tissue function

Wound Healing: Primary Intention: The extent to which cells and tissues have regenerated following intentional closure

Wound Healing: Secondary Intention: The extent to which cells and tissues in an open wound have regenerated

Goals/Evaluation Criteria

Examples Using NOC Language

- Demonstrates **Immobility Consequences: Physiological**, as evidenced by the following indicators (specify 1–5: severe, substantial, moderate, slight, or none):
    Pressure sores
    Decreased nutrition status
- Demonstrates **Risk Control**, as evidenced by the following indicators (specify 1–5: never, rarely, sometimes, often, or consistently demonstrated):
    Monitors environmental and behavioral risk factors [that contribute to Impaired skin integrity]
    Follows selected risk-control strategies
    Recognizes changes in health status [that affect skin]
- Demonstrates **Self-Mutilation Restraint** (specify 1–5: never, rarely, sometimes, often, or consistently demonstrated).
- Demonstrates **Tissue Perfusion: Peripheral**, as evidenced by the following indicators (specify 1–5: extremely, substantially, moderately, mildly, or not compromised):
    Capillary refill brisk
    Distal and proximal pulses strong and symmetric
    Skin color and sensation level normal
    Extremity temperature warm
    Localized extremity pain not present

Other Examples

Patient and family will:
- Have intact skin
- Demonstrate effective skin care routine
- Ingest foods adequate to promote skin integrity

NIC Interventions

Bed Rest Care: Promotion of comfort and safety and prevention of complications for a patient unable to get out of bed

Also see NIC Interventions for Impaired Skin Integrity, on p. 477.

Nursing Activities

All Patients at Risk

Assessments

- On admission and whenever physical condition changes, assess for risk factors that may lead to skin breakdown (e.g., bed or chair confinement, inability to move, loss of bowel or bladder control, poor nutrition, and lowered mental awareness)
- Identify sources of pressure and friction (e.g., cast, bedding, clothing)
- *(NIC) Pressure Ulcer Prevention*:
  Use an established risk assessment tool to monitor patient's risk factors (e.g., Braden scale)
  Inspect skin over bony prominences and other pressure points when repositioning or at least daily
- *(NIC) Skin Surveillance:*
  Monitor skin for the following:
  Rashes and abrasions
  Color and temperature
  Excessive dryness and moistness
  Areas of redness and breakdown

Collaborative Activities

- Refer to enterostomal therapy nurse for assistance with prevention, assessment, and treatment of skin breakdown or wounds

Other

- Use a pressure-reducing mattress (e.g., polyurethane foam pad)
- Avoid massage over bony prominences
- *(NIC) Pressure Ulcer Prevention:*
  Apply elbow and heel protectors, as appropriate
  Keep bed linens clean, dry, and wrinkle-free

Patients with Mobility/Activity Deficit

Assessments

- Assess for extent of limitations in ability to transfer or move about in bed

Other

- Pad cast edges and traction connections

  For chair-bound individuals:

- Consider postural alignment; distribution of weight, balance, and stability; and pressure relief when positioning individuals in chairs or wheelchairs
- Have patient shift weight q 15 minutes if able
- Use pressure-reducing devices for seating surfaces, do not use donut-type devices

  For bed-bound individuals:

- Avoid positioning directly on the trochanter
- Elevate the head of the bed as little and for as short a time as possible
- Use a pressure-reducing mattress or bed (e.g., foam, air, egg-crate)
- Use proper positioning, transferring, and turning techniques
- Use lifting devices to move, rather than drag, individuals during transfers and position changes
- *(NIC) Pressure Ulcer Prevention:*

  Turn q 1–2 h continuously, as appropriate

  Provide trapeze to assist patient in shifting weight frequently

  Position with pillows to elevate pressure points off the bed

  Apply elbow and heel protectors, as appropriate

Patients with Incontinence or Presence of Moisture

Assessments

- Assess need for indwelling or condom catheter
- Check for urinary or fecal incontinence q _____

Other

- Cleanse skin at time of soiling
- Individualize bathing schedule, avoid hot water, use mild cleansing agent
- Minimize skin exposure to moisture
- *(NIC) Pressure Ulcer Prevention:*

  Remove excessive moisture on the skin resulting from perspiration, wound drainage, and fecal or urinary incontinence

  Apply protective barriers, such as creams or moisture-absorbing pads, to remove excess moisture, as appropriate

  Apply transparent film occlusive dressing to areas at risk to protect skin from wetness

  Turn with care to prevent injury to fragile skin

Patients with Nutritional Deficit

Assessments

- Monitor nutritional status and food intake

Collaborative Activities

- Consult dietitian for foods high in protein, minerals, and vitamins
- Request physician order for serum albumin level, packed-cell volume, and transferrin levels

Other

- Compare actual weight to ideal body weight
- Investigate factors that compromise an apparently well-nourished individual's dietary intake (especially protein or calories) and offer support with eating
- *(NIC) Pressure Ulcer Prevention:* Ensure adequate nutrition, especially protein, vitamins B and C, iron, and calories, using supplements, as appropriate

---

SLEEP DEPRIVATION
(00096) (1998)

Definition: Prolonged periods of time without sleep (sustained natural, periodic suspension of relative unconsciousness)

Defining Characteristics

Subjective

Anxious

Daytime drowsiness

Hallucinations

Heightened sensitivity to pain

Malaise

Perceptual disorders (e.g., disturbed body sensation, delusions, feeling afloat)

Objective

Acute confusion

Agitated or combative

Apathy

Decreased ability to function

Hand tremors

Listlessness

Inability to concentrate

Irritability
Lethargy
Mild, fleeting nystagmus
Restlessness
Slowed reaction
Tiredness
Transient paranoia

Related Factors

Aging-related sleep stage shifts
Dementia
Familial sleep paralysis
Idiopathic central nervous system hypersomnolence
Inadequate daytime activity
Narcolepsy
Nightmares
Nonsleep-inducing parenting practices
Periodic limb movement (e.g., restless leg syndrome, nocturnal myoclonus)
Prolonged physical discomfort
Prolonged psychologic discomfort
Prolonged use of pharmacologic or dietary antisoporifics
Sleep apnea
Sleep terror
Sleepwalking
Sleep-related enuresis
Sleep-related painful erections
Sundowner syndrome
Sustained circadian asynchrony
Sustained environmental stimulation
Sustained inadequate sleep hygiene
Sustained unfamiliar or uncomfortable sleep environment

Suggestions for Use

Because *Sleep deprivation* represents a lack of sleep that continues over long periods of time, the defining characteristics are more varied and more severe than those for *Disturbed sleep pattern*, which is a short-term lack of sleep that might occur, for example, during a brief hospitalization. Therefore, in addition to measures to promote and restore sleep, nursing activities for *Sleep deprivation* will focus on relieving symptoms, such as paranoia, restlessness, and confusion. *Sleep deprivation* can be the etiology of other nursing diagnoses, for example, *Anxiety, Acute confusion, Disturbed thought processes, Impaired memory,* and *Disturbed sensory perception.*

Suggested Alternative Diagnoses

Activity intolerance
Confusion, acute
Fatigue
Sleep pattern, disturbed

NOC Outcomes

Rest: Extent and pattern of diminished activity for mental and physical rejuvenation

Sleep: Extent and pattern of natural periodic suspension of consciousness during which the body is restored

Symptom Severity: Extent of perceived adverse changes in physical, emotional, and social functioning

Goals/Evaluation Criteria

Examples Using NOC Language

- Demonstrates **Sleep**, as evidenced by the following indicators (specify 1–5: extremely, substantially, moderately, mildly, or not compromised):
    Feelings of rejuvenation after sleep
    Sleep pattern, quality, and routine not compromised
    Hours of sleep not compromised
    Wakeful at appropriate times

Other Examples

  The patient will:
- Report relief from symptoms of *Sleep deprivation* (e.g., confusion, anxiety, daytime drowsiness, perceptual disorders, and tiredness)
- Identify and use measures that will increase rest or sleep
- Identify factors that contribute to *Sleep deprivation* (e.g., pain, inadequate daytime activity)

NIC Interventions

Energy Management: Regulating energy use to treat or prevent fatigue and optimize function

Sleep Enhancement: Facilitation of regular sleep–wake cycles

<u>Nursing Activities</u>

See Nursing Activities for Disturbed Sleep Pattern, on pp. 491–492.

Assessments

- Assess for symptoms of *Sleep deprivation*, such as *Acute confusion*, agitation, *Anxiety*, perceptual disorders, slowed reactions, and irritability

Patient Teaching

- Teach patient and family about factors that interfere with sleep (e.g., stress, hectic lifestyle, shift work, room temperature too cold or too hot)

Collaborative Activities

- Confer with physician regarding need to revise medication regimen when it interferes with sleep
- Confer with physician regarding use of sleep medications that do not suppress rapid eye movement (REM) sleep
- Make referrals as needed for treatment of severe symptoms of *Sleep deprivation* (e.g., *Acute confusion*, agitation, or *Anxiety*)

Other

- Treat symptoms of *Sleep deprivation*, as needed (e.g., *Anxiety*, restlessness, transient paranoia, inability to concentrate); these will vary with individual patients

SLEEP PATTERN, DISTURBED
(00095) (1980, 1998)

Definition: Time-limited disruption of sleep (natural, periodic suspension of consciousness) amount and quality

<u>Defining Characteristics</u>

Subjective

Awakening earlier or later than desired

Dissatisfaction with sleep

Verbal complaints of difficulty in falling asleep

Verbal complaints of not feeling well-rested

Objective

Decreased ability to function

Decreased proportion of REM sleep (e.g., REM rebound, hyperactivity, emotional lability, agitation and impulsivity, atypical polysomnographic features)

Decreased proportion of stages 3 and 4 sleep (e.g., hyporesponsiveness, excess sleepiness, decreased motivation)

Early-morning insomnia

Increased proportion of stage 1 sleep

Less than age-normed total sleep time

Prolonged awakenings

Self-induced impairment of normal pattern

Sleep maintenance insomnia

Sleep onset greater than 30 min

Three or more nighttime awakenings

Other Possible Defining Characteristics (non-NANDA International)

Dark circles under eyes

Decreased attention span

Flat affect

Frequent daytime napping

Frequent yawning

Interrupted sleep

Irritability

Lethargy

Listlessness

Mood alterations

Ptosis of eyelid

Restlessness

Slight hand tremor

Thick speech with mispronunciation and incorrect words

Related Factors

Psychological

Aging-related sleep shifts

Anticipation

Anxiety

Biochemical agents

Body temperature

Boredom

Childhood onset

Circadian asynchrony

Daylight or darkness exposure

Daytime activity pattern

Delayed or advanced sleep phase syndrome

Depression

Dietary

Fatigue
Fear
Fear of insomnia
Frequent travel across time zones
Frequently changing sleep–wake schedule
Grief
Inadequate sleep hygiene
Loneliness
Loss of sleep partner, life change
Maladaptive conditioned wakefulness
Periodic gender-related hormonal shifts
Preoccupation with trying to sleep
Ruminative presleep thoughts
Separation from significant others
Shift work
Social schedule inconsistent with chronotype
Sustained use of antisleep agents
Temperament
Thinking about home

Environmental

Ambient temperature, humidity
Excessive stimulation
Lack of sleep privacy or control
Lighting
Medications [e.g., depressants or stimulants]
Noise
Noxious odors
Nurse [who wakens patient] for therapeutics, monitoring, lab tests
Other generated awakening
Physical restraint
Sleep partner
Unfamiliar sleep furnishings

Parental

Mother's emotional support
Mother's sleep–wake pattern
Parent–infant interaction

Physiological

Fever
Gastroesophageal reflux
Nausea
Position
Shortness of breath

Stasis of secretions
Urinary urgency
Wet

Other Possible Related Factors (Non-NANDA International)
Anxiety
Inactivity
Pain or discomfort
Unfamiliar surroundings

Suggestions for Use

Disturbed sleep pattern is used when disruption of sleep causes discomfort or interferes with the patient's desired lifestyle. *Disturbed sleep pattern* is a general diagnosis. The etiologic factors can sometimes make it specific enough to direct nursing intervention, as in *Disturbed sleep pattern related to frequent awakening of infant during the night.* When possible, the specific type of *Disturbed sleep pattern* should be identified (on the problem side of the diagnosis) in order to better direct nursing care. Following are examples of appropriate diagnoses:

Disturbed sleep pattern (early awakening) related to depression
Disturbed sleep pattern (delayed onset of sleep) related to overstimulation prior to bedtime

Suggested Alternative Diagnoses

Activity intolerance
Fatigue
Sleep deprivation

NOC Outcomes

Anxiety Control: Personal actions to eliminate or reduce feelings of apprehension and tension from an unidentifiable source
Comfort Level: Feelings of physical and psychologic ease
Pain Level: Severity of reported or demonstrated pain
Psychosocial Adjustment: Life Change: Psychosocial adaptation of an individual to a life change
Quality of Life: An individual's expressed satisfaction with current life circumstances
Rest: Extent and pattern of diminished activity for mental and physical rejuvenation
Sleep: Extent and pattern of natural periodic suspension of consciousness during which the body is restored
Well-Being: An individual's expressed satisfaction with health status

Goals/Evaluation Criteria

Examples Using NOC Language

- Patient demonstrates **Sleep**, as evidenced by the following indicators (specify 1–5: extremely, substantially, moderately, mildly, or not compromised):

    Hours of sleep not compromised

    Sleep pattern, quality, and routine not compromised

    Feelings of rejuvenation after sleep or rest

    Napping appropriate for age

    Wakeful at appropriate times

Other Examples

Patient will:

- Identify measures that will increase rest or sleep
- Demonstrate physical and psychologic well-being

NIC Interventions

Coping Enhancement: Assisting a patient to adapt to perceived stressors, changes, or threats which interfere with meeting life demands and roles

Energy Management: Regulating energy use to treat or prevent fatigue and optimize function

Sleep Enhancement: Facilitation of regular sleep–wake cycles

Nursing Activities

Assessments

- *(NIC) Sleep Enhancement:*

    Determine the effects of the patient's medications on sleep pattern

    Monitor patient's sleep pattern and note physical (e.g., sleep apnea, obstructed airway, pain or discomfort, and urinary frequency) or psychologic (e.g., fear or anxiety) circumstances that interrupt sleep

Patient/Family Teaching

- *(NIC) Sleep Enhancement:*

    Explain the importance of adequate sleep during pregnancy, illness, psychosocial stresses, etc.

    Instruct patient to avoid bedtime foods and beverages that interfere with sleep

    Instruct the patient and significant others about factors (e.g., physiologic, psychologic, lifestyle, frequent work-shift changes, rapid time-zone changes, excessively long work hours, and other environmental factors) that contribute to sleep pattern disturbances

Collaborative Activities

- Confer with physician regarding need to revise medication regimen when it interferes with sleep pattern
- *(NIC) Sleep Enhancement:* Encourage use of sleep medications that do not contain REM-sleep suppressors

Other

- Avoid loud noises and use of overhead lights during nighttime sleep, providing a quiet, peaceful environment and minimizing interruptions
- Find a compatible roommate for the patient, if possible
- Help patient identify possible underlying causes of sleeplessness, such as fear, unresolved problems, and conflicts
- Reassure patient that irritability and mood alterations are common consequences of sleep deprivation
- *(NIC) Sleep Enhancement:*

  Facilitate maintenance of patient's usual bedtime routine, presleep cues or props, and familiar objects (e.g., for children, a favorite blanket or toy, rocking, pacifier, or story; for adults, a book to read, etc.), as appropriate

  Assist patient to limit daytime sleep by providing activity that promotes wakefulness, as appropriate

  Initiate or implement comfort measures of massage, positioning, and affective touch

  Provide for naps during the day, if indicated, to meet sleep requirements

  Group care activities to minimize number of awakenings; allow for sleep cycles of at least 90 min

SLEEP, READINESS FOR ENHANCED
(00165) (2002)

Definition: A pattern of natural, periodic suspension of consciousness that provides adequate rest, sustains a desired lifestyle, and can be strengthened

Defining Characteristics

Subjective
Expresses a feeling of being rested after sleep
Expresses willingness to enhance sleep

Objective

Amount of sleep and REM sleep is congruent with developmental needs

Follows sleep routines that promote sleep habits

Occasional or infrequent use of medications to induce sleep

Related Factors

This is a wellness diagnosis; an etiology is not necessary.

Suggestions for Use

If risk factors are present, use *Risk for sleep deprivation* or *Risk for disturbed sleep pattern.*

Suggested Alternative Diagnoses

Sleep deprivation (risk for)

Sleep pattern, disturbed (risk for)

NOC Outcomes

NOC outcomes have not yet been linked to this diagnosis; however, the following may be useful:

Quality of Life: An individual's expressed satisfaction with current life circumstances

Rest: Extent and pattern of diminished activity for mental and physical rejuvenation

Sleep: Extent and pattern of natural periodic suspension of consciousness during which the body is restored

Well-Being: An individual's expressed satisfaction with health status

Goals/Evaluation Criteria

Examples Using NOC Language

- Patient demonstrates **Sleep**, as evidenced by the following indicators (specify 1–5: extremely, substantially, moderately, mildly, or not compromised):

  Hours of sleep not compromised

  Sleep pattern, quality, and routine not compromised

  Feelings of rejuvenation after sleep or rest

  Napping appropriate for age

  Wakeful at appropriate times

Other Examples

Patient will:

- Identify measures that will increase rest or sleep
- Demonstrate physical and psychologic well-being
- Obtain adequate sleep without use of medications

NIC Interventions

NIC interventions have not yet been linked to this diagnosis; however, the following may be helpful:

Energy Management: Regulating energy use to treat or prevent fatigue and optimize function

Sleep Enhancement: Facilitation of regular sleep–wake cycles

Nursing Activities

Assessments

- Assess for evidence of improvements in sleep
- *(NIC) Sleep Enhancement:*

  Determine the effects of the patient's medications on sleep pattern

  Monitor patient's sleep pattern and note physical (e.g., sleep apnea, obstructed airway, pain or discomfort, and urinary frequency) or psychologic (e.g., fear or anxiety) circumstances that interrupt sleep

Patient/Family Teaching

- *(NIC) Sleep Enhancement:*

  Instruct patient to avoid bedtime foods and beverages that interfere with sleep

  Instruct the patient and significant others about factors (e.g., physiologic, psychologic, lifestyle, frequent work-shift changes, rapid time-zone changes, excessively long work hours, and other environmental factors) that contribute to sleep pattern disturbances

Collaborative Activities

- Confer with physician regarding need to revise medication regimen when it interferes with sleep pattern
- *(NIC) Sleep Enhancement:* Encourage use of sleep medications that do not contain REM-sleep suppressors

Other

- Avoid loud noises and use of overhead lights during nighttime sleep, providing a quiet, peaceful environment and minimizing interruptions
- Find a compatible roommate for the patient, if possible
- Help patient identify and anticipate factors that can cause sleeplessness, such as fear, unresolved problems, and conflicts
- *(NIC) Sleep Enhancement:*

  Facilitate maintenance of patient's usual bedtime routine, presleep cues or props, and familiar objects (e.g., for children, a favorite blanket or toy, rocking, pacifier, or story; for adults, a book to read, etc.), as appropriate

  Assist patient to limit daytime sleep by providing activity that promotes wakefulness, as appropriate

SOCIAL INTERACTION, IMPAIRED
(00052) (1986)

Definition: Insufficient or excessive quantity or ineffective quality of social exchange

Defining Characteristics

Subjective

Family report of change of style or pattern of interaction

Verbalized discomfort in social situations

Verbalization of observed inability to receive or communicate a satisfying sense of belonging, caring, interest, or shared history

Objective

Dysfunctional interaction with peers, family, or others

Observed discomfort in social situations

Observed inability to receive or communicate a satisfying sense of belonging, caring, interest, or shared history

Observed use of unsuccessful social interaction behaviors

Related Factors

Absence of available significant others or peers

Altered thought processes

Communication barriers

Environmental barriers

Knowledge or skill deficit about ways to enhance mutuality

Limited physical mobility

Self-concept disturbance
Sociocultural dissonance
Therapeutic isolation

Other Related Factors (non-NANDA International)
Chemical dependence
Developmental disability
Psychologic impairment (specify)

Suggestions for Use

Differentiate between *Impaired social interaction* and *Social isolation*. A diagnosis of *Impaired social interaction* focuses more on the patient's social skills and abilities, whereas *Social isolation* focuses on the patient's feelings of aloneness and may not be a result of his ineffective social skills. Compare the defining characteristics and related factors in Table 9 in Suggestions for Use for *Social Isolation*, p. 501.

Suggested Alternative Diagnoses

Communication, verbal, impaired
Self-esteem, chronic or situational low
Social isolation
Thought processes, disturbed

NOC Outcomes

Child Development: 2, 4, 6, and 12 Months; 2, 3, 4, and 5 Years; Middle Childhood (6–11 Years), and Adolescence (12–17 Years): Milestones of physical, cognitive, and psychosocial progression by years of age [NOC lists each age as a separate outcome.]

Family Environment: Internal: Social climate as characterized by family member relationships and goals

Play Participation: Use of activities as needed for enjoyment, entertainment, and development by children

Role Performance: Congruence of an individual's role behavior with role expectations

Social Interaction Skills: An individual's use of effective interaction behaviors

Social Involvement: Frequency of an individual's social interactions with persons, groups, or organizations

Goals/Evaluation Criteria

Examples Using NOC Language

- Demonstrates **Play Participation** (specify 1–5: not, slightly, moderately, substantially, or totally adequate)
- Demonstrates **Social Interaction Skills** (specify 1–5: none, limited, moderate, substantial, or extensive)
- Demonstrates **Child Development**, as evidenced by the following indicators (specify 1–5: extreme, substantial, moderate, mild, or no delay from expected range). [Refer to pediatrics text or NOC manual for age-specific indicators; an exhaustive list is beyond the scope of this text.]

  2 months: Shows pleasure in interactions, especially with primary caregivers

  4 months: Recognizes parents' voices and touch

  6 months: Comforts self

  12 months: Waves bye-bye

  2 years: Interacts with adults in simple games

  3 years: Plays interactive games with peers

  4 years: Describes a recent experience

  5 years: Follows rules of interactive games with peers

  6–11 years: Plays in groups

  12–17 years: Uses social interaction skills

- Demonstrates **Role Performance**, as evidenced by the following indicators (specify 1–5: not, slightly, moderately, substantially, or totally adequate): Performance of family, community, work, friendship, and intimate role behaviors
- Demonstrates **Social Involvement**, as evidenced by the following indicators (specify 1–5: none, limited, moderate, substantial, or extensive): Interaction with close friends, neighbors, family members, and members of work group(s)

Other Examples

Patient will:

- Acknowledge the effect of own behavior on social interactions
- Demonstrate behaviors that may increase or improve social interactions
- Acquire/improve social interaction skills (e.g., disclosure, cooperation, sensitivity, assertiveness, genuineness, compromise)
- Express a desire for social contact with others
- Participate in and enjoy appropriate play

NIC Interventions

Behavior Modification: Social Skills: Assisting the patient to develop or improve interpersonal social skills

Complex Relationship Building: Establishing a therapeutic relationship with a patient who has difficulty interacting with others

Developmental Enhancement: Adolescent: Facilitating optimal physical, cognitive, social, and emotional growth of individuals during the transition from childhood to adulthood

Developmental Enhancement: Child: Facilitating or teaching parents and caregivers to facilitate the optimal gross-motor, fine-motor, language, cognitive, social, and emotional growth of preschool and school-aged children

Family Integrity Promotion: Promotion of family cohesion and unity

Family Process Maintenance: Minimization of family process disruption effects

Self-Esteem Enhancement: Assisting a patient to increase his personal judgment of self-worth

Socialization Enhancement: Facilitation of another person's ability to interact with others

Therapeutic Play: Purposeful and directive use of toys or other materials to assist children in communicating their perception and knowledge of their world and to help in gaining mastery of their environment

Nursing Activities

Assessments

- Assess established pattern of interaction between patient and others

Patient/Family Teaching

- Provide information on community resources that will assist the patient to continue with increasing social interaction after discharge

Collaborative Activities

- Confer with other disciplines and patient to establish, implement, and evaluate a plan to increase or improve the patient's interactions with others
- *(NIC) Socialization Enhancement:* Refer patient to transactional analysis group or program in which understanding of transactions can be increased, as appropriate

Other

- Assign scheduled interactions
- Identify specific behavior change
- Identify tasks that will increase or improve social interactions
- Involve supportive peers in giving feedback to patient on social interactions
- Mediate between patient and others when patient exhibits negative behavior
- *(NIC) Socialization Enhancement:*
  Encourage honesty in presenting oneself to others
  Encourage respect for the rights of others
  Encourage patience in developing new relationships
  Help patient increase awareness of strengths and limitations in communicating with others
  Use role playing to practice improved communication skills and techniques
  Request and expect verbal communication
  Give positive feedback when patient reaches out to others
  Facilitate patient input and planning of future activities

SOCIAL ISOLATION
(00053) (1982)

Definition: Aloneness experienced by the individual and perceived as imposed by others and as a negative or threatened state

Defining Characteristics

Subjective

Expressed feelings of aloneness imposed by others
Experiences feelings of differences from others
Expressed feelings of rejection
Expresses interests inappropriate to the developmental age or stage
Expresses values acceptable to the subculture but unacceptable to the dominant cultural group
Projects hostility in voice or behavior

Objective

Absence of supportive significant others (e.g., family, friends, group)

Evidence of physical or mental handicap or altered state of wellness

Inability to meet expectations of others

Inadequate or absent significant purpose in life

Inappropriate or immature activities or interests for developmental stage

Insecurity in public

No eye contact

Preoccupation with own thoughts

Repetitive meaningless actions

Sad, dull affect

Seeks to be alone or exists in a subculture

Shows behavior unacceptable to dominant cultural group

Uncommunicative

Withdrawal

Related Factors

Alterations in mental status

Alterations in physical appearance

Altered state of wellness

Factors contributing to the absence of satisfying personal relationships (e.g., delay in accomplishing developmental tasks)

Immature interests

Inability to engage in satisfying personal relationships

Inadequate personal resources

Unaccepted social behavior or values

Other Related Factors (non-NANDA International)

Chemical dependence

Psychologic impairment (specify)

Treatment-imposed isolation

Suggestions for Use

Differentiate between *Social isolation* and *Impaired social interaction*. A diagnosis of *Impaired social interaction* focuses more on the patient's social skills and abilities, whereas *Social isolation* focuses on the patient's feelings of aloneness and may not be a result of his ineffective social skills. Table 9 compares the defining characteristics and related factors of *Impaired social interaction* to *Social isolation*.

Table 9

	Impaired Social Interaction	Social Isolation
Shared Defining Characteristics	Verbalized or observed discomfort in social situations	Verbalized or observed discomfort in social situations
Differentiating Defining Characteristics	Ineffective social behaviors Feelings of rejection	Feelings of aloneness imposed by others
Related Factors	Lack of knowledge of social skills Communication barriers	Mental impairment Physical disabilities

Suggested Alternative Diagnoses

Communication, verbal, impaired
Post-trauma syndrome
Relocation stress syndrome
Social interaction, impaired
Thought processes, disturbed

NOC Outcomes

Family Environment: Internal: Social climate as characterized by family member relationships and goals

Leisure Participation: Use of restful or relaxing activities as needed to promote well-being

Loneliness: The extent of emotional, social, or existential isolation response

Mood Equilibrium: Appropriate adjustment of prevailing emotional tone in response to circumstance

Play Participation: Use of activities as needed for enjoyment, entertainment, and development by children

Social Interaction Skills: An individual's use of effective interaction behaviors

Social Involvement: Frequency of an individual's social interactions with persons, groups, or organizations

Social Support: Perceived availability and actual provision of reliable assistance from other persons

Well-Being: An individual's expressed satisfaction with health status

Goals/Evaluation Criteria

Examples Using NOC Language

- Demonstrates **Social Involvement**, as evidenced by the following indicators (specify 1–5: none, limited, moderate, substantial, or extensive):

    Reports interaction with close friends, neighbors, family members, and/or work groups

    Reports participation as member of church, club, or volunteer group

    Participates in leisure activities

Other Examples

Patient will:

- Identify and accept personal characteristics or behaviors that contribute to social isolation
- Identify community resources that will assist in decreasing social isolation after discharge
- Verbalize fewer feelings or experiences of being excluded
- Begin to establish contact with others
- Develop a mutual relationship
- Exhibit affect appropriate to situation
- Develop social skills that decrease isolation (e.g., cooperation, compromise, consideration, warmth, and engagement)
- Report increasing social support (e.g., help from others in the form of emotional help, time, money, labor, or information)

NIC Interventions

Behavior Modification: Social Skills: Assisting the patient to develop or improve interpersonal social skills

Complex Relationship Building: Establishing a therapeutic relationship with a patient who has difficulty interacting with others

Coping Enhancement: Assisting a patient to adapt to perceived stressors, changes, or threats which interfere with meeting life demands and roles

Family Integrity Promotion: Promotion of family cohesion and unity

Family Involvement Promotion: Facilitating family participation in the emotional and physical care of the patient

Mood Management: Providing for safety, stabilization, recovery, and maintenance of a patient who is experiencing dysfunctionally depressed mood or elevated mood

Recreation Therapy: Purposeful use of recreation to promote relaxation and enhancement of social skills

Self-Awareness Enhancement: Assisting a patient to explore and understand his thoughts, feelings, motivations, and behaviors

Socialization Enhancement: Facilitation of another person's ability to interact with others

Support System Enhancement: Facilitation of support to patient by family, friends, and community

Therapeutic Play: Purposeful and directive use of toys or other materials to assist children in communicating their perception and knowledge of their world and to help in gaining mastery of their environment

Nursing Activities

Also see Nursing Activities for Social Interaction, Impaired, pp. 498–499.

Other

- Assist patient to distinguish reality from perceptions
- Identify with patient those factors that may be contributing to feelings of social isolation
- Reduce stigma of isolation by respecting patient's dignity
- Reduce visitor anxiety by explaining reason for isolation precautions or equipment
- Reinforce efforts by patient, family, or friends to establish interactions
- *(NIC) Socialization Enhancement:*

  Encourage relationships with persons who have common interests and goals

  Allow testing of interpersonal limits

  Give feedback about improvement in care of personal appearance or other activities

  Confront patient about impaired judgment, when appropriate

  Encourage patient to change environment, such as going outside for walks and movies

---

SORROW, CHRONIC
(00137) (1998)

Definition: Cyclical, recurring, and potentially progressive pattern of pervasive sadness that is experienced by a client (parent, caregiver, or individual with chronic illness or disability) in response to continual loss, throughout the trajectory of an illness or disability

Defining Characteristics

Subjective

Feelings that vary in intensity, are periodic, may progress and intensify over time, and may interfere with the client's ability to reach his highest level of personal and social well-being

Client expresses one or more of the following feelings: anger, being misunderstood, confusion, depression, disappointment, emptiness, fear, frustration, guilt or self-blame, helplessness, hopelessness, loneliness, low self-esteem, recurring loss, overwhelmed

Client expresses periodic, recurrent feelings of sadness

Related Factors

Death of a loved one

Person experiences chronic physical or mental illness or disability such as: mental retardation, multiple sclerosis, prematurity, spina bifida or other birth defects, chronic mental illness, infertility, cancer, Parkinson disease

Person experiences one or more trigger events (e.g., crises in management of the illness, crises related to developmental stages and missed opportunities or milestones that bring comparisons with developmental, social, or personal norms)

Unending caregiving as a constant reminder of loss

Suggestions for Use

Compared to normal grieving that occurs in response to loss, *Chronic sorrow* does not subside with time, in part, because the loss continues unabated (as it does in a chronic disability) and the condition remains as a constant reminder of loss. *Chronic sorrow* demonstrates coping that is more effective than that which occurs with *Dysfunctional grieving*.

Several of the defining characteristics of *Chronic sorrow* are, themselves, nursing diagnoses. When more than one of the following diagnoses are present, a diagnosis of *Chronic sorrow* may be more useful: *Fear, Hopelessness, Loneliness, Chronic low self-esteem,* and *Powerlessness.*

Suggested Alternative Diagnoses

Death anxiety
Fear
Grieving, anticipatory
Grieving, dysfunctional
Hopelessness

Loneliness, risk for
Powerlessness
Self-esteem, chronic low
Spiritual distress

NOC Outcomes

Acceptance: Health Status: Reconciliation to health circumstances

Depression Control: Personal actions to minimize melancholy and maintain interest in life events

Depression Level: Severity of melancholic mood and loss of interest in life events

Grief Resolution: Adjustment to actual or impending loss

Hope: Presence of internal state of optimism that is personally satisfying and life-supporting

Mood Equilibrium: Appropriate adjustment of prevailing emotional tone in response to circumstances

Goals/Evaluation Criteria

Examples Using NOC Language

- Demonstrates **Grief Resolution**, as evidenced by the following indicators (specify 1–5: not at all, to a slight extent, to a moderate extent, to a great extent, to a very great extent):
    Verbalizes acceptance of loss
    Participates in planning funeral
    Reports decreased preoccupation with loss
    Shares loss with significant others
    Progresses through stages of grief
    Maintains grooming and hygiene

Other Examples:

Patient will:
- Express feelings of guilt, anger, or sorrow
- Identify and use effective coping strategies
- Verbalize the impact of the loss(es)
- Seek information about illness and treatment
- Identify and use available social supports, including significant others
- Work toward acceptance of the loss(es)
- Draw upon spiritual beliefs for comfort
- Maintain grooming and hygiene
- Report adequate sleep and nutrition

NIC Interventions

Coping Enhancement: Assisting a patient to adapt to perceived stressors, changes, or threats which interfere with meeting life demands and roles

Grief Work Facilitation: Assistance with the resolution of a significant loss

Hope Instillation: Facilitation of the development of a positive outlook in a given situation

Mood Management: Providing for safety, stabilization, recovery, and maintenance of a patient who is experiencing dysfunctionally depressed mood or elevated mood

Spiritual Support: Assisting the patient to feel balance and connection with a greater power

Nursing Activities

Refer to Nursing Activities for Spiritual Distress on pp. 510–511.

For patients for whom *Fear* is an etiology, refer to Nursing Activities for Fear on pp. 196–197.

For patients for whom *Chronic low self-esteem* is an etiology, refer to Nursing Activities for Self-Esteem, Chronic Low on pp. 442–443.

For patients for whom *Hopelessness* is an etiology, refer to Nursing Activities for Hopelessness on pp. 250–251.

For patients for whom *Powerlessness* is an etiology, refer to Nursing Activities for Powerlessness on pp. 389–390.

Assessments
- Assess and document the presence and source of patient's sorrow

Patient/Family Teaching
- Discuss characteristics of normal and abnormal grieving
- Provide patient and family with information about hospital and community resources, such as self-help groups

Collaborative Activities
- Initiate a patient care conference to review patient and family needs related to their stage of the grieving process and to establish a plan of care

Other
- Acknowledge the grief reactions of patient and family while continuing necessary care activities
- Discuss with patient and family the impact of the loss on the family and its functioning
- Establish a schedule for contact with patient

- Establish a trusting relationship with patient and family
- Provide a safe, secure, and private environment to facilitate patient and family grieving process
- Recognize and reinforce the strength of each family member
- *(NIC) Grief Work Facilitation:*
  Assist the patient to identify the nature of the attachment to the lost object or person
  Include significant others in discussions and decisions, as appropriate
  Encourage patient to implement cultural, religious, and social customs associated with the loss
  Encourage expression of feelings about the loss
  Answer children's questions associated with the loss
  Encourage expression of feelings in ways comfortable to the child, such as writing, drawing, or playing
  Assist the child to clarify misconceptions

SPIRITUAL DISTRESS
(00066) (1978, 2002)

Definition: Impaired ability to experience and integrate meaning and purpose in life through a person's connectedness with self, others, art, music, literature, nature, or a power greater than oneself

Defining Characteristics

Connections to self

Expresses lack of:
  Hope
  Meaning and purpose in life
  Peace and serenity
  Acceptance
  Love
  Forgiveness of self
  Courage
  Anger
  Guilt
  Poor coping

Connections with others

Expresses alienation
Refuses interactions with friends, family
Refuses interactions with spiritual leaders
Verbalizes being separated from their support system

Connections with Art, Music, Literature, Nature

Inability to express previous state of creativity (singing and listening to music and writing)

Disinterest in nature

Disinterest in reading spiritual literature

Connections with Power Greater Than Oneself

Inability to pray

Inability to participate in religious activities

Expressions of being abandoned by or having anger toward God

Inability to experience the transcendent

Requests to see a religious leader

Sudden changes in spiritual practices

Inability to be introspective or inward turning

Expresses being without hope or suffering

Related Factors

Anxiety

Chronic illness of self and others

Death and dying of self and others

Life change

Loneliness or social alienation

Pain

Self-alienation

Sociocultural deprivation

Other Related Factors (Non-NANDA International)

Discrepancy between spiritual beliefs and prescribed treatment

Suggestions for Use

(1) Spiritual well-being should be thought of in a broad sense and not limited to religion. All people are religious in the sense that they need something to give meaning to their lives. For some it is belief in God in the traditional sense; for others, it is a feeling of harmony with the universe; for still others, it may be family and children. When the patient believes that life has no meaning or purpose, in whatever sense, then *Spiritual distress* is present. (2) Some of the following suggested alternative diagnoses may lead to *Spiritual distress*.

Suggested Alternative Diagnoses

Anxiety, death

Decisional conflict

Coping, ineffective

Sorrow, chronic

Spiritual distress, risk for

NOC Outcomes

Dignified Dying: Maintaining personal control and comfort with the approaching end of life

Hope: Presence of internal state of optimism that is personally satisfying and life-supporting

Spiritual Well-Being: Personal expressions of connectedness with self, others, higher power, all life, nature, and the universe that transcend and empower the self

Goals/Evaluation Criteria

Examples Using NOC Language

- Demonstrates **Hope**, as evidenced by the following indicators (specify 1–5: none, limited, moderate, substantial, or extensive): Expression of faith, meaning in life, and inner peace
- Demonstrates **Spiritual Well-Being**, as evidenced by the following indicators (specify 1–5: extremely, substantially, moderately, mildly, or not compromised):
    Meaning and purpose in life
    Spiritual world view
    Serenity, love, and forgiveness
    Prayer, worship, or meditation
    Interaction with spiritual leaders
    Connectedness with inner self
    Connectedness with others to share thoughts, feelings, and beliefs

Other Examples

Patient will:

- Acknowledge that illness is a challenge to belief system
- Acknowledge that treatment conflicts with belief system
- Demonstrate coping techniques to deal with spiritual distress
- Express acceptance of limited religious or cultural ties
- Discuss spiritual practices and concerns
  Dying patient will:
- Express acceptance or readiness for death
- Reconcile previous relationships
- Express affection toward significant others

NIC Interventions

Spiritual Support: Assisting the patient to feel balance and connection with a greater power

Nursing Activities

Assessments

- For patients who indicate a religious affiliation, assess for direct indicators of patient's spiritual status by asking questions such as the following:

  Do you feel your faith is helpful to you? In what ways is it important to you right now?

  How can I help you carry out your faith? For example, would you like me to read your prayer book to you?

  Would you like a visit from your spiritual counselor or the hospital chaplain?

  Please tell me about any particular religious practices that are important to you.

- Make indirect assessments of the patient's spiritual status by doing the following:

  Determine patient's concept of God by observing the books at the bedside or the programs he watches on television. Also note whether the patient's life seems to have meaning, value, and purpose.

  Determine the patient's source of hope and strength. Is it God in the traditional sense, a family member, or an "inner source" of strength? Note who the patient talks about most, or ask: Who is important to you?

  Observe whether the patient seems to be praying when you enter the room, before meals, or during procedures.

  Look for items such as religious literature, rosaries, and religious get-well cards at the bedside.

  Listen for patient's thoughts about the relationship between spiritual beliefs and his state of health, particularly for statements such as: Why did God let this happen to me? or If I have faith, I will get well?

Collaborative Activities

- Communicate dietary needs (e.g., kosher food, vegetarian diet, pork-free diet) to dietitian
- Request spiritual consultation to help patient and family determine posthospitalization needs and community resources for support
- *(NIC) Spiritual Support*: Refer to spiritual advisor of patient's choice

Other

- Explain limitations that hospitalization imposes on religious observances
- Make immediate changes necessary to accommodate patient's needs (e.g., encourage patient's family or friends to bring special food)
- Provide privacy and time for patient to observe religious practices
- *(NIC) Spiritual Support:*

  Be open to patient's expressions of loneliness and powerlessness

  Use values clarification techniques to help patient clarify beliefs and values, as appropriate

  Express empathy with patient's feelings

  Listen carefully to patient's communication and develop a sense of timing for prayer or spiritual rituals

  Assure patient that nurse will be available to support patient in times of suffering

  Encourage chapel service attendance, if desired

  Provide desired spiritual articles, according to patient preference

---

SPIRITUAL DISTRESS, RISK FOR
(00067) (1998)

Definition: At risk for an altered sense of harmonious connectedness with all of life and the universe in which dimensions that transcend and empower the self may be disrupted

Risk Factors

Blocks to self-love

Energy-consuming anxiety

Inability to forgive

Loss of loved one

Low self-esteem

Maturational losses

Mental illness

Natural disasters

Physical illness

Physical or psychological stress

Poor relationships

Situational losses

Substance abuse

Suggestions for Use

See Suggestions for Use for Spiritual Distress, p. 508.

Suggested Alternative Diagnoses

Anxiety, death

Coping, ineffective

Decisional conflict
Grieving, dysfunctional
Sorrow, chronic
Spiritual distress

NOC Outcomes

Hope: Presence of internal state of optimism that is personally satisfying and life-supporting

Quality of Life: An individual's expressed satisfaction with current life circumstances

Spiritual Well-Being: Personal expressions of connectedness with self, others, higher power, all life, nature, and the universe that transcend and empower the self

Goals/Evaluation Criteria

See Goals/Evaluation Criteria for Spiritual Distress on p. 509.

NIC Interventions

Not yet identified, the following is a possible choice:

Spiritual Support: Assisting the patient to feel balance and connection with a greater power

Nursing Activities

See Nursing Activities for Spiritual Distress pp. 510–511.

Assessments

- Assess for situations that might lead to spiritual distress (e.g., low self-esteem, anxiety, lack of supportive relationships)

Other

- Institute the following measures to promote self-esteem:
    Assist patient in identifying personal strengths
    Encourage patient to verbalize concerns about close relationships
    Encourage patient and family to air feelings and to grieve
    Provide care in a nonjudgmental manner, maintaining the
        patient's privacy and dignity
- *(NIC) Spiritual Support:*
    Use values clarification techniques to help patient clarify beliefs
        and values, as appropriate
    Listen carefully to patient's communication and develop a sense
        of timing for prayer or spiritual rituals

SPIRITUAL WELL-BEING, READINESS FOR ENHANCED (00068) (1994, 2002)

Definition: Ability to experience and integrate meaning and purpose in life through a person's connectedness with self, others, art, music, literature, nature, or a power greater than oneself

Defining Characteristics

Connections to self

Desire for enhanced:

Acceptance

Courage

Forgiveness of self

Hope

Joy

Love

Meaning and purpose in life

Peace and serenity

Satisfying philosophy of life

Surrender

Heightened coping

Meditation

Connections with art, music, literature, nature

Displays creative energy (e.g., writing, poetry)

Reads spiritual literature

Sings and listens to music

Spends time outdoors

Connections with others

Provides service to others

Requests forgiveness of others

Requests interactions with friends, family

Requests interactions with spiritual leaders

Connections with power greater than self

Expresses reverence, awe

Participates in religious activities

Prays

Reports mystical experiences

Suggestions for Use

Because this is a wellness diagnosis, an etiology (e.g., related factors) is not needed. If situations exist that pose a risk to spiritual development, use *Risk for spiritual distress*.

Suggested Alternative Diagnosis

Spiritual distress, risk for

NOC Outcomes

Hope: Presence of internal state of optimism that is personally satisfying and life-supporting

Quality of Life: An individual's expressed satisfaction with current life circumstances

Spiritual Well-Being: Personal expressions of connectedness with self, others, higher power, all life, nature, and the universe that transcend and empower the self

Goals/Evaluation Criteria

Examples Using NOC Language

See Examples Using NOC Language for Spiritual Distress, p. 509.

Other examples

Patient will:

- Continue and enhance spiritual growth
- Verbalize feelings of peace and harmony with the universe
- Verbalize satisfaction with sociocultural circumstances and interpersonal relationships
- Report satisfaction with self-concept and achievement of life goals
- Indicate happiness and satisfaction with spiritual life

NIC Interventions

Hope Instillation: Facilitation of the development of a positive outlook in a given situation

Spiritual Growth Facilitation: Facilitation of growth in patient's capacity to identify, connect with, and call upon the source of meaning, purpose, comfort, strength, and hope in his life

Spiritual Support: Assisting the patient to feel balance and connection with a greater power

Nursing Activities

Also see Nursing Activities for Spiritual Distress, pp. 510–511.

Collaborative Activities

- *(NIC) Spiritual Support:* Encourage chapel service attendance, if desired

Other

- *(NIC) Spiritual Support:*
  Be open to patient's feelings about illness and death
  Assist patient to properly express and relieve anger in appropriate ways
  Be available to listen to patient's feelings
  Facilitate patient's use of meditation, prayer, and other religious traditions and rituals

---

SPONTANEOUS VENTILATION, IMPAIRED (00033) (1992)

Definition: Decreased energy reserves result in an individual's inability to maintain breathing adequate to support life

Defining Characteristics

Subjective
Dyspnea

Objective
Apprehension
Decreased cooperation
Decreased SaO_2
Decreased PO_2
Decreased tidal volume
Increased heart rate
Increased metabolic rate
Increased PCO_2
Increased restlessness
Increased use of accessory muscles

Related Factors

Metabolic factors [e.g., alkalemia, hypokalemia, hypochloremia, hypophosphatemia, anemia]
Respiratory muscle fatigue

Suggestions for Use

Impaired gas exchange is one of the defining characteristics for this label. When blood gases are altered but the patient is able to breathe without mechanical assistance, a diagnosis of *Impaired gas exchange* should be made instead of Inability to sustain spontaneous ventilation.

The author does not recommend use of this label as a nursing diagnosis. When breathing is "inadequate to support life," an emergency exists; the interventions are physician-prescribed, including resuscitation and mechanical ventilation. The nurse is accountable for monitoring changes in the patient's condition and performing interventions according to agency protocols. Goals and interventions are included in this text only because NOC and NIC standardized language includes them.

Suggested Alternative Diagnoses

Airway clearance, ineffective
Breathing patterns, ineffective
Dysfunctional ventilatory weaning response (DVWR)
Gas exchange, impaired

NOC Outcomes

Neurologic Status: Central Motor Control: Extent to which skeletal muscle activity (i.e., body movement) is coordinated by the central nervous system

Respiratory Status: Gas Exchange: Alveolar exchange of CO_2 or O_2 to maintain arterial blood gas concentrations

Respiratory Status: Ventilation: Movement of air in and out of the lungs

Vital Signs Status: Temperature, pulse, respiration, and blood pressure within expected range for the individual

Goals/Evaluation Criteria

Examples Using NOC Language

- Demonstrates **Vital Signs Status**, as evidenced by the following indicators (specify 1–5: extreme, substantial, moderate, mild, or no deviation from expected range): temperature, pulse, respirations, and blood pressure

Other Examples

Patient will:

- Have adequate energy level and muscle function to sustain spontaneous breathing
- Receive adequate nutrition prior to, during, and following weaning process
- Have arterial blood gases and oxygen saturation within acceptable range

- Demonstrate neurologic status adequate to sustain spontaneous breathing

NIC Interventions

Airway Management: Facilitation of patency of air passages

Artificial Airway Management: Maintenance of endotracheal and tracheostomy tubes and preventing complications associated with their use

Mechanical Ventilation: Use of an artificial device to assist a patient to breathe

Respiratory Monitoring: Collection and analysis of patient data to ensure airway patency and adequate gas exchange

Resuscitation: Neonate: Administering emergency measures to support newborn adaptation to extrauterine life

Ventilation Assistance: Promotion of an optimal spontaneous breathing pattern that maximizes oxygen and carbon dioxide exchange in the lungs

Vital Signs Monitoring: Collection and analysis of cardiovascular, respiratory, and body temperature data to determine and prevent complications

Nursing Activities

Assessments

- For patients requiring artificial airway: monitor tube placement, check cuff inflation q4h and whenever it is deflated and reinflated
- *(NIC) Mechanical Ventilation:*

  Monitor for impending respiratory failure

  Monitor for decrease in exhale volume and increase in inspiratory pressure in patients receiving mechanical ventilation

  Monitor the effectiveness of mechanical ventilation on patient's physiologic and psychologic status

  Monitor for adverse effects of mechanical ventilation: infection, barotrauma, and reduced cardiac output

  Monitor effects of ventilator changes on oxygenation: ABG, SaO_2, SvO_2, end-tidal CO_2, Q_{sp}/Qt, and $A\text{-}aDO_2$ levels and patient's subjective response

  Monitor degree of shunt, vital capacity, V_d/V_T, MVV, inspiratory force, FEV_1 for, and readiness to, wean from mechanical ventilation, based on agency protocol

- *(NIC) Respiratory Monitoring:*
  Note location of trachea
  Auscultate breath sounds, noting areas of decreased or absent ventilation and presence of adventitious sounds
  Determine the need for suctioning by auscultating for crackles and rhonchi over major airways
  Monitor for increased restlessness, anxiety, and air hunger
  Monitor for crepitus, as appropriate

Patient/Family Teaching

- Instruct patient and family about weaning process and goals, including the following:
  How patient may feel as process evolves
  Participation required by patient
  Reasons why weaning is necessary
- *(NIC) Mechanical Ventilation:* Instruct the patient and family about the rationale and expected sensations associated with use of mechanical ventilators

Collaborative Activities

- *(NIC) Mechanical Ventilation:*
  Consult with other health care personnel in selection of a ventilator mode
  Administer muscle-paralyzing agents, sedatives, and narcotic analgesics, as appropriate

Other

- Initiate calming techniques, as appropriate
- *(NIC) Mechanical Ventilation:*
  Initiate setup and application of the ventilator
  Ensure that ventilator alarms are on
  Provide patient with a means for communication (e.g., paper and pencil or alphabet board)
  Perform suctioning, based on presence of adventitious sounds or increased ventilatory pressures
  Provide routine oral care

For patients requiring an artificial airway:

- Provide artificial airway management according to agency procedures and protocols, which may include the following:
  Provide oral care at least q4h
  Rotate endotracheal tube from side to side daily
  Tape endotracheal tube securely; change tapes or ties q24h

Administer sedation, utilize mitts or wrist restraints, if necessary, to prevent unplanned extubation

Clean stoma and tracheal cannula q4h (according to agency protocol)

Suction oropharynx, as needed

NOTE: For in-depth information about artificial airway management, refer to med/surg text, nursing techniques/skills manual, or agency protocols

For neonates requiring resuscitation:

- Refer to maternity or pediatric nursing text for full details of resuscitation procedure
- Have resuscitation equipment available at birth
- Calmly explain procedures to parents to minimize anxiety
- Prepare for neonatal transfer or transport

For patients requiring ventilatory weaning:

- Refer to Nursing Activities for Ventilatory Weaning Response, Dysfunctional (DVWR), pp. 615–617.

SUDDEN INFANT DEATH SYNDROME, RISK FOR (00156) (2002)

Definition: Presence of risk factors for sudden death of an infant under 1 year of age

Risk Factors

Modifiable

Delayed or nonattendance of prenatal care

Infant overheating or overwrapping

Infants placed to sleep in the prone or side-lying position

Pre- and postnatal infant smoke exposure

Soft underlayment or loose articles in the sleep environment

Potentially Modifiable

Low birth weight

Prematurity

Young maternal age

Nonmodifiable

Male gender

Ethnicity (e.g., African American or Native American race of mother)

Seasonality of sudden infant death syndrome (SIDS) deaths (higher in winter and fall months)

SIDS mortality peaks between infant aged 2 to 4 months

Suggestions for Use

Use the most specific label that matches the patient's defining characteristics. This label is more specific than *Risk for injury*, for example. Note that risk factors for *Risk for SIDS* are limited to the sleep environment, except for prenatal and nonmodifiable factors; whereas *Risk for suffocation* includes risk factors throughout the entire environment. It also is applicable to children older than one year.

Suggested Alternative Diagnoses

Injury, risk for
Suffocation, Risk for

NOC Outcomes

NOC has not yet linked outcomes to this diagnosis; however, the following may be useful:

Knowledge: Infant Care: Extent of understanding conveyed about caring for a baby 0–12 months

Respiratory Status: Ventilation: Movement of air in and out of the lungs

Risk Control: Actions to eliminate or reduce actual, personal, and modifiable health threats

Risk Detection: Actions taken to identify personal health threats

Goals/Evaluation Criteria

Examples Using NOC Language

- Demonstrates **Risk Control**, as evidenced by the following indicators (specify 1–5: never, rarely, sometimes, often, or consistently demonstrated):

    Monitors personal behavior risk factors
    Adjusts risk control strategies as needed
    Commits to risk control strategies

Other Examples

Parent will:

- Identify appropriate safety factors that protect individual or child from SIDS
- Place infant to sleep in supine position
- Verbalize knowledge of safe mattress and bed linens
- Avoid smoking during pregnancy

NIC Interventions

NIC has not yet linked interventions to this diagnosis; however, the following may be useful:

Teaching: Infant Safety: Instruction on safety during first year of life

Nursing Activities

Assessments

- Assess sleeping arrangements for safety (e.g., no featherbed mattresses or pillows in infant crib)
- Assess prenatally for risk factors such as young maternal age, smoking

Patient/Family Teaching

- Provide educational materials related to strategies and counter-measures for preventing SIDS and to emergency resuscitation measures for dealing with it
- *(NIC) Environmental Management: Safety:* Provide patient with emergency phone numbers (e.g., ambulance, 911)
- Teach family to not expose infant to second-hand smoke
- Teach to position infant supine for sleeping.
- Teach to not use featherbed or other fluffy type mattresses, blankets, or pillows in infant's bed

Collaborative Activities

- Refer patient to educational classes in the community (e.g., CPR)

SUFFOCATION, RISK FOR
(00036) (1980)

Definition: Accentuated risk of accidental suffocation (i.e., inadequate air available for inhalation)

Risk Factors

Internal (Individual)

Cognitive or emotional difficulties
Disease or injury process
Lack of safety education
Lack of safety precautions
Reduced motor abilities
Reduced olfactory sensation

External (Environmental)

Children left unattended in bathtubs or pools

Children playing with plastic bags or inserting small objects into their mouths or noses

Discarded or unused refrigerators or freezers without removed doors

Household gas leaks

Low-strung clothesline

Pacifier hung around infant's head

Person who eats large mouthfuls of food

Pillow placed in an infant's crib

Propped bottle placed in an infant's crib

Smoking in bed

Use of fuel-burning heaters not vented to outside

Vehicle warming in closed garage

Suggestions for Use

Use the most specific label that matches the patient's defining characteristics. This label is more specific than *Risk for injury* or *Risk for trauma,* for example.

Suggested Alternative Diagnoses

Injury, risk for

Trauma, risk for

NOC Outcomes

Aspiration Control: Personal actions to prevent the passage of fluid and solid particles into the lung

Respiratory Status: Ventilation: Movement of air in and out of the lungs

Risk Control: Actions to eliminate or reduce actual, personal, and modifiable health threats

Risk Detection: Actions taken to identify personal health threats

Safety Behavior: Home Physical Environment: Individual or caregiver actions to minimize environmental factors that might cause physical harm or injury in the home

Goals/Evaluation Criteria

Examples Using NOC Language

- Demonstrates **Safety Behavior: Home Physical Environment**, as evidenced by the following indicators (specify 1–5: not, slightly, moderately, substantially, or totally adequate):

    Safe disposal of hazardous materials

    Removal of unused refrigerator and freezer doors

    Provision of age-appropriate toys

Other Examples

Parent will:

- Identify appropriate safety factors that protect individual or child from suffocation
- Recognize signs of substance abuse or addiction
- Verbalize knowledge of emergency procedures

NIC Interventions

Airway Management: Facilitation of patency of air passages

Aspiration Precautions: Prevention or minimization of risk factors in the patient at risk for aspiration

Environmental Management: Safety: Monitoring and manipulation of the physical environment to promote safety

Respiratory Monitoring: Collection and analysis of patient data to ensure airway patency and adequate gas exchange

Teaching: Infant Safety: Instruction on safety during first year of life

Nursing Activities

Assessments

- *(NIC) Environmental Management: Safety:* Identify safety hazards in the environment (i.e., physical, biologic, and chemical)
- *(NIC) Respiratory Monitoring:*
  Monitor rate, rhythm, depth, and effort of respirations
  Monitor for hoarseness and voice changes every hour in patients with facial burns
  Institute resuscitation efforts, as needed

Patient/Family Teaching

- Provide educational materials related to strategies and countermeasures for preventing suffocation and to emergency measures for dealing with it
- Provide information on environmental hazards and characteristics (e.g., stairs, windows, cupboard locks, swimming pools, streets, gates)
- *(NIC) Environmental Management: Safety:* Provide patient with emergency phone numbers (e.g., health department, environmental services, EPA [Environmental Protection Agency], and police)

Collaborative Activities

- Refer parent to educational classes in the community (CPR), first aid, swimming classes

- *(NIC) Environmental Management: Safety:* Notify agencies authorized to protect the environment (e.g., health department, environmental services, EPA, and police)

Other

- *(NIC): Airway Management:* Position the patient to maximize ventilation potential
- *(NIC) Environmental Management: Safety:* Modify the environment to minimize hazards and risks

SUICIDE, RISK FOR
(00150) (2000)

Definition: At risk for self-inflicted, life-threatening injury

Risk Factors

Behavioral

Buying a gun

Giving away possessions

History of prior suicide attempt

Impulsiveness

Making or changing a will

Marked changes in behavior, attitude, school performance

Stockpiling medicines

Sudden euphoric recovery from major depression

Verbal

States desire to die and end it all

Threats of killing oneself

Situational

Adolescents living in nontraditional settings (e.g., juvenile detention center, prison, half-way house, group home)

Economic instability

Living alone

Loss of autonomy or independence

Presence of gun in home

Relocation, institutionalization

Retired

Psychological

Abuse in childhood

Alcohol and substance use or abuse

Family history of suicide

Gay or lesbian youth
Guilt
Psychiatric illness or disorder (e.g., schizophrenia, bipolar disorder)

Demographic

Age: elderly, young adult males, adolescents
Divorced, widowed
Gender: male
Race: Caucasian, Native American

Physical

Chronic pain
Physical illness
Terminal illness

Social

Cluster suicides
Disrupted family life
Grief, bereavement
Helplessness
Hopelessness
Legal or disciplinary problem
Loneliness
Loss of important relationship
Poor support systems
Social isolation

Suggestions for Use

When risk factors for suicide (e.g., suicidal ideation, suicidal plan) are present, use *Risk for Suicide* instead of *Risk for Self-Directed Violence,* which is less specific.

Suggested Alternative Diagnoses

Risk for self-directed violence
Risk for self-mutilation

NOC Outcomes

NOC outcomes have not yet been linked to this nursing diagnosis; however, the following may be useful:

Depression Control: Personal actions to minimize melancholy and maintain interest in life events

Depression Level: Severity of melancholic mood and loss of interest in life events

Distorted Thought Control: Self-restraint of disruption in perception, thought processes, and thought content

Impulse Control: Self-restraint of compulsive or impulsive behavior

Risk Control: Actions to eliminate or reduce actual, personal, and modifiable health threats

Suicide Self-Restraint: Ability to refrain from gestures and attempts at killing self

Will to Live: Desire, determination, and effort to survive

Goals/Evaluation Criteria

Examples Using NOC Language

- *Risk for suicide* is diminished, as demonstrated by Depression Control, Depression Level, Distorted Thought Control, Impulse Control, Risk Control, Suicide Self-Restraint, and Will to Live
- Demonstrates **Suicide Self-Restraint**, as evidenced by the following indicators (specify 1–5):
    Seeks help when feeling self-destructive
    Verbalizes suicidal ideas if present
    Refrains from gathering means for suicide
    Does not give away possessions
    Does not require treatment for suicidal gestures or attempts
    Does not attempt suicide

Other Examples

- Verbalizes the desire to live
- Verbalizes feelings of anger
- Contacts agreed-upon persons if suicidal thoughts occur

NIC Interventions

NIC interventions have not yet been developed for this diagnosis; however the following may be useful:

Anger Control Assistance: Facilitation of the expression of anger in an adaptive nonviolent manner

Area Restriction: Limitation of patient mobility to a specified area for purposes of safety or behavior management

Behavior Management: Self-Harm: Assisting the patient to decrease or eliminate self-mutilating or self-abusive behaviors

Environmental Management: Violence Prevention: Monitoring and manipulation of the physical environment to decrease the potential for violent behavior directed toward self, others, or environments

Suicide Prevention: Reducing risk of self-inflicted harm with intent to end life

Surveillance: Safety: Purposeful and ongoing collection and analysis of information about the patient and the environment for use in promoting and maintaining patient safety

Nursing Activities

Assessments

- As often as indicated, but at least daily, assess and document patient's potential for suicide (specify intervals)
- Assess for behaviors that signal thoughts or plans for suicide (e.g., giving away possessions)
- *(NIC) Suicide Prevention:*

  Monitor for medication side effects and desired outcomes

  Search the newly hospitalized patient and personal belongings for weapons or potential weapons during inpatient admission procedure, as appropriate

  Search environment routinely and remove dangerous items to maintain it as hazard free

  Monitor patient during use of potential weapons (e.g., razor)

  Observe, record, and report any change in mood or behavior that may signify increasing suicidal risk and document results of regular surveillance checks

  Conduct mouth checks following medication administration to ensure that patient is not "cheeking" the medications for later overdose attempt

Patient/Family Teaching

- Teach limit-setting techniques to family
- Teach family and significant others to recognize behaviors signaling an increase in risk (e.g., verbal expressions such as "I'm going to kill myself," or "I wish I could just be gone"; withdrawal)
- Teach visitors about restricted items (e.g., razors, scissors, plastic bags)
- *(NIC) Suicide Prevention:*

  Explain suicide precautions and relevant safety issues to the patient, family, and significant others (e.g., purpose, duration, behavioral expectations and behavioral consequences)

  Involve family in discharge planning (e.g., illness and medication teaching, recognition of increasing suicidal risk, patient's plan for dealing with thoughts of harming self, community resources)

Collaborative Activities

- Confer with physician on use of appropriate restraining measures when necessary to prevent injury to self
- Initiate a multidisciplinary patient care conference to develop a plan of care, or when modifying suicide precautions
- *(NIC) Suicide Prevention:*

    Refer patient to mental health care provider (e.g., psychiatrist or psychiatric or mental health advanced practice nurse) for evaluation and treatment of suicide ideation and behavior, as needed

    Consider hospitalization of patient who is at serious risk for suicidal behavior

    Administer medications as appropriate to decrease anxiety, agitation, or psychosis and to stabilize mood

    Assist patient to identify network of supportive persons and resources (e.g., clergy, family, providers)

    Communicate risk and relevant safety issues to other care providers

Other

- Institute suicide precautions, as needed (e.g., 24-hr attendant)
- Reassure patient that you will protect him against suicidal impulses until he is able to regain control by: (1) observing patient constantly (even though privacy is lost), (2) checking patient frequently, and (3) taking the suicidal ideation seriously
- Encourage patient to verbalize anger
- Discuss with patient and family the role of anger in self-harm
- Require patient to wear a hospital gown instead of own clothing if there is risk that he may leave the building
- Use restraint and seclusion, as needed; but place in least restrictive environment that still allows for the necessary level of observation
- Conduct room searches according to institutional policy
- *(NIC) Suicide Prevention:*

    Contract (verbally or in writing) with patient, as appropriate, for no self-harm for a specified period of time, recontracting at specified time intervals

    Interact with the patient at regular intervals to convey caring and openness and to provide an opportunity for the patient to talk about feelings

    Avoid repeated discussion of past suicide history by keeping discussions present- and future-oriented

Limit access to windows, unless locked and shatterproof, as appropriate

Consider strategies to decrease isolation and opportunity to act on harmful thoughts (e.g., use of a sitter)

SURGICAL RECOVERY, DELAYED
(00100) (1998)

Definition: Extension of the number of postoperative days required for individuals to initiate and perform on their own behalf activities that maintain life, health, and well-being

Defining Characteristics

Difficulty in moving about

Evidence of interrupted healing of surgical area (e.g., red, indurated, draining, immobile)

Fatigue

Loss of appetite with or without nausea

Perception more time is needed to recover

Postpones resumption of work or employment activities

Report of pain or discomfort

Requires help to complete self-care

Related Factors

To be developed

Suggestions for Use

The defining characteristics for this diagnosis represent several other nursing diagnoses: *Impaired skin integrity, Risk for imbalanced nutrition, Nausea, Impaired mobility, Self-care deficit, Fatigue,* and *Pain.* If only one or two of the defining characteristics are present, use those individual diagnoses. If several are present, *Delayed surgical recovery* may be used. Note, however, that this label is not yet fully developed.

Suggested Alternative Diagnoses

Activity intolerance

Fatigue

Impaired mobility

Impaired skin integrity

Pain

Risk for imbalanced nutrition: less than body requirements
Self-care deficit

NOC Outcomes

Endurance: Extent that energy enables a person to sustain activity

Immobility Consequences: Physiological: Extent of compromise in physiological functioning due to impaired physical mobility

Nutritional Status: Extent to which nutrients are available to meet metabolic needs

Pain Level: Severity of reported or demonstrated pain

Self-Care: Activities of Daily Living (ADLs): Ability to perform the most basic physical tasks and personal care activities

Wound Healing: Primary Intention: The extent to which cells and tissues have regenerated following intentional closure

Goals/Evaluation Criteria

The patient will:

- Recognize and cope effectively with surgery-related anxiety
- Regain presurgery energy level, as evidenced by rested appearance, ability to concentrate, and statements that exhaustion is not present
- Regain presurgery mobility
- Demonstrate healing of surgical incision: edges approximated and no drainage, redness, or induration
- Experience timely resolution of pain, progressing to oral analgesics by (date), and requiring no pain medications by (date)
- Meet all discharge criteria by the date of expected stay for his particular surgery

NIC Interventions

Bed Rest Care: Promotion of comfort and safety and prevention of complications for a patient unable to get out of bed

Energy Management: Regulating energy use to treat or prevent fatigue and optimize function

Incision Site Care: Cleansing, monitoring, and promotion of healing in a wound that is closed with sutures, clips, or staples

Nutrition Management: Assisting with or providing a balanced dietary intake of foods and fluids

Nutrition Therapy: Administration of food and fluids to support metabolic processes of a patient who is malnourished or at high risk for becoming malnourished

Nutritional Monitoring: Collection and analysis of patient data to prevent or minimize malnourishment

Pain Management: Alleviation of pain or a reduction in pain to a level of comfort that is acceptable to the patient

Self-Care Assistance: Assisting another to perform activities of daily living

Surveillance: Purposeful and ongoing acquisition, interpretation, and synthesis of patient data for clinical decision making

Wound Care: Prevention of wound complications and promotion of wound healing

Nursing Activities

NOTE: The following nursing activities are general because the nursing diagnosis is nonspecific. It does not specify any particular type of surgery, and it includes several different nursing diagnoses (see the preceding Suggestions for Use).

NOTE: For more specific nursing activities, refer to Nursing Activities for the nursing diagnoses *Activity intolerance, Fatigue, Nausea, Impaired mobility, Impaired skin integrity, Pain, Risk for imbalanced nutrition: less than body requirements*, and *Self-care deficit*.

Assessments

- Monitor nature and location of pain
- Assess patient's self-care abilities (e.g., consider mobility, sedation, and level of consciousness)
- *(NIC) Surveillance:*

  Select appropriate patient indices for ongoing monitoring, based on patient's condition

  Establish the frequency of data collection and interpretation, as indicated by status of the patient

  Monitor neurologic status

  Monitor vital signs, as appropriate

  Monitor for signs and symptoms of fluid and electrolyte imbalance

  Monitor tissue perfusion, as appropriate

  Monitor for infection, as appropriate

  Monitor nutritional status, as appropriate

  Monitor gastrointestinal function, as appropriate

  Monitor elimination patterns, as appropriate

  Monitor for bleeding tendencies in high-risk patient

  Note type and amount of drainage from tubes and orifices and notify the physician of significant changes

- *(NIC) Energy Management:*

  Determine causes of fatigue (e.g., treatments, pain, and medications)

  Monitor patient for evidence of excess physical and emotional fatigue

  Monitor cardiorespiratory response to activity (e.g., tachycardia, other dysrhythmias, dyspnea, diaphoresis, pallor, hemodynamic pressures, and respiratory rate)

  Monitor or record patient's sleep pattern and number of sleep hours

- *(NIC) Nutrition Management:* Ascertain patient's food preferences
- *(NIC) Wound Care:* Inspect the wound with each dressing change

Patient Teaching

- *(NIC) Energy Management:* Teach patient and significant other techniques of self-care that will minimize oxygen consumption (e.g., self-monitoring and pacing techniques for performance of activities of daily living)
- *(NIC) Incision Site Care:*

  Instruct the patient how to minimize stress on the incision site

  Instruct the patient on how to care for the incision during bathing or showering

  Teach the patient and the family how to care for the incision, including signs and symptoms of infection

Collaborative Activities

- *(NIC) Nutrition Management:* Determine—in collaboration with dietitian, as appropriate—number of calories and type of nutrients needed to meet nutrition requirements
- *(NIC) Surveillance:*

  Analyze physician orders in conjunction with patient status to ensure safety of the patient

  Obtain consultation from the appropriate health care worker to initiate new treatment or change existing treatments

Other

- Ensure that the patient receives appropriate analgesic care
- Consider cultural influences on pain response
- Reduce or eliminate factors that precipitate or increase the pain experience (e.g., fear, fatigue, monotony, and lack of knowledge)
- Provide assistance until patient is fully able to assume self-care

- Encourage independence but intervene when patient is unable to perform activities
- Compare current status with previous status to detect improvements and deterioration in patient's condition
- *(NIC) Energy Management:*

  Determine what and how much activity is required to build endurance

  Use passive and active range-of-motion exercises to relieve muscle tension

  Avoid care activities during scheduled rest periods

  Institute appropriate treatment, using standing protocols
- *(NIC) Wound Care:*

  Provide incision site care, as needed

  Administer IV site care, as appropriate

  Maintain patency of any drainage tubes

  Bandage appropriately

  Position to avoid placing tension on the wound, as appropriate

---

SWALLOWING, IMPAIRED
(00103) (1986, 1998)

Definition: Abnormal functioning of the swallowing mechanism associated with deficits in oral, pharyngeal, or esophageal structure or function

Defining Characteristics

Pharyngeal Phase Impairment

Abnormality in pharyngeal phase by swallow study

Altered head positions

Choking, coughing, or gagging

Delayed swallow

Food refusal

Gurgly voice quality

Inadequate laryngeal elevation

Multiple swallows

Nasal reflux

Recurrent pulmonary infections

Unexplained fevers

Esophageal Phase Impairment

Abnormality in esophageal phase by swallow study

Acidic-smelling breath

Bruxism

Complaints of "something stuck"

Food refusal or volume limiting

Heartburn or epigastric pain

Hematemesis

Hyperextension of head or arching during or after meals

Nighttime coughing or awakening

Observed evidence of difficulty in swallowing (e.g., stasis of food in oral cavity, coughing or choking)

Odynophagia

Regurgitation of gastric contents or wet burps

Repetitive swallowing or ruminating

Unexplained irritability surrounding mealtime

Vomiting

Vomitus on pillow

Oral Phase Impairment

Abnormality in oral phase of swallow study

Coughing, choking, gagging before a swallow

Food falls from mouth

Food pushed out of mouth

Inability to clear oral cavity

Incomplete lip closure

Lack of chewing

Lack of tongue action to form bolus

Long meals with little consumption

Nasal reflux

Piecemeal deglutition

Pooling in lateral sulci

Premature entry of bolus

Sialorrhea or drooling

Slow bolus formation

Weak suck, resulting in inefficient nippling

<u>Related Factors</u>

Congenital Deficits

Upper airway anomalies

Failure to thrive or protein energy malnutrition

Conditions with significant hypotonia

Respiratory disorders

History of tube feeding

Behavioral feeding problems

Self-injurious behavior

Neuromuscular impairment (e.g., decreased or absent gag reflex, decreased strength or excursion of muscles involved in mastication, perceptual impairment, facial paralysis)

Mechanical obstruction (e.g., edema, tracheostomy tube, tumor)

Congenital heart disease

Cranial nerve involvement

Neurological Problems

Upper airway anomalies

Laryngeal abnormalities

Achalasia

Gastroesophageal reflux disease

Acquired anatomic defects

Cerebral palsy

Internal or external traumas

Tracheal, laryngeal, esophageal defects

Traumatic head injury

Nasal or nasopharyngeal cavity defects

Oral cavity or oropharynx abnormalities

Premature infants

Suggestions for Use

Impaired swallowing may be associated with a variety of medical conditions (e.g., cerebral palsy, CVA, Parkinson disease, malignancies affecting the brain, reconstructive surgery of the head and neck, and decreased consciousness from anesthesia or other causes). It may also be related to *Fatigue.*

Suggested Alternative Diagnoses

Aspiration, risk for

Infant feeding pattern, ineffective

NOC Outcomes

Aspiration Control: Personal actions to prevent the passage of fluid and solid particles into the lung

Swallowing Status: Extent of safe passage of fluids or solids from the mouth to the stomach

Swallowing Status: Esophageal Phase: Adequacy of the passage of fluids or solids from the pharynx to the stomach

Swallowing Status: Oral Phase: Adequacy of preparation, containment, and posterior movement of fluids or solids in the mouth for swallowing

Swallowing Status: Pharyngeal Phase: Adequacy of the passage of fluids or solids from the mouth to the esophagus

Goals/Evaluation Criteria

Examples Using NOC Language

- Demonstrates **Swallowing Status**, as evidenced by the following indicators (specify 1–5: extremely, substantially, moderately, mildly, or not compromised):

   Maintains food in mouth

   Chewing ability

   Delivery of bolus to hypopharynx is commensurate with swallow reflex

   Ability to clear oral cavity

   Choking, coughing, or gagging not present

   Normal swallow effort

   Comfort with swallowing

Other Examples

   Patient will:

- Identify emotional or psychologic factors that interfere with swallowing
- Tolerate food ingestion without choking or aspiration
- Have no impairment of facial and throat muscles, swallowing, tongue movement, or gag reflex

NIC Interventions

Aspiration Precautions: Prevention or minimization of risk factors in the patient at risk for aspiration

Positioning: Deliberative placement of the patient or a body part to promote physiological or psychological well-being

Swallowing Therapy: Facilitating swallowing and preventing complications of impaired swallowing

Nursing Activities

Assessments

- Evaluate family's comfort level
- *(NIC) Aspiration Precautions:*

   Monitor level of consciousness, cough reflex, gag reflex, and swallowing ability

   Monitor for signs and symptoms of aspiration

- *(NIC) Swallowing Therapy:*

   Monitor patient's tongue movements while eating

Monitor for sealing of lips during eating, drinking, and swallowing

Check mouth for pocketing of food after eating

Monitor body hydration (e.g., intake, output, skin turgor, and mucous membranes)

Patient/Family Teaching

- *(NIC) Swallowing Therapy:*

Instruct patient to reach for particles of food on lips or chin with tongue

Instruct patient and caregiver on emergency measures for choking

Collaborative Activities

- Consult dietitian for food that can be easily swallowed
- *(NIC) Aspiration Precautions:* Request medication in elixir form
- *(NIC) Swallowing Therapy:*

Collaborate with other members of health care team (e.g., occupational therapist, speech pathologist, and dietitian) to provide continuity in patient's rehabilitative plan

Collaborate with speech therapist to instruct patient's family about swallowing exercise regimen

Other

- Reassure patient during episodes of choking
- *(NIC) Aspiration Precautions:*

Position upright 90 degrees or as far as possible

Keep tracheal cuff inflated

Keep suction setup available

Feed in small amounts

Avoid liquids or use thickening agent

Cut food into small pieces

Break or crush pills before administration

- *(NIC) Swallowing Therapy:*

Provide mouth care, as needed

Provide or use assistive devices, as appropriate

Avoid use of drinking straws

Assist patient to position head in forward flexion in preparation for swallowing (chin tuck)

Acknowledge patient's embarrassment regarding impaired swallowing

Involve family during ingestion of food or medications to provide support and reassurance

Assist patient to place food at back of mouth and on unaffected side

THERAPEUTIC REGIMEN MANAGEMENT: COMMUNITY, INEFFECTIVE (00081) (1994)

Definition: Pattern of regulating and integrating into community processes programs for treatment of illness and the sequelae of illness that are unsatisfactory for meeting health-related goals

Defining Characteristics

Deficits in people and programs to be accountable for illness care of aggregates

Deficits in advocates for aggregates

Deficits in community activities for secondary and tertiary prevention

Illness symptoms above the norm expected for the number and type of population

Number of health care resources are insufficient for the incidence or prevalence of illness(es)

Unavailable health care resources for illness care

Unexpected acceleration of illness(es)

Related Factors

To be developed by NANDA International

Related Factors (Non-NANDA International)

Lack of community programs for disease prevention, smoking cessation, alcohol abuse, and so forth

Complex population needs

Ineffective communication among subgroups and community

Failure of society to value the community and subgroups

Failure of community and subgroups to value self

Government policies

Suggestions for Use

This diagnosis is appropriate for a community in which one or more groups are underserved, perhaps because of insufficient resources, ineffective management of available resources, exposure to risk factors such as toxic chemicals, and so forth. This diagnosis is more narrowly focused on health care delivery than is

Ineffective community coping, which describes the general adaptation and problem-solving processes of the community.

Suggested Alternative Diagnoses

Community coping, ineffective

NOC Outcomes

Community Competence: The ability of a community to collectively problem solve to achieve goals

Community Health Status: The general state of well-being of a community or population

Goals/Evaluation Criteria

The community will:

- Identify needed resources
- Budget resources for illness prevention and care
- Identify factors affecting the community's ability to meet health care needs of specific aggregates
- Obtain advocates who are accountable for health care of specific aggregates
- Develop plans for prevention and treatment of illnesses
- Experience a trend in illness symptoms toward the norm for that illness

NIC Interventions

Community Health Development: Facilitating members of a community to identify a community's health concerns, mobilize resources, and implement solutions

Environmental Management: Community: Monitoring and influencing of the physical, social, cultural, economic, and political conditions that affect the health of groups and communities

Health Policy Monitoring: Surveillance and influence of government and organization regulations, rules, and standards that affect nursing systems and practices to ensure quality care of patients

Program Development: Planning, implementing, and evaluating a coordinated set of activities designed to enhance wellness, or to prevent, reduce, or eliminate one or more health problems of a group or community

Nursing Activities

Assessments

- *(NIC) Environmental Management: Community:*
  Initiate screening for health risks from the environment
  Monitor status of known health risks
- *(NIC) Health Policy Monitoring:* Assess implications and requirements of proposed policies and standards for quality patient care

Teaching

- *(NIC) Environmental Management: Community:* Conduct educational programs for targeted risk groups
- *(NIC) Health Policy Monitoring:* Acquaint policy makers with implications of current and proposed policies and standards for patient welfare
- *(NIC) Program Development:* Educate members of the planning group regarding the planning process, as appropriate

Collaborative Activities

- *(NIC) Environmental Management: Community:*
  Participate in multidisciplinary teams to identify threats to safety in the community
  Collaborate in the development of community action programs
  Coordinate services to at-risk groups and communities
  Work with environmental groups to secure appropriate governmental regulations

Other

- *(NIC) Health Policy Monitoring:*
  Review proposed policies and standards in organizational, professional, and governmental literature and in the popular media
  Promote governmental policy to reduce specified risks
  Identify and resolve discrepancies between health policies and standards and current nursing practice
  Lobby policy makers to make changes in health policies and standards to benefit patients
  Testify in organizational, professional, and public forums to influence the formulation of health policies and standards that benefit patients
  Assist consumers of health care to be informed of current and proposed changes in health policies and standards and the implications for health outcomes

- *(NIC) Environmental Management: Community:* Encourage neighborhoods to become active participants in community safety
- *(NIC) Program Development:*

  Assist the group or community in identifying significant health needs or problems

  Convene a task force, including appropriate community members, to examine the priority need or problem

  [Develop goals, objectives, methods, and a time frame for implementing the program]

  Gain acceptance for the program by the target group, providers, and related groups

  Plan for evaluation of the program

  Evaluate the program for relevance, efficiency, and cost-effectiveness

  Modify and refine the program

THERAPEUTIC REGIMEN MANAGEMENT, EFFECTIVE (00082) (1994)

Definition: Pattern of regulating and integrating into daily living a program for treatment of illness and its sequelae that are satisfactory for meeting specific health goals

Defining Characteristics

Subjective

Verbalized desire to manage the treatment of illness and prevention of sequelae

Verbalized intent to reduce risk factors for progression of illness and sequelae

Objective

Appropriate choices of daily activities for meeting the goals of a treatment or prevention program

Illness symptoms are within a normal range of expectation

Suggestions for Use

This diagnosis does not need to include related factors because it is a wellness diagnosis. The definition is almost identical to *Effective therapeutic regimen management,* but the defining characteristics are slightly different.

Suggested Alternative Diagnoses

Therapeutic regimen management, readiness for enhanced

NOC Outcomes

Adherence Behavior: Self-initiated action taken to promote wellness, recovery, and rehabilitation

Compliance Behavior: Actions taken on the basis of professional advice to promote wellness, recovery, and rehabilitation

Family Participation in Professional Care: Family involvement in decision-making, delivery, and evaluation of care provided by health care personnel

Knowledge: Treatment Regimen: Extent of understanding conveyed about a specific treatment regimen

Participation: Health Care Decisions: Personal involvement in selecting and evaluating health care options

Risk Control: Actions to eliminate or reduce actual, personal, and modifiable health threats

Symptom Control: Personal actions to minimize perceived adverse changes in physical and emotional functioning

Goals/Evaluation Criteria

Examples Using NOC Language

- Demonstrates **Adherence Behavior**, as evidenced by the following indicators (specify 1–5: never, rarely, sometimes, often, or consistently demonstrated):

    Uses health-related information from a variety of sources to develop health strategies

    Provides rationale for adopting a regimen

    Describes rationale for deviating from a recommended regimen

    Performs self-monitoring

- Demonstrates **Participation: Health Care Decisions**, as evidenced by the following indicator (specify 1–5: never, rarely, sometimes, often, or consistently demonstrated): Evaluates satisfaction with health care outcomes

- Demonstrates **Risk Control**, as evidenced by the following indicators (specify 1–5: never, rarely, sometimes, often, or consistently demonstrated):

    Monitors environmental and personal behavior risk factors

    Participates in screening for associated health problems and identified risks

Other Examples

Patient will:

- Describe and follow prescribed health regimens (e.g., diet, exercise)
- Change or modify health regimen as directed by health provider
- Report symptom control

NIC Interventions

Anticipatory Guidance: Preparation of patient for an anticipated developmental or situational crisis

Behavior Modification: Promotion of a behavior change

Decision-Making Support: Providing information and support for a patient who is making a decision regarding health care

Family Involvement Promotion: Facilitating family participation in the emotional and physical care of the patient

Health Education: Developing and providing instruction and learning experiences to facilitate voluntary adaptation of behavior conducive to health in individuals, families, groups, or communities

Health System Guidance: Facilitating a patient's location and use of appropriate health services

Mutual Goal Setting: Collaborating with patient to identify and prioritize care goals, then developing a plan for achieving those goals

Patient Contracting: Negotiating an agreement with a patient that reinforces a specific behavior change

Risk Identification: Analysis of potential risk factors, determination of health risks, and prioritization of risk reduction strategies for an individual or group

Self-Modification Assistance: Reinforcement of self-directed change initiated by the patient to achieve personally important goals

Teaching: Procedure/Treatment: Preparing a patient to understand and mentally prepare for a prescribed procedure or treatment

Nursing Activities

Assessments

- Assess patient's knowledge of health promotion and disease prevention
- Identify patient's usual methods of coping and problem solving

Patient/Family Teaching

- Help patient to plan for the future by providing information on the usual course of the patient's illness
- Teach stress management techniques
- *(NIC) Health System Guidance:*

  Explain the immediate health care system, how it works, and what the patient and family can expect

  Inform the patient of accreditation and state health department requirements for judging the quality of a facility

  Give written instructions for purpose and location of health care activities, as appropriate

  Inform patient how to access emergency services by telephone and vehicle, as appropriate

Collaborative Activities

- Offer information on community resources specific to health goals of the patient (e.g., support groups)
- *(NIC) Health System Guidance:* Identify and facilitate communication among health care providers and patient and family, as appropriate

Other

- Help patient to identify and prepare for upcoming developmental milestones, role changes, or situational crises
- Help patient to identify situational obstacles that interfere with adherence to therapeutic regimen
- Plan to visit patient at strategic developmental or situational times
- *(NIC) Health System Guidance:* Encourage the patient and family to ask questions about services and charges

THERAPEUTIC REGIMEN MANAGEMENT; FAMILY, INEFFECTIVE (00080) (1994)

Definition: Pattern of regulating and integrating into family processes a program for treatment of illness and the sequelae of illness that is unsatisfactory for meeting specific health goals

Defining Characteristics

Subjective

Verbalized desire to manage the treatment of illnesses and prevention of the sequelae

Verbalized difficulty with regulation and integration of one or more effects or prevention of complications

Verbalizes that family did not take action to reduce risk factors for progression of illness and sequelae

Objective

Acceleration [expected or unexpected] of illness symptoms of a family member

Inappropriate family activities for meeting the goals of a treatment or prevention program

Lack of attention to illness and its sequelae

Related Factors

Complexity of health care system

Complexity of therapeutic regimen

Decisional conflicts

Economic difficulties

Excessive demands made on individual or family

Family conflict

Suggestions for Use

Use this diagnosis for families who are motivated to follow a therapeutic regimen but who are having difficulty doing so. It is not appropriate for families who are not interested in adhering to the treatment program. This diagnosis is more narrowly focused than *Interrupted family processes* or *Ineffective family coping*, both of which include problems other than managing the family's treatment program. It is difficult to differentiate this label from *Ineffective management of therapeutic regimen* because individuals typically are a part of a family.

Suggested Alternative Diagnoses

Coping: family, disabled

Family processes, interrupted

Health maintenance, ineffective

Management of therapeutic regimen, ineffective

NOC Outcomes

Family Functioning: Ability of the family to meet the needs of its members through developmental transitions

Family Health Status: Overall health status and social competence of family unit

Family Participation in Professional Care: Family involvement in decision making, delivery, and evaluation of care provided by health care personnel

Goals/Evaluation Criteria

The family will:
- Indicate a desire to manage the therapeutic regimen or program
- Identify factors interfering with adhering to the therapeutic regimen
- Adjust usual activities as needed to incorporate the treatment programs of family members (e.g., diet, school activities)
- Experience a decrease in illness symptoms among family members

NIC Interventions

Family Involvement Promotion: Facilitating family participation in the emotional and physical care of the patient

Family Mobilization: Utilization of family strengths to influence patient's health in a positive direction

Family Process Maintenance: Minimization of family process disruption effects

Nursing Activities

Also see Nursing Activities for Management of Therapeutic Regimen, Ineffective on pp. 550–551.

Assessments
- Assess present status of family coping and processes
- Assess family members' levels of understanding of illness, complications, and recommended treatments
- Assess family members' readiness to learn
- Identify family cultural influences and health beliefs
- *(NIC) Family Involvement:*
  Identify family members' capabilities for involvement in care of patient
  Determine physical, emotional, and educational resources of primary caregiver
  Monitor family structure and roles
  Identify individual family members' understanding and beliefs about the situation
  Determine level of patient dependency on family, as appropriate for age or illness
  Identify and respect family's coping mechanisms

Patient/Family Teaching

- Teach family time management and organizational skills
- Provide caregivers with skills needed for patient's therapy
- Teach strategies for maintaining or restoring patient's health
- Teach strategies for care of a dying patient
- *(NIC) Family Involvement:* Facilitate family understanding of the medical aspects of illness

Collaborative Activities

- Help family to identify community health care resources
- Refer family to family support groups

Other

- Involve family in discussion of strengths and resources
- Assist patient and family to establish realistic goals
- Assist family members to plan and implement patient therapies and lifestyle changes
- Support maintenance of family routines and rituals in hospital (e.g., private meals together, family discussions)
- Discuss family's plans for child care when parents must be absent
- Plan patient home care activities to decrease disruption of family routine
- *(NIC) Family Involvement:*
  Encourage care by family members during hospitalization, when appropriate
  Encourage family members to keep or maintain family relationships, as appropriate
  Assist primary caregiver to acquire needed care delivery supplies
  Support primary caregiver in the use of relief services opportunities

---

THERAPEUTIC REGIMEN MANAGEMENT, INEFFECTIVE (00078) (1992)

Definition: Pattern of regulating and integrating into daily living a program for treatment of illness and the sequelae of illness that is unsatisfactory for meeting specific health goals

Defining Characteristics

Subjective

Choices of daily living ineffective for meeting the goals of a treatment or prevention program

[Statements that patient and family] did not take action to include treatment regimens in daily routines

[Statements that patient and family] did not take action to reduce risk factors for progression of illness and sequelae

Verbalized desire to manage the treatment of illness and prevention of sequelae

Verbalized difficulty with regulation and integration of one or more prescribed regimens for treatment of illness and its effects or prevention of complications

Objective

Acceleration [expected or unexpected] of illness symptoms

Related Factors

Complexity of health care system
Complexity of therapeutic regimen
Decisional conflicts
Family conflict
Family patterns of health care
Inadequate number and types of cues to action
Knowledge deficits
Mistrust of regimen or health care personnel
Perceived barriers
Perceived benefits
Perceived seriousness
Perceived susceptibility
Powerlessness
Social support deficits

Suggestions for Use

Use this diagnosis for patients who wish to follow a therapeutic regimen and are motivated to do so but are having difficulty with it. For example, this diagnosis is appropriate for a patient who is trying to lose weight and has the necessary information but finds it difficult to adhere to a low-calorie diet because her business requires her to eat out frequently. It is not appropriate for an obese patient who is not interested in dieting or losing weight.

Suggested Alternative Diagnoses

Adjustment, impaired
Denial, ineffective
Health maintenance, ineffective
Noncompliance (specify)

NOC Outcomes

Compliance Behavior: Actions taken on the basis of professional advice to promote wellness, recovery, and rehabilitation

Knowledge: Treatment Regimen: Extent of understanding conveyed about a specific treatment regimen

Participation: Health Care Decisions: Personal involvement in selecting and evaluating health care options

Treatment Behavior: Illness or Injury: Personal actions to palliate or eliminate pathology

Goals/Evaluation Criteria

Refer to Goals/Evaluation Criteria for Management of Therapeutic Regimen, Effective pp. 542–543.

Other Examples

Patient will:

- Develop and follow plan to achieve therapeutic regimen
- Identify obstacles that interfere with adherence to the therapeutic regimen
- Avoid risk-taking behaviors
- Recognize and report symptoms of change in disease status
- Use therapeutic equipment and devices correctly

NIC Interventions

Behavior Modification: Promotion of a behavior change

Decision-Making Support: Providing information and support for a patient who is making a decision regarding health care

Health System Guidance: Facilitating a patient's location and use of appropriate health services

Mutual Goal Setting: Collaborating with patient to identify and prioritize care goals, then developing a plan for achieving those goals

Patient Contracting: Negotiating an agreement with a patient that reinforces a specific behavior change

Self-Modification Assistance: Reinforcement of self-directed change initiated by the patient to achieve personally important goals

Self-Responsibility Facilitation: Encouraging a patient to assume more responsibility for own behavior

Teaching: Disease Process: Assisting the patient to understand information related to a specific disease process

Teaching: Procedure/Treatment: Preparing a patient to understand and mentally prepare for a prescribed procedure or treatment

Nursing Activities

Assessments

- Assess patient's level of understanding of illness, complications, and recommended treatments to determine knowledge deficit
- Interview patient and family to determine problem areas in integrating treatment regimen into lifestyle
- *(NIC) Self-Modification Assistance:*

  Appraise the patient's reasons for wanting to change

  Appraise the patient's present knowledge and skill level in relationship to the desired change

  Appraise the patient's social and physical environment for extent of support of desired behaviors

Patient/Family Teaching

- Identify essential treatments
- Offer information on community resources specific to health goals of patient (e.g., support groups)
- Assist patient to identify situational obstacles that interfere with adherence to therapeutic regimen
- Provide information on illness, complications, and recommended treatments
- *(NIC) Self-Modification Assistance*: Instruct the patient on how to move from continuous reinforcement to intermittent reinforcement

Collaborative Activities

- Collaborate with other health care providers to determine how to modify therapeutic regimen without jeopardizing patient's health

Other

- Assist patient to develop realistic plan to achieve adherence to therapeutic regimen. Plan should include the following:

  Identification of modifications or adaptations in ADLs

  Identification of support systems to achieve therapeutic goals

  Identification of actions patient and family are willing to take (e.g., dietary changes, exercise modification, sleep pattern changes, medication and treatment schedules, sexual activity modifications, role changes)

- Provide coaching and support to motivate patient's continued adherence to therapy
- *(NIC) Self-Modification Assistance:*

Encourage the patient to examine personal values and beliefs and satisfaction with them

Assist the patient in identifying a specific goal for change

Assist the patient in identifying target behaviors that need to change to achieve the desired goal

Explore with the patient potential barriers to change behavior

Identify with the patient the most effective strategies for behavior changes

Encourage the patient to identify appropriate, meaningful reinforcers and rewards

Foster moving toward primary reliance on self-reinforcement versus family or nurse rewards

Assist the patient in identifying the circumstances or situations in which the behavior occurs (e.g., cues or triggers)

Explain to the patient the importance of self-monitoring in attempting behavior change

THERAPEUTIC REGIMEN MANAGEMENT, READINESS FOR ENHANCED (00162) (2002)

Definition: A pattern of regulating and integrating into daily living a program(s) for treatment of illness and its sequelae that is sufficient for meeting specific health goals and can be strengthened

Defining Characteristics

Subjective

Expresses desire to manage the treatment of illness and prevention of sequelae

Expresses little to no difficulty with regulation and integration of one or more prescribed regimens for treatment of illness or prevention of complications

Objective

Choices of daily living are appropriate for meeting the goals of treatment or prevention

Describes reduction of risk factors for progression of illness and
sequelae

No unexpected acceleration of illness symptoms

Suggestions for Use

This diagnosis does not need to include related factors because
it is a wellness diagnosis. The definition is almost identical to
Effective therapeutic regimen management, but the defining characteristics are slightly different. Although NANDA International
includes both in its taxonomy, there is likely a great deal of overlapping in the situations in which they can be used.

Suggested Alternative Diagnoses

Therapeutic regimen management, effective

NOTE: For standardized and other goals and nursing interventions refer to *Effective therapeutic regimen management* on pp.
542–544.

THERMOREGULATION, INEFFECTIVE
(00008) (1986)

Definition: Temperature fluctuation between hypothermia and
hyperthermia

Defining Characteristics

Objective

Cyanotic nail beds

Cool skin

Fluctuations in body temperature above or below normal range

Flushed skin

Hypertension

Increased respiratory rate

Pallor (moderate)

Piloerection

Reduction in body temperature below normal range

Seizures or convulsions

Shivering (mild)

Slow capillary refill

Tachycardia

Warm to touch

Related Factors

Aging
Fluctuating environmental temperature
Immaturity
Trauma or illness

Suggestions for Use

This label is most appropriate for patients who are especially vulnerable to environmental conditions (e.g., newborns and the elderly).

Suggested Alternative Diagnoses

Body temperature, risk for imbalanced
Hyperthermia
Hypothermia

NOC Outcomes

Thermoregulation: Balance among heat production, heat gain, and heat loss
Thermoregulation: Neonate: Balance among heat production, heat gain, and heat loss during the neonatal period

Goals/Evaluation Criteria

For specific patient outcomes and evaluation criteria, refer to Goals/Evaluation Criteria for Hyperthermia, p. 252, Hypothermia, p. 255, and Risk for Imbalanced Body Temperature, p. 43.

NIC Interventions

Newborn Care: Management of neonate during the transition to extrauterine life and subsequent period of stabilization
Temperature Regulation: Attaining or maintaining body temperature within a normal range
Temperature Regulation: Intraoperative: Attaining or maintaining desired intraoperative body temperature

Nursing Activities

Nursing interventions focus on teaching for prevention of *Ineffective thermoregulation* and on maintaining a normal body temperature by manipulating external factors, such as clothing and room temperature. Refer to Nursing Activities for Risk for

Altered Body Temperature, pp. 44–45; Hyperthermia, pp. 253–254, and Hypothermia, pp. 256–257.

THOUGHT PROCESSES, DISTURBED
(00130) (1976, 1996)

Definition: Disruption in cognitive operations and activities [e.g., conscious thought, reality orientation, problem solving, and judgment]

Defining Characteristics

Subjective
Cognitive dissonance
Inaccurate interpretation of environment
Inappropriate nonreality-based thinking

Objective
Distractibility
Egocentricity
Hyper- or hypovigilance
Memory deficit or problems

Related Factors

To be developed

Non-NANDA International Related Factors
Mental disorders (specify)
Organic mental disorders (specify)
Personality disorders (specify)
Substance abuse

Suggestions for Use

This diagnosis is a result of mental or personality or chronic organic disorders that may be exacerbated by situational crises. It may be the etiology of other problems, such as *Self-care deficit, Impaired home maintenance, Risk for injury,* and *Ineffective management of therapeutic regimen.*

Suggested Alternative Diagnoses

Communication, impaired verbal
Confusion, acute or chronic
Environmental interpretation syndrome, impaired

Sensory perception, disturbed: auditory, gustatory, kinesthetic, olfactory, tactile, visual

NOC Outcomes

Cognitive Ability: Ability to execute complex mental processes
Cognitive Orientation: Ability to identify person, place, and time
Concentration: Ability to focus on a specific stimulus
Decision Making: Ability to choose between two or more alternatives
Distorted Thought Control: Self-restraint of disruption in perception, thought processes, and thought content
Identity: Ability to distinguish between self and non-self and to characterize one's essence
Information Processing: Ability to acquire, organize, and use information
Memory: Ability to cognitively retrieve and report previously stored information
Neurologic Status: Consciousness: Extent to which an individual arouses, orients, and attends to the environment

Goals/Evaluation Criteria

Examples Using NOC Language

- Demonstrates **Cognitive Orientation**, as evidenced by the following indicators (specify 1–5: never, rarely, sometimes, often, or consistently demonstrated): Identifies self; significant other; current place; and correct day, month, year, and season
- Demonstrates appropriate **Decision Making** (specify 1–5: never, rarely, sometimes, often, or consistently demonstrated)
- Demonstrates **Identity**, as evidenced by the following indicators (specify 1–5: never, rarely, sometimes, often, or consistently demonstrated):
    Verbalizes clear sense of personal identity
    Differentiates self from environment and other human beings
    Recognizes interpersonal versus intrapersonal conflicts
- Demonstrates **Neurologic Status: Consciousness**, as evidenced by the following indicators (specify 1–5: extremely, substantially, moderately, mildly, or not compromised):
    Opens eyes to external stimuli
    Obeys commands
    Attends to environmental stimuli

Other Examples

Patient and family will:

- Accurately recall immediate, recent, and remote information
- Correctly identify familiar people and objects
- Demonstrate logical, organized thought processes
- Compare and contrast two items
- Not be easily distracted
- Perform serial subtractions from 100 by 7s or 3s
- Spell simple words backward
- Respond appropriately to environmental and communication cues (e.g., auditory, written)
- Not act on hallucinations or delusions

NIC Interventions

Analgesic Administration: Use of pharmacologic agents to reduce or eliminate pain

Anxiety Reduction: Minimizing apprehension, dread, foreboding, or uneasiness related to an unidentified source of anticipated danger

Cerebral Perfusion Promotion: Promotion of adequate perfusion and limitation of complications for a patient experiencing or at risk for inadequate cerebral perfusion

Cognitive Restructuring: Challenging a patient to alter distorted thought patterns and view self and the world more realistically

Cognitive Stimulation: Promotion of awareness and comprehension of surroundings by utilization of planned stimuli

Decision-Making Support: Providing information and support for a patient who is making a decision regarding health care

Delusion Management: Promoting the comfort, safety, and reality orientation of a patient experiencing false, fixed beliefs that have little or no basis in reality

Dementia Management: Provision of a modified environment for the patient who is experiencing a chronic confusional state

Environmental Management: Safety: Monitoring and manipulation of the physical environment to promote safety

Hallucination Management: Promoting the safety, comfort, and reality orientation of a patient experiencing hallucinations

Memory Training: Facilitation of memory

Neurologic Monitoring: Collection and analysis of patient data to prevent or minimize neurologic complications

Reality Orientation: Promotion of patient's awareness of personal identity, time, and environment

Nursing Activities

Assessments

- Assess and document patient's orientation to person, place, time, and situation q _____
- *(NIC) Delusion Management:*
  Monitor self-care ability
  Monitor physical status of patient
  Monitor delusions for presence of content that is self-harmful or violent
  Monitor cognitive functioning, using a standardized assessment tool
  Monitor carefully for physiologic causes of increased confusion that may be acute and reversible
  Monitor patient for medication side effects and desired therapeutic effects

Patient/Family Teaching

- *(NIC) Delusion Management:*
  Educate family and significant others about ways to deal with patient who is experiencing delusions
  Provide illness teaching to patient and significant others if delusions are illness-based (e.g., delirium, schizophrenia, or depression)

Collaborative Activities

- Identify community resources
- Involve social services for additional support
- *(NIC) Delusion Management:* Administer antipsychotic and antianxiety medications on a routine and as-needed basis

Other

- Post schedule of activities in room
- Call patient by preferred name
- Refer to calendar and clock often
- Use familiar items from home provided by family
- Provide positive feedback and reinforcement of appropriate behavior
- Provide support to patient and family during patient's periods of disorientation

- *(NIC) Delusion Management:*

  Avoid arguing about false beliefs; state doubt matter-of-factly

  Focus discussion on the underlying feelings, rather than the content of the delusion ("It appears as if you may be feeling frightened")

  Encourage patient to verbalize delusions to caregivers before acting on them

  Provide recreational, diversional activities that require attention or skill

  Decrease excessive environmental stimuli, as needed

  Assign consistent caregivers on a daily basis

- *(NIC) Dementia Management:*

  Provide a low-stimulation environment (e.g., quiet, soothing music; nonvivid and simple, familiar patterns in décor; performance expectations that do not exceed cognitive-processing ability; and dining in small groups)

  Identify and remove potential dangers in environment for patient

  Prepare for interaction with eye contact and touch, as appropriate

  Give one simple direction at a time

  Speak in a clear, low, warm, and respectful tone of voice

  Provide unconditional positive regard

  Use distraction, rather than confrontation, to manage behavior

  Provide cues—such as current events, seasons, location, and names—to assist orientation

  Label familiar photos with names of the individuals in the photos

  Assist family to understand it may be impossible for patient to learn new material

  Limit number of choices patient has to make, so not to cause anxiety

---

TISSUE INTEGRITY, IMPAIRED
(00044) (1986, 1998)

Definition: Damage to mucous membrane, corneal, integumentary, or subcutaneous tissues

Defining Characteristics

Objective

Damaged or destroyed tissue (e.g., corneal, mucous membrane, integumentary, or subcutaneous)

Related Factors

Altered circulation

Chemical irritants (e.g., body excretions and secretions, medications)

Fluid deficit or excess

Impaired physical mobility

Knowledge deficit

Mechanical factors (e.g., pressure, shear, friction)

Nutritional deficit or excess

Radiation (including therapeutic radiation)

Thermal factors (e.g., temperature extremes)

Suggestions for Use

1. If tissue integrity is at risk because of immobility and if other systems are also at risk, consider using *Risk for disuse syndrome*.

2. If the necessary defining characteristics are present, use the more specific problems of *Impaired oral mucous membrane* or *Impaired skin integrity*. *Impaired tissue integrity* should be used only when the damage is to tissue other than the skin and mucous membranes.

3. Do not use *Impaired tissue integrity* to rename a surgical incision or ostomy.

Suggested Alternative Diagnoses

Disuse syndrome, risk for

Oral mucous membrane, impaired

Skin integrity, impaired

Surgical recovery, delayed

NOC Outcomes

Tissue Integrity: Skin and Mucous Membranes: Structural intactness and normal physiologic function of skin and mucous membranes

Wound Healing: Primary Intention: The extent to which cells and tissues have regenerated following intentional closure

Wound Healing: Secondary Intention: The extent to which cells and tissues in an open wound have regenerated

Goals/Evaluation Criteria

Also refer to Goals/Evaluation Criteria for Impaired Skin Integrity, pp. 476–477.

Examples Using NOC Language

- Demonstrates **Tissue Integrity**, as evidenced by the following indicators (specify 1–5: extremely, substantially, moderately, mildly, or not compromised):
    Tissue texture and thickness in expected range
    Tissue perfusion

Other Examples

- No signs or symptoms of infection

NIC Interventions

Eye Care: Prevention or minimization of threats to eye or visual integrity

Incision Site Care: Cleansing, monitoring, and promotion of healing in a wound that is closed with sutures, clips, or staples

Oral Health Maintenance: Maintenance and promotion of oral hygiene and dental health for the patient at risk for developing oral or dental lesions

Pressure Ulcer Prevention: Prevention of pressure ulcers for a patient at high risk for developing them

Wound Care: Prevention of wound complications and promotion of wound healing

Nursing Activities

For specific nursing activities, refer to the following nursing diagnoses:

Infection, risk for (pp. 277–278)
Oral mucous membrane, impaired (pp. 345–346)
Sensory perception, disturbed (visual) (pp. 466–467)
Skin integrity, impaired (pp. 482–484)
Skin integrity, risk for impaired (pp. 477–479)
Tissue perfusion, ineffective (peripheral) (pp. 577–578)

TISSUE PERFUSION, INEFFECTIVE (SPECIFY: CARDIOPULMONARY, CEREBRAL, GASTROINTESTINAL, AND RENAL) (00024)(1980, 1998)

Definition: Decrease in oxygen resulting in the failure to nourish the tissues at the capillary level

Defining Characteristics

Cardiopulmonary

Subjective
Chest pain
Dyspnea
Sense of impending doom

Objective
Abnormal arterial blood gases
Altered respiratory rate outside of acceptable parameters
Arrhythmias
Bronchospasms
Capillary refill greater than 3 s
Chest retraction
Nasal flaring
Use of accessory muscles

Cerebral

Objective
Altered mental status
Behavioral changes
Changes in motor response
Changes in pupillary reactions
Difficulty in swallowing
Extremity weakness or paralysis
Speech abnormalities

Gastrointestinal

Subjective
Abdominal pain or tenderness
Nausea

Objective
Abdominal distention
Hypoactive or absent bowel sounds

Renal

Objective
Altered BP outside of acceptable parameters
Diminished arterial pulsations
Elevation in BUN/creatinine ratio
Hematuria
Oliguria or anuria
Skin color pale on elevation

Related Factors

Altered affinity of hemoglobin for oxygen

Decreased hemoglobin concentration in blood

Enzyme poisoning

Exchange problems

Hypervolemia

Hypoventilation

Impaired transport of the oxygen across alveolar or capillary membrane

Interruption of flow, arterial

Interruption of flow, venous

Mechanical reduction of venous or arterial blood flow

Mismatch of ventilation with blow flow

Suggestions for Use

With the exception of *Ineffective peripheral tissue perfusion,* I do not recommend use of this diagnosis. The following Suggested Alternative Diagnoses offer alternative labels that specifically address responses to impaired perfusion of renal, cerebral, cardiopulmonary, and gastrointestinal tissue. Altered tissue perfusion can be used appropriately as an etiology for other diagnoses (e.g., *Acute confusion related to Altered cerebral tissue perfusion*).

Ineffective cardiopulmonary, cerebral, gastrointestinal, and renal tissue perfusion actually represent medical diagnoses or conditions. The outcomes and interventions for ineffective tissue perfusion are medical/surgical treatments. The nurse's role is to monitor and detect changes in the patient's condition. Therefore, nursing care may be better directed by the use of other nursing diagnoses or collaborative problems. However, because NOC and NIC have linked outcomes and interventions to this diagnosis, this text also includes them.

Suggested Alternative Diagnoses

Cardiopulmonary

Activity intolerance

Activity intolerance, risk for

Breathing pattern, ineffective

Cardiac output, decreased

Dysfunctional ventilatory weaning response (DVWR)

Fatigue

Gas exchange, impaired

Spontaneous ventilation, inability to sustain

Cerebral

Communication, impaired: verbal

Confusion, acute or chronic

Injury, risk for

Sensory or perceptual alterations: (auditory, gustatory, kinesthetic, olfactory, visual)

Gastrointestinal

Infection; risk for

Pain, acute

Pain, chronic

Renal

Fluid volume excess

Fluid volume imbalance, risk for

NOC Outcomes

Cardiopulmonary Tissue Perfusion

Cardiac Pump Effectiveness: Extent to which blood is ejected from the left ventricle per minute to support systemic perfusion pressure

Circulation Status: Extent to which blood flows unobstructed, unidirectionally, and at an appropriate pressure through large vessels of the systemic and pulmonary circuits

Tissue Perfusion: Cardiac: Extent to which blood flows through the coronary vasculature and maintains heart function

Tissue Perfusion: Peripheral: Extent to which blood flows through the small vessels of the extremities and maintains tissue perfusion

Vital Signs Status: Temperature, pulse, respiration, and BP within expected range for the individual

Cerebral Tissue Perfusion

Circulation Status: Extent to which blood flows unobstructed, unidirectionally, and at an appropriate pressure through large vessels of the systemic and pulmonary circuits

Neurologic Status: Extent to which the peripheral and central nervous systems receive, process, and respond to internal and external stimuli

Neurological Status: Consciousness: Extent to which an individual arouses, orients, and attends to the environment

Neurological Status: Central Motor Control: Extent to which skeletal muscle activity (body movement) is coordinated by the central nervous system

Tissue Perfusion: Cerebral: Extent to which blood flows through the cerebral vasculature and maintains brain function

Gastrointestinal Tissue Perfusion

Bowel Elimination: Ability of the gastrointestinal tract to form and evacuate stool effectively

Circulation Status: Extent to which blood flows unobstructed, unidirectionally, and at an appropriate pressure through large vessels of the systemic and pulmonary circuits

Electrolyte and Acid–Base Balance: Balance of electrolytes and nonelectrolytes in the intra- and extracellular compartments of the body

Fluid Balance: Balance of water in the intra- and extracellular compartments of the body

Hydration: Amount of water in the intra- and extracellular compartments of the body

Tissue Perfusion: Abdominal Organs: Extent to which blood flows through the small vessels of the abdominal viscera and maintains organ function

Renal Tissue Perfusion

Circulation Status: Extent to which blood flows unobstructed, unidirectionally, and at an appropriate pressure through the large vessels of the systemic and pulmonary circuits

Electrolyte and Acid–Base Balance: Balance of electrolytes and nonelectrolytes in the intra- and extracellular compartments of the body

Fluid Balance: Balance of water in the intra- and extracellular compartments of the body

Hydration: Amount of water in the intra- and extracellular compartment of the body

Tissue Perfusion: Abdominal Organs: Extent to which blood flows through the small vessels of the abdominal viscera and maintains organ function

Urinary Elimination: Ability of the urinary system to filter wastes, conserve solutes, and collect and discharge urine in a healthy pattern

Goals/Evaluation Criteria

Cardiopulmonary

Examples Using NOC Language

- Demonstrates **Cardiac Pump Effectiveness, Cardiac Tissue Perfusion**, and **Peripheral Tissue Perfusion**
- Demonstrates **Circulation Status**, as evidenced by the following indicators (specify 1–5: extremely, substantially, moderately, mildly, or not compromised):

  Systolic BP, diastolic BP, pulse pressure, mean BP, CVP, and pulmonary wedge pressure in expected ranges

  Peripheral pulses strong and symmetrical

  Peripheral edema and ascites not present

  Heart rate, cardiac index, blood gases, and ejection fraction in expected ranges

  Abnormal heart sounds not present

  Angina not present

  No adventitious breath sounds, neck vein distention, pulmonary edema, or large vessel bruits

  Extreme fatigue not present

  Orthostatic hypotension not present

Cerebral

Examples Using NOC Language

- Demonstrates **Circulation Status**, as evidenced by the following indicators (specify 1–5: extremely, substantially, moderately, mildly, or not compromised):

  Systolic and diastolic BP in expected ranges

  Orthostatic hypotension not present

  Large-vessel bruits not present

- Demonstrates **Cognitive Ability**, as evidenced by the following indicators (specify 1–5: extremely, substantially, moderately, mildly, or not compromised):

  Communicates clearly and appropriately for age and ability

  Demonstrates attentiveness, concentration, and orientation

  Demonstrates recent and remote memory

  Processes information

  Makes appropriate decisions

Other Examples

Patient will:

- Have intact central and peripheral nervous systems
- Demonstrate intact cranial sensorimotor function

- Exhibit intact autonomic functioning
- Have pupils equal and reactive
- Be free from seizure activity
- Not experience headache

Gastrointestinal

Examples Using NOC Language

- Demonstrates **Bowel Elimination**, as evidenced by the following indicators (specify 1–5: extremely, substantially, moderately, mildly, or not compromised):

  Stool color, amount, odor, and consistency WNL

  Visible peristalsis, painful cramps, and bloating not present

  Bowel sounds not compromised

- Demonstrates **Circulation Status**, as evidenced by the following indicators (specify 1–5: extremely, substantially, moderately, mildly, or not compromised):

  Systolic and diastolic BP in expected ranges

  Peripheral tissue perfusion not compromised

  Neck vein distention not present

- Demonstrates **Electrolyte and Acid–Base Balance**, as evidenced by the following indicators (specify 1–5: extremely, substantially, moderately, mildly, or not compromised):

  Mental alertness, cognitive orientation, and muscle strength not compromised

  Lab tests in expected range (e.g., serum Na^+, K^+, Cl^-, Ca^+, Mg^+, bicarbonate)

- Demonstrates **Fluid Balance**, as evidenced by the following indicators (specify 1–5: extremely, substantially, moderately, mildly, or not compromised):

  Neck vein distention not present

  Adventitious breath sounds not present

  24-hr intake and output balanced

- Demonstrates **Hydration**, as evidenced by the following indicators (specify 1–5: extremely, substantially, moderately, mildly, or not compromised):

  Ascites and peripheral edema not present

  Abnormal thirst not present

  Moist mucous membranes

  Fever not present

  Urine output WNL

  Hematocrit WNL

Other Examples

- Demonstrates adequate food, fluid, and nutrient intake
- Reports sufficient energy
- Displays body mass and weight in expected range

Renal

Examples Using NOC Language

- Demonstrates **Circulation Status**, as evidenced by the following indicators (specify 1–5: extremely, substantially, moderately, mildly, or not compromised):

   Systolic and diastolic BP in expected ranges

   Peripheral tissue perfusion not compromised
- Demonstrates **Electrolyte and Acid–Base Balance**, as evidenced by the following indicators (specify 1–5: extremely, substantially, moderately, mildly, or not compromised):

   Mental alertness, cognitive orientation, and muscle strength not compromised

   Lab tests in expected range (e.g., serum Na^+, K^+, Cl^-, Ca^+, Mg^+, bicarbonate, BUN, creatinine)
- Demonstrates **Fluid Balance**, as evidenced by the following indicators (specify 1–5: extremely, substantially, moderately, mildly, or not compromised):

   Neck vein distention not present

   Adventitious breath sounds not present

   24-hr intake and output balanced
- Demonstrates **Hydration**, as evidenced by the following indicators (specify 1–5: extremely, substantially, moderately, mildly, or not compromised):

   Ascites and peripheral edema not present

   Abnormal thirst not present

   Moist mucous membranes

   Fever not present

   Urine output within normal limits

   Hematocrit within normal limits

Other Examples

- Urine odor and color in expected range
- Urine clear
- Laboratory tests within normal limits (e.g., urine specific gravity, glucose, ketone, pH, and protein levels and microscopic results)
- Arterial PCO_2 within normal limits

NIC Interventions

Cardiopulmonary

Cardiac Care: Acute: Limitation of complications for a patient recently experiencing an episode of an imbalance between myocardial oxygen supply and demand, resulting in impaired cardiac function

Circulatory Care: Arterial Insufficiency: Promotion of arterial circulation

Circulatory Care: Venous Insufficiency: Promotion of venous circulation

Respiratory Monitoring: Collection and analysis of patient data to ensure airway patency and adequate gas exchange

Shock Management: Cardiac: Promotion of adequate tissue perfusion for a patient with severely compromised pumping function of the heart

Cerebral

Cerebral Perfusion Promotion: Promotion of adequate perfusion and limitation of complications for a patient experiencing or at risk for inadequate cerebral perfusion

Circulatory Care: Arterial Insufficiency: Promotion of arterial circulation

Circulatory Care: Venous Insufficiency: Promotion of venous circulation

Intracranial Pressure (ICP) Monitoring: Measurement and interpretation of patient data to regulate intracranial pressure

Neurologic Monitoring: Collection and analysis of patient data to prevent or minimize neurologic complications

Peripheral Sensation Management: Prevention or minimization of injury or discomfort in the patient with altered sensation

Gastrointestinal

Fluid/Electrolyte Management: Regulation and prevention of complications from altered fluid or electrolyte levels

Gastrointestinal Intubation: Insertion of a tube into the gastrointestinal tract

Nutrition Management: Assisting with or providing a balanced dietary intake of foods and fluids

Renal

Fluid Management: Promotion of fluid balance and prevention of complications resulting from abnormal or undesired fluid levels

Fluid/Electrolyte Management: Regulation and prevention of complications from altered fluid or electrolyte levels

Hemodialysis Therapy: Management of extracorporeal passage of the patient's blood through a dialyzer

Hemofiltration Therapy: Cleansing of acutely ill patient's blood via a hemofilter controlled by the patient's hydrostatic pressure

Peritoneal Dialysis Therapy: Administration and monitoring of dialysis solution in and out of the peritoneal cavity

Nursing Activities

Cardiopulmonary

Assessments

- Monitor chest pain (e.g., intensity, duration, and precipitating factors)
- Observe for ST changes on ECG
- Monitor cardiac rate and rhythm
- Auscultate heart and lung sounds
- Monitor coagulation studies (e.g., prothrombin time [PT], partial thromboplastin time [PTT], and platelet counts)
- Weigh patient daily
- Monitor electrolyte values associated with dysrhythmias (e.g., serum potassium and magnesium)
- *(NIC) Circulatory Care (Arterial and Venous Insufficiency):*
  Perform a comprehensive appraisal of peripheral circulation (e.g., check peripheral pulses, edema, capillary refill, color, and temperature of extremity)
  Monitor fluid status, including intake and output
  Evaluate peripheral edema and pulses
- *(NIC) Respiratory Monitoring:*
  Monitor for increased restlessness, anxiety, and air hunger
  Note changes in SaO_2, SvO_2, and changes in ABG values, as appropriate

Patient/Family Teaching

- Instruct the patient to avoid performing Valsalva maneuver (e.g., do not strain during bowel movement)

- Explain restrictions on caffeine, sodium, cholesterol, and fat intake
- Explain rationale for eating small, frequent meals

Collaborative Activities

- Administer medications according to order or protocols (e.g., analgesics, anticoagulants, nitroglycerin, vasodilators, diuretic, and positive inotropic and contractility medications)

Other

- Reassure patient and family that call bells, lights, and pages will be answered promptly
- Promote rest (e.g., limit visitors, control environmental stimuli)
- Do not take rectal temperatures
- *(NIC) Circulatory Care (Venous Insufficiency)*
    Apply antiembolism stockings (e.g., elastic or pneumatic stockings), if appropriate

Cerebral

Assessments

- Monitor the following:
- Vital signs: temperature, BP, pulse, and respirations
- PO_2, PCO_2, pH, and bicarbonate levels
- $PaCO_2$, SaO_2, and hemoglobin levels to determine delivery of oxygen to tissues
- Pupil size, shape, symmetry, and reactivity
- Diplopia, nystagmus, blurred vision, and visual acuity
- Headache
- Level of consciousness and orientation
- Memory, mood, and affect
- Cardiac output
- Corneal, cough, and gag reflexes
- Muscle tone, motor movement, gait, and proprioception
- *(NIC) Intracranial Pressure (ICP) Monitoring:*
    Monitor patient's Intracranial pressure and neurological response to care activities
    Monitor cerebral perfusion pressure
    Note patient's change in response to stimuli
- *(NIC) Peripheral Sensation Management:*
    Monitor for paresthesia: numbness and tingling
    Monitor fluid status, including intake and output

Collaborative Activities

- Maintain hemodynamic parameters (e.g., systemic arterial pressure) within prescribed range
- Administer medications to expand intravascular volume, as ordered
- Induce hypertension to maintain cerebral perfusion pressure, as ordered
- Administer osmotic and loop diuretics, as ordered
- Elevate head of bed from 0–45 degrees, depending on patient's condition and medical orders

Other

- *(NIC) Circulatory Care (Venous Insufficiency)*: Apply antiembolism stockings (e.g., elastic or pneumatic stockings), if appropriate

Gastrointestinal

Assessments

- Monitor vital signs
- Monitor serum electrolyte levels
- Monitor for manifestations (e.g., neuromuscular) of electrolyte imbalance
- Monitor cardiac rhythm
- Keep accurate record of fluid intake and output
- Assess for signs of altered fluid and electrolyte balance (e.g., dry mucous membranes, cyanosis, and jaundice)
- *(NIC) Nutrition Management:*
  Monitor recorded intake for nutritional content and calories
  Weigh patient at appropriate intervals

Collaborative Activities

- Administer supplemental electrolytes, as ordered
- *(NIC) Nutrition Management:*
  Determine—in collaboration with dietitian, as appropriate—number of calories and type of nutrients needed to meet nutrition requirements
  Insert gastrointestinal tube, if needed (consult agency procedure manual or fundamentals text)
  Monitor gastric output and administer nasogastric replacement, per order
  Restrict food or fluid intake, if appropriate.

Renal

Assessments

- *(NIC) Fluid Management:*

  Observe hydration status (e.g., moist mucous membranes, adequacy of pulses, and orthostatic blood pressure)

  Monitor lab results relevant for fluid balance (e.g., hematocrit, BUN, albumin, total protein, serum osmolality, and urine specific gravity)

  Monitor lab results for fluid retention (e.g., increased specific gravity, increased BUN, decreased hematocrit, and increased urine osmolality)

  Observe for signs of fluid overload or retention (e.g., crackles, elevated CVP or pulmonary capillary wedge pressure, edema, neck vein distention, and ascites)

  Maintain accurate intake and output record

  Monitor vital signs

  Monitor patient's response to prescribed electrolyte therapy

  Weigh daily and monitor trends

  For hemodialysis patients:
- Monitor serum electrolyte levels
- Monitor blood pressure
- Weigh patient before and after procedure
- Monitor BUN, serum creatinine, serum electrolytes, and hematocrit levels between dialysis treatments
- Assess for signs of dialysis disequilibrium syndrome (e.g., headache, nausea and vomiting, hypertension, and altered level of consciousness)
- Observe for dehydration, muscle cramps, or seizure activity
- Assess for bleeding at the dialysis access site or elsewhere
- Observe for transfusion reaction, if appropriate
- Assess patency of arteriovenous fistula (e.g., palpate for pulse, auscultate for bruit)
- Assess mental status (e.g., consciousness, orientation)
- Monitor clotting times

  For peritoneal dialysis patients:
- Assess temperature, orthostatic BP, apical pulse, respirations, and lung sounds before dialysis
- Weigh patient daily
- Measure and record abdominal girth
- Note BUN, serum electrolyte, creatinine, pH, and hematocrit levels prior to dialysis and periodically during the procedure

- During instillation and dwell periods, observe for respiratory distress
- Record amount and type of dialysate instilled, dwell time, and amount and appearance of the drainage
- Monitor for signs of infection at exit site and in peritoneum

Patient/Family Teaching

- Explain all procedures and expected sensations to patient
- Explain the need for fluid restrictions, as needed

For dialysis patients:
- Teach patient signs and symptoms that indicate the need to contact a physician (e.g., fever, bleeding)
- Teach procedure to patients having home dialysis

Collaborative Activities

- Administer diuretics, as ordered
- Notify physician if signs and symptoms of fluid volume excess worsen

For hemodialysis patients:
- Administer heparin according to protocol and adjust dosage

Other

- Distribute prescribed fluid intake appropriately over 24-hr period
- Maintain fluid and diet restrictions (e.g., low sodium, no salt), as ordered

For hemodialysis patients:
- Do not perform venipunctures or take blood pressures on the arm with a fistula

For peritoneal dialysis patients:
- Use strict aseptic technique at all times
- Warm dialysate to body temperature before dialysis
- Place in semi-Fowler position and slow instillation rate if respiratory distress occurs

TISSUE PERFUSION (PERIPHERAL), INEFFECTIVE (00024) (1980, 1998)

Definition: Decrease in oxygen resulting in the failure to nourish the tissues at the capillary level

[**NOTE:** NANDA International includes *Ineffective peripheral tissue perfusion* with *Ineffective tissue perfusion (cerebral/gastrointestinal/renal)*.]

Defining Characteristics

Altered sensations
Altered skin characteristics (e.g., hair, nails, moisture)
Bruits
Blood pressure changes in extremities
Claudication
Delayed healing
Diminished arterial pulsations
Edema
Positive Homan sign
Skin color pale on elevation; does not return on lowering the leg
Skin discolorations
Skin temperature changes
Weak or absent pulses

Related Factors

Altered affinity of hemoglobin for oxygen
Decreased hemoglobin concentration in blood
Enzyme poisoning
Exchange problems
Hypervolemia
Hypoventilation
Hypovolemia
Impaired transport of the oxygen across alveolar or capillary membrane
Interruption of arterial flow
Interruption of venous flow
Mechanical reduction of venous or arterial blood flow
Mismatch of ventilation with blow flow
Table 10 provides help in identifying Ineffective tissue perfusion (peripheral)

Table 10

Objective Data	Chances that characteristics will be present in given diagnosis	Chances that characteristics will not be explained by any other diagnosis
Skin temperature: cold extremities	High	Low
Skin color: dependent blue or purple	Moderate	Low
Pale on elevation, color does not return on lowering leg	High	High
Diminished arterial pulsations	High	High
Skin quality shining	High	Low
Lack of lanugo; round scars covered with atrophied skin	High	Moderate
Gangrene	Low	High
Slow-growing, dry, brittle nails	High	Moderate
Claudication	Moderate	High
Blood pressure changes in extremities	Moderate	Moderate
Bruits	Moderate	Moderate
Slow healing of lesions	High	Low

Suggestions for Use

Because some of the nursing interventions are different, it is usually important to determine whether *Ineffective peripheral tissue perfusion* is of arterial or venous origin.

Suggested Alternative Diagnoses

Injury, risk for
Peripheral neurovascular dysfunction, risk for
Skin integrity, risk for impaired
Tissue integrity, impaired

NOC Outcomes

Sensory Function: Cutaneous: Extent to which the stimulation of the skin is sensed in an impaired area

Tissue Integrity: Skin and Mucous Membranes: Structural intactness and normal physiologic function of skin and mucous membranes

Tissue Perfusion: Peripheral: Extent to which blood flows through the small vessels of the extremities and maintains tissue function

Goals/Evaluation Criteria

Examples Using NOC Language

- Demonstrates **Fluid Balance**, as evidenced by the following indicators (specify 1–5: extremely, substantially, moderately, mildly, or not compromised):

    BP in expected range

    Peripheral pulses palpable

    Peripheral edema not present

    Skin hydration

- Demonstrates **Tissue Integrity: Skin and Mucous Membranes**, as evidenced by the following indicators (specify 1–5: extremely, substantially, moderately, mildly, or not compromised):

    Tissue temperature, sensation, elasticity, hydration, pigmentation, color, and thickness

    Tissue lesion-free

- Demonstrates **Tissue Perfusion: Peripheral**, as evidenced by the following indicators (specify 1–5: extremely, substantially, moderately, mildly, or not compromised):

    Proximal and distal peripheral pulses strong and symmetrical

    Sensation level normal

    Muscle function intact

    Skin intact, color normal

    Extremity temperature warm

    Localized extremity pain not present

Other Examples

    Patient will:

- Be able to describe plan for care at home

NIC Interventions

Circulatory Care: Arterial Insufficiency: Promotion of arterial circulation

Circulatory Care: Venous Insufficiency: Promotion of venous circulation

Embolus Care: Peripheral: Limitation of complications for a patient experiencing, or at risk for, occlusion of peripheral circulation

Neurologic Monitoring: Collection and analysis of patient data to prevent or minimize neurologic complications

Peripheral Sensation Management: Prevention or minimization of injury or discomfort in the patient with altered sensation

Skin Surveillance: Collection and analysis of patient data to maintain skin and mucous membrane integrity

Nursing Activities

Assessments

- *(NIC) Circulatory Care (Arterial and Venous):*
  Perform a comprehensive appraisal of peripheral circulation (e.g., check peripheral pulses, edema, capillary refill, color, and temperature of extremity)

  Assess degree of discomfort or pain

  Monitor fluid status, including intake and output

- *(NIC) Peripheral Sensation Management:*
  Monitor [peripherally] sharp or dull or hot or cold discrimination

  Monitor for paresthesia: numbness, tingling, hyperesthesia, and hypoesthesia

  Monitor for thrombophlebitis and deep vein thrombosis

  Monitor fit of bracing devices, prosthesis, shoes, and clothing

  Monitor position of body parts while bathing, sitting, lying, or changing position

  Examine skin daily for alteration in skin integrity

Patient/Family Teaching

Instruct patient and family about:

- Avoiding extremes of temperature to extremities
- The importance of adhering to diet and medication regimen
- Reportable signs and symptoms that may require notification of physician
- *(NIC) Circulatory Care (Arterial and Venous):*
  Proper foot care

  The importance of prevention of venous stasis (e.g., not crossing legs, elevating feet without bending knees, and exercise)

Collaborative Activities

- Give pain medications, notify physician if pain is unrelieved
- *(NIC) Circulatory Care (Arterial and Venous):* Administer antiplatelet or anticoagulant medications, as appropriate

Other

- Avoid chemical, mechanical, or thermal trauma to involved extremity

- Discourage smoking and use of stimulants
- *(NIC) Circulatory Care: Arterial:*
  Lower extremity to improve arterial circulation, as appropriate
- *(NIC) Circulatory Care: Venous:*
  Apply antiembolism stockings (e.g., elastic or pneumatic stockings), if appropriate
  Elevate affected limb 20 degrees or greater above the level of the heart to improve venous return, as appropriate
  Encourage passive or active range-of-motion exercises during bed rest, as appropriate
- *(NIC) Peripheral Sensation Management:*
  Avoid or carefully monitor use of heat or cold, such as heating pads, hot-water bottles, and ice packs
  Place cradle over affected body parts to keep bedclothes off affected areas
  Discuss or identify causes of abnormal sensations or sensation changes

TRANSFER ABILITY, IMPAIRED
(00090) (1998)

Definition: Limitation of independent movement between two nearby surfaces [specify level of independence]

Defining Characteristics

Objective
Impaired ability to transfer:
  From bed to chair and chair to bed
  On or off a toilet or commode
  Between uneven levels
  From chair to car or car to chair
  From chair to floor or floor to chair
  From standing to floor or floor to standing

Other Defining Characteristics (Non-NANDA International)
Cognitive impairment
Decreased muscle strength, control, or mass
Depressive mood state or anxiety
Developmental delay
Intolerance to activity, decreased strength and endurance
Joint stiffness or contractures
Lack of physical or social environmental supports

Limited cardiovascular endurance

Loss of integrity of bone structures

Medications

Musculoskeletal impairment

Neuromuscular impairment

Pain

Prescribed movement restrictions

Reluctance to initiate movement

Sedentary lifestyle or disuse or deconditioning

Selective or generalized malnutrition

Sensoriperceptual impairments

Related Factors

To be developed

Suggestions for Use

(1) Use *Impaired transfer ability* to describe individuals with limited ability for independent physical movement, such as decreased ability to move arms or legs or generalized muscle weakness, or when nursing interventions will focus on restoring mobility and function or preventing further deterioration. Do not use this label to describe temporary conditions that cannot be changed by the nurse (e.g., traction, prescribed bedrest, or permanent paralysis). When the patient's transfer ability cannot be improved, this label should be used as a related or risk factor for other nursing diagnoses, such as *Risk for falls*. (2) Specify level of mobility, using the same criteria as for *Impaired physical mobility*.

Level 0: Is completely independent

Level 1: Requires use of equipment or device

Level 2: Requires help from another person for assistance, supervision, or teaching

Level 3: Requires help from another person and equipment or device

Level 4: Is dependent; does not participate in activity

(3) See Suggestions for Use for Impaired Physical Mobility on p. 307.

Suggested Alternative Diagnoses

Disuse syndrome, risk for

Falls, risk for

Injury, risk for

Mobility: bed, impaired

Mobility: physical, impaired
Mobility: wheelchair, impaired
Self-care deficit
Walking, impaired

NOC Outcomes

Balance: Ability to maintain body equilibrium
Body Positioning: Self-Initiated: Ability to change own body positions
Mobility Level: Ability to move purposefully
Muscle Function: Adequacy of muscle contraction needed for movement
Transfer Performance: Ability to change body locations

Goals/Evaluation Criteria

- The patient will perform full range of motion of all joints
- The patient will transfer:
    From bed to chair or bed to standing
    To and from a toilet or commode
    From wheelchair to car or car to wheelchair
    From standing to floor or floor to standing

NIC Interventions

Exercise Promotion: Strength Training: Facilitating regular resistive muscle training to maintain or increase muscle strength
Exercise Therapy: Ambulation: Promotion and assistance with walking to maintain or restore autonomic and voluntary body functions during treatment and recovery from illness or injury
Exercise Therapy: Balance: Use of specific activities, postures, and movements to maintain, enhance, or restore balance
Exercise Therapy: Joint Mobility: Use of active or passive body movement to maintain or restore joint flexibility
Exercise Therapy: Muscle Control: Use of specific activity or exercise protocols to enhance or restore controlled body movement
Positioning: Wheelchair: Placement of a patient in a properly selected wheelchair to enhance comfort, promote skin integrity, and foster independence
Teaching: Psychomotor Skill: Preparing a patient to perform a psychomotor skill
Transport: Moving a patient from one location to another

Nursing Activities

Assessments

- Perform ongoing assessment of patient's transfer ability
- Assess need for assistance from home health agency or other placement service and assess need for durable medical equipment
- Assess vision, hearing, and proprioception
- *(NIC) Exercise Therapy: Muscle Control:*

  Determine patient's readiness to engage in activity or exercise protocol

  Determine accuracy of body image

  Monitor patient's emotional, cardiovascular, and functional responses to exercise protocol

  Monitor patient's self-exercise for correct performance

Patient/Family Teaching

- Instruct in active or passive range-of-motion exercises
- Give step-by-step directions
- Provide written information and diagrams
- Give frequent feedback to prevent formation of bad habits
- Provide information about assistive devices that may help with transfers
- Teach home caregivers how to incorporate balance and strength exercises into ADLs
- *(NIC) Exercise Therapy: Muscle Control:*

  Provide step-by-step cueing for each motor activity during exercise or ADLs

  Instruct patient to recite each movement as it is being performed

Collaborative Activities

- Use occupational and physical therapy as resources in developing plan to maintain or increase transfer mobility, plan should include balance and muscle-strengthening exercises

Other

- Position call light or button within easy reach
- Provide positive reinforcement during activities
- Implement pain control measures before beginning exercises or physical therapy
- Be sure care plan includes number of personnel needed to transfer patient
- Assist patient to transfer, as needed

- *(NIC) Exercise Therapy: Muscle Control:*
  Dress patient in nonrestrictive clothing
  Assist to maintain trunk or proximal joint stability during motor activity
  Reorient patient to movement functions of the body
  Incorporate ADLs into exercise protocol, if appropriate
  Assist patient to prepare and maintain a progress graph or chart to motivate adherence with exercise protocol

---

TRAUMA, RISK FOR
(00038) (1980)

Definition: Accentuated risk of accidental tissue injury (e.g., wound, burn, fracture)

Risk Factors
External (*Environmental*)

High-crime neighborhood and vulnerable clients; pot handles facing toward front of stove; use of thin or worn pot holders; knives stored uncovered; inappropriate call-for-aid mechanisms for bedresting client; inadequately stored combustibles or corrosives (e.g., matches, oily rags, lye); highly flammable children's toys or clothing; obstructed passageways; high beds; large icicles hanging from the roof; snow or ice collected on stairs, walkways; overexposure to sun, sunlamps, radiotherapy; overloaded electrical outlets; overloaded fuse boxes; play or work near vehicle pathways (e.g., driveways, laneways, railroad tracks); playing with fireworks or gunpowder; guns or ammunition stored unlocked; contact with rapidly moving machinery, industrial belts, or pulleys; litter or liquid spills on floors or stairways; defective appliances; bathing in very hot water (e.g., unsupervised bathing of young children); bathtub without handgrip or antislip equipment; children playing with matches, candles, cigarettes, sharp-edged toys; children playing without gates at the top of the stairs; delayed lighting of gas burner or oven; contact with intense cold; grease waste collected on stoves; children riding in the front seat in car; driving a mechanically unsafe vehicle; driving after partaking of alcoholic beverages or drugs; nonuse or misuse of seat restraints; driving at excessive speeds; driving without necessary visual aids; entering unlighted rooms; experimenting with chemical or gasoline; exposure to dangerous machinery; faulty electrical plugs; frayed wires; unanchored electric wires; contact with acids or alkalis; unsturdy or absent stair rails; use of unsteady ladders or chairs; use of cracked dishware or glasses; wearing plastic apron or flowing clothes around open flame; unscreened fires or heaters; unsafe window protection in homes with young children; sliding on coarse bed linen or struggling within bed restraints; misuse of necessary headgear for motorized cyclists or young children carried on adult bicycles; potential igniting gas leaks; unsafe road or road-crossing conditions; slippery floors (e.g., wet or highly waxed); smoking in bed or near oxygen; unanchored rugs

Internal (Individual)

Weakness, poor vision, balancing difficulties, reduced temperature or tactile sensation, reduced large or small muscle coordination, reduced hand-eye coordination, lack of safety education, lack of safety precautions, insufficient finances to purchase safety equipment or effect repairs, cognitive or emotional difficulties, history of previous trauma

Suggestions for Use

Use a more specific diagnosis when possible.

Suggested Alternative Diagnoses

Aspiration, risk for
Home maintenance, impaired
Falls, risk for
Injury, risk for
Perioperative positioning injury, risk for
Poisoning, risk for

NOC Outcomes

Knowledge: Personal Safety: Extent of understanding conveyed about preventing unintentional injuries

Safety Behavior: Fall Prevention: Individual or caregiver actions to minimize risk factors that might precipitate falls

Safety Behavior: Home Physical Environment: Individual or caregiver actions to minimize environmental factors that might cause physical harm or injury in the home

Safety Behavior: Personal: Individual or caregiver efforts to control behaviors that might cause physical injury

Safety Status: Falls Occurrence: Number of falls in the past week

Safety Status: Physical Injury: Severity of injuries from accidents and trauma

Tissue Integrity: Skin and Mucous Membranes: Structural intactness and normal physiological function of skin and mucous membranes

Goals/Evaluation Criteria

Examples Using NOC Language

- Demonstrates **Safety Behavior: Home Physical Environment**, as evidenced by the following indicators (specify 1–5: not, slightly, moderately, substantially, or totally adequate):

  Smoke detector maintenance

  Provision of accessible telephone

  Disposal of unused medicines

  Storage of firearms to prevent accidents

  Arrangement of furniture to reduce risks

  Removal of unused refrigerator and freezer doors

  Provision of age-appropriate toys

  Use of electrical outlet covers

  Placement of window guards as needed

- Practices **Safety Behavior: Fall Prevention**, as evidenced by the following indicators (specify 1–5: not, slightly, moderately, substantially, or totally adequate):

  Correct use of assistive devices

  Placement of barriers to prevent falls

  Placement of handrailings, as needed

  Elimination of clutter, spills, glare from floors

  Taking down rugs

  Arrangement for removal of snow and ice from walking surfaces

  Use of rubber mats and grab bars in tub or shower

  Use of precautions when taking medications that increase risk for falls

  Use of vision-correcting devices

Other Examples

- Patient will avoid physical injury

NIC Interventions

Environmental Management: Safety: Monitoring and manipulation of the physical environment to promote safety

Pressure Management: Minimizing pressure to body parts

Skin Surveillance: Collection and analysis of patient data to maintain skin and mucous membrane integrity

Teaching: Infant Safety: Instruction on safety during the first year of life

Teaching: Toddler Safety: Instruction on safety during the second and third years of life

Vehicle Safety Promotion: Assisting individuals, families, and communities to increase awareness of measures to reduce unintentional injuries in motorized and nonmotorized vehicles

Nursing Activities

Assessments

- *(NIC) Environmental Management: Safety:*
  Identify the safety needs of the patient based on level of physical and cognitive function and past history of behavior
  Identify safety hazards in the environment (i.e., physical, biological, and chemical)

Patient/Family Teaching

- Instruct patient and family in safety measures specific to risk area
- Provide educational materials related to strategies for prevention of trauma
- Provide information on environmental hazards and characteristics (e.g., stairs, windows, cupboard locks, swimming pools, streets, or gates)

Collaborative Activities

- Refer to educational classes in the community (e.g., CPR, first aid, or swimming)
- *(NIC) Environmental Management: Safety:* Assist patient in relocating to safer environment (e.g., referral for housing assistance)

Other

- *(NIC) Environmental Management: Safety:*
  Modify the environment to minimize hazards and risk
  Provide adaptive devices (e.g., step stools and handrails) to increase the safety of the environment
  Use protective devices (e.g., restraints, side rails, locked doors, fences, and gates) to physically limit mobility or access to harmful situations

UNILATERAL NEGLECT
(00123) (1986)

Definition: Lack of awareness and attention to one side of the body

Defining Characteristics

Objective
Consistent inattention to stimuli on affected side
Does not look toward affected side
Inadequate self-care
Leaves food on plate on affected side
Inadequate positioning or safety precautions in regard to the affected side

Related Factors

Effects of disturbed perceptual abilities (e.g., hemianopsia)
Neurologic illness or trauma
One-sided blindness

Other Related Factors (Non-NANDA International)
Anesthesia of one side of the body (i.e., hemianesthesia)
Blindness in half of the field of vision in one or both eyes (i.e., hemianopia)
Paralysis of one side of body (i.e., hemiplegia)
Real or pretended ignorance of presence of paralysis (i.e., anosognosia)
Weakness of one side of body (i.e., hemiparesis)

Suggestions for Use

Unilateral neglect may occur with medical conditions such as brain injuries, cerebral aneurysms or tumors, and cerebrovascular accidents. There are usually other nursing diagnoses associated with the pathophysiology of *Unilateral neglect*, for example, those in the following section, Suggested Alternative Diagnoses.

Suggested Alternative Diagnoses

Anxiety
Injury, risk for
Self-care deficit
Sensory perception, disturbed

NOC Outcomes

Body Image: Positive perception of own appearance and body functions

Body Positioning: Self-Initiated: Ability to change own body positions

Self-Care: Activities of Daily Living (ADLs): Ability to perform the most basic physical tasks and personal care activities

Goals/Evaluation Criteria

Examples Using NOC Language

- Demonstrates **Body Image**, as evidenced by the following indicators (specify 1–5: never, rarely, sometimes, often, or consistently positive):

    Positive internal picture of self

    Congruence between body reality, body ideal, and body presentation

    Adjustment to changes in body function

- Performs **Self-Care: Activities of Daily Living (ADLs)**, as evidenced by the following indicators (specify 1–5: dependent; does not participate, requires assistive person and device; requires assistive person, independent with assistive device; or completely independent): eating, dressing, toileting, bathing, grooming, hygiene, ambulation, and transfer

Other Examples

Patient will:

- Be able to change own body positions (specify: lying to sitting, sitting to lying, kneeling to standing, and so forth)
- Acknowledge extent of deficit
- Modify behavior and environment to accommodate deficit
- Demonstrate improving perception of environment
- Not experience falls or other accidents

NIC Interventions

Self-Care Assistance: Assisting another to perform activities of daily living

Unilateral Neglect Management: Protecting and safely reintegrating the affected part of the body while helping the patient adapt to disturbed perceptual abilities

Nursing Activities

Assessments

- Assess the nature and extent of deficit
- *(NIC) Unilateral Neglect Management:* Monitor for abnormal responses to three primary types of stimuli: sensory, visual, and auditory

Patient/Family Teaching

- Explain and reinforce nature and extent of deficit to patient and family
- Provide information about community resources
- *(NIC) Unilateral Neglect Management:* Instruct caregivers on the cause, mechanisms, and treatment of unilateral neglect

Collaborative Activities

- *(NIC) Unilateral Neglect Management:* Consult with occupational and physical therapists concerning timing and strategies to facilitate reintegration of neglected body parts and function

Other

- Provide visual, olfactory, and tactile stimulation
- *(NIC) Unilateral Neglect Management:*
  Provide realistic feedback about patient's perceptual deficit
  Touch unaffected shoulder when initiating conversation
  Place food and beverages within field of vision and turn plate, as necessary
  Rearrange the environment to use the right or left visual field, such as positioning personal items, television, or reading materials within view on unaffected side
  Gradually move personal items and activity to affected side as patient demonstrates an ability to compensate for neglect
  Assist patient to bathe and groom affected side first as patient demonstrates an ability to compensate for neglect
  Keep side rail up on affected side, as appropriate
  Ensure that affected extremities are properly and safely positioned
  Include family in rehabilitation process to support the patient's efforts and assist with care, as appropriate

URINARY ELIMINATION, IMPAIRED
(00016) (1973)

Definition: Disturbance in urine elimination

Defining Characteristics

Subjective
Dysuria
Urgency
Objective
Frequency
Hesitancy
Incontinence
Nocturia
Retention

Related Factors

Multiple causality, including anatomic obstruction, sensory or motor impairment, urinary tract infection

Suggestions for Use

Use a more specific label when possible. For specific patient outcomes, evaluation criteria, and nursing interventions, refer to the following Section, Suggested Alternative Diagnoses.

Suggested Alternative Diagnoses

Urinary incontinence, functional
Urinary incontinence, reflex
Urinary incontinence, stress
Urinary incontinence, total
Urinary incontinence, urge
Urinary incontinence, urge, risk for
Urinary retention

NOC Outcomes

Urinary Continence: Control of the elimination of urine
Urinary Elimination: Ability of the urinary system to filter wastes, to conserve solutes, and to collect and discharge urine in a healthy pattern

Goals/Evaluation Criteria

Examples Using NOC Language

- Demonstrates **Urinary Continence**, as evidenced by the following indicators (specify 1–5: never, rarely, sometimes, often, or consistently positive):

    Able to toilet independently

    Absence of urinary tract infection ($<$ 100,000 WBC)

    Voids $>$ 150 cc each time

    Predictable pattern to passage of urine

Other Examples

- Urine continence
- Demonstration of adequate knowledge of medications that affect urinary function
- Urinary elimination not compromised:

    Urine odor, amount, and color in expected range

    No hematuria

    Passes urine without pain, hesitancy, or urgency

    BUN, serum creatinine, and specific gravity WNL

    Urine proteins, glucose, ketones, pH, and electrolytes WNL

NIC Interventions

Urinary Bladder Training: Improving bladder function for those with urge incontinence by increasing the bladder's ability to hold urine and the patient's ability to suppress urination

Urinary Elimination Management: Maintenance of an optimum urinary elimination pattern

Urinary Incontinence Care: Assistance in promoting continence and maintaining perineal skin integrity

Nursing Activities

Also refer to Nursing Activities for the preceding Suggested Alternative Diagnoses.

Assessments

- *(NIC) Urinary Elimination Management:*

    Monitor urinary elimination, including frequency, consistency, odor, volume, and color, as appropriate

    Obtain midstream voided specimen for urinalysis, as appropriate

Patient/Family Teaching

- *(NIC) Urinary Elimination Management:*

    Teach patient signs and symptoms of urinary tract infection

    Instruct patient and family to record urinary output, as appropriate

Instruct patient to respond immediately to urge to void

Teach patient to drink 8 oz of liquid with meals, between meals, and in early evening

Collaborative Activities

• *(NIC) Urinary Elimination Management*: Refer to physician if signs and symptoms of urinary tract infection occur

---

URINARY ELIMINATION, READINESS FOR ENHANCED (00166) (2002)

Definition: A pattern of urinary functions that is sufficient for meeting elimination needs and can be strengthened

Defining Characteristics

Subjective

Expresses willingness to enhance urinary elimination

Objective

Urine is straw colored with no odor

Specific gravity is within normal limits

Amount of output is within normal limits for age and other factors

Positions self for emptying of bladder

Fluid intake is adequate for daily needs

Suggestions for Use

None

Suggested Alternative Diagnoses

None

NOC Outcomes

Not yet developed; however, the following may be useful:

Urinary Elimination: Ability of the urinary system to filter wastes, to conserve solutes, and to collect and discharge urine in a healthy pattern

Goals/Evaluation Criteria

Examples Using NOC Language

• Demonstrates **Urinary Elimination**, as evidenced by the following indicators (specify 1–5: extremely, substantially, moderately, mildly, or not compromised):

Free of urine leakage between voidings [5]

Empties bladder completely [5]
Absence of postvoid residual >100–200 cc [5]
Fluid intake in expected range [5]

Other Examples

Patient will:

- Describe plan for enhancing urinary function
- Remain free of urinary tract infection
- Have a balanced 24-hr intake and output
- Report normal amount and characteristics of urine
- Demonstrate adequate knowledge of medications that affect urinary function
- Experience normal urinary elimination:
    Urine odor, amount, and color in expected range
    No hematuria
    Passes urine without pain, hesitancy, or urgency
    BUN, serum creatinine, and specific gravity within normal limits
    Urine proteins, glucose, ketones, pH, and electrolytes within normal limits

NIC Interventions

Not yet developed; however, the following may be useful:

Urinary Elimination Management: Maintenance of an optimum urinary elimination pattern

Nursing Activities

Assessments

- Identify and document patient's bladder evacuation pattern
- Inquire about use of prescription and nonprescription medications with anticholinergic or alpha agonist properties
- *(NIC) Urinary Elimination Management:*
    Monitor urinary elimination, including frequency, consistency, odor, volume, and color, as appropriate

Patient/Family Teaching

- Provide information about normal urinary functioning
- Provide information about fluid requirements, regular voiding, and so forth
- *(NIC) Urinary Elimination Management:*
    Teach patient signs and symptoms of urinary tract infection
    Instruct patient to respond immediately to urge to void
    Teach patient to drink 8 oz of liquid with meals, between meals, and in early evening

Other

- Assist to make plan for improving urinary function
- Encourage oral intake of fluids: ____ cc for day; ____ cc for evening; _____ cc for nights

---

URINARY INCONTINENCE, FUNCTIONAL
(00020) (1986, 1998)

Definition: Inability of usually continent person to reach toilet in time to avoid unintentional loss of urine

Defining Characteristics

Able to completely empty bladder

Amount of time required to reach toilet exceeds length of time between sensing urge and uncontrolled voiding

Loss of urine before reaching toilet

May only be incontinent in early morning

Senses need to void

Related Factors

Altered environmental factors

Impaired cognition

Impaired vision

Neuromuscular limitations

Psychologic factors

Weakened supporting pelvic structures

Suggestions for Use

None

Suggested Alternative Diagnoses

Urinary incontinence, reflex

Urinary incontinence, stress

Urinary incontinence, total

Urinary incontinence, urge

Self-care deficit: toileting

Urinary elimination, impaired

Urinary retentions

NOC Outcomes

Tissue Integrity: Skin and Mucous Membranes: Structural intactness and normal physiological function of skin and mucous membranes

Urinary Continence: Control of the elimination of urine

Urinary Elimination: Ability of the urinary system to filter wastes, to conserve solutes, and to collect and discharge urine in a healthy pattern

Goals/Evaluation Criteria

Examples Using NOC Language

- Demonstrates **Urinary Continence**, as evidenced by the following indicators (specify 1–5: never, rarely, sometimes, often, or consistently demonstrated):

    Recognizes urge to void

    Adequate time to reach toilet between urge and evacuation of urine

    Underclothing dry during day

    Underclothing or bedding dry during night

    Able to toilet independently

    Predictable pattern to passage of urine

Other Examples

Patient will:

- Use adaptive equipment to help with clothing and transfers when incontinence is related to impaired mobility

NIC Interventions

Perineal Care: Maintenance of perineal skin integrity and relief of perineal discomfort

Prompted Voiding: Promotion of urinary continence through the use of timed verbal toileting reminders and positive social feedback for successful toileting

Urinary Elimination Management: Maintenance of an optimum urinary elimination pattern

Urinary Habit Training: Establishing a predictable pattern of bladder emptying to prevent incontinence for persons with limited cognitive ability who have urge, stress, or functional incontinence

Urinary Incontinence Care: Assistance in promoting continence and maintaining perineal skin integrity

Nursing Activities

Assessments

- *(NIC) Urinary Incontinence Care:*

    Identify multifactorial causes of incontinence (e.g., urinary output, voiding pattern, cognitive function, preexistent urinary problems, postvoid residual, and medications)

    Monitor urinary elimination, including frequency, consistency, odor, volume, and color

    Obtain urine for culture and sensitivity testing, as needed

Patient/Family Teaching

- Discuss with patient and family ways to modify environment to reduce number of wetness episodes, consider the following strategies:

    Improving environmental lighting to enhance vision

    Installing raised toilet seat and hand rails

    Providing bedside commode, bedpan, and handheld urinal

    Removing loose rugs

- Instruct patient and family in prompted voiding routine (frequent reminders) based on patient's pattern of toileting to decrease wetness episodes

- Instruct patient and family in skin care and hygiene routine to prevent skin breakdown

- Offer strategies for bladder management during activities away from home

- *(NIC) Urinary Incontinence Care:*

    Explain etiology of problem and rationale for actions

    Discuss procedures and expected outcomes with patient

    Instruct patient and family to record urinary output and pattern, as appropriate

    Instruct patient to drink a minimum of 1500 ml fluids a day

Collaborative Activities

- Consult with physical and occupational therapy for assistance with manual dexterity

- *(NIC) Urinary Incontinence Care:* Refer to urinary continence specialist, as appropriate

Other

- *(NIC) Urinary Habit Training:*

    Establish interval of initial toileting schedule, based on voiding pattern

    Toilet patient or remind patient to void at prescribed intervals

Use power of suggestion (e.g., running water or flushing toilet) to assist patient to void

Avoid leaving patient on toilet for more than 5 min

Reduce toileting interval by one-half hour if more than three incontinence episodes in 24 hr

Increase toileting interval by 1 hr if patient is unable to void at two or more scheduled toileting times

Increase the toileting interval by 1 hr if patient has no incontinence episodes for three days until optimal 4-hr interval is achieved

- *(NIC) Urinary Incontinence Care:*

Assist to develop and maintain a sense of hope

Modify clothing and environment to provide easy access to toilet [e.g., obtain clothing that is easily removed; substitute elastic waistbands and Velcro for zippers, buttons, snap devices, and hooks, whenever feasible]

Provide protective garments, as needed

Cleanse genital skin area at regular intervals

Provide positive feedback for any decrease in episodes of incontinence

Schedule diuretic administration to have least impact on lifestyle

URINARY INCONTINENCE, REFLEX
(00018) (1986, 1998)

Definition: Involuntary loss of urine occurring at somewhat predictable intervals when a specific bladder volume is reached

Defining Characteristics

Subjective

Incomplete emptying with lesion above sacral micturition center

No sensation of bladder fullness

No sensation of urge to void

No sensation of voiding

Sensation of urgency without voluntary inhibition of bladder contraction

Sensations associated with full bladder, such as sweating, restlessness, and abdominal discomfort

Objective

Complete emptying with lesion above pontine micturition center

Predictable pattern of voiding

Unable to cognitively inhibit or initiate voiding

Related Factors

Neurological impairment above level of sacral micturition center or pontine micturition center

Tissue damage from radiation cystitis, inflammatory bladder conditions, or radical pelvic surgery

Suggestions for Use

None

Suggested Alternative Diagnoses

Urinary incontinence, functional

Urinary incontinence, stress

Urinary incontinence, total

Urinary incontinence, urge

Self-care deficit: toileting

Urinary elimination, impaired

Urinary retention

NOC Outcomes

Neurological Status: Autonomic: Extent to which the autonomic nervous system coordinates visceral function

Tissue Integrity: Skin and Mucous Membranes: Structural intactness and normal physiological function of skin and mucous membranes

Urinary Continence: Control of the elimination of urine

Urinary Elimination: Ability of the urinary system to filter wastes, to conserve solutes, and to collect and discharge urine in a healthy pattern

Goals/Evaluation Criteria

Also see NOC examples for Urinary Incontinence, Functional p. 594.

Examples Using NOC Language

- Demonstrates **Urinary Continence**, as evidenced by the following indicators (specify 1–5: never, rarely, sometimes, often, or consistently demonstrated):

    Voids in appropriate receptacle

    Voids > 150 ml each time

    Absence of urinary tract infection (< 100,000 WBC)

Other Examples

Patient will:

- Be free of skin breakdown
- Demonstrate intermittent self-catheterization procedure

NIC Interventions

Perineal Care: Maintenance of perineal skin integrity and relief of perineal discomfort

Urinary Bladder Training: Improving bladder function for those with urge incontinence by increasing the bladder's ability to hold urine and the patient's ability to suppress urinarion

Urinary Catheterization, Intermittent: Regular periodic use of a catheter to empty the bladder

Urinary Elimination Management: Maintenance of an optimum urinary elimination pattern

Urinary Habit Training: Improving bladder function for those with urge incontinence by increasing the bladder's ability to hold urine and the patient's ability to suppress urination

Urinary Incontinence Care: Assistance in promoting continence and maintaining perineal skin integrity

Nursing Activities

Assessments

- Assess for ability to recognize urge to void
- Identify voiding pattern (either voiding after specified intake or voiding after a specified interval)
- Monitor technique of patient and caregivers who perform intermittent catheterization
- For patients undergoing intermittent catheterization, monitor color, odor, and clarity of urine and perform frequent urinalysis to monitor for infection
- Determine patient's readiness and ability to perform intermittent self-catheterization
- *(NIC) Urinary Habit Training*: Keep a continence specification record for three days to establish voiding pattern

Patient/Family Teaching

- Teach patient and family reportable signs and symptoms of autonomic dysreflexia, such as severe hypertension, severe headache, diaphoresis above level of injury, tachycardia of sudden onset

- Teach patient, family, and caregivers technique for clean intermittent catheterization
- Teach signs and symptoms of urinary tract infection (e.g., fever, chills, flank pain, hematuria, and change in consistency and odor of urine)

Collaborative Activities

- Refer to enterostomal therapy nurse for instruction in clean intermittent self-catheterization, as appropriate
- Administer antibacterial therapy, per medical order, at initiation of intermittent catheterization

Other

- Assist patient in maintaining adequate hygiene and skin care routine, consider the following strategies:
    Applying moisture barrier ointment or skin sealant
    Keeping skin dry
    Using collection device for urine
- Consider condom catheter collection device with leg bag
- Remind the patient to try to hold urine until scheduled elimination time
- Maintain fluid intake of approximately 2000 ml/day

For intermittent urinary catheterization:
- Provide quiet room and privacy for procedure
- Use clean or sterile technique (per protocol) for catheterization
- Determine catheterization schedule, based on assessment of voiding patterns
- If output of > 300 ml is obtained (for adults), catheterize more frequently
- *(NIC) Urinary Habit Training:*
    Establish interval of initial toileting schedule, based on voiding pattern
    Toilet patient or remind patient to void at prescribed intervals
    Use power of suggestion (e.g., running water or flushing toilet) to assist patient to void
    Avoid leaving patient on toilet for more than 5 min
    Reduce toileting interval by one-half hour if more than three incontinence episodes occur in 24 hr
    Increase toileting interval by 1 hr if patient is unable to void at two or more scheduled toileting times
    Increase the toileting interval by 1 hr if patient has no incontinence episodes for three days until optimal 4-hr interval is achieved

URINARY INCONTINENCE, STRESS
(00017) (1986)

Definition: Loss of less than 50 ml of urine occurring with increased abdominal pressure

Defining Characteristics

Subjective
Reported dribbling with increased abdominal pressure
Urinary urgency

Objective
Observed dribbling with increased abdominal pressure
Urinary frequency (more often than every 2 hr)

Related Factors

Degenerative changes in pelvic muscles and structural supports associated with increased age
High intra-abdominal pressure (e.g., obesity, gravid uterus)
Incompetent bladder outlet
Overdistention between voidings
Weak pelvic muscles and structural supports

Suggestions for Use

None

Suggested Alternative Diagnoses

Urinary incontinence, functional
Urinary incontinence, reflex
Urinary incontinence, total
Urinary incontinence, urge
Self-care deficit: toileting
Urinary elimination, impaired
Urinary retention

NOC Outcomes

Tissue Integrity: Skin and Mucous Membranes: Structural intactness and normal physiological function of skin and mucous membranes
Urinary Continence: Control of the elimination of urine
Urinary Elimination: Ability of the urinary system to filter wastes, to conserve solutes, and to collect and discharge urine in a healthy pattern

Goals/Evaluation Criteria

Also see NOC examples for Urinary Incontinence, Functional p. 594.

Examples Using NOC Language

- Demonstrates **Urinary Continence**, as evidenced by the following indicators (specify 1–5: never, rarely, sometimes, often, or consistently demonstrated): No urine leakage with increased abdominal pressure (e.g., sneezing, laughing, lifting)

Other Examples

Patient will:
- Describe a plan for treating the stress incontinence
- Maintain a voiding frequency of more than q2h

NIC Interventions

Perineal Care: Strengthening and training the levator ani and urogenital muscles through voluntary, repetitive contraction to decrease stress, urge, or mixed types of urinary incontinence

Pelvic Muscle Exercise: Strengthening the levator ani and urogenital muscles through voluntary, repetitive contraction to decrease stress, urge, or mixed incontinence

Urinary Elimination Management: Maintenance of an optimum urinary elimination pattern

Urinary Incontinence Care: Instituting a program to promote continence and to maintain perineal skin integrity

Nursing Activities

See Nursing Activities for Urinary Incontinence, Functional pp. 595–596.

Patient/Family Teaching

- Instruct patient in hygiene and skin care measures
- Teach self-administration of oral or topical estrogens to ameliorate symptoms
- Teach techniques that strengthen the sphincter and structural supports of the bladder (e.g., pelvic muscle exercises, urine stop-and-start exercises)
- Inform patient that it may require several weeks of exercising to obtain improvement

Collaborative Activities

- Consult with physician regarding surgical or medical management of incontinent episodes

Other

- Assist patient to select appropriate garment or pad for short-term incontinence management
- Give positive feedback for doing pelvic floor exercises
- (NIC) Urinary Incontinence Care: Limit ingestion of bladder irritants (e.g., cola, coffee, tea, and chocolate)

URINARY INCONTINENCE, TOTAL
(00021) (1986)

Definition: Continuous and unpredictable loss of urine

Defining Characteristics

Subjective

Unawareness of incontinence

Objective

Constant flow of urine occurs at unpredictable times without distention or uninhibited bladder contractions or spasms

Lack of perineal or bladder-filling awareness

Nocturia

Unsuccessful incontinence refractory treatments

Related Factors

Anatomic (fistula)

Independent contraction of detrusor reflex due to surgery

Neurologic dysfunction causing triggering of micturition at unpredictable times

Neuropathy preventing transmission of reflex indicating bladder fullness

Trauma or disease affecting spinal cord nerves

Suggestions for Use

None

Suggested Alternative Diagnoses

Self-care deficit: toileting

Urinary elimination, impaired

Urinary incontinence, functional

Urinary incontinence, reflex

Urinary incontinence, stress

Urinary incontinence, urge

Urinary retention

NOC Outcomes

Tissue Integrity: Skin and Mucous Membranes: Structural intactness and normal physiological function of skin and mucous membranes

Urinary Continence: Control of the elimination of urine

Urinary Elimination: Ability of the urinary system to filter wastes, to conserve solutes, and to collect and discharge urine in a healthy pattern

Goals/Evaluation Criteria

Also see NOC examples for Urinary Incontinence, Functional p. 594.

Examples Using NOC Language

- Demonstrates **Urinary Continence**, as evidenced by the following indicators (specify 1–5: never, rarely, sometimes, often, or consistently demonstrated):

    Responds in timely manner to urge

    Absence of urinary tract infection ($< 100,000$ WBC)

Other Examples

Patient and family will:

- Maintain adequate skin integrity
- Describe a plan of care for indwelling (i.e., Foley) catheter at home

NIC Interventions

Perineal Care: Maintenance of perineal skin integrity and relief of perineal discomfort

Urinary Elimination Management: Maintenance of an optimum urinary elimination pattern

Urinary Incontinence Care: Institution of a program to promote continence and to maintain perineal skin integrity

Nursing Activities

See Nursing Activities for Urinary Incontinence, Functional on pp. 595–596.

Assessments

- Assess patient for presence of fistula (i.e., urethral, vaginal, rectovaginal)
- Assess patient for skin breakdown and maintenance of adequate hygiene and skin care routine

Patient/Family Teaching

- Instruct patient and family in use of indwelling catheter management at home
- Instruct patient and family to report signs and symptoms of urinary tract infection (e.g., fever, chills, flank pain, hematuria, and change in consistency and odor of urine)

Collaborative Activities

- Consult physician about use of indwelling catheter

Other

- For skin care, consider the following measures:
  Ensure skin is adequately dried
  Apply moisture barrier, ointment, or skin sealant
- *NIC Urinary Incontinence Care:* Limit fluids for 2–3 hrs before bedtime, as appropriate

---

URINARY INCONTINENCE, URGE
(00019) (1986)

Definition: Involuntary passage of urine occurring soon after a strong sense of urgency to void

Defining Characteristics

Subjective
Bladder contraction or spasm
Objective
Frequency (voiding more often than every 2 hr)
Inability to reach toilet in time
Nocturia (urination more than two times per night)
Urinary urgency
Voiding in small amounts (less than 100 ml) or in large amounts (more than 500 ml)

Related Factors

Alcohol
Caffeine
Decreased bladder capacity (e.g., history of pelvic inflammatory disease, abdominal surgery, indwelling urinary catheter)
Increased fluid intake
Increased urine concentration

Irritation of bladder stretch receptors, causing spasm (e.g., bladder infection)

Overdistention of bladder

Suggestions for Use

None

Suggested Alternative Diagnoses

Self-care deficit: toileting

Urinary elimination, impaired

Urinary incontinence, functional

Urinary incontinence, reflex

Urinary incontinence, stress

Urinary incontinence, total

Urinary retention

NOC Outcomes

Tissue Integrity: Skin and Mucous Membranes: Structural intactness and normal physiological function of skin and mucous membranes

Urinary Continence: Control of the elimination of urine

Urinary Elimination: Ability of the urinary system to filter wastes, to conserve solutes, and to collect and discharge urine in a healthy pattern

Goals/Evaluation Criteria

Also see NOC examples for Urinary Incontinence, Functional p. 594.

Examples Using NOC Language

• Demonstrates **Urinary Continence**, as evidenced by the following indicators (specify 1–5: never, rarely, sometimes, often, or consistently demonstrated):

Responds in timely manner to urge

Free of medications that interfere with urinary control

Maintains environment barrier-free to independent toileting

Urine passes without urgency

Other Examples

Patient will:

• Describe bladder management program to restore satisfactory urinary elimination pattern

• Have less frequent incontinent episodes

NIC Interventions

Perineal Care: Maintenance of perineal skin integrity and relief of perineal discomfort

Urinary Elimination Management: Maintenance of an optimum urinary elimination pattern

Urinary Habit Training: Establishing a predictable pattern of bladder emptying to prevent incontinence for persons with limited cognitive ability who have urge, stress, or functional incontinence

Urinary Incontinence Care: Institution of a program to promote continence and to maintain perineal skin integrity

Nursing Activities

See Nursing Activities for Urinary Incontinence, Functional pp. 595–596.

Patient/Family Teaching

- Instruct patient regarding techniques that will increase bladder capacity, such as initiating pelvic floor raising when feeling the urge to void and using a bladder-training schedule that lengthens the time between voids
- *(NIC) Urinary Incontinence Care:*
  Explain etiology of problem and rationale for actions
  Discuss procedures and expected outcomes with patient

Collaborative Activities

- Consult with physical and occupational therapists for assistance with manual dexterity
- Consult with physician regarding: (1) antispasmodic and anticholinergic medications and (2) medical management (e.g., electrostimulation therapy, investigation of underlying irritative or inflammatory bladder disorders, and surgical therapy)

Other

- Assist patient to void prior to sleep and encourage nighttime voids to reduce urgency
- Provide bedpan, bedside commode, and urinal nearby to encourage frequent voiding episodes

URINARY INCONTINENCE: URGE, RISK FOR (00022) (1998)

Definition: At risk for involuntary loss of urine associated with a sudden, strong sensation of urinary urgency

Risk Factors

Detrusor hyperreflexia from cystitis, urethritis, tumors, renal calculi, central nervous system disorders above pontine micturition center

Detrusor muscle instability with impaired contractility

Effects of medications, caffeine, or alcohol

Ineffective toileting habits

Involuntary sphincter relaxation

Small bladder capacity

Suggestions for Use

None

Suggested Alternative Diagnoses

Incontinence, urinary, urge

NOC Outcomes

Urinary Continence: Control of the elimination of urine

Urinary Elimination: Ability of the urinary system to filter wastes, to conserve solutes, and to collect and discharge urine in a healthy pattern

Goals/Evaluation Criteria

See Goals/Evaluation Criteria for Urinary Incontinence, Urge p. 605.

NIC Interventions

Urinary Bladder Training: Improving bladder function for those with urge incontinence by increasing the bladder's ability to hold urine and the patient's ability to suppress urination

Urinary Elimination Management: Maintenance of an optimum urinary elimination pattern

Urinary Habit Training: Establishing a predictable pattern of bladder emptying to prevent incontinence for persons with limited cognitive ability who have urge, stress, or functional incontinence

Nursing Activities

Assessments

- Assess for risk factors (see Risk Factors above)
- Evaluate environment for barriers to timely toileting
- Assess patient's self-care abilities and mobility
- *(NIC) Urinary Incontinence Care*: Monitor urinary elimination, including frequency, consistency, odor, volume, and color

Patient/Family Teaching

- Instruct patient regarding techniques that will increase bladder capacity, such as initiating pelvic floor raising when feeling the urge to void and using a bladder-training schedule that lengthens the time between voids
- Discuss with patient and family ways to modify environment to remove obstacles and improve self-care ability, consider the following strategies:

  Improving environmental lighting to enhance vision

  Installing a raised toilet seat and hand rails

  Providing a bedside commode, bedpan, and handheld urinal

  Using assistive devices (e.g., wheelchairs, canes, walkers, and nonskid walking shoes)

Collaborative Activities

- Consult with physical and occupational therapists for assistance with manual dexterity

Other

- Obtain clothing that is easily removed
- Substitute elastic waistbands and Velcro for zippers, buttons, snap devices, and hooks, whenever feasible
- Assist patient to void prior to sleep and encourage nighttime voids to reduce urgency
- Discourage use of bladder irritants, such as caffeine, alcohol, citrus juices, carbonated drinks, cigarette smoke, and certain spicy foods

URINARY RETENTION
(00023) (1986)

Definition: Incomplete emptying of the bladder

Defining Characteristics

Subjective
Dysuria
Sensation of bladder fullness
Objective
Bladder distention
Dribbling
Overflow incontinence
Residual urine
Small, frequent voiding or absence of urine output

Related Factors

Blockage
High urethral pressure caused by weak detrusor
Inhibition of reflex arc
Strong sphincter

Suggestions for Use

None

Suggested Alternative Diagnoses

Urinary incontinence, functional
Urinary incontinence, stress
Urinary incontinence, urge
Urinary elimination, impaired

NOC Outcomes

Urinary Continence: Control of the elimination of urine
Urinary Elimination: Ability of the urinary system to filter wastes, to conserve solutes, and to collect and discharge urine in a healthy pattern

Goals/Evaluation Criteria

Examples Using NOC Language

- Demonstrates **Urinary Continence**, as evidenced by the following indicators (specify 1–5: never, rarely, sometimes, often, or consistently positive):

    Free of urine leakage between voidings

Empties bladder completely
Absence of postvoid residual >100–200 cc
Fluid intake in expected range

Other Examples

Patient will:

- Demonstrate bladder evacuation by clean intermittent self-catheterization procedure
- Describe plan of care at home
- Remain free of urinary tract infection
- Report a decrease in bladder spasms
- Have a balanced 24-hr intake and output

NIC Interventions

Urinary Bladder Training: Improving bladder function for those with urge incontinence by increasing the bladder's ability to hold urine and the patient's ability to suppress urination

Urinary Catheterization: Insertion of a catheter into the bladder for temporary or permanent drainage of urine

Urinary Catheterization: Intermittent: Regular periodic use of a catheter to empty the bladder

Urinary Elimination Management: Maintenance of an optimum urinary elimination pattern

Urinary Retention Care: Assistance in relieving bladder distention

Nursing Activities

Assessments

- Identify and document patient's bladder evacuation pattern
- *(NIC) Urinary Retention Care:*

  Monitor use of nonprescription agents with anticholinergic or alpha agonist properties

  Monitor effects of prescribed pharmaceuticals, such as calcium channel blockers and anticholinergics

  Monitor intake and output

  Monitor degree of bladder distention by palpation and percussion

Patient/Family Teaching

- Instruct patient in reportable signs and symptoms of urinary tract infection (e.g., fever, chills, flank pain, hematuria, and change in consistency and odor of urine)
- *(NIC) Urinary Retention Care:* Instruct patient and family to record urinary output, as appropriate

Collaborative Activities

- Refer to enterostomal therapy nurse for instruction in clean intermittent self-catheterization q4–6 hours while awake.
- *(NIC) Urinary Retention Care:* Refer to urinary continence specialist, as appropriate

Other

- Establish a bladder-evacuation training program
- Space fluids throughout the day to ensure adequate intake without bladder overdistention
- Encourage oral intake of fluids: ____ cc for day; ____ cc for evening; ____ cc for nights
- *(NIC) Urinary Retention Care:*

  Provide privacy for elimination

  Use the power of suggestion by running water or flushing the toilet

  Stimulate the reflex bladder by applying cold to the abdomen, stroking the inner thigh, or running water

  Provide enough time for bladder emptying (10 min)

  Use spirits of wintergreen in bedpan or urinal

  Provide Crede maneuver, as necessary

  Catheterize for residual, as appropriate

  Insert urinary catheter, as appropriate

VENTILATORY WEANING RESPONSE, DYSFUNCTIONAL (DVWR) (00034) (1992)

Definition: Inability to adjust to lowered levels of mechanical ventilator support that interrupts and prolongs the weaning process

Defining Characteristics

Nurses have defined three levels of DVWR in which these defining characteristics occur in response to weaning (Logan & Jenny, 1991).

Mild DVWR

Subjective

Breathing discomfort

Expressed feelings of increased need for oxygen

Fatigue

Queries about possible machine malfunction

Warmth

Objective

Increased concentration on breathing

Restlessness

Slight increase in respiratory rate from baseline

Warmth

Moderate DVWR

Subjective

Apprehension

Objective

Color changes; pale, slight cyanosis

Decreased air entry on auscultation

Diaphoresis

Eye widening (wide-eyed look)

Hypervigilance to activities

Inability to cooperate

Inability to respond to coaching

Baseline increase in respiratory rate < 5 breaths per minute

Slight increase from baseline BP < 20 mmHg

Slight increase from baseline heart rate < 20 BPM

Slight respiratory accessory muscle use

Severe DVWR

Objective

Adventitious breath sounds, audible airway secretions

Agitation

Cyanosis

Decreased level of consciousness

Deterioration in ABG from current baseline data

Discoordinated breathing with the ventilator

Full respiratory accessory muscle use

Increase from baseline BP > 20 mmHg

Increase from baseline heart rate > 20 BPM

Paradoxical abdominal breathing

Profuse diaphoresis

Respiratory rate increases significantly from baseline

Shallow, gasping breaths

Related Factors

Physiological

Inadequate nutrition

Ineffective airway clearance

Sleep pattern disturbance

Uncontrolled pain or discomfort

Situational

Adverse environment (e.g., noisy, active environment, negative events in the room, low nurse–patient ratio, extended nurse absence from bedside, unfamiliar nursing staff)

History of multiple unsuccessful weaning attempts

History of ventilator dependence > 1 week

Inadequate social support

Inappropriate pacing of diminished ventilator support

Uncontrolled episodic energy demands or problems

Psychological

Anxiety: moderate, severe

Decreased motivation

Decreased self-esteem

Fear

Hopelessness

Insufficient trust in the nurse

Knowledge deficit of the weaning process

Patient perceived inefficacy about the ability to wean

Patient role

Powerlessness

Suggestions for Use

DVWR is concerned specifically with patient responses to separation from the mechanical ventilator. Other respiratory diagnoses may also occur during weaning, for example, *Ineffective airway clearance, Ineffective breathing pattern,* and *Impaired gas exchange.* This diagnostic label does not include the reasons for the weaning problems. If you do not know the etiology of the *DVWR,* use unknown etiology.

Suggested Alternative Diagnoses

Airway clearance, ineffective

Breathing pattern, ineffective

Gas exchange, impaired

NOC Outcomes

Anxiety Control: Personal actions to eliminate or reduce feelings of apprehension and tension from an unidentifiable source

Respiratory Status: Gas Exchange: Alveolar exchange of CO_2 or O_2 to maintain ABG concentrations

Respiratory Status: Ventilation: Movement of air in and out of the lungs

Vital Signs Status: Temperature, pulse, respiration, and BP within expected range for the individual

Goals/Evaluation Criteria

Examples Using NOC Language

- Demonstrates **Vital Signs Status**, as evidenced by the following indicators (specify 1–5: extreme, substantial, moderate, mild, or no deviation from expected range): temperature, apical and radial pulse rate, respiration rate, and systolic and diastolic BP
- Demonstrates **Respiratory Status: Gas Exchange**, as evidenced by the following indicators (specify 1–5: extremely, substantially, moderately, mildly, or not compromised):

    Neurologic status in expected range

    Chest x-ray findings in expected range

    PaO_2, $PaCO_2$, arterial pH, and O_2 saturation WNL
- Demonstrates **Respiratory Status: Ventilation**, as evidenced by the following indicators (specify 1–5: extremely, substantially, moderately, mildly, or not compromised):

    Restlessness, cyanosis, and fatigue not present

    Accessory muscle use not present

    Chest retraction not present

    Shortness of breath and dyspnea not present

Other Examples

Patient will:

- Achieve established weaning goals
- Be physiologically stable for weaning process
- Be psychologically and emotionally ready for weaning process

NIC Interventions

Airway Management: Facilitation of patency of air passages

Artificial Airway Management: Maintenance of endotracheal and tracheostomy tubes and preventing complications associated with their use

Mechanical Ventilation: Use of an artificial device to assist a patient to breathe

Mechanical Ventilatory Weaning: Assisting the patient to breathe without the aid of a mechanical ventilator

Respiratory Monitoring: Collection and analysis of patient data to ensure airway patency and adequate gas exchange

Ventilation Assistance: Promotion of an optimal spontaneous breathing pattern that maximizes oxygen and carbon dioxide exchange in the lungs

Vital Signs Monitoring: Collection and analysis of cardiovascular, respiratory, and body temperature data to determine and prevent complications

Nursing Activities

Assessments

- Assess patient's readiness to wean by considering the following respiratory indicators:

    ABG stable with PaO_2 > 60 on 40–60% oxygen

    Maximum inspiratory force > −20 cm H_2O so independent respiration can be initiated

    Unassisted tidal volume > 5 ml/kg ideal body weight

    Vital capacity > 13 ml/kg ideal body weight

    Stable spontaneous respiratory rate < 30 breaths per minute

    Cough effective enough to handle secretions

    Length of time on ventilator

- Assess patient's readiness to wean by considering the following nonrespiratory indicators:

    Absence of constipation, diarrhea, or ileus

    Absence of fever and infection

    Adequate nutritional status as evidenced by acceptable serum albumin and transferrin and midarm muscle circumference > 15th percentile

    Adequate rest and sleep

    Hemoglobin and hematocrit WNL for patient

    Improvements in body strength and endurance

    Normal BP for patient

    Psychologic and emotional readiness

    Satisfactory fluid and electrolyte balance

    Stable heart rate and rhythm

    Tolerable pain or discomfort level

- Determine why previous weaning attempts were unsuccessful, if applicable

- Monitor patient's response to current medications and correlate response with weaning goals

- *(NIC) Mechanical Ventilatory Weaning:*

  Monitor degree of shunt, vital capacity, V_d/V_t, mandatory minute ventilation (MMV), inspiratory force, and FEV_1 for readiness to wean from mechanical ventilation, based on agency protocol

  Monitor for signs of respiratory muscle fatigue (e.g., abrupt rise in $PaCO_2$ level; rapid, shallow ventilation; and paradoxical abdominal wall motion), hypoxemia, and tissue hypoxia while weaning is in process

Patient/Family Teaching

- Instruct patient and family in weaning process and goals, which should include:

  How patient may feel as process evolves

  Participation of family

  Participation required by patient

  What patient can expect from nurse

  Reasons why weaning is necessary

- *(NIC) Mechanical Ventilatory Weaning:* Assist the patient to distinguish spontaneous breaths from mechanically delivered breaths

Collaborative Activities

- Discuss weaning process and goals with physician and respiratory care practitioner, including patient's present and preexisting medical conditions

- *(NIC) Mechanical Ventilatory Weaning:* Collaborate with other health team members to optimize patient's nutritional status, ensuring that 50% of the diet's nonprotein calorie source is fat, rather than carbohydrate

Other

- Encourage self-care to increase sense of control and participation in own care

- Normalize ADLs to patient's tolerance level

- Establish a trusting relationship that instills patient's confidence in nurse to assist patient with weaning process

- Establish effective methods of communication between patient and others (e.g., writing, blinking eyes, squeezing hand)

- Initiate weaning process by:

  Checking equipment to make sure it is attached to oxygen and that settings are correct

  Checking for presence of bilateral breath sounds

  Checking tubing for kinks and excessive moisture

Checking vital signs and patient for indicators of nontolerance or fatigue q5–15 minutes

Documenting weaning process and patient's tolerance

Explaining procedure to patient and family

Measuring and recording baseline respiratory rate, heart rate, BP, ECG rhythm, lung sounds, vital capacity, tidal volume, inspiratory force, and saturated oxygen via pulse oximeter

Preoxygenating, hyperinflating, suctioning, and reoxygenating patient prior to weaning

Providing a quiet environment during weaning time

Providing diversions such as television or radio

Sitting patient in an upright position to decrease abdominal pressure on the diaphragm and allow for better lung expansion

Starting the weaning time when patient has rested and is awake and alert

Staying with patient during weaning time to provide coaching and reassurance

Understanding the rationale for weaning orders (e.g., use of continuous positive airway pressure [CPAP], synchronized intermittent mandatory ventilation [SIMV], pressure support ventilation [PSV], and MMV, or T-piece)

- Reconnect patient to ventilator at preweaning settings if indicators of nontolerance occur
- Document in nursing care plan those strategies that promote success with weaning process to ensure consistency (e.g., communication method with patient, family participation, and coaching methods)
- *(NIC) Mechanical Ventilatory Weaning:*

Alternate periods of weaning trials with sufficient periods of rest and sleep

Avoid delaying return of patient with fatigued respiratory muscles to mechanical ventilation

Set a schedule to coordinate other patient care activities with weaning trials

Use relaxation techniques, as appropriate

VIOLENCE: OTHER-DIRECTED,
RISK FOR (00138) (1980, 1996)

Definition: At risk for behaviors in which an individual demonstrates that he can be physically, emotionally, or sexually harmful to others

Risk Factors

Objective

Availability or possession of weapon(s)

Body language: rigid posture, clenching of fists and jaw, hyperactivity, pacing, breathlessness, threatening stances

Cognitive impairment (e.g., learning disabilities, attention-deficit disorder, decreased intellectual functioning)

Cruelty to animals

Fire setting

History of childhood abuse

History of drug or alcohol abuse

History of violence against others (e.g., hitting someone, kicking someone, spitting at someone, scratching someone, throwing objects at someone, biting someone, attempted rape, rape, sexual molestation, urinating or defecating on a person)

History of threats of violence (e.g., verbal threats against property, verbal threats against person, social threats, cursing, threatening notes or letters, threatening gestures, sexual threats)

History of violence, indirect (e.g., tearing off clothes, ripping objects off walls, writing on walls, urinating on floor, defecating on floor, stamping feet, temper tantrum, running in corridors, yelling, throwing objects, breaking a window, slamming doors, sexual advances)

History of violent antisocial behavior (e.g., stealing, insistent borrowing, insistent demand for privileges, insistent interruption of meetings, refusal to eat, refusal to take medication, ignoring instructions)

History of witnessing family violence

Impulsivity

Motor vehicle offenses (e.g., frequent traffic violations, use of a motor vehicle to release anger)

Neurologic impairment (e.g., positive EEG, CAT or MRI, head trauma, positive neurologic findings, seizure disorders)

Pathological intoxication

Prenatal and perinatal complications or abnormalities

Psychotic symptomatology (e.g., auditory, visual, command hallucinations; paranoid delusions; loose, rambling, or illogical
thought processes)

Suicidal behavior

Other Risk Factors (Non-NANDA International)

Arrest or conviction pattern

Catatonic excitement

History of abuse by spouse

Manic excitement

Toxic reactions to medications

Suggestions for Use

Use this diagnosis for patients who need nursing interventions
for the purpose of protecting others and preventing or decreasing
violent episodes. The diagnosis *Disabled family coping* may be
more useful for situations in which there is domestic violence. If
the need is to focus on *Anxiety* or *Low self-esteem,* consider using
those suggested alternative diagnoses.

Suggested Alternative Diagnoses

Anxiety

Coping: family, compromised

Coping, ineffective

Self-esteem, chronic low

Self-esteem, situational low

NOC Outcomes

Abusive Behavior Self-Control: Self-restraint of own behaviors to
avoid abuse and neglect of dependents or significant others

Aggression Control: Self-restraint of assaultive, combative, or
destructive behavior toward others

Distorted Thought Control: Self-restraint of disruption in perception, thought processes, and thought content

Impulse Control: Self-restraint of compulsive or impulsive behavior

Risk Control: Alcohol Use: Actions to eliminate or reduce alcohol
use that poses a threat to health

Risk Control: Drug Use: Actions to eliminate or reduce drug use
that poses a threat to health

ls/Evaluation Criteria

mples Using NOC Language

Demonstrates **Aggression Control**, as evidenced by the following indicators (specify 1–5: never, rarely, sometimes, often, or consistently demonstrated):

> Refrains from:
> Verbal outbursts
> Striking others
> Violating others' personal space
> Harming others; harming animals
> Destroying property
> Identifies when angry, frustrated, or feeling aggressive
> Vents negative feelings [e.g., anger, frustration] appropriately

- Demonstrates **Impulse Control**, as evidenced by the following indicators (specify 1–5: never, rarely, sometimes, often, or consistently demonstrated):

> Identifies feelings or behaviors that lead to impulsive actions
> Identifies consequences of impulsive actions to self or others
> Avoids high-risk environments and situations
> Verbalizes control of impulses

Other Examples

Patient will:
- Identify factors that precipitate violent behaviors
- Identify alternative ways to cope with problems
- Identify support systems in the community
- Not abuse others physically, emotionally, or sexually

NIC Interventions

Abuse Protection Support: Identification of high-risk, dependent relationships and actions to prevent further infliction of physical or emotional harm

Anger Control Assistance: Facilitation of the expression of anger in an adaptive nonviolent manner

Environmental Management: Violence Prevention: Monitoring and manipulation of the physical environment to decrease the potential for violent behavior directed toward self, others, or environment

Impulse Control Training: Assisting the patient to mediate impulsive behavior through application of problem-solving strategies to social and interpersonal situations

Nursing Activities

Assessments

- Identify behaviors that signal impending violence against others, specify behaviors
- *(NIC) Anger Control Assistance:* Monitor potential for inappropriate aggression and intervene before its expression
- *(NIC) Environmental Management: Violence Prevention:*
  Monitor the safety of items being brought to the environment by visitors
  Monitor patient during use of potential weapons (e.g., razor)

Patient/Family Teaching

- *(NIC) Anger Control Assistance:* Instruct on use of calming measures (e.g., time-outs and deep breaths)

Collaborative Activities

- Clarify use of 72-hr hold for evaluation and treatment in psychiatric unit in the event of abuse against others
- Confer with physician on use of appropriate restraining measures when necessary to prevent injury to others
- Follow hospital or agency policy regarding legal responsibility for reporting abuse to authorities
- Initiate a multidisciplinary patient care conference to develop a plan of care

Other

- Encourage patient to verbalize anger
- Identify situations that provoke violence, specify situations
- Provide positive feedback when patient adheres to behavior limits
- *(NIC) Anger Control Assistance:*
  Use a calm, reassuring approach
  Limit access to frustrating situations until patient is able to express anger in an adaptive manner
  Encourage patient to seek assistance of nursing staff or responsible others during periods of increasing tension
  Prevent physical harm if anger is directed at self or others (e.g., restrain and remove potential weapons)
  Provide physical outlets for expression of anger or tension (e.g., punching bag, sports, clay, and writing in a journal)
  Identify consequences of inappropriate expression of anger
  Establish expectation that patient can control his behavior

Assist in developing appropriate methods of expressing anger to others (e.g., assertiveness and use of feeling statements)
- *(NIC) Environmental Management: Violence Prevention:*
Assign single room to patient with potential for violence toward others
Place patient in a room near nursing station
Limit access to windows, unless locked and shatterproof, as appropriate
Place patient in least restrictive environment that allows for necessary level of observation
Maintain a designated safe area (e.g., seclusion room) for patient to be placed when violent
Provide plastic, rather than metal, clothes hangers, as appropriate
Provide paper dishes and plastic utensils at meals

VIOLENCE: SELF-DIRECTED, RISK FOR
(00140) (1994)

Definition: At risk for behaviors in which an individual demonstrates that he can be physically, emotionally, or sexually harmful to self

Risk Factors

Age 15–19
Age over 45
Behavioral clues (e.g., writing forlorn love notes, directing angry messages at a significant other who has rejected the person, giving away personal items, taking out a large life insurance policy)
Conflictual interpersonal relationships
Emotional status (e.g., hopelessness, despair, increased anxiety, panic, anger, hostility)
Employment (e.g., unemployed, recent job loss or failure)
Family background (e.g., chaotic or conflictual, history of suicide)
History of multiple suicide attempts
Marital status (e.g., single, widowed, divorced)
Mental health (e.g., severe depression, psychosis, severe personality disorder, alcoholism, or drug abuse)
Occupation (e.g., executive, administrator or owner of business, professional semiskilled worker)
People who engage in autoerotic sexual acts
Personal resources (e.g., poor achievement, poor insight, affect unavailable and poorly controlled)

Physical health (e.g., is hypochondriac, chronic, or terminal illness)

Sexual orientation (e.g., bisexual [active], homosexual [inactive])

Social resources (e.g., poor rapport, socially isolated, unresponsive family)

Suicidal ideation (frequent, intense, prolonged)

Suicidal plan (clear and specific, lethality, method and availability of destructive means)

Verbal clues (e.g., talking about death, better off without me, asking questions about lethal dosages and drugs)

Suggestions for Use

If the specific risk factors for *Risk for self-mutilation* or *Risk for suicide* are present, the more specific nursing diagnosis should be used instead of *Risk for self-directed violence.*

Suggested Alternative Diagnoses

Self-mutilation, risk for

Suicide, Risk for

NOC Outcomes

Depression Control: Personal actions to minimize melancholy and maintain interest in life events

Depression Level: Severity of melancholic mood and loss of interest in life events

Distorted Thought Control: Self-Restraint of disruption in perception, thought processes, and thought content

Impulse Control: Self-restraint of compulsive or impulsive behavior

Self-Mutilation Restraint: Ability to refrain from intentional self-inflicted injury (nonlethal)

Suicide Self-Restraint: Ability to refrain from gestures and attempts at killing self

Goals/Evaluation Criteria

Examples Using NOC Language

- Demonstrates **Impulse Control**, as evidenced by the following indicators:

    Vents negative feelings appropriately

    Identifies feelings or behaviors that lead to impulsive actions

    Identifies consequences of impulsive actions to self or others

    Avoids high-risk environments and situations

    Verbalizes control of impulses

Other Examples

Patient will:

- Identify alternative ways to cope with problems
- Identify support systems in the community
- Report a decrease in suicidal thoughts
- Not attempt suicide
- Not harm self

NIC Interventions

Anger Control Assistance: Facilitation of the expression of anger in an adaptive nonviolent manner

Behavior Management: Self-Harm: Assisting the patient to decrease or eliminate self-mutilating or self-abusive behaviors

Environmental Management: Violence Prevention: Monitoring and manipulation of the physical environment to decrease the potential for violent behavior directed toward self, others, or environment

Hope Instillation: Facilitation of the development of a positive outlook in a given situation

Impulse Control Training: Assisting the patient to mediate impulsive behavior through application of problem-solving strategies to social and interpersonal situation

Suicide Prevention: Reducing risk of self-inflicted harm with intent to end life

Nursing Activities

Assessments

- Assess and document patient's potential for suicide q _____
- Identify behaviors that signal impending violence against self, specify behaviors
- *(NIC) Environmental Management: Violence Prevention:*
  Monitor the safety of items being brought to the environment by visitors
  Monitor patient during use of potential weapons (e.g., razor)

Patient/Family Teaching

- *(NIC) Anger Control Assistance:* Instruct on use of calming measures (e.g., time-outs and deep breaths)

Collaborative Activities

- Clarify use of 72-hr hold for evaluation and treatment in psychiatric unit in the event of abuse against self

- Confer with physician on use of appropriate restraining measures when necessary to prevent injury to self
- Initiate a multidisciplinary patient care conference to develop a plan of care

Other

- Institute suicide precautions, as needed (e.g., 24-hr attendant)
- Reassure patient that you will protect him against own suicidal impulses until able to regain control by: (1) constantly observing patient, (2) frequently checking patient, and (3) taking patient's suicidal ideation seriously
- Discuss with patient and family the role of anger in self-harm
- Encourage patient to verbalize anger
- *(NIC) Anger Control Assistance:*
  Use a calm, reassuring approach
  Limit access to frustrating situations until patient is able to express anger in an adaptive manner
  Encourage patient to seek assistance of nursing staff or responsible others during periods of increasing tension
  Prevent physical harm if anger is directed at self (e.g., restrain and remove potential weapons)
  Provide physical outlets for expression of anger or tension (e.g., punching bag, sports, clay, and writing in a journal)
  Establish expectation that patient can control his behavior
- *(NIC) Environmental Management: Violence Prevention:*
  Place patient with potential for self-harm with a roommate to decrease isolation and opportunity to act on self-harm thoughts, as appropriate
  Place patient in a room near nursing station
  Limit access to windows, unless locked and shatterproof, as appropriate
  Place patient in least restrictive environment that allows for necessary level of observation
  Apply mitts, splints, helmets, or restraints to limit mobility and ability to initiate self-harm, as appropriate
  Provide plastic, rather than metal, clothes hangers, as appropriate
  Provide paper dishes and plastic utensils at meals

WALKING, IMPAIRED
(00088) (1998)

Definition: Limitation of independent movement within the environment on foot [specify level]

Defining Characteristics

Impaired ability to:
>Climb stairs
>Navigate curbs
>Walk on an incline or decline
>Walk on uneven surfaces
>Walk required distances

Related Factors

>To be developed

Non-NANDA International Related Factors
Altered cellular metabolism
Cognitive impairment
Cultural beliefs regarding age-appropriate activity
Decreased muscle strength, control, or mass
Depressive mood state or anxiety
Developmental delay
Intolerance to activity, decreased strength and endurance
Joint stiffness or contractures
Lack of knowledge regarding value of physical activity
Lack of physical or social environmental supports
Limited cardiovascular endurance
Loss of integrity of bone structures
Medications
Musculoskeletal impairment
Neuromuscular impairment
Pain
Reluctance to initiate movement
Sedentary lifestyle, disuse, or deconditioning
Selective or generalized malnutrition
Sensoriperceptual impairments

Suggestions for Use

As with other mobility diagnoses, the author recommends specifying the patient's functional level, as follows:

Level 0: Completely independent

Level 1: Requires use of equipment or device

Level 2: Requires help from another person for assistance, supervision, or teaching

Level 3: Requires help from another person and equipment or device

Level 4: Dependent; does not participate in activity

Use *Impaired walking* to describe individuals with limited ability for independent physical movement or generalized muscle weakness or when nursing interventions will focus on restoring mobility and function or preventing further deterioration. An example of an appropriate diagnosis would be *Impaired walking related to ineffective management of chronic pain secondary to rheumatoid arthritis.* If immobility problems in addition to *Impaired Walking* exist, consider using *Impaired Physical Mobility.*

Do not use this label to describe temporary immobility that cannot be changed by the nurse (e.g., traction, prescribed bed rest) or permanent paralysis. *Impaired walking* may be used effectively as the etiology of a nursing diagnosis, for example, *Self-care deficit: toileting related to impaired walking* +4.

Suggested Alternative Diagnoses

Disuse syndrome, risk for

Injury, risk for

Mobility, physical, impaired

Self-care deficit

Transfer ability, impaired

NOC Outcomes

Ambulation: Walking: Ability to walk from place to place

Endurance: Extent that energy enables a person to sustain activity

Joint Movement: Active: Range of motion of joints with self-initiated movement

Mobility Level: Ability to move purposefully

Self-Care: Activities of Daily Living (ADLs): Ability to perform the most basic physical tasks and personal care activities

Goals/Evaluation Criteria

Examples Using NOC Language

- Will not have *Impaired Walking,* as demonstrated by: Ambulation: Walking, Endurance, Active Joint Movement, Mobility Level, and Self-Care: Activities of Daily Living (ADLs)

- Demonstrates **Mobility Level**, as evidenced by the following indicators (specify 1–5: dependent, does not participate, requires assistive person and device, requires assistive person, is independent with assistive device, or is completely independent):

  Balance performance

  Body positioning performance

  Muscle and joint movement

  Transfer performance

  Ambulation: walking

Other Examples

Patient will:

- Bear weight and walk with adequate gait
- Walk a distance appropriate to his overall condition
- Demonstrate correct use of assistive devices (e.g., crutches, cane) with supervision
- Request assistance with mobilization activities, as needed
- Perform ADLs independently with assistive devices (specify activity and device)

NIC Interventions

Energy Management: Regulating energy use to treat or prevent fatigue and optimize function

Exercise Therapy, Ambulation: Promotion and assistance with walking to maintain or restore autonomic and voluntary body functions during treatment and recovery from illness or injury

Exercise Therapy, Joint Mobility: Use of active or passive body movement to maintain or restore joint flexibility

Self-Care Assistance: Assisting another to perform activities of daily living

Nursing Activities

Assessments

Assessment is an ongoing process to determine the performance level at which the patient's mobility is impaired.

Level 1 Nursing Activities

- Provide positive reinforcement during activities
- Collaborate with physical therapist in developing strength, balance, and flexibility exercises
- Assess need for assistance from home health agency and need for durable medical equipment

- *(NIC) Exercise Therapy: Ambulation:*

  Monitor patient's use of crutches or other walking aids

  Instruct patient how to position self throughout the transfer process

  Apply or provide assistive device (e.g., cane, walker, or wheelchair) for ambulation if the patient is unsteady

  Assist patient to use footwear that facilitates walking and prevents injury

  Encourage independent ambulation within safe limits

Level 2 Nursing Activities

- Assess patient's learning needs regarding _____ (specify)
- Assess need for assistance from home health agency and need for durable medical equipment
- Instruct and encourage patient in active or passive range-of-motion exercises
- Instruct patient regarding weight-bearing status
- Instruct patient regarding correct body alignment
- Instruct and encourage patient to use a trapeze or weights to enhance and maintain strength of upper extremities
- Use occupational and physical therapy as resources in developing a plan for maintaining or increasing mobility
- Provide positive reinforcement during activities
- Supervise all mobilization attempts
- *(NIC) Exercise Therapy: Ambulation:*

  Instruct patient and caregiver about safe transfer and ambulation techniques

  Assist patient to stand and ambulate specified distance with specified number of staff

Levels 3 and 4 Nursing Activities

- Use occupational and physical therapy as resources in planning patient care activities
- Encourage patient and family to view limitations realistically
- Provide positive reinforcement during activities
- Develop a plan to include the following:

  Perform passive range-of-motion (PROM) or assisted range-of-motion (AROM) exercises, as indicated

  Type of assistive device

  Number of personnel needed to mobilize patient

  Schedule of activities

  Maximization of patient's mobility, given necessary constraints

- Assess patient motivation level for overcoming limitations
- Administer analgesics before beginning exercises or walking, as needed
- *(NIC) Exercise Therapy: Ambulation:*
  Use a gait belt to assist with transfer and ambulation, as needed

---

WANDERING

(00154) (2000)

Definition: Meandering, aimless, or repetitive locomotion that exposes the individual to harm; frequently incongruent with boundaries, limits, or obstacles

Defining Characteristics

Objective

Following behind or shadowing a caregiver's locomotion

Frequent or continuous movement from place to place, often revisiting the same destinations

Fretful locomotion or pacing

Getting lost

Haphazard locomotion

Hyperactivity

Inability to locate significant landmarks in a familiar setting

Locomotion into unauthorized or private spaces

Locomotion that cannot be easily dissuaded or redirected

Long periods of locomotion without an apparent destination

Periods of locomotion interspersed with periods of nonlocomotion (e.g., sitting, standing, sleeping)

Persistent locomotion in search of missing or unattainable people or places

Scanning, seeking, or searching behaviors

Trespassing

Related Factors

Cognitive impairment (specifically: memory and recall deficits, disorientation, poor visuoconstructive [or visuospatial] ability, language [primarily expressive] defects)

Cortical atrophy

Premorbid behavior (e.g., outgoing, sociable personality; premorbid dementia)

Separation from familiar people and places

Sedation

Emotional state, especially frustration, anxiety, boredom, or depression (agitation)

Over- or understimulating social or physical environment

Physiological state or need (e.g., hunger or thirst, pain, urination, constipation)

Time of day

Suggestions for Use

Wandering may occur as a result of psychosocial diagnoses such as *Confusion* and *Disturbed thought processes.* If defining characteristics of *Wandering* are present, it should be used instead of the broader diagnoses.

Suggested Alternative Diagnoses

Confusion, acute

Confusion, chronic

Environmental interpretation syndrome, impaired

Injury, risk for

Thought processes, disturbed

NOC Outcomes

NOC outcomes have not yet been developed; however, the following may be useful:

Cognitive Ability: Ability to execute complex mental processes

Information Processing: Ability to acquire, organize, and use information

Safety Status: Physical Injury: Severity of injuries from accidents and trauma

Symptom Severity: Extent of perceived adverses changes in physical, emotional, and social functioning

Goals/Evaluation Criteria

Examples Using NOC Language

- Demonstrates **Safety Status: Physical Injury,** as evidenced by the following indicators (specify 1–5: severe, substantial, moderate, slight, or none):

    Skin abrasions

    Bruises

    Lacerations

    Burns

    Open head injuries

Extremity [or other] fractures

Extremity [or back] sprains

Dental injuries

- Demonstrates **Cognitive Ability,** as evidenced by the following indicators (specify 1–5: extremely, substantially, moderately, mildly, or not compromised):

Demonstrates control over selected events

Processes information

Demonstrates immediate, recent, and remote memory

Makes appropriate decisions

Attentiveness

Other Examples

Patient will:

- Not wander into unauthorized or private places
- Not become lost
- Not leave the building (if institutionalized)
- Walk only on agreed-upon safe route

NIC Interventions

NIC interventions have not been developed for *Wandering;* however, the following may be useful:

Anxiety Reduction: Minimizing apprehension, dread, foreboding, or uneasiness related to an unidentified source of anticipated danger

Area Restriction: Limitation of patient mobility to a specified area for purposes of safety or behavior management

Calming Technique: Reducing anxiety in patient experiencing acute distress

Delirium Management: Provision of a safe and therapeutic environment for the patient who is experiencing an acute confusional state

Dementia Management: Provision of a modified environment for the patient who is experiencing a chronic confusional state

Elopement Precautions: Minimizing the risk of a patient leaving a treatment setting without authorization when departure presents a threat to the safety of patient or others

Environmental management: Manipulation of the patient's surroundings for therapeutic benefit

Surveillance: Safety: Purposeful and ongoing collection and analysis of information about the patient and the environment for use in promoting and maintaining patient safety

Nursing Activities

Assessments

- Assess for factors that create the risk for *Wandering* (e.g., confusion, agitation, anxiety)
- *(NIC) Environmental Management:*
  Identify the safety needs of patient, based on level of physical and cognitive function and past history of behavior
- *(NIC) Elopement Precautions:*
  Monitor patient for indicators of elopement potential (e.g., verbal indicators, loitering near exits, multiple layers of clothing, disorientation, separation anxiety, and homesickness)
- *(NIC) Dementia Management:*
  Determine type and extent of cognitive deficit(s), using standardized assessment tool

Patient/Family Teaching

- Explain to family and friends how best to interact with a confused person or a person with delirium or dementia
- Explain to the family the purpose or precautions such as area restriction, identification bands, increased supervision, gates, physical restraints, and so forth
- Provide information about ways to make the home safe for the patient

Collaborative Activities

- *(NIC) Elopement Precautions:*
  Clarify the legal status of patient (e.g., minor or adult and voluntary or court-ordered treatment)
  Communicate risk to other care providers

Other

- Use locks or gates on doors and windows, or electronic buzzers at property boundaries.
- Notify neighbors about the patient's wandering, and give them instructions for notifying if they see the person wandering
- Avoid restraints, if possible; use pressure-sensitive alarms instead (e.g., chair or bed sensors)
- Provide a consistent, familiar environment (e.g., avoid room changes and unfamiliar people)
- Mark patient's boundaries clearly (e.g., with brightly colored tape on the floor, signs on the door, and so forth)

- *(NIC) Dementia Management:*
  Provide space for safe pacing and wandering
  Place identification bracelet on patient
- *(NIC) Elopement Precautions:*
  Familiarize patient with environment and routine to decrease anxiety
  Limit patient to a physically secure environment (e.g., locked or alarmed doors at exits and locked windows), as needed
  Increase supervision or surveillance when patient is outside secure environment (e.g., hold hands and increase staff-to-patient ratio)
  Record physical description (e.g., height, weight, eye, hair, and skin color, and any distinguishing characteristics [for reference, should patient elope])
- *(NIC) Environmental Management:* Remove environmental hazards (e.g., loose rugs and small, movable furniture)

Clinical Conditions Guide to Nursing Diagnoses and Collaborative Problems

Medical Conditions
Surgical Conditions
Psychiatric Conditions
Antepartum and Postpartum Conditions
Newborn Conditions
Pediatric Conditions

This section contains lists of potential complications (also called multidisciplinary problems and collaborative problems) and nursing diagnoses associated with selected conditions (e.g., medical, surgical, childbearing). However, because nursing diagnoses represent human responses, and because human beings respond in infinite ways, any nursing diagnosis could occur with any disease process or condition. In a sense, then, all nursing diagnoses on these lists are potential diagnoses. When using these lists, keep in mind that for each condition (e.g., congestive heart failure): (1) every patient with that condition must be monitored for the associated complications, (2) a patient may have nursing diagnoses that are not included in the list, and (3) the list may include many nursing diagnoses that the patient does not have.

For the nursing diagnoses in this section, the etiologies (which follow "related to") are stated in broad, general terms. Etiologies, like problems, are highly individual. Therefore, when writing a nursing diagnosis, use the list as a starting point and expand the etiology to fully describe that patient's pathophysiology, disease process, situation, or other related factors. The format used for collaborative problems is adapted from Carpenito (1997b, pp. 28–29), for example, Potential Complication (PC) of burns: Hypovolemic shock.

Some patient teaching is required for every patient. Therefore, the nursing diagnosis Deficient knowledge is not listed for any of the clinical conditions in this section. It is assumed that all clients, regardless of disease or medical diagnosis, will be assessed for Deficient knowledge.

Also note that almost every patient is at risk for the nursing diagnosis Ineffective individual management of therapeutic regimen related to lack of knowledge of disease process, therapies, and self-care. This text includes that diagnosis only in situations where the processes, therapies, and so forth are complex, or where the patient could be expected to lack the abilities to manage for other reasons (e.g., memory loss, confusion).

MEDICAL CONDITIONS

Acquired immune deficiency syndrome (AIDS)

Arthritis

Autoimmune disorders

Blood disorders

Burns

Cancer

Cardiac disorders (angina/coronary insufficiency, myocardial infarction, congestive heart failure, pericarditis/endocarditis)

Chest trauma

Dying patient

Endocrine disorders (Cushing disease, diabetes mellitus, hypoglycemia, hyperthyroidism, hypothyroidism)

Gastrointestinal disorders (inflammation, bleeding, ulcers, abdominal pain)

Immobilized patient

Liver disease

Neurologic disorders (cerebrovascular accident, other)

Obesity

Pancreatitis

Renal failure, acute

Renal failure, chronic

Respiratory disorders, acute (pneumonia, pulmonary edema, pulmonary embolism)

Respiratory disorders, chronic

Urologic disorders

Vascular disease

Acquired Immune Deficiency Syndrome (AIDS)

Potential Complications (Collaborative Problems)

PC of AIDS: Human immunodeficiency virus [HIV] wasting syndrome, malignancies (e.g., Kaposi sarcoma, lymphoma), meningitis, opportunistic infections (e.g., candidiasis, cytomegalovirus, herpes, Pneumocystis carinii pneumonia)

Nursing Diagnoses

Activity intolerance Related factors: Fatigue, weakness, medication side effects, fever, malnutrition, *Impaired gas exchange* (secondary to lung infections or malignancy)

Airway clearance, ineffective Related factors: Decreased energy or fatigue, respiratory infections, tracheobronchial secretions, pulmonary malignancy, pneumothorax

Anxiety Related factors: Uncertain future, perception of effects of disease and treatments on lifestyle

Body image, disturbed Related factors: Chronic illness, lesions of KS, alopecia, weight loss, changes in sexuality

Caregiver role strain (actual/risk for) Related and risk factors: Illness severity of the care receiver, unpredictable illness course or instability in the care receiver's health, duration of caregiving required, inadequate physical environment for providing care, lack of respite and recreation for caregiver, complexity and number of caregiving tasks

Confusion, acute or chronic Related factors: Infection of CNS (e.g., toxoplasmosis), CMV infection, KS, lymphoma, progress of HIV

Coping: family, compromised/disabled (also consider *Family processes, interrupted*) Related factors: Inadequate or incorrect information or understanding by family member or close friend, chronic illness, chronically unresolved feelings

Coping, ineffective Related factor: Personal vulnerability in a situational crisis (e.g., terminal illness)

Diarrhea Related factors: Medication, diet, infections

Deficient diversional activity Related factors: Frequent or lengthy medical treatments, long-term hospitalization, prolonged bed rest

Fatigue Related factors: Disease process, overwhelming psychologic or emotional demands

Fear Related factors: *Powerlessness,* real threat to own well-being, possibility of disclosure, possibility of death

Fluid volume, deficient Related factors: Inadequate fluid intake secondary to oral lesions, *Diarrhea*

Grieving, anticipatory/dysfunctional Related factors: Impending death or impending changes in lifestyle, loss of body function, changes in appearance, abandonment by significant others

Home maintenance, impaired Related factors: Inadequate support systems, lack of knowledge, lack of familiarity with community resources

Hopelessness Related factors: Deteriorating physical condition, poor prognosis

Infection, risk for Risk factor: Cellular immunodeficiency

Infection transmission, risk for (non-NANDA International) Risk factor: Contagious nature of body fluids

Injury (falls), risk for Related factors: *Fatigue*, weakness, cognitive changes, encephalopathy, neuromuscular changes

Therapeutic regimen management, ineffective Related factors: Complexity of medication regimen; *Deficient knowledge* of disease, medications, and community resources; depression; illness or malaise

Nutrition, imbalanced: less than body requirements Related factors: Difficulty in swallowing, loss of appetite, oral and esophageal lesions, gastrointestinal malabsorption, increased metabolic rate, *Nausea*

Oral mucous membrane, impaired Risk factors: Compromised immune system, opportunistic infections (e.g., candidiasis, herpes)

Pain, [acute] Related factors: Progression of disease process, medication side effects, lymphedema secondary to KS, headaches secondary to CNS infection, peripheral neuropathy, severe myalgias

Powerlessness Related factors: Terminal illness, treatment regimen, unpredictable nature of disease

Self-care deficit: (specify) Related factors: Decreased strength and endurance; *Activity intolerance; Confusion, acute/chronic*

Self-esteem, low (chronic, situational) Related factors: Chronic illness, situational crisis

Sensory/perception, disturbed (auditory/visual) Related factors: Hearing loss secondary to medications, visual loss related to CMV infection

Sexuality patterns, ineffective Related factors: Safer sex practices, fear of HIV transmission, abstinence, impotence secondary to medications

Skin integrity, impaired Related factors: Tissue and muscle wasting secondary to altered nutritional state, perineal excoriation secondary to *Diarrhea* and lesions (e.g., candidiasis, herpes), *Impaired physical mobility*, KS lesions

Sleep pattern, disturbed Related factors: *Pain*, night sweats, medication regimen, medication side effects, *Anxiety*, depression, drug withdrawal (e.g., heroin, cocaine)

Social isolation Related factors: Stigma, others' fear of contracting disease, own fear of HIV transmission, cultural and religious mores, physical appearance, *Self-esteem* and *Body image, disturbed*

Spiritual distress Related factors: Challenged belief and value system, test of spiritual beliefs

Violence, risk for self-directed Risk factor: Suicidal ideation, *Hopelessness*

Arthritis

Includes but is not limited to rheumatoid arthritis, osteoarthritis, juvenile rheumatoid arthritis, gouty arthritis, and septic arthritis

Potential Complications (Collaborative Problems)

PC of arthritis: Fibrous or bony ankylosis, joint contractures, neuropathy

PC of corticosteroids (intra-articular injections): Intra-articular infection, joint degeneration

PC of corticosteroids (systemic administration): Cushing syndrome, hyperglycemia, delayed wound healing, osteoporosis, muscle wasting, hypertension, edema, congestive heart failure, hypokalemia, depressed immune response, peptic ulcers, renal failure, growth retardation (children), psychotic reactions, cataract formation, atherosclerosis, thrombophlebitis

PC of nonsteroidal anti-inflammatory medications: Gastric ulceration or bleeding, nephropathy

Nursing Diagnoses

Body image, disturbed Related factors: Chronic illness, joint deformities, *Impaired physical mobility*

Coping, ineffective Related factors: Personal vulnerability in a situational crisis (e.g., new diagnosis of illness, declining health), unpredictable exacerbations

Family processes, interrupted Related factors: Change in family roles, disability of family member, lack of support system

Fatigue Related factors: *Pain,* overwhelming psychologic or emotional demands, systemic inflammation, anemia

Home maintenance, impaired Related factors: *Impaired physical mobility, Fatigue, Pain*

Therapeutic regimen management, ineffective Related factors: *Deficient knowledge* of medication and therapies, forgetful about taking medications because of *Impaired memory,* reliance on quackery

Pain, acute/chronic Related factors: Progression of joint abnormalities, inflammation

Mobility: physical, impaired Related factors: Stiffness, *Pain,* joint ankylosis, contractures, decreased muscle strength

Powerlessness Related factors: Incurable nature of the disease, not feeling better even when following therapeutic regimen

Self-care deficit: (specify) Related factors: Musculoskeletal impairment, *Pain, Impaired physical mobility, Fatigue*

Sexuality patterns, ineffective Related factors: *Fatigue, Pain, Impaired physical mobility*

Sleep pattern, disturbed Related factor: *Pain*

Social interaction, impaired Related factors: *Fatigue,* difficulty ambulating

<u>Autoimmune Disorders</u>

Include but are not limited to systemic lupus erythematosus (SLE), scleroderma, rheumatic fever, glomerulonephritis, and multiple sclerosis

Potential Complications (Collaborative Problems)

PC of lupus erythematosus: Vasculitis, pericarditis, pleuritis, cerebral infarction, hemolytic anemia, glomerulonephritis

PC of glomerulonephritis or renal failure: Ascites, anasarca, sepsis

PC of corticosteroid therapy: Cushing syndrome, hyperglycemia, delayed wound healing, osteoporosis, muscle wasting, hypertension, edema, congestive heart failure, hypokalemia, depressed immune response, peptic ulcers, renal failure, growth retardation (children), psychotic reactions, cataract formation, atherosclerosis, thrombophlebitis

Nursing Diagnoses

Activity intolerance Related factors: *Anxiety, Acute/chronic pain,* weakness, *Fatigue*

Adjustment, impaired Related factors: Necessity for major lifestyle or behavior change

Body image, disturbed Related factors: Chronic illness, *Chronic pain*, rash, lesions, ulcers, purpura, mottling of hands, alopecia, and altered body function

Caregiver role strain Related and risk factors: Illness severity of care receiver, duration of caregiving required, lack of respite and recreation for caregiver, complexity and number of caregiving tasks

Coping: family, compromised See *Family processes*

Coping, ineffective Related factors: Personal vulnerability in a situational crisis (e.g., declining health), unpredictable course of disease, exacerbations

Diversional activity, deficient Related factors: Long-term hospitalization, frequent or lengthy treatments, forced inactivity

Family processes, interrupted Related factors: Chronic illness or disability, complex therapies, change in family roles, hospitalization or change in environment, disability of family member

Fatigue Related factors: Increased energy needs secondary to chronic inflammation, altered body chemistry, effects of medication therapy

Fear Related factors: Environmental stressors or hospitalization, *Powerlessness*, real or imagined threat to own well-being

Fluid volume excess Related factor: Decreased urine output secondary to sodium retention or glomerulonephritis

Grieving, anticipatory/dysfunctional Related factors: Potential loss of body function, potential loss of social role, terminal illness, chronic illness

Home maintenance, impaired Related factors: *Pain, Impaired physical mobility*

Hopelessness Related factors: Failing or deteriorating physical condition, long-term stress

Incontinence, functional, urinary Related factor: *Impaired physical mobility*

Infection, risk for Risk factors: Immunosuppression, chronic disease, pharmaceutical agents, secondary to glomerulonephritis

Therapeutic regimen management, ineffective Related factors: *Deficient knowledge* (disease process, balanced rest and exercise, symptoms of exacerbations and complications, medications and treatment, community resources)

Mobility: physical, impaired Related factors: *Pain*, medically prescribed limitations, (joint) changes, neuromuscular impairment

Noncompliance Related factors: Denial of illness, negative perception or consequences of treatment regimen, perceived benefits of continued illness

Nutrition, imbalanced: less than body requirements Related factors: Difficulty in chewing, *Impaired swallowing*, loss of appetite, *Nausea*, and vomiting

Oral mucous membrane, impaired Related factors: Pathophysiology of the disease, medication side effects

Pain Related factors: Inflammation of connective tissues, blood vessels, and mucous membranes

Powerlessness Related factors: Unpredictability of chronic, terminal disease; complex treatment regimen; physical and psychologic changes associated with the disease

Protection, ineffective Related factor: Corticosteroid therapy

Role performance, ineffective Related factors: Chronic illness, *Chronic pain*

Self-care deficit: (specify) Related factors: Decreased strength and endurance, *Pain, Activity intolerance*, stiffness, *Fatigue*

Self-esteem, low (chronic, situational) Related factors: Chronic illness, *Chronic pain*, *Ineffective role performance*, inability to achieve developmental tasks because of disabling condition

Sensory perception, disturbed (visual, kinesthetic, tactile) Related factor: Disease process

Sexuality patterns, ineffective Related factors: *Fatigue*, *Pain*, *Impaired physical mobility*

Skin integrity, impaired (actual/risk for) Related and risk factors: Rashes, lesions, medications, altered circulation, *Impaired physical mobility*, photosensitivity, edema

Sleep pattern, disturbed Related factors: *Pain* and discomfort, *Anxiety*, inactivity

Social interaction, impaired Related factors: *Self-esteem, low* (*chronic, situational*) limited physical mobility, *Fatigue*, embarrassment over appearance

Social isolation Related factor: Others' response to appearance

Blood Disorders

Include but are not limited to anemias, polycythemia, and coagulation disorders

Potential Complications (Collaborative Problems)

PC of anemias: Cardiac failure, iron overload, bleeding, infection

PC of coagulation disorders: Hemorrhage, thrombus formation, renal failure, congestive heart failure

Nursing Diagnoses

Activity intolerance Related factors: Insufficient oxygen transport secondary to low red blood cell count, pulmonary congestion, tissue hypoxia, *Acute pain*, *Fatigue*, decreased strength and endurance

Anxiety Related factors: Lack of knowledge of disease and treatments, uncertainty of outcome

Constipation Related factors: Atrophy of mucosa, medication (iron) side effects

Diarrhea Related factors: Atrophy of mucosa

Family processes, interrupted Related factors: Hospitalization or change in environment, illness or disability of family member

Fear Related factors: Environmental stressors or hospitalization, treatments

Injury (bleeding), risk for Risk factors: Abnormal blood profile, sickle cells, decreased hemoglobin, thrombocytopenia, splenomegaly

Infection, risk for Risk factors: Decreased resistance secondary to abnormal white blood cells

Nutrition, imbalanced: less than body requirements Related factors: Loss of appetite secondary to sore mouth, *Nausea*

Oral mucous membrane, impaired Related factors: Atrophy of GI mucosa, tissue hypoxia, papillary atrophy, and inflammatory changes (pernicious anemia)

Pain Related factor: Altered body function (e.g., bleeding in joint spaces)

Protection, ineffective See *Injury, risk for*

Tissue perfusion, ineffective (peripheral) Related factors: Deficit or malfunction of RBCs, hyperviscosity (in polycythemia)

Burns

Potential Complications (Collaborative Problems)

PC of burns: Hypovolemic shock, hypervolemia, paralytic ileus, renal failure, sepsis, stress ulcers

Nursing Diagnoses

Airway clearance, ineffective Related factors: Tracheal edema, decreased pulmonary ciliary action

Anxiety Related factors: Suddenness of injury, pain from injury and treatments, uncertainty of prognosis, immobility

Aspiration, risk for Risk factors: Presence of tracheostomy or endotracheal tube, tube feeding, *Impaired swallowing*, hindered elevation of upper body

Body image, disturbed Related factors: Physical impairment, scarring, contractures

Body temperature, risk for imbalanced Risk factor: Dehydration secondary to *Impaired skin integrity*

Breathing pattern, ineffective Related factor: *Pain*

Caregiver role strain Related factors: Illness severity of care receiver, duration of caregiving required, lack of respite and recreation for caregiver, complexity and number of caregiving tasks

Constipation Related factors: Decreased activity, medications (e.g., narcotic analgesics)

Coping: family, ineffective Related factors: See *Family processes, interrupted*

Disuse syndrome, risk for Risk factor: Severe *Pain*

Diversional activity, deficient Related factors: Monotony of long-term hospitalization, separation from family, *Social isolation*

Family processes, interrupted Related factors: Long-term, complex therapies; long-term hospitalization; change in environment; separation from family members; critical nature of injury

Fatigue Related factors: Overwhelming psychologic or emotional demands

Fear Related factors: Environmental stressors or hospitalization, painful procedures, threat of dying, projected effects of injury on lifestyle and relationships

Fluid volume, deficient Related factor: Abnormal fluid loss (e.g., intravascular to interstitial fluid shift)

Gas exchange, impaired Related factors: Smoke inhalation, heat damage to lungs, carbon monoxide poisoning

Hypothermia Related factor: Loss of epithelial tissue

Infection, risk for Risk factors: Tissue destruction (loss of skin barrier), impaired immune response, invasive procedures, and other increased environmental exposures

Management of therapeutic regimen: family (or individual), ineffective
Related factors: *Deficient knowledge* of wound care, exercise and other
therapies, nutrition, pain management, and signs and symptoms of complications

Mobility: physical, impaired Related factors: *Pain*, edema, dressings,
splints, wound contractures

Nutrition, imbalanced: less than body requirements Related factors: Difficulty swallowing, high metabolic rate needed for wound healing

Pain Related factors: Burn injury, exposed nerve endings, treatments

Powerlessness Related factor: Inability to control situation (e.g., due to
treatment regimen, health care environment, *Pain*)

Self-care deficit: (specify) Related factors: *Pain*, dressings, splints,
enforced immobility, *Activity intolerance*, decreased strength and
endurance, limited range of motion

Self-esteem, low (chronic, situational) Related factors: *Body image, disturbed*, loss of role responsibilities, loss of functional abilities, delay in
achieving developmental tasks secondary to effects of injury

Sensory perception, disturbed: auditory, gustatory, kinesthetic, olfactory, tactile, visual (specify) Related factors: Sensory deficit, sensory
overload (environmental), stress, *Sleep deprivation*, protective isolation, enforced immobility

Sleep pattern, disturbed (or sleep deprivation) Related factors: *Pain, Anxiety*, dressings, splints, invasive lines

Social isolation Related factors: Separation from family, infection control
measures, embarrassment over appearance, response of others to
appearance

Tissue perfusion, ineffective (peripheral): Related factor: Constriction
from circumferential burns

Cancer

NOTE: Nursing diagnoses depend greatly upon the location, type,
and stage of the cancer.

Potential Complications (Collaborative Problems)

PC of cancer: Cachexia, electrolyte imbalance, pathological fractures,
hemorrhage, malnutrition (negative nitrogen balance), metastasis to vital
organs (e.g., brain, bones, kidneys, lungs, liver), spinal cord compression,
superior vena cava syndrome

PC of chemotherapy: Anaphylactic reaction, anemia, CNS toxicity, congestive heart failure, electrolyte imbalance, hemorrhagic cystitis, leukopenia, necrosis at IV site, renal failure, thrombocytopenia

PC of narcotic medications: Depressed respiration, consciousness and
blood pressure; cardiovascular collapse; profound brain damage; biliary
spasm

PC of radiation therapy: Increased intracranial pressure, myelosuppression, inflammation, fluid and electrolyte imbalances

Nursing Diagnoses

Activity intolerance Related factors: See *Fatigue*

Adjustment, impaired Related factors: Necessity for major lifestyle changes, incomplete grieving

Airway clearance, ineffective Related factors: Tracheobronchial obstruction; ineffective cough secondary to decreased energy, *Fatigue*, and *Pain*; increased viscosity of secretions

Anxiety Related factors: Unfamiliar hospital environment, uncertainty of prognosis, lack of knowledge about cancer and treatment, threat of death, threat of or change in role functioning, inadequate pain relief

Body image, disturbed Related factors: Hair loss, edema, blebs and blisters, petechiae, erythema

Bowel incontinence Related factors: Decreased awareness of need to defecate, disease process, loss of rectal sphincter control

Breathing pattern, ineffective Related factors: Medications, *Chronic pain, Fatigue*, anemia

Caregiver role strain Related factors: Illness severity of care receiver, duration of caregiving required, lack of respite and recreation for caregiver, complexity and number of caregiving tasks

Constipation Related factors: Decreased activity, dietary changes, medications (e.g., narcotic analgesics, chemotherapy), radiation therapy, painful defecation

Coping, Ineffective Related factors: Personal vulnerability in a maturational crisis (e.g., terminal illness in childhood) or in a situational crisis (e.g., terminal illness)

Decisional conflict Related factors: Lack of relevant information, multiple or divergent sources of information, multiple treatment choices, lack of support system

Diarrhea Related factors: Dietary changes, impaction, radiation, chemotherapy (specify), antibiotics, stress

Disuse syndrome, risk for Risk factors: Severe *Pain*, altered level of consciousness

Falls, risk for Risk factors: Weakness, Sensory perception, disturbed, *Disturbed thought processes, Confusion*

Family processes, interrupted Related factors: Change in family roles, complex therapies, hospitalization or change in environment, illness or disability of family member, separation of family members, fears associated with the diagnosis, financial effects of illness

Fatigue Related factors: *Pain*, disease process, overwhelming psychologic or emotional demands, malnutrition, hypoxia/*Impaired gas exchange*

Fear Related factors: Real or imagined threat to own well-being, environmental stressors or hospitalization, impending death, fear of pain

Fluid volume, deficient Related factors: Inadequate fluid intake (e.g., altered ability to obtain fluids, weakness, *Fatigue*, anorexia, *Nausea*, depression), abnormal fluid loss (e.g., vomiting, diarrhea)

Grieving, anticipatory/dysfunctional Related factors: Terminal illness, impending loss of body function, effects of cancer on lifestyle, withdrawal from or of others

Home maintenance, impaired Related factors: Lack of support system, inadequate finances, *Deficient knowledge* regarding community and other supports, *Acute/chronic confusion, Disturbed thought processes, Disturbed sensory perception*

Hopelessness Related factors: Failing or deteriorating physical condition, long-term stress, lost spiritual belief, overwhelming functional losses, impending death

Infection, risk for Risk factors: Immunosuppression, neutropenia, pharmaceutical agents

Mobility: physical, impaired Related factors: Decreased strength and endurance, musculoskeletal impairment, neuromuscular impairment, *Pain*, sedation, *Fatigue*, edema, enforced immobility (e.g., for chemotherapy infusions)

Nausea Related factors: Side effects of chemotherapy and other medications, stress, *Pain*, difficulty swallowing

Nutrition, imbalanced: less than body requirements Related factors: Difficulty in swallowing, *Nausea*, vomiting, loss of appetite, changes in taste, isolation, *Anxiety*, stress, *Impaired oral mucous membrane, Fatigue*, increased metabolic demands of the tumor

Oral mucous membrane, impaired Related factors: Chemotherapy, radiation to head and neck, *Imbalanced nutrition: less than body requirements*, inadequate hydration, immunosuppression

Pain, acute/chronic Related factors: Ongoing tissue destruction (i.e., localizations), infection, stomatitis, chemotherapy

Powerlessness Related factor: Terminal illness, feelings of inability to change the progression of events, uncertainty about prognosis and treatments

Role performance, ineffective Related factors: *Chronic pain,* treatment side effects

Self-care deficit: (specify) Related factors: Developmental disability, maturational age, *Pain, Activity intolerance, Fatigue*, depression

Sexual dysfunction/Sexuality patterns, ineffective Related factors: *Pain*, change in body image, *Fear* (patient or partner), *Fatigue* from treatments or disease, lack of privacy

Skin integrity, impaired Related factors: Radiation, chemotherapy, allergic reactions to medications, loss of muscle and subcutaneous tissue secondary to poor nutritional status, immunologic deficit, *Impaired physical mobility* secondary to weakness

Sleep pattern, disturbed/Sleep deprivation Related factors: *Anxiety*, emotional state, medical treatment regimen, *Pain*, pruritus

Social interaction, impaired Related factors: Fear of rejection, actual rejection by others, *Self-esteem, low (chronic, situational),* therapeutic isolation (e.g., secondary to radiation or protective isolation)

Spiritual distress Related factors: Test of spiritual beliefs, challenged belief and value system, unresolved conflicts, *Dysfunctional grieving*

Swallowing, impaired Related factors: Irritated oropharyngeal cavity, mechanical obstruction, head and neck radiation

Thought processes, disturbed Related factors: Chemotherapy, toxicity, cerebellar localization

Cardiac Disorders

Potential Complications (Collaborative Problems)

PC of angina/coronary insufficiency: Myocardial infarction

PC of congestive heart failure: Cardiogenic shock, deep vein thrombosis, hepatic failure, acute pulmonary edema, renal failure

PC of digitalis administration: Toxicity

PC of dysrhythmias: Decreased cardiac output, causing decreased myocardial perfusion, causing heart failure; severe atrioventricular conduction blocks; thromboemboli formation; ventricular fibrillation

PC of myocardial infarction (chest pain, arrhythmias): Cardiogenic shock, dysrhythmia, thromboembolism, pulmonary edema, pulmonary embolism, pericarditis

PC of pericarditis/endocarditis: Congestive heart failure, emboli (e.g., pulmonary, cerebral, renal, spleen, coronary), cardiac tamponade, valvular stenosis

Nursing Diagnoses

Angina/Coronary Insufficiency

Activity intolerance Related factors: *Anxiety*, arrhythmias, *Pain*, lack of exercise or conditioning due to fear of pain

Anxiety Related factors: Chest pain, threat to self-concept, change in role functioning

Breathing pattern, ineffective Related factors: *Acute Pain, Anxiety*

Denial, ineffective Related factors: *Fear* of effects of diagnosis on lifestyle, *Fear* of heart attack

Falls, risk for Risk factors: Dizziness and hypotension secondary to vasodilator, calcium channel blockers, and opiate analgesic medications

Family processes, interrupted Related factors: Change in family roles, hospitalization, inability of family member to perform usual roles

Fear Related factors: Environmental stressors or hospitalization, unknown future

Nausea Related factors: Side effects of calcium channel blockers and opiate analgesics, *Pain*

Noncompliance Related factors: Denial of illness, negative side effects of medications, negative perception of treatment regimen, perceived benefits of continued illness, dysfunctional patient or provider relationship

Pain Related factors: Myocardial ischemia, headache secondary to vasodilators

Role performance, ineffective Related factors: Chronic illness, treatment side effects, *Fear* of heart attack

Sexual dysfunction/Sexuality patterns, ineffective Related factors: *Pain*, Fear of pain, *Low self-esteem (chronic, situational)*

Sleep pattern, disturbed Related factors: *Pain* and discomfort, *Anxiety*

Myocardial Infarction (Chest Pain, Arrhythmias)

Activity intolerance Related factors: *Acute Pain*, weakness/*Fatigue* because of insufficient oxygen secondary to cardiac ischemia

Anxiety Related factors: Severe *Pain*, threat to or change in health status, anticipated change in role functioning, unknown outcome, unfamiliar environment

Cardiac output, decreased Related factors: Dysfunctional electrical conduction, increased ventricular workload, ventricular ischemia, ventricular damage

Constipation Related factors: Decreased peristalsis secondary to medications (e.g., opiate analgesics), decreased activity, NPO or soft diet

Coping, Ineffective Related factors: Personal vulnerability to situational crisis (e.g., new diagnosis of illness, declining health)

Death anxiety Related factors: *Fear* of dying

Denial, ineffective Related factors: *Fear* of consequences of disease on roles, lifestyle, and so forth

Family processes, interrupted Related factors: Inability of patient to assume family roles, hospitalization, separation of family members

Fear Related factors: *Pain*, unknown future, real or imagined threat to own well-being, strange (e.g., hospital) environment, *Fear* of death

Fluid volume excess Related factor: Decreased kidney perfusion secondary to heart failure

Gas exchange, impaired Related factor: Decreased cardiac output, decreased pulmonary blood supply secondary to pulmonary hypertension or congestive heart failure

Grieving, dysfunctional Related factors: Actual or perceived losses resulting from illness

Home maintenance, impaired Related factors: *Pain, Fear* of pain, *Activity intolerance, Fear* of another heart attack

Nausea Related factors: Severe chest pain, side effect of medications

Pain Related factor: Myocardial ischemia

Powerlessness Related factors: Treatment regimen, hospital environment, anticipated lifestyle changes

Role performance, ineffective Related factors: Situational crisis, treatment side effects, *Pain, Fear* of pain, *Activity intolerance*

Self-care deficit: (specify) Related factors: *Pain, Activity intolerance*

Self-esteem, low (chronic, situational) Related factors: Treatment side effects, perceived or actual role changes

Sexual dysfunction/Sexuality patterns, ineffective Related factors: *Fear* of pain, *Activity intolerance, Low self-esteem (chronic, situational),* disease-related role changes

Sleep deprivation/Sleep pattern, disturbed Related factors: Strange (e.g., hospital) environment, *Pain*, treatments

Congestive Heart Failure

Activity intolerance Related factors: Weakness due to prolonged bed rest or sedentary lifestyle, *Fatigue*, insufficient oxygenation secondary to *decreased cardiac output*

Anxiety Related factors: Shortness of breath, dyspnea, progressive nature of disease

Anxiety, death Related factor: Possibility of dying

Family processes, interrupted Related factors: Hospitalization or change in environment, illness or disability of family member

Fatigue Related factors: Inadequate oxygenation secondary to decreased cardiac output, difficulty sleeping

Fear See *Anxiety*

Fluid volume excess Related factors: *Decreased cardiac output;* reduced glomerular filtration; increased antidiuretic hormone (ADH) production, causing sodium or water retention

Gas exchange, impaired Related factors: Alveolar capillary membrane changes, fluid in alveoli, decreased pulmonary blood supply

Home maintenance, impaired Related factors: *Fatigue*, shortness of breath, clouded sensorium secondary to insufficient oxygen

Hopelessness Related factors: Failing or deteriorating physical condition, lack of energy for coping

Therapeutic regimen management, ineffective Related factors: *Deficient knowledge* (cardiac function or disease process, diet, activity exercise, medications, signs and symptoms of complications, and self-care), *Impaired memory*, *Fatigue*

Nutrition, imbalanced: less than body requirements Related factors: *Nausea*, anorexia secondary to venous congestion of gastrointestinal tract, *Fatigue*

Powerlessness Related factors: Chronic illness, progressive nature of illness

Self-care deficit: (specify) Related factors: *Fatigue*, dyspnea

Skin integrity, impaired Related factors: *Ineffective peripheral tissue perfusion, Impaired physical mobility*, edema

Sleep deprivation/Sleep pattern, disturbed Related factors: *Anxiety*, nocturia, inability to assume preferred sleep position because of nocturnal dyspnea

Pericarditis/Endocarditis

Activity intolerance Related factors: Inadequate oxygenation secondary to restriction of cardiac filling, causing reduced cardiac output

Anxiety Related factors: *Pain*, change in health status, threat of death

Breathing pattern, ineffective Related factors: *Acute Pain* secondary to inflammation

Cardiac output, decreased Related factors: Restriction of cardiac filling or ventricular contractility, effusion, dysrhythmias, increased ventricular workload

Fear See *Anxiety*

Pain Related factors: Effusion, tissue inflammation

Chest Trauma

Includes but is not limited to hemothorax and pneumothorax

Potential Complications (Collaborative Problems)

PC of chest trauma: Flail chest, hemothorax, pneumothorax, tension pneumothorax, and mediastinal shift

Nursing Diagnoses

Breathing pattern, ineffective Related factors: *Acute Pain, Anxiety*

Dysfunctional ventilatory weaning response (DVWR) Related factors: *Anxiety*, history of ventilator dependence > one week, inappropriate pacing of diminished ventilatory support, uncontrolled episodic energy demands or problems

Fear Related factors: Real or imagined threat to own well-being, sudden injury, unknown extent of or prognosis for injury

Mobility: physical, impaired Related factors: *Pain*/discomfort, presence of chest tubes, IV lines

Pain Related factor: Chest injury

Self-care deficit: (specify) Related factors: *Pain*/discomfort, presence of tubes and lines

Sleep deprivation/Sleep pattern, disturbed Related factors: *Pain* and discomfort, medical regimen

Spontaneous ventilation, impaired Related factors: Injury to thoracic cage or lung tissue, flail chest

Dying Patient

Nursing Diagnoses

Activity intolerance Related factors: *Chronic pain*, weakness, *Fatigue* secondary to disease process, medications, or inadequate intake of calories

Adjustment, impaired Related factor: Incomplete grieving over loss of physical or role function

Airway clearance, ineffective Related factors: Decreased energy, *Fatigue, Pain*, tracheobronchial obstruction

Anxiety, death Related factors: Imminence of death, lack of resolution

Bowel incontinence Related factors: Loss of sphincter control, decreased awareness of need to defecate

Caregiver role strain Related factors: Illness severity of the care receiver, inability to change outcome for the patient, inadequate physical environment for providing care, lack of respite and recreation for caregiver, complexity and amount of caregiving tasks

Communication, impaired verbal Related factors: Inability to speak, inability to speak clearly

Coping: family, compromised Related factor: Family member's temporary preoccupation with own emotional conflicts and personal suffering

Coping, ineffective Related factor: Personal vulnerability to situational crisis (terminal illness)

Denial, ineffective Related factors: *Fear* of dying, *Fear* of effect on others

Family processes, interrupted Related factors: Change in family roles, hospitalization or change in environment, illness or disability of family member, separation of family members

Fatigue Related factors: Disease process, overwhelming psychologic or emotional demands, decreased intake of nutrients for energy

Fear Related factors: *Powerlessness*, environmental stressors or hospitalization, *Fear* of pain, *Fear* of the unknown, *Fear* of dying

Grieving, anticipatory Related factor: Impending death of self

Grieving, dysfunctional Related factors: *Ineffective denial*, unresolved family issues, loss of faith (e.g., *Spiritual distress*), lack of support system

Hopelessness Related factors: Failing or deteriorating physical condition, lack of social or family support, loss of spiritual belief

Incontinence, urinary, functional/total Related factors: Disorientation, *Impaired mobility*, neurologic dysfunction

Nutrition, imbalanced: less than body requirements Related factors: *Impaired swallowing*, loss of appetite, *Nausea* and vomiting

Oral mucous membrane, impaired Related factors: Chemotherapy, inability to perform oral hygiene or obtain fluids, radiation to head and neck

Pain Related factors: Specific to patient's cause of death

Powerlessness Related factors: Inability to change outcome of terminal illness, loss of independence, overwhelming treatment regimen

Self-care deficit: (specify) Related factors: *Pain* and discomfort, *Activity intolerance*, decreased strength and endurance

Skin integrity, impaired Related factors: *Impaired physical mobility, Urinary/Bowel incontinence,* radiation therapy, poor nutritional status, dehydration

Sleep pattern, disturbed Related factors: *Pain* and discomfort, *Anxiety*

Social isolation Related factors: Medical condition, alteration in physical appearance

Sorrow, chronic Related factors: See *Grieving*

Spiritual distress Related factors: Challenged belief and value system, separation from religious and cultural ties, test of spiritual beliefs

Endocrine Disorders

Include but are not limited to Cushing disease, diabetes mellitus, hyperthyroidism, hypothyroidism, hypoglycemia, and pancreatic tumors

Potential Complications (Collaborative Problems)

PC of Cushing disease: Hypertension, congestive heart failure, potassium and sodium imbalance, psychosis, hyperglycemia, osteoporosis

PC of diabetes mellitus: Ketoacidosis, coma, hypoglycemia, infections, coronary artery disease, peripheral vascular disease, retinopathy, neuropathy, nephropathy

PC of hyperthyroidism: Thyroid storm, heart disease, exophthalmos

PC of hypothyroidism: Arteriosclerotic heart disease, myxedema coma, psychosis

PC of repeated or prolonged hypoglycemia: Neuropathy, retinal hemorrhage, CVAs, personality changes, intellectual damage

Nursing Diagnoses

Cushing Disease

Activity intolerance Related factors: Muscle weakness secondary to protein wasting, hyperglycemia, and potassium depletion; congestive heart failure

Body image, disturbed Related factors: Change in appearance (e.g., moon face, virilism in women, acne) secondary to disease process and medication therapy, changes in social involvement

Infection, risk for Risk factors: Skin and capillary fragility, negative nitrogen balance, compromised immune response, hyperglycemia, lowered resistance to stress, poor wound healing

Injury, risk for Risk factors: Fractures secondary to osteoporosis, hypertension secondary to sodium and water retention

Therapeutic regimen management, ineffective Related factors: *Deficient knowledge* (disease process, therapeutic diet, diagnostic tests, surgical treatment, self-administration of steroids, indications of need to call physician)

Nutrition, imbalanced: less than body requirements Related factors: Disturbance of carbohydrate metabolism, increased resistance to insulin

Skin integrity, impaired Related factors: Decreased connective tissue, edema secondary to sodium and water retention, thinning and dryness of the skin

Self-care deficit: (specify) Related factors: *Fatigue*, generalized weakness, demineralization of bones

Sexuality patterns, ineffective Related factors: Impotence, cessation of menses, loss of libido secondary to excessive adrenocorticotropic hormone (ACTH) production

Thought processes, disturbed Related factors: Increased levels of glucocorticoids and ACTH

Diabetes Mellitus/Hypoglycemia

Coping: family, compromised/disabling Related factors: Complex self-care regimen, chronic disease, inability to predict future, inadequate or incomplete information/understanding, changes required in family functioning

Fear Related factors: Effects on lifestyle, need for self-injections, diabetes complications

Infection, risk for Risk factors: Decreased leukocyte function, delayed healing, impaired circulation

Injury, risk for Risk factors: Impaired vision, hypoglycemia, impaired tactile sensation

Therapeutic regimen management, ineffective Related factors: *Deficient knowledge* (disease process, diet and exercise balance, self-monitoring and self-medication, foot care, signs and symptoms of complications, community resources)

Noncompliance Related factors: Complexity of self-care and medical regimen, chronicity of disease, denial

Nutrition, imbalanced: less than body requirements Related factors: Inability to utilize glucose, resulting in weight loss, muscle weakness, and thirst

Powerlessness Related factors: Perceived inability to prevent complications such as blindness and amputations

Sensory perception, disturbed (tactile, visual) Related factors: Glucose, insulin, or electrolyte imbalance, peripheral neurovascular changes

Sexual dysfunction/Sexuality patterns, ineffective Related factors: Impotence secondary to peripheral neuropathy, psychologic conflicts (male), psychologic stressors, frequent genitourinary problems (female)

Hyperthyroidism

Anxiety Related factor: CNS irritability

Comfort, altered (heat intolerance) (non-NANDA International) Related factor: Increased metabolic rate

Diarrhea Related factor: Increased peristalsis secondary to increased metabolic rate

Fatigue Related factors: Increased energy requirements, CNS irritability

Hyperthermia, risk for: Risk factor: Inability to compensate for excess thyroid activity

Nutrition, imbalanced: less than body requirements Related factors: Hypermetabolic rate, constant activity, inability to ingest enough calories, vomiting, *Diarrhea*

Tissue integrity, impaired [corneal] Related factors: Periorbital edema, reduced ability to blink, eye dryness, corneal abrasions or ulcerations

Hypothyroidism

Activity intolerance Related factors: Apathy, weakness, inadequate oxygen and decreased energy secondary to decreased metabolic rate

[Comfort, altered (cold intolerance)] Related factor: Slowed metabolic rate

Constipation Related factors: Decreased activity and decreased peristalsis secondary to decreased metabolic rate

Fatigue Related factors: See *Activity intolerance*

Hypothermia Related factor: Decreased metabolic rate

Injury, risk for Risk factors: Hypersensitivity to sedatives, narcotics, and anesthetics secondary to decreased metabolic rate

Mobility: physical, impaired Related factors: *Fatigue*, weakness, mucin deposits in joints and interstitial spaces, changes in reflexes and coordination

Nutrition, imbalanced: more than body requirements Related factor: Intake greater than body needs secondary to decreased metabolic rate

Skin integrity, impaired Related factors: Dryness and edema secondary to movement of fluid into interstitial spaces

Social interaction, impaired Related factors: Weakness, apathy, changes in appearance, depression

Gastrointestinal Disorders

Potential Complications (Collaborative Problems)

PC of GI inflammatory diseases (e.g., diverticulitis): GI bleeding, anal fissure, fluid and electrolyte imbalances, anemia, intestinal obstruction, fistula, abscess, perforation

PC of GI bleeding: Hypovolemic shock, anemia

PC of peptic ulcers: Perforation, pyloric obstruction, hemorrhage

Nursing Diagnoses

GI Inflammation (e.g., Diverticulitis, Inflammatory Bowel Disease)

Constipation Related factors: Inadequate ingestion of dietary fiber, narrowing of intestinal lumen secondary to scar tissue

Coping, ineffective Related factors: Chronic condition, no definitive treatment, *Chronic pain*, *Disturbed sleep pattern*, ostomy

Diarrhea Related factors: Inflammation of GI tract, malabsorption

Fluid volume, deficient Related factors: *Diarrhea*, vomiting, decreased fluid intake

Nutrition, imbalanced: less than body requirements Related factors: *Diarrhea*, *nausea* and abdominal cramping associated with eating, ulcers of the mucous membrane, decreased absorption of nutrients

Pain, chronic Related factors: Inflammation or obstruction of GI tract, hyperperistalsis

GI Bleeding

Activity intolerance Related factor: Weakness/*Fatigue* secondary to anemia or blood loss

Coping, ineffective Related factor: Personal vulnerability to situational crisis (e.g., acute illness)

Fatigue Related factors: Disease process, low hemoglobin level

Fear Related factor: Real or imagined threat to own well-being

Fluid volume, deficient Related factor: Abnormal fluid loss (e.g., emesis, diarrhea)

Nutrition, imbalanced: less than body requirements Related factors: Loss of appetite, *Nausea* and vomiting

Ulcers

Constipation Related factors: Effects of antacids and anticholinergics

Diarrhea Related factor: Effects of magnesium-containing antacids

Pain, acute/chronic Related factors: Lesions secondary to increased gastric secretions

Abdominal Pain/Irritable Bowel Syndrome

Anxiety Related factors: Necessity for frequent bowel movements, *Diarrhea*, *Pain*, chronicity of the condition

Constipation Related factors: Decreased activity, decreased fluid intake, dietary changes, medications (specify)

Diarrhea Related factors: Dietary changes, increased intestinal motility, medications (specify), alcohol intake, smoking, *Fatigue*, cold drinks

Fluid volume, deficient Related factors: Abnormal fluid loss (specify), inadequate fluid intake, abnormal blood loss (specify), excessive continuous consumption of alcohol

Nutrition, imbalanced: less than body requirements Related factors: Loss of appetite, *Nausea*, vomiting, food intolerance, fear of precipitating *Diarrhea*

Pain, acute Related factors: Injury, noxious stimulus (e.g., fruits, alcohol)

Pain, chronic Related factors: Specific to patient

Sleep deprivation/Sleep pattern, disturbed Related factors: *Pain* and discomfort, *Anxiety*, *Diarrhea*

Immobilized Patient

Potential Complications (Collaborative Problems)

PC of immobility: Contractures; joint ankylosis; osteoporosis; thrombophlebitis, embolus; hypostatic pneumonia; renal calculi

Nursing Diagnoses

Activity intolerance Related factors: Generalized weakness, *Fatigue*, compromised circulatory or respiratory system

Constipation Related factors: Decreased activity, decreased colon motility secondary to increased adrenaline production

Coping, ineffective Related factor: Personal vulnerability to a situational crisis (specify), inability to perform usual role functions, dependence on others, *Low self-esteem* (*chronic, situational*)

Disuse syndrome, risk for Risk factors: Paralysis, mechanical immobilization, prescribed immobility, severe *Pain*, altered level of consciousness

Diversional activity, deficient Related factor: Prolonged bed rest

Dysreflexia, autonomic Related factor: Spinal cord injury T7 or above

Incontinence, urinary functional/total Related factor: Neurologic impairment

Mobility: physical, impaired Related factors: Decreased strength and endurance; *Activity Intolerance; Pain*; neuromuscular, musculoskeletal, and cognitive impairment; depression, severe *Anxiety*

Self-care deficit: (specify) Related factors: *Pain, Activity intolerance*, decreased strength and endurance, prescribed immobility

Skin integrity, impaired Related factors: *Impaired physical mobility*, atrophy of dermis and subcutaneous tissues, loss of skin turgor, impaired circulation

Sleep pattern, disturbed Related factors: Lack of physical activity, *Pain* and discomfort, inability to change positions independently or assume usual sleep position

Urinary retention Related factors: Decreased muscle tone of bladder, inability to relax the perineal muscles, embarrassment of using bedpan, lack of privacy, unnatural position for urination

Liver Disease

Includes but is not limited to cirrhosis and hepatitis

Potential Complications (Collaborative Problems)

PC of liver disease: Anemia; hepatic encephalopathy; glomerulonephritis, renal failure; esophageal varices; GI bleeding, hemorrhage; hypokalemia; negative nitrogen balance; disseminated intravascular coagulation (DIC)

Nursing Diagnoses

Activity intolerance Related factors: Weakness, extreme *Fatigue* secondary to bed rest, impaired respiratory function secondary to ascites

Anxiety Related factors: Unknown prognosis of the disease, uncertainty of the future, alcohol withdrawal

Body image, disturbed Related factors: Change in appearance (e.g., jaundice, ascites), chronic illness

Breathing patterns, ineffective Related factor: Pressure on diaphragm secondary to ascites

Confusion, acute Related factors: Alcohol abuse, inability of liver to detoxify certain substances, increased serum ammonia level

Coping, ineffective Related factor: Personal vulnerability to situational crisis (e.g., new diagnosis of illness, declining health)

Diarrhea Related factors: Dietary changes, inability to metabolize fats, stress

Family processes, interrupted Related factors: Change in family roles, illness or disability of family member

Fatigue Related factors: Disease process, malnutrition

Fear Related factor: Real or imagined threat to own well-being

Fluid volume excess Risk factors: Malnutrition, portal hypertension, sodium retention

Infection, risk for Risk factors: Hypoproteinemia, enlarged spleen, leukopenia

Injury, risk for Risk factors: Continued intake of hepatotoxins (e.g., alcohol), decreased prothrombin and coagulation factors

Therapeutic regimen management, ineffective Related factors: *Deficient knowledge* (e.g., disease process, nutritional needs, symptoms of complications, effects of alcohol), lack of motivation to stop drinking

Mobility: physical, impaired Related factor: Weakness secondary to prolonged bed rest

Nutrition, imbalanced: less than body requirements Related factors: Loss of appetite; *Nausea*; vomiting; bile stasis; decreased absorption and storage of fat-soluble vitamins; impaired fat, glucose, and protein metabolism; *Diarrhea*

Pain, acute/chronic Related factors: Ascites, liver enlargement

Self-care deficit: (specify) Related factors: *Pain, Fatigue, Activity intolerance*

Self-esteem, low (chronic, situational) Related factors: Chronic illness, situational crisis, *Disturbed body image,* inability to stop drinking alcohol

Skin integrity, impaired Related factors: Physical immobility; itching secondary to jaundice, edema, and ascites

Thought processes, disturbed Related factors: See *Confusion*

Neurologic Disorders

Include but not limited to CVA (stroke), multiple sclerosis, amyotrophic lateral sclerosis, brain tumors, Guillain-Barré, syndrome, myasthenia gravis, seizure disorders, Alzheimer disease, coma, head injury, cerebral thrombosis, and transient ischemic attack. Associated psychiatric diagnoses include CNS infections (e.g., tertiary neurosyphilis, viral encephalitis, Jakob-Creutzfeldt disease), brain trauma, Huntington chorea, Parkinson disease, and meningitis

Potential Complications (Collaborative Problems)

PC of cerebrovascular accident (stroke): Increased intracranial pressure, respiratory infection, brain stem failure, cardiac dysrhythmias

PC of brain tumor: Increased intracranial pressure, paralysis, hyperthermia, sensory-motor changes

PC of other neurologic disorders (e.g., multiple sclerosis): Pneumonia, respiratory failure, renal failure

Nursing Diagnoses

CVA (Stroke)

NOTE: Nursing diagnoses for CVA will vary depending upon the location and severity of the lesion. CVA can have mild to severe effects.

Activity intolerance Related factors: *Anxiety, Fatigue,* weakness, deconditioning secondary to immobility, neuromuscular deficits

Airway clearance, ineffective Related factors: Decreased energy, *Fatigue,* decreased cough and gag reflexes, muscle paralysis

Aspiration, risk for Risk factors: Reduced level of consciousness, *Impaired swallowing,* depressed cough and gag reflexes

Body image, disturbed Related factors: Chronic illness, diminished physical function, loss of control over body

Caregiver role strain Related factors: Illness severity of care receiver, duration of caregiving required, lack of respite and recreation for caregiver, complexity and number of caregiving tasks, elderly caregiver

Communication, impaired verbal Related factors: Aphasia, dysarthria, inability to speak, inability to speak clearly

Constipation Related factors: Decreased activity, medications (specify), weak abdominal muscles

Disuse syndrome, risk for Risk factors: Altered level of consciousness, paralysis

Falls, risk for Risk factors: *Impaired physical mobility, Disturbed sensory perception*

Family processes, interrupted Related factors: Hospitalization or change in environment, separation of family members, illness or disability of family member, change in family roles

Fluid volume, deficient Related factors: Decreased access to, intake of, or absorption of fluids secondary to weakness, impaired motor functions (e.g., swallowing), impaired cognition and level of consciousness

Grieving, dysfunctional Related factors: Actual loss (e.g., of function), chronic illness, inability to fulfill usual roles

Home maintenance, impaired Related factors: Home environment obstacles; inadequate support system; lack of familiarity with community resources; sensorimotor or cognitive deficits; caregiver's lack of knowledge of reality orientation, skin care, and so forth

Hopelessness Related factor: Failing or deteriorating physical condition

Incontinence, urinary, functional Related factors: Cognitive impairment, inability to reach toilet secondary to *Impaired physical mobility*

Incontinence, urinary, total Related factors: Loss of bladder tone or sphincter control; inability to perceive need to void, secondary to neurologic dysfunction

Memory, impaired Related factor: Residual effects of CVA

Mobility: physical, impaired Related factors: Neuromuscular impairment (e.g., weakness, paresthesia, flaccid paralysis, spastic paralysis) secondary to damage of upper motor neurons, perceptual impairment, cognitive impairment

Nutrition, imbalanced: less than body requirements Related factors: Difficulty chewing, *Impaired swallowing*, inability to prepare food secondary to mobility deficits

Powerlessness Related factors: Treatment regimen, chronic disease

Relocation stress syndrome Related factors: Change in environment or location (e.g., transfer to long-term care facility), *Anxiety*, depression

Self-care deficit: (specify) Related factors: Neuromuscular impairment, decreased strength and endurance, *Activity intolerance*, decreased range of motion, weakness secondary to disease and immobility

Sensory perception, disturbed: (specify: auditory, gustatory, kinesthetic, olfactory, tactile, visual) Related factors: Altered sensory reception, transmission, or integration, secondary to hypoxia and compression or displacement of brain tissue

Skin integrity, impaired Related factors: Altered sensation, *Impaired mobility*, incontinence of stool or urine, poor nutritional status

Social interaction, impaired Related factors: *Impaired verbal communication, Impaired physical mobility*, embarrassment about disabilities

Swallowing, impaired Related factors: Muscle paralysis secondary to damaged upper motor neurons, impaired perception or level of consciousness

Unilateral neglect (specify side) Related factors: *Disturbed sensory perception (visual)* with perceptual loss of corresponding body segment

Other Neurologic Disorders

Activity intolerance Related factors: *Acute/Chronic pain*, weakness and *Fatigue*

Airway clearance, ineffective Related factor: Decreased energy and *Fatigue*, neuromuscular weakness

Anxiety Related factors: Change in health status, threat to or change in role functioning, change in interaction patterns, seriousness of condition, threat to self-concept, separation from support system

Aspiration, risk for Risk factors: *Impaired swallowing*, presence of tracheostomy or endotracheal tube, reduced level of consciousness, depressed cough and gag reflexes, tube feedings, hindered elevation of upper body

Breathing pattern, ineffective Related factors: Neuromuscular paralysis or weakness, decreased energy and *Fatigue*

Caregiver role strain Related factors: Complex, long-term needs of patient

Communication, impaired verbal Related factors: Psychologic impairment, aphasia, inability to speak, inability to speak clearly, tracheostomy, muscle weakness

Constipation Related factors: Decreased activity, inability to ingest adequate fiber

Coping, ineffective Related factor: Personal vulnerability to situational crisis (e.g., new diagnosis of illness, declining health, terminal illness)

Disuse syndrome, risk for Risk factors: Paralysis, altered level of consciousness

Diversional activity, deficient Related factors: Forced inactivity, long-term hospitalization

Family processes, interrupted Related factors: Change in family roles; change in family structure; cognitive and emotional changes of family member; hospitalization or change in environment; *Impaired verbal communication*, secondary to CNS changes

Fatigue Related factors: Disease process, immobility

Fear Related factor: Real threat to well-being (see *Anxiety*)

Fluid volume, deficient Related factors: Inadequate fluid intake, vomiting secondary to increased intracranial pressure

Grieving, anticipatory or dysfunctional Related factors: Functional losses, role changes, uncertain prognosis, inability to change outcome of disease process

Home maintenance, impaired Related factors: *Activity intolerance*, effects of debilitating disease, home environment obstacles, inadequate support system, insufficient family organization or planning, psychologic impairment, lack of familiarity with community resources

Hopelessness Related factors: Failing or deteriorating physical condition, perception of having no way to improve situation

Incontinence, urinary, functional Related factors: Cognitive impairment; *Impaired physical mobility; Confusion acute/chronic*; disorientation; lack of sphincter control; spastic bladder

Incontinence, urinary, total Related factor: Neurologic dysfunction (see *Functional urinary incontinence*)

Injury (e.g., falls), risk for Risk factors: Sensory dysfunction (e.g., visual disturbances), cognitive, and psychomotor deficits secondary to compression or displacement of brain tissue, muscular weakness, unsteady gait

Mobility: physical, impaired Related factors: Neuromuscular impairment, decreased strength and endurance, *Pain*/discomfort, medically prescribed treatment, muscle rigidity, tremors

Nutrition, imbalanced: less than body requirements Related factors: Difficulty chewing secondary to cranial nerve involvement, *Impaired swallowing*, psychologic impairment, loss of appetite, *Fatigue*

Pain, acute/chronic Related factors: Neurologic injury, headache secondary to displaced brain tissue or increased intracranial pressure

Powerlessness See *Hopelessness*

Role performance, ineffective Related factors: Chronic illness, treatment side effects, brain changes

Self-care deficit: (specify) Related factors: *Pain* (e.g., headache, joint pain), decreased strength and endurance, sensory-motor impairments, cognitive deficits, *Fatigue,* paralysis

Sexual dysfunction/Sexuality patterns, ineffective Related factors: Loss of perineal sensation, *Fatigue*, decreased libido, *Low self-esteem* (*chronic, situational*), *Impaired physical mobility*

Skin integrity, impaired Related factors: Physical immobilization, impaired circulation

Social interaction, impaired Related factors: Communication barriers, *Low self-esteem* (*chronic, situational*), extended hospitalization, *Impaired physical mobility,* embarrassment

Spontaneous ventilation, impaired Related factors: Impaired neuromuscular function, pressure on brain stem

Swallowing, impaired Related factors: Impairment of laryngeal or pharyngeal neuromuscular function; impaired sensory transmission, reception, or integration secondary to cerebellar lesions

Thought processes, disturbed Related factors: Chronic organic disorder, pressure on brain tissue

Urinary retention Related factor: Sensory or motor impairment

Violence: self-directed or directed at others, risk for Risk factor: Organic mental disorder

Obesity

Nursing Diagnoses

Activity intolerance Related factors: Sedentary lifestyle, exertional discomfort (e.g., shortness of breath)

Coping, Ineffective Related factors: Personal vulnerability in situational crisis, use of food to cope with stressors

Family processes, interrupted Related factor: Effects of weight-loss therapy on family relationships

Health maintenance, ineffective Related factor: Lack of ability to make deliberate and thoughtful judgments about exercise, nutrition, and so forth

Health-seeking behaviors (specify) Related factors: Specific to patient

Mobility: physical, impaired Related factor: Decreased strength and endurance

Nutrition, imbalanced: more than body requirements Related factors: Eating disorder, lack of physical exercise, decreased metabolic requirements, lack of basic nutritional knowledge

Self-esteem, low (chronic, situational) Related factors: Responses of peers and family to obesity, negative view of self as compared to societal ideal, *Disturbed body image*

Sexuality patterns, ineffective Related factors: *Disturbed body image*, difficulty assuming sexual positions, rejection by partner

Social interaction, impaired Related factors: Self-concept disturbance, feelings of embarrassment, actual rejection by others because of appearance

Pancreatitis

Potential Complications (Collaborative Problems)

PC of pancreatitis: Coma, delirium tremens, hemorrhage, hypovolemic shock, hypocalcemia, hyperglycemia or hypoglycemia, psychosis, pleural effusion or respiratory failure

Nursing Diagnoses

Activity intolerance Related factors: *Acute Pain*, weakness/*Fatigue*, malnutrition

Anxiety Related factors: Change in health status, unfamiliar environment, *Fear* of reccurrence of *Pain*

Breathing patterns, ineffective Related factors: Abdominal distention, ascites, *Pain*, pleural effusion, respiratory failure

Coping, ineffective Related factors: Alcohol abuse, severity of illness, chronicity of illness

Denial, ineffective Related factors: Failure to acknowledge alcohol abuse or dependency (see *Ineffective coping*)

Diarrhea Related factor: Excessive fats in stools secondary to insufficient pancreatic enzymes

Family processes, dysfunctional: alcoholism Related factors: Hospitalization or change in environment, change in family roles, alcohol abuse by family member or patient

Fear Related factor: Real or imagined threat to own well-being (see *Anxiety*)

Fluid volume, deficient Related factors: Abnormal fluid loss (e.g., nasogastric suctioning, vomiting, fever, diaphoresis), inadequate fluid intake (e.g., NPO status), fluid shifts (e.g., into retroperitoneal space), bleeding

Infection, risk for Related factors: Stasis and shifts of body fluids (e.g., retroperitoneal effusion), change in pH of fluids, immunosuppression, chronicity of disease, *Imbalanced nutritional status*

Therapeutic regimen management, ineffective Related factors: *Deficient knowledge* (e.g., related to disease process, treatments, therapeutic diet, follow-up care, alcohol treatment programs, signs and symptoms of addiction), impaired judgment secondary to alcohol abuse

Noncompliance Related factors: Negative perception of treatment regimen, dysfunctional relationship between patient and provider, poor judgment secondary to alcohol abuse

Nutrition, imbalanced: less than body requirements Related factors: Loss of appetite, *Nausea*/vomiting, decreased ability to digest foods secondary to loss of insulin and digestive enzymes, chemical dependence, NPO status, nasogastric suctioning

Pain Related factors: Inflammation of pancreas and surrounding tissue, pancreatic duct obstruction, interruption of blood supply, pleural effusion, pancreatic enzymes in peritoneal tissues, nasogastric suctioning

Self-care deficit: (specify) Related factors: *Pain*/discomfort, *Activity intolerance*, *Confusion*

Renal Failure, Acute

Potential Complications (Collaborative Problems)

PC of renal failure: Electrolyte imbalance, fluid overload, metabolic acidosis, pericarditis, platelet dysfunction, secondary infections

Nursing Diagnoses

Activity intolerance Related factors: Increased energy requirements (e.g., fever, inflammation), decreased energy production, inadequate nutrition, anemia

Anxiety Related factors: Unknown prognosis, severity of illness

Cardiac output, decreased Related factor: Increased ventricular workload secondary to volume overload

Confusion See *Thought processes, disturbed*

Environmental interpretation syndrome, impaired See *Thought processes, disturbed*

Fear Related factors: Environmental stressors or hospitalization, *Powerlessness*, threat to own well-being, threat to child's well-being, severity of illness, multisystem effects

Fluid volume excess Related factors: Changes in renal vascular supply resulting in ischemia, tubular necrosis, decreased glomerular filtration rate

Infection, risk for Risk factors: Invasive procedures, disease process, lowered resistance, malnutrition

Nutrition, imbalanced: less than body requirements Related factors: Anorexia, *Nausea* and vomiting, dietary restrictions, change in taste, loss of smell, stomatitis, increased metabolic needs

Oral mucous membrane, impaired Related factors: Extracellular fluid depletion, stomatitis

Skin integrity, impaired Related factors: Poor skin turgor secondary to extracellular fluid, *Diarrhea*

Thought processes, disturbed Related factors: Decreased cerebral perfusion, accumulation of toxic wastes

Renal Failure, Chronic

Potential Complications (Collaborative Problems)

PC chronic renal failure: Anemia, congestive heart failure, fluid and electrolyte imbalance, fluid overload, hyperparathyroidism, infections, medication toxicity, metabolic acidosis, GI bleeding, pericarditis, cardiac tamponade, pleural effusion, pulmonary edema, uremia

Nursing Diagnoses

Activity intolerance Related factors: Weakness or *Fatigue* secondary to anemia, inadequate oxygenation secondary to cardiac or pulmonary complications

Body image, disturbed Related factors: *Delayed growth and development*, treatment side effects, chronic illness, surgery (e.g., insertion of hemodialysis blood access or peritoneal catheter, amputations), kidney transplant

Breathing pattern, ineffective Related factors: Anemia, volume overload, pressure of dialysate on diaphragm

Caregiver role strain Related factors: Complexity, amount, and duration of caregiving tasks; illness severity; situational stressors within the family; caregiver's health, knowledge, skills, experience, competing role commitments, and coping styles; isolation, lack of opportunity for respite and recreation

Comfort, altered (non-NANDA International) Related factors: Pruritus, fluid retention, vomiting, urate or calcium phosphate crystals on skin

Confusion, acute/chronic Related factors: Uremic encephalopathy, inadequate oxygenation secondary to cardiac or respiratory complications, anemia

Constipation Related factors: Restriction of fluids and fiber-rich foods, decreased activity, presence of phosphate-binding agents, medications

Coping: family, disabled Related factors: Chronically unresolved feelings, chronic illness and uncertain future of patient, complexity of home care (e.g., home dialysis)

Coping, ineffective Related factors: Personal vulnerability in situational crisis (e.g., new diagnosis of chronic illness, declining health, terminal illness), inability to concentrate, short attention span, and impaired reasoning secondary to central nervous system involvement

Diversional activity, deficient Related factor: Frequent or lengthy medical treatments, lack of energy and mobility to participate

Falls, risk for Risk factors: Impaired mobility, sensory impairment, hypotension, weakness

Fatigue Related factors: Altered renal function, inactivity, inadequate nutrition (see *Activity intolerance*).

Fear Related factors: Environmental stressors/hospitalization, *Powerlessness*, real or imagined threat to well-being

Fluid volume, deficient Related factors: Abnormal fluid loss (e.g., vomiting), abnormal blood loss secondary to hemodialysis procedure, inadequate fluid intake, compensatory diuresis of dilute urine secondary to decreased ability to concentrate urine, inability of tubules to reabsorb sodium, shifts between blood and dialysate

Fluid volume excess Related factors: Increased fluid intake secondary to excess sodium intake, sodium retention, hyperglycemia, *Noncompliance* with fluid restriction, shifts between blood and dialysate

Grieving, dysfunctional Related factors: Chronic illness, loss, terminal illness, separation from significant others, loss of role function

Hopelessness Related factors: Failing or deteriorating physical condition, lack of social supports, long-term stress, inability to change progression of disease

Infection, risk for Risk factors: Immunosuppression, malnutrition, invasive therapy (e.g., dialysis)

Memory, impaired Related factor: Neurologic changes

Mobility: physical, impaired Related factors: Decreased strength and endurance secondary to anemia, cardiac or respiratory complications, musculoskeletal impairment (e.g., fractures secondary to osteoporosis), neuromuscular impairment

Noncompliance Related factors: Denial of illness, dysfunctional relationship between patient and provider, negative perception or consequence of treatment regimen, perceived benefits of continued illness

Nutrition, imbalanced: less than body requirements Related factors: Loss of appetite, *Nausea* or vomiting, dietary restrictions, stomatitis, loss of taste or smell secondary to cranial nerve changes

Powerlessness Related factors: Treatment regimen, inability to change progressive course of the disease

Self-care deficit: (specify) Related factors: Depression, *Pain* and discomfort, *Activity intolerance,* neuromuscular impairment, musculoskeletal impairment

Self-esteem, low (chronic, situational) See *Body image, disturbed*

Sexual dysfunction Related factors: *Low self-esteem* (*chronic, situational*), impotence, loss of libido, *Activity intolerance*

Skin integrity, impaired Related factors: Edema, dry skin, pruritus, impaired venous circulation secondary to surgical creation of hemodialysis blood access, impaired arterial circulation secondary to hypertension, hyperglycemia

Therapeutic regimen management, ineffective Related factors: *Deficient knowledge* (e.g., related to disease, dietary restrictions, medications, signs and symptoms of complications, community resources), complexity of regimen, *Acute/chronic confusion* and *Impaired memory* secondary to disease process

Respiratory Disorders, Acute

Potential Complications (Collaborative Problems)

PC of pneumonia: Lung tissue necrosis

PC of pulmonary edema: Right-sided heart failure, anasarca, multiple organ system failure

PC of pulmonary embolism: pulmonary infarction with necrosis

Nursing Diagnoses

Pneumonia

Activity intolerance Related factor: Weakness and *Fatigue*

Anxiety Related factors: Threat to or change to health status, dyspnea

Fluid volume, deficient Related factors: Factors affecting fluid needs (e.g., fever)

Gas exchange, impaired Related factors: Decreased functional lung tissue secondary to consolidation, increased secretions

Nutrition, imbalanced: less than body requirements Related factor: Loss of appetite

Pain Related factors: Injury, difficulty breathing

Self-care deficit: (specify) Related factors: *Pain* and discomfort, *Activity intolerance*

Sleep deprivation/Sleep pattern, disturbed Related factors: Dyspnea, *Pain*

Pulmonary Edema

Activity intolerance Related factors: Imbalance between oxygen supply and demand, weakness and *Fatigue*

Cardiac output, decreased Related factors: Increased ventricular workload

Fatigue See *Activity intolerance*

Fear Related factors: Environmental stressors or hospitalization

Fluid volume excess Related factor: Decreased urine output secondary to pulmonary edema

Nutrition, imbalanced: less than body requirements Related factor: Loss of appetite

Self-care deficit: (specify) Related factors: *Pain* and discomfort, *Activity intolerance*

Sleep deprivation/Sleep pattern, disturbed Related factor: Dyspnea

Pulmonary Embolism

Activity intolerance Related factors: *Acute Pain*, imbalance between oxygen supply and demand

Fear Related factor: Real or imagined threat to own well-being

Gas exchange, impaired Related factor: Decreased pulmonary blood supply secondary to pulmonary embolus

Self-care deficit: (specify) Related factors: *Pain* and discomfort, *Activity intolerance*

Respiratory Disorders, Chronic

Includes but is not limited to asthma, COPD, and chronic restrictive pulmonary disease.

Potential Complications (Collaborative Problems)

PC of chronic pulmonary disease: Hypoxemia, right-sided heart failure, respiratory infection, spontaneous pneumothorax

Nursing Diagnoses

Activity intolerance Related factors: Dyspnea, weakness and *Fatigue*, inadequate oxygenation, *Anxiety*, *Disturbed sleep pattern*

Airway clearance, ineffective Related factors: Tracheobronchial obstruction, excessive and tenacious secretions, ineffective cough secondary to decreased energy and *Fatigue*

Anxiety Related factors: Dyspnea, *Fear* of suffocation, smoking cessation

Caregiver role strain Related factors: Illness severity of the care receiver, unpredictable course of the illness, amount and duration of caregiving required, inadequate physical environment for providing care, lack of respite and recreation for caregiver

Communication, impaired verbal Related factor: Dyspnea

Coping, ineffective Related factors: Personal vulnerability in situational crisis (e.g., declining health), difficulty of smoking cessation

Family processes, interrupted Related factors: Change in family roles or structure, hospitalization or change in environment, chronic illness or disability of family member

Fear See *Anxiety*

Fluid volume, deficient Related factors: Inadequate fluid intake secondary to difficulty in breathing, fluid loss secondary to fever and diaphoresis

Health maintenance, ineffective Related factors: Health beliefs, lack of social supports, difficulty with smoking cessation

Home maintenance, impaired Related factors: *Fatigue*, *Activity intolerance*, lack of social support

Nutrition, imbalanced: less than body requirements Related factors: Loss of appetite, *Nausea* and vomiting, decreased energy, dyspnea

Powerlessness Related factors: Treatment regimen, chronic illness, lifestyle changes, loss of control (e.g., "too late" to improve lung function)

Self-care deficit: (specify) Related factors: Decreased strength and endurance, *Activity intolerance*

Sexual dysfunction/Sexuality patterns, ineffective Related factors: Dyspnea, lack of energy, relationship changes

Sleep pattern, disturbed Related factors: *Anxiety*, medical regimen (e.g., pulmonary treatments), inability to assume usual sleep position because of dyspnea, unfamiliar hospital environment, cough

Ventilatory weaning response, dysfunctional (DVWR) Related factors: *Ineffective airway clearance*, patient perceived inefficacy about the ability to wean, *Fear* of suffocation, lack of motivation, *Anxiety*, inappropriate pacing of diminished ventilator support, history of ventilator dependence > one week, history of multiple unsuccessful weaning attempts

Urologic Disorders

Include but are not limited to cystitis, glomerulonephritis, pyelonephritis, and urolithiasis

Potential Complications (Collaborative Problems)

PC of cystitis: Renal infection, ulceration of bladder

PC of urolithiasis: Pyelonephritis, renal insufficiency

PC of pyelonephritis: Chronic pyelonephritis, bacteremia, renal insufficiency

Nursing Diagnoses

Diarrhea Related factor: Stimulation of renal or intestinal reflexes

Fluid volume, deficient Related factors: Fever, vomiting, *Diarrhea* secondary to stimulation of renal or intestinal reflexes

Hyperthermia Related factors: Inflammatory process, increased metabolic rate

Incontinence, urinary, urge Related factors: Bladder irritation, dysuria, pyuria, frequency

Nutrition, imbalanced: less than body requirements Related factors: Anorexia secondary to fever, *Nausea*, vomiting, and *Pain*

Pain Related factors: Inflammation of bladder or renal tissues; headache; muscular pain; abdominal pain; distention, trauma, and smooth-muscle spasms; and edema in renal tissue (in urolithiasis)

Vascular Disease

Includes but is not limited to deep vein thrombosis, hypertension, stasis ulcers, varicosities, peripheral vascular disease, and thrombophlebitis

Potential Complications (Collaborative Problems)

PC of varicose veins: Vascular rupture, hemorrhage, venous stasis ulcers, cellulitis

PC of peripheral arterial disease: Arterial thrombosis, CVA, hypertension, ischemic ulcers, cellulitis

PC of deep vein thrombosis: Chronic leg edema, stasis ulcers, pulmonary embolism

Nursing Diagnoses

Activity intolerance Related factors: *Pain*, claudication

Body image, disturbed Related factors: Chronic illness, appearance of legs

Injury, risk for Risk factors: Sensory dysfunction, *Impaired physical mobility*

Pain Related factors: Tissue ischemia secondary to decreased peripheral circulation, engorgement or distention of veins

Role performance, ineffective Related factor: *Chronic Pain*

Self-esteem, low (chronic, situational) Related factor: Chronic illness (see *Disturbed body image*

Skin integrity, impaired Related factors: Draining wound, tissue ischemia secondary to impaired circulation, physical immobilization, ankle or leg edema, decreased sensation secondary to chronic atherosclerosis

Tissue perfusion, ineffective (peripheral) Related factors: Impaired venous circulation, impaired arterial circulation

SURGICAL CONDITIONS

Abdominal surgery

Breast surgery

Chest surgery

Craniotomy

Ear surgery

Eye surgery

Musculoskeletal surgery

Neck surgery

Rectal surgery

Skin graft

Spinal surgery

Urologic surgery

Vascular surgery

Abdominal Surgery

Includes but is not limited to appendectomy, cholecystectomy, colectomy, colon resection, colostomy, gastrectomy, gastric resection, gastroenterostomy, abdominal hysterectomy with or without salpingo-oophorectomy, ileostomy, laparotomy, lysis of adhesions, Marshall-Marchetti-Krantz operation, ovarian cystectomy, salpingotomy, small bowel resection, splenectomy, vagotomy, and hiatal hernia repair

Potential Complications (Collaborative Problems)

PC of general anesthesia: Stasis pneumonia

PC of surgery: Dehiscence, evisceration, fistula formation, hemorrhage, paralytic ileus, peritonitis, pulmonary embolism, renal failure, surgical trauma (e.g., to ureter, bladder, or rectum), thrombophlebitis, urinary retention

Nursing Diagnoses

Airway clearance, ineffective See *Breathing pattern, ineffective*

Anxiety Related factors: Surgical procedure, preoperative procedures (e.g., IV insertion, Foley catheter, fluid restrictions), postoperative procedures (e.g., coughing and deep breathing, NPO status)

Aspiration, risk for Risk factors: Decreased motility and depressed cough and gag reflexes secondary to anesthesia or analgesics, presence of endotracheal tube, incomplete lower esophageal sphincter, GI tubes, increased intragastric pressure, increased gastric residual, delayed gastric emptying, hindered elevation of upper body

Body image, disturbed Related factors: Surgery (e.g., ostomy), situational crisis, treatment side effects, cultural or spiritual factors

Breathing pattern, ineffective Related factors: *Pain*, immobility, postanesthesia state

Caregiver role strain Related factors: Illness severity of care receiver, discharge of family member with significant home care needs, past history of poor relationship between caregiver and care receiver

Constipation Related factors: Decreased activity, decreased fluid and fiber intake, lack of privacy, change in daily routine, decreased peristalsis secondary to anesthetic, narcotic analgesics

Delayed surgical recovery Related factors: Infection, ileus, poor preoperative health, chronic illnesses, poor nutritional status

Fear Related factors: Environmental stressors or hospitalization, real or imagined threat to own well-being, unpredictable outcome of surgical procedure, general anesthesia, surgical outcome, *Pain*

Fluid volume, deficient Related factors: Abnormal blood loss, abnormal fluid loss (e.g., vomiting), failure of regulatory mechanisms

Infection, risk for Risk factors: Stasis of body fluids, altered peristalsis, suppressed inflammatory response, invasive procedures and lines, surgical incision, urinary catheter

Nutrition, imbalanced: less than body requirements Related factors: Loss of appetite, *Nausea* or vomiting, diet restrictions, increased protein and vitamin requirements for healing

Oral mucous membrane, impaired Related factors: Mouth breathing and NPO status secondary to nasogastric tube

Pain Related factors: Incision, abdominal distention, immobility

Perioperative positioning injury, risk for Risk factors: Advanced age, disorientation, edema, emaciation, muscle weakness, obesity, sensory or perceptual disturbances due to anesthesia

Sexual dysfunction or Ineffective sexuality patterns Related factors: *Pain*, health-related transitions, *Disturbed body image,* altered body function or structure, reaction of partner (e.g., to ostomy or hysterectomy), physiologic impotence or inadequate vaginal lubrication secondary to the surgery

Skin integrity, impaired Related factors: Mechanical factors, *Impaired physical mobility* secondary to pain and invasive lines, excretions and secretions, poor nutritional state, altered sensation

Social isolation Related factors: Embarrassment about odors, appearance, or appliance (e.g., ostomy pouch); reaction of others to appearance and odors

Tissue perfusion, ineffective (gastrointestinal) Related factors: Interruption of arterial flow, exchange problems, hypervolemia, hypovolemia

Breast Surgery

Includes but is not limited to breast augmentation, mastectomy, reconstruction, lumpectomy, and biopsy

Potential Complications (Collaborative Problems)

PC of breast surgery: Cellulitis, lymphedema, hematoma, seroma

Nursing Diagnoses

Anxiety Related factors: Threat to self-concept, threat to or change in health status, threat to or change in interaction patterns with significant others, situational or maturational crisis

Body image, disturbed Related factors: Surgery, treatment side effects, cultural or spiritual factors pertaining to changes in breast and sexuality

Coping, ineffective Related factors: Changes in appearance, concern over others' reaction, loss of function, diagnosis of cancer

Family processes, interrupted Related factors: Complex therapies (e.g., radiation, chemotherapy), hospitalization or change in environment, reactions of significant others to disfigurement

Fear Related factors: Disease process or prognosis (e.g., cancer), *Powerlessness*

Grieving, anticipatory/dysfunctional Related factors: Loss of body part or function, change in appearance

Mobility: physical, impaired Related factors: Decreased range of motion of shoulder or arm secondary to lymphedema, nerve or muscle damage, or *Pain*

Pain Related factors: Surgical procedure, paresthesia

Self-care deficit: dressing/grooming Related factors: *Pain* and discomfort, neuromuscular impairment

Sexuality patterns, ineffective Related factors: *Pain*, altered body function or structure, illness, medical treatment, *Disturbed body image*, *Low self-esteem* (*chronic, situational*), reaction of significant other

Chest Surgery

Includes but is not limited to biopsy, cardiopulmonary bypass, coronary artery bypass, lobectomy, and thoracotomy

Potential Complications (Collaborative Problems)

PC of coronary artery bypass graft: Cardiovascular insufficiency, respiratory insufficiency, renal insufficiency

PC of thoracotomy: Atelectasis, cardiac dysrhythmias, hemorrhage, pneumonia, pneumothorax, hemothorax, mediastinal shift, pulmonary edema, pulmonary embolus, subcutaneous emphysema, thrombophlebitis

PC of chest surgery: Myocardial infarction

Nursing Diagnoses

Activity intolerance Related factors: Imbalance between oxygen supply and demand, *acute Pain*, weakness and *Fatigue*, narcotic analgesics, loss of alveolar ventilation

Breathing pattern, ineffective Related factors: Ineffective cough secondary to decreased energy and *Fatigue*, *acute Pain*, increased tracheobronchial secretions

Cardiac output, decreased Related factors: Dysfunctional electrical conduction, ventricular ischemia, ventricular damage, diminished circulating volume, increased systemic vascular resistance

Communication, impaired verbal Related factor: Intubation

Coping, ineffective Related factors: Personal vulnerability in situational crisis (specify), inability to perform usual roles, loss of body function (e.g., respiratory), temporary dependence, need for changes in lifestyle

Family processes, interrupted Related factors: Fear of death or disability, disruption of family processes, stressful environment (e.g., intensive care unit, hospital)

Fear Related factors: Environmental stressors or hospitalization, threat to own well-being, *Fear* of complications after being transferred out of intensive care unit

Gas exchange, impaired Related factors: Decreased functional lung tissue secondary to pneumonia or lung resection, respiratory distress syndrome, ventilation–perfusion imbalance

Infection, risk for Risk factor: Collection of fluid in thoracic cavity

Mobility, physical, impaired Related factors: Limited arm or shoulder movement secondary to muscle dissection and prescribed position restrictions, *Pain*

Noncompliance Related factors: Denial of illness, negative perception of treatment regimen, difficulty with smoking cessation

Pain Related factors: Surgical incisions, chest tubes, immobility

Role performance, ineffective Related factors: Surgery, treatment side effects, dependent role during recuperation, uncertain future

Self-care deficit: (specify) Related factors: *Pain* and discomfort, *Activity intolerance* secondary to inadequate oxygenation, *Impaired physical mobility* (arms, shoulders)

Self-esteem, low (chronic, situational) Related factors: Changes in lifestyle, symbolic meaning of the heart, inability to perform usual roles

Sleep deprivation/Sleep pattern, disturbed Related factors: *Pain* and discomfort, unfamiliar surroundings, medically prescribed treatments (e.g., nebulizer)

Ventilatory weaning response, dysfunctional (DVWR) Related factors: Uncontrolled *Pain* and discomfort, moderate to severe *Anxiety*, *Fear*, history of ventilatory dependence > one week

Craniotomy

Includes but is not limited to acoustic neuroma removal, cerebral aneurysm clipping, cerebral bleed, and cerebral trauma

Potential Complications (Collaborative Problems)

PC of craniotomy: Cardiac dysrhythmias, cerebral or cerebellar dysfunction, cerebrospinal fluid leaks, cranial nerve impairment, fluid and

electrolyte imbalance, GI bleeding, hemorrhage, hematomas, hydrocephalus, hygromas, hyperthermia/hypothermia, hypoxemia, meningitis
or encephalitis, seizures, residual neurologic defects

Nursing Diagnoses

Activity intolerance Related factors: Weakness and *Fatigue*, *Pain*, *Sleep
deprivation*, decreased level of consciousness

Airway clearance, ineffective Related factors: Tracheobronchial secretions, increased intracranial pressure

Aspiration, risk for Risk factor: Cranial nerve dysfunction

Body image, disturbed Related factors: Surgery, treatment side effects
(e.g., difficulty speaking, appearance)

Breathing pattern, ineffective Related factors: Depression of respiratory
center, neuromuscular paralysis or weakness, cranial nerve dysfunction, airway obstruction secondary to neck edema

Caregiver role strain Related factors: Illness severity of care receiver, discharge of family member with significant home care needs, unpredictable
illness course, psychologic or cognitive problems in care receiver

Confusion, acute/chronic See *Thought processes, disturbed*

Communication, impaired verbal Related factors: Aphasia, dysarthria,
Acute confusion, intubation

Disuse syndrome, risk for Risk factors: Paralysis, prescribed or mechanical immobilization, decreased level of consciousness

Environmental interpretation syndrome, impaired See *Thought processes,
disturbed*

Fear Related factors: Environmental stressors or hospitalization, *Powerlessness*, threat to own well-being, seriousness of surgery, possibility of
dying

Fluid volume excess Related factor: Decreased urine output secondary to
renal dysfunction

Incontinence, bowel Related factor: Decreased level of consciousness

Incontinence, urinary, functional Related factors: Cognitive impairment,
disorientation, *Impaired physical mobility*

Incontinence, urinary, total Related factors: Neuropathy preventing trans-
missions of reflex indicating bladder fullness, neurologic dysfunction
causing triggering of micturition at unpredictable times, independent
contraction of detrusor reflex due to surgery

Injury (contractures), risk for Risk factors: Sensory dysfunction, *Impaired
physical mobility*

Memory, impaired Related factors: Brain tissue hypoxia or loss secondary
to disease or surgery

Mobility, physical, impaired Related factors: Neuromuscular impairment,
perceptual or cognitive impairment, depression, severe *Anxiety*

Nutrition, imbalanced: less than body requirements Related factor:
Inability to eat secondary to decreased level of consciousness

Pain Related factors: Surgical procedure, paresthesia

Role performance, ineffective Related factors: Surgery, psychologic
impairment, treatment side effects, visual and speech disturbances,
seizures, memory loss

Self-care deficit: (specify) Related factors: *Activity intolerance*, neuromuscular impairment, altered level of consciousness, *Disturbed sensory perception, Pain*, weakness

Sensory perception, disturbed: (specify) Related factors: Altered sensory reception, transmission, or integration; sensory deficit; sensory overload

Swallowing, impaired Related factors: Cranial nerve dysfunction; altered sensory reception, transmission, or integration; neuromuscular impairment

Therapeutic regimen management, ineffective Related factors: *Acute* or *chronic confusion*; *Impaired memory* and judgment secondary to residual effects on brain tissue; lack of social support

Thought processes, disturbed Related factors: Increased intracranial pressure, *Sleep deprivation,* brain tissue loss secondary to cerebral edema, hypoxia or surgical resection

Tissue perfusion, ineffective (cerebral) Related factors: Interruption of arterial blood flow, increased intracranial pressure

Ear Surgery

Includes but is not limited to myringotomy, reconstruction, and stapedectomy

Potential Complications (Collaborative Problems)

PC of ear surgery: Facial paralysis, hearing loss, infection

Nursing Diagnoses

Communication, impaired verbal Related factor: Hearing loss

Falls, risk for Risk factors: Vertigo, nystagmus

Infection, risk for Risk factors: Exposure to upper respiratory infections, invasive procedures

Pain Related factors: Inflammation, tissue trauma, edema, presence of surgical packing

Self-care deficit: (specify) Related factor: *Activity intolerance* secondary to dizziness and loss of balance

Sensory perception, disturbed (auditory) Related factors: Sensory deficit, sensory overload, surgical packing, edema, disturbance of middle-ear structures

Trauma, risk for Risk factor: Displacement of prosthesis secondary to increased middle-ear pressure

Eye Surgery

Includes but is not limited to blepharoplasty, cataract removal, cryosurgery for retinal detachment, iridectomy, iridotomy, and lens implant

Potential Complications (Collaborative Problems)

PC of eye surgery: Bleeding, endophthalmus, hyphema (i.e., blood in anterior chamber of the eye), increased intraocular pressure, infection, lens implant dislocation, macular edema, retinal detachment, secondary glaucoma

Nursing Diagnoses

Body image, disturbed Related factor: Change in appearance (enucleation)

Falls, risk for Risk factors: Unsafe ambulation secondary to limited vision, eye patches, unfamiliar environment

Fear Related factor: Real or imagined threat to own well-being (e.g., permanent loss of vision)

Mobility: physical, impaired Related factors: Medically prescribed treatment and positioning, impaired vision

Self-care deficit: (specify) Related factors: Eye patches, impaired vision

Sensory perception, disturbed (visual) Related factor: Sensory deficit secondary to eye patches or impaired vision

Musculoskeletal Surgery

Includes but is not limited to amputation, arthrotomy, bunionectomy, casts, hip pinning, hip prosthesis, open reduction or internal fixation of fracture, shoulder repair, total ankle replacement, total hip replacement, total knee replacement, and traction

Potential Complications (Collaborative Problems)

PC of amputation: Edema of the stump

PC of fractures: Fat embolus, nonunion of bone, reflex sympathetic dystrophy

PC of fractures and casts: Compartmental syndrome

PC of fractures and musculoskeletal surgery: Deep vein thrombosis, nerve damage

PC of joint replacement surgery: Joint dislocation or displacement of prosthesis

PC of musculoskeletal surgery: Flexion contractures, hematoma, hemorrhage, infection, pulmonary embolism, sepsis, stress fractures, synovial herniation,

PC of total hip replacement: Femoral head necrosis

Nursing Diagnoses

Activity intolerance Related factors: *Pain*, weakness, *Sleep deprivation*

Anxiety Related factors: Lack of knowledge of surgery and postoperative routines (e.g., physical therapy, walking with crutches), threat to self-concept, threat to or change in role functioning

Body image, disturbed Related factors: Surgery (e.g., loss of limb), loss of functional abilities (e.g., need to use wheelchair), fear of others' response to appearance

Confusion, acute Related factors: Hypoxemia, medications (e.g., opiate analgesics), infection, impaction

Constipation Related factors: Decreased activity, dietary changes, medication (e.g., opiates, anesthetics)

Coping, ineffective Related factors: *Pain, Self-care deficits*, long-term and debilitating nature of disease

Disuse syndrome, risk for Risk factor: Prescribed immobilization

Diversional activity, deficient Related factors: Prolonged bed rest, institutionalization

Falls, risk for Risk factors: Unfamiliarity of assistive devices (e.g., crutches), weakness secondary to surgery and immobility

Grieving, anticipatory/dysfunctional Related factors: Loss of limb, changes in lifestyle, loss of ability to perform usual roles

Home maintenance, impaired Related factors: Barriers (e.g., stairs) and hazards (e.g., throw rugs), Activity intolerance

Infection, risk for Risk factors: Inadequate primary defense secondary to exposure of joint, broken skin

Injury (contractures), risk for Risk factors: Immobility secondary to *Pain* or weakness

Mobility: physical, impaired Related factors: *Pain*, stiffness, decreased strength

Pain Related factors: Muscle cramps, paresthesia, inflammation, surgical procedure, joint destruction, phantom limb pain

Peripheral neurovascular dysfunction, risk for Related factors: Fractures, mechanical compression, orthopedic surgery, trauma, immobilization, casts and traction devices

Self-care deficit: (specify) Related factors: *Pain, Activity intolerance, Impaired physical mobility,* decreased strength and endurance

Skin integrity, impaired Related factors: Mechanical factors, prescribed physical immobilization, *Impaired physical mobility*, impaired circulation, altered sensation, casts and other appliances, edema (e.g., of stump)

Sleep deprivation/Sleep pattern, disturbed Related factors: *Pain* and discomfort, unfamiliar surroundings, medically induced regimen, inability to assume usual sleep position

Therapeutic regimen management, ineffective Related factors: Lack of knowledge of disease process, surgical treatment, self-care, complex rehabilitation regimen, alterations in lifestyle, insufficient energy to perform exercises

Tissue perfusion, ineffective (peripheral) Related factors: Reduced arterial or venous blood flow, trauma to blood vessels, edema, dislocation of prosthesis

Neck Surgery

Includes but is not limited to carotid endarterectomy, laryngectomy, parathyroidectomy, radical neck dissection, thyroidectomy, tonsillectomy, and tracheostomy

Potential Complications (Collaborative Problems)

PC of neck surgery: Airway obstruction, aspiration, cerebral infarction, cranial nerve damage (e.g., facial, hypoglossal, glossopharyngeal, vagus), fistula formation (e.g., between hypopharynx and skin), hemorrhage, hypertension, hypotension, infection, local nerve impairment, thyroid storm, tracheal stenosis, vocal cord paralysis

PC radical neck dissection: Flap rejection

PC thyroidectomy/parathyroidectomy: Hypoparathyroidism, causing hypocalcemia and tetany

Nursing Diagnoses

Activity intolerance Related factors: Imbalance between oxygen supply and demand, *Anxiety, Pain,* weakness secondary to limited mobility, *Fatigue* secondary to accelerated metabolic rate (e.g., thyroidectomy)

Airway clearance, ineffective Related factors: Decreased energy, edema, *Pain*, tracheobronchial obstruction, increased tracheobronchial secretions, edema of the glottis, tracheal compression secondary to hemorrhage, presence of tracheostomy tube

Anxiety See *Fear*

Aspiration, risk for Risk factors: Depressed cough or gag reflexes, presence of tracheostomy or endotracheal tube, *Impaired swallowing*, hindered elevation of upper body, removal of epiglottis (in partial laryngectomy), loss of normal reflexes and excessive secretions secondary to surgery

Body image, disturbed Related factors: Changes in appearance secondary to surgery, depression, treatment side effects

Breathing pattern, ineffective Related factors: *Anxiety*, decreased energy, accidental decannulation

Communication, impaired verbal Related factors: *Acute confusion*, inability to speak, inability to speak clearly secondary to *Pain* and edema, tracheostomy, laryngectomy, weak or hoarse voice secondary to trauma to laryngeal nerve

Coping, ineffective Related factors: Personal vulnerability in situational crisis (specify), inability to speak, disfigurement, inadequate support system (see *Body image, disturbed*)

Falls, risk for Risk factors: Sensory dysfunction, integrative dysfunction, vascular insufficiency, altered mobility

Fear Related factors: Real or imagined threat to own well-being (e.g., fear of suffocation), unfamiliarity with environment and pre- and postoperative routines

Fluid volume, deficient Related factors: Loss of fluid through abnormal routes, hypermetabolic state, decreased intake secondary to *Pain* and *Impaired swallowing*

Grieving, anticipatory/dysfunctional Related factors: Actual loss of function, change in appearance, threat of dying

Infection, risk for Risk factors: Tissue destruction and increased environmental exposure, loss of normal filtration systems in the mouth and nose secondary to use of artificial airway, immunosuppression secondary to chemotherapy and malignancies

Mobility: physical, impaired Related factors: Limited shoulder and head movement secondary to removal of muscles and nerves, flap graft reconstruction

Nutrition, imbalanced: less than body requirements Related factors: *Pain, Impaired swallowing*, loss of appetite, *Nausea* and vomiting, loss of sense of smell, cachexia secondary to malignancy, accelerated metabolic rate (e.g., from thyroidectomy)

Oral mucous membrane, impaired Related factors: Inadequate oral hygiene, tubes, surgery in oral cavity, infection, radiation therapy to head and neck

Pain Related factor: Surgical procedure, edema, tracheostomy tube irritation

Role performance, ineffective Related factors: Surgery, treatment side effects, *Impaired physical mobility*

Self-esteem, low (chronic, situational) See *Body image, disturbed*

Skin integrity, impaired Related factors: Mechanical factors, radiation, altered nutritional state

Social isolation Related factors: Difficulty communicating, embarrassment and concern over others' response to disfigurement, avoidance by others

Swallowing, impaired Related factors: Irritated oropharyngeal cavity, mechanical obstruction, edema, cranial nerve damage

Tissue integrity, impaired Related factors: Nutritional deficit, irritants, mechanical factors (e.g., tracheostomy tube), radiation

Ventilatory weaning response, dysfunctional (DVWR) Related factors: *Ineffective airway clearance,* lack of motivation secondary to malaise, moderate to severe *Anxiety, Fear,* uncontrolled episodic energy demands or problems

Rectal Surgery

Includes but is not limited to fissurectomy, hemorrhoidectomy, pilonidal cystectomy, and polypectomy

Potential Complications (Collaborative Problems)

PC of rectal surgery: Hemorrhage, infection, stricture formation

Nursing Diagnoses

Constipation Related factors: Dietary changes, decreased motility secondary to medication and inactivity, *Fear* of painful defecation

Incontinence, bowel Related factor: Loss of sphincter integrity

Infection, risk for Risk factors: Loss of primary line of defense secondary to surgery, fecal contamination

Pain Related factors: Surgical procedure, passage of stool

Skin Graft

Includes but is not limited to excision of lesion with flap, excision of lesion with full-thickness graft, excision of lesion with split-thickness graft, and excision of lesion with synthetic graft

Potential Complications (Collaborative Problems)

PC of skin graft: Edema, flap necrosis, hematoma, infection

Nursing Diagnoses

Body image, disturbed Related factor: Results of reconstructive surgery not as anticipated by patient

Constipation Related factor: Decreased activity secondary to prescribed positioning

Diversional activity, deficient Related factors: Prolonged bed rest, prescribed positioning

Fear Related factors: Real or imagined threat to own well-being, fear of flap failure, fear of others' reactions to appearance

Mobility: physical, impaired Related factors: *Pain* and discomfort, prescribed position

Pain Related factors: Surgical procedure, paresthesia

Peripheral neurovascular dysfunction, risk for Risk factors: Immobilization, burns, edema

Tissue perfusion, ineffective (specify) Related factors: Restricted blood flow secondary to edema, blood clot, or tension on the flap

Spinal Surgery

Includes but is not limited to Harrington rod implant, laminectomy, Luque rod implant, and spinal fusion

Potential Complications (Collaborative Problems)

PC of laminectomy/spinal fusion: Displacement of bone graft

PC of spinal surgery: Bladder and bowel dysfunction, cerebrospinal fistula, hematoma, hemorrhage, infection, nerve root injury, paralytic ileus, sensorineural impairments, spinal cord edema or injury

Nursing Diagnoses

Activity intolerance Related factors: *Fear* of damaging surgical site, *Pain*, weakness and *Fatigue*, sedentary lifestyle, enforced inactivity

Caregiver role strain Related factors: Premature birth and congenital defect, developmental delay or retardation of the care receiver–caregiver, duration of caregiving required

Constipation Related factors: Decreased activity, medications (e.g., opiates), inability to assume normal position for defecation, change in daily routine, temporary loss of parasympathetic function innervating the bowels

Falls, risk for Risk factors: Sensory dysfunction, loss of balance, muscle weakness secondary to recent inactivity, vertigo secondary to postural hypotension

Mobility: physical, impaired Related factors: *Pain*, neuromuscular impairment, stiffness in fused area, prescribed activity and position limitations

Nutrition, imbalanced: more than body requirements Related factors: increased appetite when pain subsides, sedentary lifestyle, decreased activity

Pain, acute/chronic Related factors: Bed rest, muscle cramps, paresthesia, surgical procedure (e.g., graft site), inflammation, localized edema, muscle spasms

Peripheral neurovascular dysfunction Related factors: Fractures, mechanical compression, trauma, immobilization

Self-care deficit: (specify) Related factors: Prescribed postoperative immobility, *Pain*

Skin integrity, impaired Related factors: Prescribed activity restrictions, diminished or interrupted blood flow secondary to edema, hematoma, or hypovolemia

Urinary retention Related factors: Swelling in operative area, inability to assume usual position for voiding

Urologic Surgery

Includes but is not limited to cystocele repair, rectocele repair, removal of bladder tumor, cystoscopy, nephrectomy, penile implant, percutaneous nephrostomy, retroperitoneal lymphadenotomy, prostatectomy, transurethral resection of the prostate, ureterolithotomy, urostomy, and vasectomy

Potential Complications (Collaborative Problems)

PC of prostate resection/prostatectomy: Retrograde ejaculation

PC of urologic surgery: Bladder neck constriction, bladder perforation (intraoperative), epididymitis, hemorrhage, paralytic ileus, urethral stricture, urinary tract infection

PC of urostomy/nephrostomy: Stomal necrosis, stenosis, obstruction

Nursing Diagnoses

Anxiety Related factors: Threat to self-concept, change in health status, change in body appearance or function, threat to or change in role functioning, threat to or change in interaction pattern

Body image, disturbed Related factors: Surgery, depression, treatment side effects (e.g., impotence), appearance of ostomy (e.g., urostomy)

Grieving, anticipatory/dysfunctional Related factor: Potential loss of body parts or function

Incontinence, urinary, stress Related factors: Incompetent bladder outlet, overdistention between voidings, weak pelvic muscles and structural supports

Incontinence, urinary, urge Related factors: Decreased bladder capacity, surgery, irritation of bladder stretch receptors causing spasms, overdistention of bladder

Infection, risk for Risk factors: Stasis of body fluids, change in pH of secretions, suppressed inflammatory response, tissue destruction and increased environmental exposure, invasive procedures and lines (e.g., catheters, irrigation, suprapubic drains)

Mobility: physical, impaired Related factor: *Pain*

Pain Related factors: Muscle cramps, surgical procedure, coughing and deep breathing (e.g., renal surgeries), bladder spasms, back and leg pain, clot in drainage devices (e.g., from transurethral resection)

Sexual dysfunction Related factors: Side effects of surgery, *Pain*, altered body function or structure, *Disturbed body image*, reaction of partner to ostomy, erectile dysfunction (male), inadequate vaginal lubrication (female)

Social isolation Related factors: Concern about others' reaction to ostomy, worry about odor and leaking from appliance

Urinary retention Related factors: Inhibition of reflex arc, blockage secondary to edema or inflammation

Vascular Surgery

Includes but is not limited to aortic aneurysm resection, aortoiliac bypass graft, embolectomy, femoroiliac bypass graft, portacaval shunt, sympathectomy, and vein ligation

Potential Complications (Collaborative Problems)

PC of aortic aneurysm resection: Renal failure, myocardial infarction, hemorrhage, emboli, spinal cord ischemia, congestive heart failure, rupture of suture line

PC of vascular surgery: Cardiac dysrhythmia, compartmental syndrome, failure of anastomosis, infection, lymphocele, occlusion of graft

Nursing Diagnoses

Activity intolerance Related factors: *Anxiety, Pain*, weakness secondary to inactivity, imbalance between oxygen supply and demand

Caregiver role strain Related factors: Illness severity of care receiver, unpredictable illness course or instability in the care receiver's health, complexity and amount of caregiving tasks

Fear Related factor: Real or imagined threat to own well-being (e.g., surgery, failure of graft, loss of limb, death)

Fluid volume, deficient Related factors: Loss of fluid through abnormal routes, medications, third spacing, hematoma, diuresis secondary to contrast media given for angiography

Fluid volume excess Related factor: Decreased urine output secondary to heart failure

Grieving, anticipatory/dysfunctional Related factor: Potential loss of body part or function

Injury, risk for Risk factors: Tissue hypoxia, abnormal blood profile, *Impaired mobility*

Mobility: physical, impaired Related factors: *Pain*, nerve injury secondary to ischemia

Pain, acute/chronic Related factors: Surgical procedure, increased tissue perfusion to previously ischemic tissue, peripheral nerve ischemia, paresthesias

Peripheral neurovascular dysfunction, risk for Risk factors: Immobilization, vascular obstruction

Sexual dysfunction Related factors: Impotence and retrograde ejaculation secondary to aortic aneurysm resection

Tissue integrity, impaired Related factors: Chronically compromised peripheral tissue perfusion, decreased activity postoperatively, multiple surgical procedures

Tissue perfusion, ineffective: (specify) Related factors: Interruption of venous blood flow, exchange problems, graft occlusion, edema, compartmental syndrome, inadequate anticoagulation, progressive arterial disease

PSYCHIATRIC CONDITIONS

Assaultive patient

Borderline personality

Eating disorders

Mania

Paranoia

Phobias

Psychosis

Severe depression

Substance abuse

Suicide

Withdrawn patient

Assaultive Patient

Associated psychiatric diagnoses include but are not limited to bipolar disorder, manic; disorganized schizophrenia; substance use disorders; organic mental disorders; drug-induced psychoses; personality disorders; panic disorder; and post-traumatic stress disorder.

Nursing Diagnoses

Coping: defensive Related factors: Psychologic impairment (specify), situational crisis (specify), neurologic alteration, other physical factors (specify)

Post-trauma syndrome Related factors: Abuse, incest, rape, participation in combat

Self-esteem, chronic low Related factors: Psychologic impairment (specify), repeatedly unmet expectations

Self-esteem, situational low Related factor: Situational crisis (specify)

Sensory perception, disturbed: (specify) Related factors: Alcohol or substance abuse (specify); altered sensory reception, transmission, or integration; sensory deficit (specify); sensory overload (specify)

Social interaction, impaired Related factors: Developmental disability, communication barriers, psychologic impairment (specify)

Thought processes, disturbed Related factors: Mental disorder (specify), organic mental disorder (specify), personality disorder (specify), substance abuse

Violence: self-directed or directed at others, risk for Risk factors: Manic excitement, panic states, rage reaction, history of violence, drug or alcohol intoxication or withdrawal, temporal lobe epilepsy, paranoid ideation, organic brain syndrome, arrest or conviction pattern, toxic reaction to medications, command hallucinations

Borderline Personality

Nursing Diagnoses

Anxiety Related factors: Threat to or change in role functioning, situational crises (specify), maturational crisis (specify), unmet needs, change in environment, threat to or change in interaction patterns, unconscious conflict about values or beliefs, negative self-talk, post-traumatic experience

Coping: family, disabled Related factors: Conflicting coping styles, highly ambivalent family relationships, chronically unresolved feelings (specify), role changes, and ongoing family disorganization secondary to patient's illness

Coping, ineffective Related factors: Personal vulnerability in situational or maturational crisis (specify); procrastination, stubbornness, and inefficiency in performing social roles; unrealistic perceptions; unmet expectations; disregard for social norms; inadequate support system; no assertion or recognition of own needs; poor impulse control; mood shifts, use of splitting and projection

Identity, personal, disturbed Related factors: Situational crises, psychologic impairment (e.g., borderline personality disorder), developmental impairment

Powerlessness Related factor: Pattern of helplessness

Role performance, ineffective Related factors: Situational crises, psychologic impairment (e.g., borderline personality disorder)

Self-esteem, chronic low Related factors: Psychologic impairment (e.g., borderline personality disorder), repeatedly unmet expectations of others, inability to meet role expectations, learned helplessness

Self-Mutilation, risk for Risk factors: Inability to cope with increased psychologic or physiologic tension in a healthy manner; feelings of depression, rejection, self-hatred, separation anxiety, guilt, and depersonalization; fluctuating emotions; drug or alcohol abuse; history of self-injury; history of physical, emotional, or sexual abuse

Sexuality patterns, ineffective Related factors: Conflict with sexual orientation, sexual abuse, impaired relationship with significant person

Social interaction, impaired Related factors: Psychologic impairment (e.g., borderline personality disorder), low self-esteem, misinterpretation of internal or external stimuli, hypervigilance in social situations, dysfunctional interactions, withdrawal, inability to maintain attachments, fear of abandonment

Suicide, risk for Risk factors: Suicidal ideation, substance abuse, despair, anger or rage

Violence: self-directed or directed at others, risk for Risk factors: Rage reaction, suicidal ideation, history of self-mutilation, substance abuse (specify)

Eating Disorders

Associated psychiatric diagnoses are limited to anorexia nervosa and bulimia.

Potential Complications (Collaborative Problems)

PC of eating disorders: Amenorrhea, anemia, dysrhythmias

Nursing Diagnoses

Activity intolerance Related factor: Weakness and *Fatigue* secondary to malnutrition

Anxiety Related factors: Threat to self-concept, worry about being overweight, change in environment, situational or maturational crises, unmet needs

Body image, disturbed Related factors: Eating disorder (see *Anxiety*), dysfunctional family system

Constipation Related factors: Less than adequate amounts of fiber and bulk-forming foods in diet, chronic use of medication and enemas, inadequate fluid intake

Coping: family, disabled Related factors: Arbitrary disregard for patient's needs, chronically unresolved feelings (specify guilt, anxiety, hostility, despair, and so forth), conflicting coping styles, highly ambivalent family relationships, effect of marital discord on family members

Coping, ineffective Related factors: Personal vulnerability in a maturational or situational crisis (specify), feelings of loss of control, inaccurate perception of weight status, *Anxiety* about maturing body

Fluid volume, deficient Related factors: Extreme weight loss, self-induced vomiting, abuse of laxatives or diuretics

Noncompliance Related factors: Denial of illness, negative perception of treatment regimen, perceived benefits of continued illness

Nutrition, imbalanced: less than body requirements Related factors: Psychologic impairment (e.g., bulimia, anorexia), refusal to eat, self-induced vomiting, laxative abuse, need for more calories because of physical exertion (e.g., excessive exercising)

Self-esteem, chronic low Related factors: Psychologic impairment (specify), repeatedly unmet expectations, perception of self as fat

Sexuality patterns, ineffective Related factors: Ineffective or absent role models, *Disturbed body image*, impaired relationship with significant other, *Chronic or situational low self-esteem*

Social interaction, impaired Related factor: Psychologic impairment (e.g., anorexia, bulimia), fear and mistrust of relationships

Therapeutic regimen management, ineffective Related factors: *Decisional conflict*, family conflict, mistrust of regimen or health care personnel, denial of illness, perceived lack of benefits of treatment, *Powerlessness*

Mania

Associated psychiatric diagnoses include but are not limited to bipolar disorders (manic, mixed), schizophrenia (undifferentiated type, catatonic type), schizoaffective disorder, and substance use disorders.

Potential Complications (Collaborative Problems)

PC of lithium therapy: Lithium toxicity

Nursing Diagnoses

Anxiety Related factors: Change in role functioning, change in environment, change in interaction patterns, unmet needs, threats to self-concept

Communication, impaired verbal Related factors: Hyperactivity, pressured speech

Coping, defensive Related factors: Ideas of grandiosity, self-importance, or abilities secondary to feelings of inferiority

Coping, ineffective Related factor: Personal vulnerability in a situational crisis (specify)

Family processes, interrupted Related factors: Illness or disability of family member, exhaustion of family members, situational crises (e.g., financial difficulty, role changes), patient's euphoria and grandiose ideas, manipulative behavior, limit testing, patient's refusal to take responsibility for own actions

Fluid volume, deficient Related factors: Inadequate fluid intake secondary to manic behaviors, medication-induced *Diarrhea* and vomiting, polyuria

Health maintenance, ineffective Related factors: Significant alteration in communication skills, lack of ability to make deliberate and thoughtful judgments

Injury, risk for Risk factors: Orientation; drugs (e.g., alcohol, caffeine, nicotine); cognitive, affective, and psychomotor factors

Nutrition, imbalanced: less than body requirements Related factor: Inadequate intake to balance excessive (i.e., manic) activity

Personal identity, disturbed Related factor: Psychologic impairment (specify)

Role performance, ineffective Related factor: Psychologic impairment (specify), see *Interrupted family processes*

Sensory perception, disturbed (specify) Related factors: *Sleep deprivation*, endogenous chemical alteration, stress

Sleep pattern, disturbed Related factors: Psychologic impairment (specify), inability to recognize *Fatigue* and need for sleep, hyperactivity, denial of need to sleep

Social interaction, impaired Related factors: Psychologic impairment (specify), others' unwillingness to tolerate patient's behaviors

Suicide, risk for Risk factors: Impulsive behavior, delusional thinking, command hallucinations, impaired reality testing

Thought processes, disturbed Related factor: Mental disorder (specify), delusions, hallucinations, euphoria, flight of ideas

Violence: self-directed or directed at others, risk for Risk factors: Manic excitement, rage reaction, history of violence, irritability, impulsive behavior, delusional thinking, command hallucinations, impaired reality testing

Paranoia

Associated psychiatric diagnoses include but are not limited to schizophrenia (undifferentiated type, paranoid type), mood disorders (major depression [e.g., single episode, recurrent]), bipolar disorders (e.g., mixed, manic, depressed), schizoaffective disorder, paranoid disorders, substance abuse disorders, organic mental disorders, and personality disorders.

Nursing Diagnoses

Anxiety (severe) Related factors: Failure to master developmental task of trust versus mistrust, delusions

Coping, defensive Related factor: Psychologic impairment (specify)

Coping, ineffective Related factors: Personal vulnerability in situational crisis, use of projection to control fears and anxieties

Family processes, interrupted Related factors: Illness or disability of family member, temporary or long-term family disorganization, exhausted family patient's behaviors

Fear Related factor: Imagined threat to own well-being

Health maintenance, ineffective Related factors: Significant alteration in communication skills, lack of ability to make deliberate and thoughtful judgments

Noncompliance Related factors: Denial of illness, negative perception of treatment regimen, mistrust of caregivers

Powerlessness Related factors: Health care environment, treatment regimen, feelings of inadequacy, maladaptive interpersonal relationships (e.g., use of force, abusive relationships), *Situational or chronic low self-esteem*, feelings that he has no control over situations

Self-esteem, low (chronic, situational) Related factors: Psychologic impairment (specify), failure of relationships, feelings of *Powerlessness*

Sexuality patterns, ineffective Related factors: Impaired relationship with significant other secondary to manipulative, violent, or other unacceptable behaviors; conflicts with sexual orientation

Sleep pattern, disturbed Related factors: Psychologic impairment, *Fear* of danger, hypervigilance

Social interaction, impaired Related factors: Psychologic impairment (specify), delusions, suspiciousness, *Fear* and mistrust of others

Thought processes, disturbed Related factors: Mental disorder (specify), organic mental disorder (specify), personality disorder (specify), poor reality testing secondary to mistrust of others, delusions, hallucinations

Violence: self-directed or directed at others, risk for Risk factors: Panic states, drug or alcohol intoxication or withdrawal, delusions, feelings of *Anxiety,* perceived danger

Phobias

Associated psychiatric diagnoses include but are not limited to agoraphobia, simple phobia, and social phobia.

Nursing Diagnoses

Anxiety Related factors: Threat to or change in role functioning, change in environment, threat to self-concept, threat to or change in interaction pattern, unmet needs

Coping, ineffective Related factor: Personal vulnerability in situational or maturational crisis (specify)

Diversional activity, deficient Related factors: Impaired perception of reality, fear of loss of control if dreaded object or situation is encountered

Fear Related factors: Real or imagined threat to own well-being, learned irrational response to objects or situations

Role performance, ineffective Related factors: Psychologic impairment (e.g., phobic disorder), inability to perform role behaviors secondary to irrational fears

Social interaction, impaired Related factors: Psychologic impairment (e.g., phobic disorder), *Fear* of encountering dreaded object or situation, *Fear* of loss of control

Social isolation Related factors: Psychologic impairment (e.g., phobic disorder), others' reactions to irrational behaviors

Psychosis

Associated psychiatric diagnoses include but are not limited to schizophrenia (disorganized, catatonic, paranoid, and undifferentiated types) schizophreniform disorder; bipolar disorders (mixed, manic, and depressed) organic mental disorders; substance abuse disorders; and medical conditions.

Nursing Diagnoses

Anxiety (severe, panic) Related factors: Continuation of maladaptive coping learned early in life, unconscious conflicts, unmet needs, threats to self-concept

Communication, impaired verbal Related factors: Psychologic impairment (specify), incoherent or illogical speech, medication side effects

Coping: family, disabled Related factors: Long-term pattern of multiple stressors, significant others exhausted by prolonged illness

Health maintenance, ineffective Related factors: Lack of ability to make deliberate and thoughtful judgments

Home maintenance, impaired Related factors: Psychologic impairment (specify), *Disturbed thought processes*, impaired judgment or decision making

Noncompliance Related factors: Denial of illness, negative perception of treatment regimen, *Disturbed thought processes*, responding to delusions and hallucinations

Personal identity, disturbed Related factors: Psychologic impairment (specify), psychologic conflicts, childhood abuse, underdeveloped ego, threats to self-concept, threats to physical integrity

Self-care deficit: (specify) Related factors: Psychologic impairment (specify), severe *Anxiety*, *Disturbed thought processes*, inability to make decisions, feelings of worthlessness, lack of energy

Self-mutilation, risk for Risk factors: Fluctuating emotions, command hallucinations, patients in psychotic state—frequently males in young adulthood

Sensory perception, disturbed (auditory, visual) Related factors: Escalating *Anxiety*, withdrawal

Social interaction, impaired Related factor: Psychologic impairment (specify)

Thought processes, disturbed Related factors: Mental disorder (specify), organic mental disorder (specify), dementia, delirium

Violence: self-directed or directed at others, risk for Risk factors: Paranoid ideation, suicidal ideation, history of violence, substance abuse (specify), responding to delusions and hallucinations

Severe Depression

Associated psychiatric diagnoses include but are not limited to bipolar disorder (depressed) and major depression.

Nursing Diagnoses

Activity intolerance Related factors: Weakness and *Fatigue*, depression, inadequate nutrition

Anxiety Related factors: Psychologic conflicts, unmet needs, unconscious values/goals conflicts, change in role functioning, change in interaction patterns, threat to self-concept

Constipation Related factors: Decreased activity, lack of exercise, inadequate intake of fiber and fluids, medications (specify)

Coping: family, disabled Related factors: Role conflicts, marital discord secondary to long-term depression (see *Interrupted family processes*)

Coping, ineffective Related factors: Personal vulnerability in situational or maturational crisis, guilt, *Low self-esteem*, feelings of rejection, unconscious conflicts

Family processes, interrupted Related factors: Illness or disability of family member, changes in roles or responsibilities, family disorganization, *Impaired verbal communication*, difficulty accepting or receiving help

Grieving, dysfunctional Related factors: Actual loss (specify), anticipated loss (specify), perceived loss (specify), unresolved grief secondary to prolonged *Ineffective denial*, repressed feelings

Health maintenance, ineffective Related factors: Lack of ability to make deliberate and thoughtful judgments, significant alteration in communication skills, lack of energy, feelings of worthlessness

Home maintenance, impaired Related factors: Psychologic impairment (specify), inability to concentrate, impaired decision making, lack of energy

Hopelessness Related factors: Long-term stress, lack of social supports, abandonment by others

Injury, risk for Risk factors: Orientation; drugs (e.g., alcohol, caffeine, nicotine); cognitive, affective, and psychomotor factors; electroconvulsive therapy and anesthesia effects on cardiovascular and respiratory systems; medication side effects such as sedation or blurred vision

Nutrition, imbalanced: less than body requirements Related factors: Psychologic impairment (specify), loss of appetite, feelings of worthlessness, emotional stress or *Anxiety*

Powerlessness Related factors: Psychologic impairment (specify), negative beliefs about own abilities, past failures, lack of energy, feelings of worthlessness

Role performance, ineffective Related factors: Psychologic impairment (specify), lack of energy, *Powerlessness*, helplessness

Self-care deficit: (specify) Related factors: Depression, lack of energy

Self-esteem, chronic low Related factors: Psychologic impairment (specify), repeatedly unmet expectations, past failures, feelings of worthlessness

Sexuality patterns, ineffective Related factors: *Chronic or situational low self-esteem*, lack of energy, loss of interest, decreased sex drive

Sleep pattern, disturbed Related factors: *Anxiety*, psychologic impairment (e.g., depression), decreased serotonin, daytime inactivity, naps, difficulty falling asleep at night, hypersomnia, early awakening

Social interaction, impaired Related factors: Psychologic impairment (depression), failure to initiate interactions secondary to decreased energy or inertia, poor self-concept, lack of social skills, feelings of worthlessness

Social isolation Related factors: Others' responses to depressed mood, *Disturbed thought processes*, lack of social skills, feelings of unworthiness

Thought processes, disturbed Related factors: Mental disorder (specify), overgeneralizing, negative thinking, dichotomous thinking

Violence: self-directed, risk for Risk factors: Suicidal ideation or intent secondary to feelings of worthlessness and *Hopelessness*, loneliness

Substance Abuse

Associated psychiatric diagnoses include alcohol or drug intoxication, withdrawal and dependence.

Potential Complications (Collaborative Problems)

PC of alcoholism: Delirium tremens

PC of substance abuse: Hallucinations, hypertension, sepsis, toxic overdose

PC of substance abuse or withdrawal: Seizures

Nursing Diagnoses

Anxiety Related factors: Change in health status, change in role functioning, situational crisis, unmet needs, *Impaired memory*, loss of control, fear of withdrawal, legal implications

Coping: family, compromised/disabled Related factors: Temporary family disorganization and role changes, unrealistic expectations and demands, lack of mutual decision-making skills, inadequate information or understanding by family member, arbitrary disregard for patient's needs, chronically unresolved feelings (specify guilt, anxiety, hostility, despair, and so forth), conflicting coping styles, inconsistent limit setting, highly ambivalent family relationships, violence

Coping, ineffective Related factors: Personal vulnerability in situational or maturational crisis (specify), anger, denial, dependence, inability to manage stressors

Decisional conflict (specify) Related factor: Chemical dependence

Denial, ineffective Related factors: Feelings of vulnerability, ambivalence about withdrawal, inability to cope without alcohol or drugs, *Anxiety, Fear*

Diarrhea Related factors: Excessive alcohol or drug intake, withdrawal

Family processes, dysfunctional: alcoholism Related factor: Alcohol abuse by a family member

Fluid volume, deficient Related factors: Excessive, continuous consumption of alcohol, vomiting, *Diarrhea*

Home maintenance, impaired Related factors: Insufficient family organization or planning, psychologic impairment (e.g., substance abuse), decreased motivation, *Disturbed thought processes*, depression, severe *Anxiety*

Injury, risk for Risk factors: Orientation; affective factors; impaired judgment; *Confusion, acute/chronic*; delirium; substance intoxication

Memory, impaired Related factor: Organic brain damage

Noncompliance Related factors: Denial of illness, negative perception of treatment regimen, inability to ask for or accept help, lack of social support, inability to cope with stressors without alcohol or drugs

Nutrition, imbalanced: less than body requirements Related factors: Chemical dependence (specify), anorexia, hypermetabolism secondary to stimulants, no money for food

Nutrition, imbalanced: more than body requirements Related factor: Increased appetite secondary to drug taking (e.g., marijuana)

Parenting, impaired Related factors: Dysfunctional relationship between parents, change in marital status, psychologic impairment (substance abuse) (see *Family coping* and *Family processes*)

Post-trauma syndrome Related factors: Abuse, accidents, assault, disaster, epidemic, incest, kidnapping, torture, terrorism, participation in combat

Powerlessness Related factors: Pattern of helplessness, failed attempts to abstain, changes in personal or social life

Role performance, ineffective Related factor: Psychologic impairment (e.g., substance abuse)

Self-esteem, chronic low Related factors: Repeatedly unmet expectations, guilt, failed withdrawal, ambivalence

Sensory perception, disturbed (auditory, kinesthetic, tactile, visual) Related factors: Alcohol intoxication, substance intoxication (specify)

Sexual dysfunction/Sexuality patterns, ineffective Related factors: *Chronic or situational low self-esteem*, impotence, loss of libido secondary to substance abuse, neurologic damage, debilitation from drug use, embarrassment about changes in appearance (e.g., testicular atrophy, spider angiomas)

Sleep pattern, disturbed Related factors: Chemical dependence (specify, e.g., stimulants), nightmares, difficulty sleeping at night secondary to sleeping during the day

Social interaction, impaired Related factors: Chemical dependence (specify), inability to focus on others, emotional immaturity, aggressiveness, *Anxiety*

Social isolation Related factors: Others' responses to impulsive behaviors, avoidance behaviors and anger, job loss, perceived difference from others

Violence: self-directed or directed at others, risk for Risk factors: Substance intoxication (specify), substance withdrawal (specify), disorientation, impaired judgment, altered perceptions, poor impulse control

Suicide

Risk for suicide actually represents a nursing diagnosis that can be associated with any of the psychiatric diagnoses (e.g., schizophrenia, substance abuse). The following nursing diagnoses may also occur for patients who are suicidal.

Nursing Diagnoses

Anxiety Related factors: Threat to self-concept, threat to or change in role functioning, situational or maturational crises, unmet needs, changes in social supports

Coping, ineffective Related factors: Personal vulnerability in situational or maturational crisis (specify)

Decisional conflict Related factors: Perceived threat to value system, lack of support system

Hopelessness Related factors: Abandonment, lack of social supports, lost spiritual belief

Personal identity, disturbed Related factor: Situational crisis (specify)

Post-trauma syndrome Related factors: Abuse, accidents, assault, disaster, epidemic, incest, kidnapping, terrorism, torture, catastrophic illness or accident, participation in combat

Rape-trauma syndrome Related factor: Patient's biopsychosocial response to event

Self-esteem, chronic low Related factors: Psychologic impairment (specify), repeatedly unmet expectations

Self-mutilation, risk for Risk factors: Inability to cope with increased psychologic or physiologic tension in a healthy manner; feelings of depression, rejection, self-hatred, separation anxiety, guilt, and depersonalization; fluctuating emotions; drug or alcohol abuse

Sensory perception, disturbed: (specify) Related factor: Alcohol or substance abuse (specify)

Spiritual distress Related factor: Challenged beliefs and values systems

Thought processes, disturbed Related factors: Mental disorders (specify), organic mental disorders (specify), personality disorders (specify), substance abuse

Violence: self-directed, risk for Risk factors: History of suicide attempt, command hallucinations, battered women, panic states, history of abuse by others, suicidal ideation, substance abuse

Withdrawn Patient

Associated psychiatric diagnoses include but are not limited to major depression; schizophrenia: disorganized, catatonic, paranoid, and undifferentiated types; schizophreniform disorder; phobic disorders; schizoid personality disorder; avoidant personality disorder; substance use disorders; and organic mental disorders.

Nursing Diagnoses

Anxiety Related factors: Threat to or change in role functioning, real or perceived threat to physical self or to self-concept, unconscious conflicts (e.g., values, beliefs), negative self-talk, feelings of apprehension and uneasiness, altered perceptions

Communication, impaired verbal Related factors: Psychologic impairment (specify), refusal to speak or make eye contact

Coping, ineffective Related factor: Personal vulnerability in situational or maturational crisis (specify)

Diversional activity, deficient Related factors: Lack of motivation, deficit in social skills, impaired perception of reality

Family processes, interrupted Related factors: Illness or disability of family member, inability to communicate secondary to withdrawal

Fear Related factors: *Powerlessness*, real or imagined threat to own well-being

Grieving, dysfunctional Related factors: Actual loss (specify), anticipated loss (specify), perceived loss (specify)

Health maintenance, ineffective Related factors: Lack of ability to make thoughtful and deliberate judgments, significant alteration in communication skills, lack of awareness of environment and own needs

Parenting, impaired Related factors: Psychologic impairment (specify), situational crisis (specify), see *Interrupted family processes*

Personal identity, disturbed Related factor: Psychologic impairment (specify)

Role performance, ineffective Related factor: Psychologic impairment (specify)

Self-esteem, low (chronic, situational) Related factor: Psychologic impairment (specify)

Self-mutilation, risk for Risk factors: Inability to cope with increased psychologic or physiologic tension in a healthy manner; feelings of depression, rejection, self-hatred, separation anxiety, guilt, and depersonalization; need for sensory stimuli

Social interaction, impaired Related factors: Psychologic impairment (specify), *Fear* of social situations, *Anxiety*, depression

Social isolation Related factors: Psychologic impairment (specify), others' difficulty communicating with patient

Thought processes, disturbed Related factors: Mental disorders (specify), organic mental disorders (specify), personality disorders (specify)

Antepartum and Postpartum Conditions

Abortion, spontaneous or induced

Change in birthing plans

Gestational diabetes

Hyperemesis gravidarum

Maternal infection

Painful breast

Perinatal loss

Postpartum care, uncomplicated

Preeclampsia

Suppression of preterm labor

Uterine bleeding

Abortion, Spontaneous or Induced

Potential Complications (Collaborative Problems)

PC of abortion: Hemorrhage, infection

Nursing Diagnoses

Anxiety Related factors: Threat to health status, ambivalence, *Deficient knowledge* regarding procedures and postprocedural care, unfamiliar sights and sounds, *Fear* of implications for future pregnancies

Coping, ineffective Related factors: Unresolved feelings (e.g., guilt) about elective abortion; societal, moral, religious, and family conflicting values; unresolved feelings over loss of baby

Decisional conflict Related factors: Values conflicts, inadequate support system

Family processes, interrupted Related factors: Effects of elective procedure or spontaneous loss on relationships, inability of family members to agree on decisions, adolescent identity conflicts, preexisting personal or marital conflicts

Grieving, anticipatory/dysfunctional Related factors: Perinatal loss, perceived or actual loss of cultural or religious approval

Health maintenance, ineffective Related factor: *Deficient knowledge* (e.g., of contraception, "safer sex")

Infection, risk for Risk factors: Invasive procedures, traumatized tissue, incomplete expulsion of uterine contents

Pain Related factor: Strong uterine contractions

Powerlessness Related factors: Treatment regimen, inability to change the course of events or prevent the loss, perception that there are limited or no options

Self-esteem, low (chronic, situational) Related factors: Unmet expectations for pregnancy, unmet expectations for child, preexisting *Low self-esteem*

Sexual dysfunction/Sexuality patterns, ineffective Related factors: *Low Self-esteem*, fear of pregnancy, unstable relationship with significant others, *Disturbed body image*

Spiritual distress Related factors: Test of spiritual beliefs, unresolved feelings about elective abortion, inability to find meaning in spontaneous abortion

Change in Birthing Plans

May include any deviation from a couple's original birthing plans. Such a change may include but is not limited to use of analgesia, anesthesia, or forceps; limitation of visitors; episiotomy, and cesarean birth.

Nursing Diagnoses

Family processes, interrupted Related factors: Unmet expectations for childbirth, situational crisis (e.g., fetal distress), separation of family members (e.g., emergency hysterectomy secondary to uterine rupture)

Fear Related factors: Real or imagined threat to child or to own well-being, unfamiliar equipment, urgency of emergency procedures

Pain Related factors: Surgery, episiotomy, uterine contractions, invasive procedures

Parent/infant/child attachment, risk for impaired Risk factors: Unmet expectations for childbirth, separation of family members

Powerlessness Related factors: Complication threatening pregnancy, perceived inability to effect outcome of situation, inability to cope with overwhelming uterine contractions

Self-esteem, low (chronic, situational) Related factors: Unmet expectations for childbirth (e.g., inability to "tolerate" uterine contractions, inability to deliver vaginally)

Gestational Diabetes

Potential Complications (Collaborative Problems)

PC of gestational diabetes: Anemia, dystocia, fetal morbidity or mortality, hydramnios, ketoacidosis, pregnancy-induced hypertension, pyelonephritis

Nursing Diagnoses

Family processes, interrupted Related factors: Hospitalization or change in environment, illness or disability of family member, inadequate finances

Fear Related factors: Environmental stressors or hospitalization, *Powerlessness*, real or imagined threat to own well-being, real or imagined threat to child, implications for future pregnancies

Infection (urinary tract infection, vaginitis), risk for Risk factors: Favorable environment for bacterial growth secondary to glycosuria

Injury, risk for (maternal or fetal) Risk factors: Hypoglycemia, hyperglycemia

Nutrition, imbalanced: less than body requirements Related factors: Inadequate intake to support increased calorie needs of pregnancy, secondary to limited exposure to basic nutritional knowledge; *Nausea*

Nutrition, imbalanced: more than body requirements Related factors: Limited exposure to new basic nutritional knowledge, imbalance between intake and available insulin

Sensory perception, disturbed (visual) Related factor: Increase in diabetic retinopathy

Hyperemesis Gravidarum

Potential Complications (Collaborative Problems)

PC of hyperemesis: Bleeding secondary to hypothrombinemia, fetal death, fluid and electrolyte imbalance, hypotension, negative nitrogen balance, peripheral neuropathy

Nursing Diagnoses

Activity intolerance Related factors: Inadequate nutrition, dehydration, decreased activity

Coping, ineffective Related factors: Personal vulnerability during health crisis, projected role changes, worry about safety of fetus

Family processes, interrupted Related factors: Hospitalization or change in environment, illness or disability of family member, threats to job security (of patient or spouse), need for child care for siblings

Fatigue See *Activity intolerance*

Fear Related factor: Real or imagined threat to child

Fluid volume, deficient Related factors: Inadequate fluid intake secondary to *Nausea*, abnormal fluid loss secondary to vomiting

Nutrition, imbalanced: less than body requirements Related factors: Limited intake of nutrients secondary to *Nausea*, loss of nutrients secondary to vomiting

Parenting, risk for impaired See *Role performance, ineffective*

Powerlessness Related factors: Complications threatening pregnancy, perceived or actual inability to change the course of events

Role performance, ineffective Related factors: Unmet expectations for pregnancy, *Nausea*, hospitalization

Self-esteem, low (chronic, situational) Related factors: Unmet expectations for pregnancy, inability to meet role demands (e.g., work, mother, spouse)

Maternal Infection

Includes but is not limited to active genital herpes, amnionitis, AIDS, and hepatitis B

Potential Complications (Collaborative Problems)

PC of infection: Fetal morbidity or mortality, sepsis

Nursing Diagnoses

Activity intolerance Related factors: Disease process, malaise

Body image, disturbed Related factors: Pregnancy, odors and lesions secondary to infection, precautions regarding hand washing and spread of infection

Breastfeeding, interrupted Related factors: Maternal illness, maternal medications that are contraindicated for the infant

Diversional activity, deficient See *Risk for loneliness*

Family processes, interrupted Related factors: Change in family roles, hospitalization or change in environment, unresolved feelings about how the infection was acquired

Fear Related factor: Real or imagined threat to child

Infection, risk for Risk factor: Presence of lesions (e.g., herpes) predispose patient to secondary infections

Infection (transmission), risk for Risk factor: Contagious nature of disease (e.g., herpes, hepatitis B)

Loneliness, risk for Related factor: Therapeutic isolation

Pain Related factors: Cesarean birth, infection, lesions

Parenting, impaired Risk factor: Delayed parent–infant attachment secondary to need for infection precautions

Self-esteem, low (chronic, situational) Related factors: Cesarean birth, inability to assume new role, inability to fulfill usual role requirements (e.g., wife, mother, worker)

Social interaction, impaired Related factor: Therapeutic isolation

Painful Breast

Includes but is not limited to sore, cracked nipples, engorgement, and mastitis.

Potential Complications (Collaborative Problems)

PC of cracked nipples: engorgement: Mastitis

PC of mastitis: Abscess

Nursing Diagnoses

Breastfeeding, ineffective See *Interrupted breastfeeding*

Breastfeeding, interrupted Related factors: *Pain*, engorgement; sore, cracked nipples; mastitis; maternal medications that are contraindicated for the infant

Health maintenance, ineffective Related factors: Limited exposure to information about breast hygiene, care of nipples, treatments, or signs and symptoms of infection

Pain Related factors: Sore nipples, breast engorgement, edema and inflammation of breast tissues

Parent/infant/child attachment, risk for impaired Risk factors: *Pain*, unmet expectations

Role performance, ineffective Related factors: Assumption of new role, unmet expectations for childbirth, *Pain* and discomfort, Interrupted breastfeeding

Skin integrity (nipples), impaired Related factors: Inadequate breast care, improper positioning of baby at breast, incorrect sucking by infant

Perinatal Loss

Includes but is not limited to less-than-perfect baby, miscarriage, stillbirth, adoption, and elective abortion

Nursing Diagnoses

Coping: family, compromised/disabled Related factor: Chronically unresolved feelings about loss

Coping, ineffective Related factor: Personal vulnerability in a situational crisis

Family processes, interrupted Related factors: Illness or disability of baby, fetal demise, stillbirth, lack of adequate support system, *Dysfunctional*

grieving, conflicting styles of grieving among family members, guilt, blaming

Fear Related factors: Real or imagined threat to child, environmental stressors or hospitalization, *Powerlessness*, implications for future pregnancies

Grieving, anticipatory Related factors: Imminent loss of child, anticipated loss of perfect child

Grieving, dysfunctional Related factors: Inability to resolve feelings about actual or anticipated loss of child or of perfect child, marital discord, lack of support system

Parenting, impaired Related factors: Interruption in bonding process, unrealistic expectations of self or partner (see *Interrupted family processes*)

Powerlessness Related factors: Complication threatening pregnancy, inability to change course of events

Role performance, ineffective Related factors: *Dysfunctional grieving* secondary to loss of child, birth of less-than-perfect baby, guilt, blame

Self-esteem, low (chronic, situational) Related factors: Unmet expectations for child, feelings of failure (e.g., to produce a perfect child)

Sexual dysfunction Related factors: Medically imposed restrictions, *Fear* of harming fetus, *Chronic or situational low self-esteem*, *Fear* of another pregnancy

Spiritual distress Related factors: Test of spiritual beliefs, intense suffering

Postpartum Care, Uncomplicated

Potential Complications (Collaborative Problems)

PC of Childbirth: Hematoma; hemorrhage secondary to uterine atony, retained placental fragments, lacerations; infection or sepsis

Nursing Diagnoses

Anxiety Related factors: Changes in role functioning, inexperience

Body image, disturbed Related factors: Lack of or inaccurate information about body's adjustment after delivery, change in body appearance (e.g., striae)

Breastfeeding, effective Related factors: Basic breastfeeding knowledge, normal breast structure, normal infant oral structure, gestational age of more than 34 weeks, supportive resources, maternal confidence

Breastfeeding, ineffective Related factors: *Interrupted breastfeeding*, inexperience, cultural influences, breast engorgement, infant factors (e.g., inability to latch on or suck)

Constipation Related factors: *Fear* of painful defecation, decreased peristalsis after delivery, decreased activity, decreased fluid intake, effects of analgesics, decreased tone of abdominal muscles

Family processes, interrupted Related factors: Transition in family roles, change in family structure, lack of adequate support systems

Health maintenance, ineffective Related factors: *Deficient knowledge* (e.g., hygiene, contraception, nutrition, infant care, symptoms of complications), lack of support from partner

Home maintenance, impaired Related factors: Inadequate support system, lack of organizational skills, *Ineffective coping*

Incontinence, urinary, stress Related factor: Tissue trauma during delivery

Nutrition, imbalanced: less than body requirements Related factor: Lack of basic nutritional knowledge concerning lactation

Pain Related factors: Episiotomy, sore nipples, breast engorgement, hemorrhoids, sore muscles, uterine contractions (afterpains)

Parent/infant/child attachment, risk for impaired See *Impaired parenting*

Parenting, impaired Related factors: Lack of knowledge or skill regarding effective parenting; unrealistic expectations of self, infant, and partner; unwanted child; no role models; inexperience

Role performance, ineffective Related factor: Assumption of new role

Sexuality patterns, ineffective Related factors: *Pain, Fear* of pain, *Disturbed body image,* demands of infant, lack of sleep

Sleep pattern, disturbed Related factors: Excessive social demands, role demands (e.g., frequent breastfeeding), *Pain, Anxiety,* exhilaration and excitement

Urinary retention Related factors: Local tissue edema, effects of medication/anesthesia, *Pain,* inability to assume normal voiding position secondary to effects of epidural anesthesia or analgesia

Preeclampsia

Preeclampsia is sometimes referred to as toxemia of pregnancy, pregnancy-induced hypertension, pregnancy related hypertension, and eclampsia (when seizures occur).

Potential Complications (Collaborative Problems)

PC of magnesium sulfate therapy Magnesium toxicity

PC of PRH: Cerebral edema, coma, fetal morbidity or mortality, HELLP syndrome (hemolysis, elevated liver enzymes, low platelet count), hypertension (malignant), pulmonary edema, renal insufficiency or damage, seizures

PC of malignant hypertension Uncontrolled hypertension: cerebral hemorrhage

PC of seizures: Precipitous birth, fetal bradycardia, placental separation

Nursing Diagnoses

Activity intolerance Related factors: Imbalance between oxygen supply and demand; lethargy, weakness, and *Fatigue* secondary to prescribed bed rest and magnesium sulfate side effects; preeclampsia

Body image, disturbed Related factors: Changes in appearance related to pregnancy and edema

Breathing pattern, ineffective Related factor: Side effects of magnesium sulfate

Constipation Related factors: Side effects of magnesium sulfate, decreased activity, decreased intake of fiber

Diversional activity, deficient Related factor: Prolonged bed rest

Family processes, interrupted Related factors: Hospitalization or change in environment, illness or disability of family member, enforced bed rest, role changes

Fear Related factors: Changes in birthing plans, real or imagined threat to child (e.g., premature labor), environmental stressors or hospitalization, threat to own well-being

Fluid volume, deficient (intravascular) Related factors: Intercompartmental fluid shifts secondary to loss of plasma proteins and decreased plasma colloid osmotic pressure

Fluid volume excess (extracellular tissues) Related factors: Sodium and water retention, fluid shift into extracellular spaces secondary to decreased plasma colloid osmotic pressure

Home maintenance, impaired Related factors: Inadequate support system, *Deficient knowledge*, inability to perform usual roles

Injury, risk for (maternal and fetal) Risk factors: Seizure activity, inadequate placental perfusion, falls secondary to vertigo or postural hypotension, visual disturbances, fetal distress secondary to inadequate placental perfusion

Nausea Related factor: Side effect of magnesium sulfate

Noncompliance Related factors: Unable to comply with bed rest secondary to perceived demands of role (e.g., care of siblings), perceived negative effects of medical regimen (e.g., unpalatable diet), perception that condition is not serious secondary to having no subjectively unpleasant symptoms, *Deficient knowledge* (e.g., related to disease, treatments, symptom relief, dietary restrictions)

Nutrition, imbalanced: less than body requirements Related factors: Lack of basic nutritional knowledge, loss of appetite, *Nausea* and vomiting, drowsiness secondary to medications

Pain Related factors: Epigastric (precursor to eclampsia), headache secondary to magnesium sulfate administration

Sensory perception, disturbed (visual) Related factor: Alterations precede eclampsia

Tissue perfusion, ineffective: cerebral, renal, placental Related factors: Vasospasm (spiral arteries), edema, decreased intravascular volume

Suppression of Preterm Labor

Potential Complications (Collaborative Problems)

PC of preterm labor: Preterm delivery of infant, pulmonary edema (secondary to tocolytic medications)

PC of magnesium sulfate therapy: Magnesium toxicity

Nursing Diagnoses

Anxiety Related factors: Outcome of pregnancy, side effects of tocolytics, insufficient time to prepare for labor or infant care

Diversional activity, deficient Related factor: Prolonged bed rest

Family processes, interrupted Related factors: Illness or disability of family member, change in family roles, lack of adequate support systems, enforced bed rest

Fear Related factor: Possibility of early labor and delivery

Home maintenance, impaired Related factors: Inadequate support system, enforced bed rest

Management of therapeutic regimen, ineffective Related factors: *Deficient knowledge*, excessive demands made on individual or family, social support deficits

Nausea Related factor: Side effects of tocolytic medications

Pain (headache) Related factor: Side effects of magnesium sulfate

Powerlessness Related factors: Complications threatening pregnancy, lack of improvement despite complying with bed rest and medication regimen

Self-esteem, low (chronic, situational) Related factors: Unmet expectations for childbirth, inability to fulfill usual roles

Sexual dysfunction Related factors: Medically imposed restrictions, *Fear* of harming fetus, *Fear* of causing uterine contractions

Sleep pattern, disturbed Related factors: Frequency of medication and monitoring

Uterine Bleeding

This includes but is not limited to the following conditions: (1) Antepartal bleeding may result from first trimester spotting, placenta previa, abruptio placentae, uterine rupture, or hydatidiform mole; (2) postpartal bleeding may be a consequence of postpartum hemorrhage or shock or uterine atony.

Potential Complications (Collaborative Problems)

PC of uterine bleeding: Anemia, disseminated intravascular coagulation, fetal death, renal failure, sepsis, shock

Nursing Diagnoses

Breastfeeding, interrupted Related factors: Maternal illness, *Fatigue,* Activity intolerance, activities of caregivers

Cardiac output, decreased Related factor: Hypovolemia

Diversional activity, deficient Related factors: Prolonged bed rest or activity limitations

Family processes, interrupted Related factors: Change in family roles, patient's inability to assume usual role, hospitalization or change in environment

Fear Related factors: Threat to the pregnancy or baby, threat to own well-being, *Powerlessness*, environmental stressors or hospitalization, implications for future pregnancies

Grieving, anticipatory Related factors: Possible loss of pregnancy and expected child, possible effect on future childbearing abilities secondary to intractable postpartum hemorrhage

Home maintenance, impaired Related factors: Inadequate support system, prescribed bed rest, *Activity intolerance* secondary to blood loss and anemia

Infection, risk for Risk factors: Traumatized tissue, invasive procedures, blood loss, partial separation of placenta

Mobility: physical, impaired Related factors: Increased bleeding in response to activity, presence of lines (e.g., IV, urinary catheter, fetal monitor)

Pain Related factors: Surgical procedure, uterine contractions, collection of blood between placenta and uterine wall

Powerlessness Related factors: Complications threatening pregnancy or future pregnancies

Self-care deficit: (specify) Related factors: Medically imposed restrictions, *Activity intolerance* secondary to blood loss

Self-esteem, low (chronic, situational) Related factors: Unmet expectations for childbirth, inability to perform usual role functions

Sexual dysfunction Related factors: Medically imposed restrictions, *Fear* of harming fetus, *Fear* of starting labor or increasing bleeding

Tissue perfusion, ineffective [placental] Related factors: Imbalance between oxygen supply and demand to the fetus secondary to hypovolemia, hypotension, placental separation

---

Newborn Conditions

Congenital anomalies

Drug withdrawal

Feeding problems

High-risk infant

Hyperbilirubinemia

Hypoglycemia

Hypothermia

Low birth weight/small for gestational age

Normal newborn

Respiratory distress

Congenital Anomalies

Include but are not limited to infants with serious congenital anomalies (e.g., congenital heart disease, meningomyelocele, choanal atresia, tracheoesophageal fistula)

Potential Complications (Collaborative Problems)

PC of congenital heart disease: Congestive heart failure, dysrhythmias

PC of meningomyelocele: Hydrocephalus, neurovascular deficits below lesion

PC of tracheoesophageal fistula Aspiration pneumonia, choking

Nursing Diagnoses

Activity intolerance Related factor: Imbalance between oxygen supply and demand

Aspiration, risk for Risk factor: Secondary to tracheoesophageal fistula

Breastfeeding, ineffective Related factors: Infant *Fatigue*, inadequate sucking reflex, interrupted or infrequent feeding, difficulty breathing, secondary to cardiac anomaly

Breastfeeding, interrupted Related factor: Infant illness

Breathing pattern, ineffective Related factors: Decreased energy or *Fatigue* secondary to cardiac anomaly, aspiration pneumonia

Cardiac output, decreased Related factors: Increased ventricular workload, hypovolemia, cardiac anomaly (specify)

Caregiver role strain Related factors: Illness severity of the infant; premature birth or congenital defect; unpredictable illness course; situational stressors within the family; complexity and duration of caregiving; caregiver's health; lack of developmental readiness, knowledge, skills, or experience; competing role commitments; ineffective coping styles; isolation; limited opportunity for respite and recreation

Development, risk for delayed See *Growth, risk for delayed*

Family processes, interrupted Related factors: Unmet expectations for child, separation of family members, illness or disability of infant, immaturity of parents, lack of resources, lack of social supports, lack of knowledge

Fatigue Related factor: Disease process (e.g., cardiac anomaly, aspiration pneumonia)

Fear Related factor: Real threat to child

Gas exchange, impaired Related factors: Decreased pulmonary blood supply secondary to pulmonary hypertension, congestive heart failure, respiratory distress syndrome, decreased functional lung tissue secondary to respiratory distress syndrome, atelectasis

Grieving, anticipatory Related factor: Anticipatory loss of child

Growth, risk for delayed Risk factors: Congenital anomaly, fetal distress, prematurity, unhealthy maternal lifestyle during pregnancy, serious illness, delayed bonding secondary to infant's condition or parent's unmet expectations

Infant feeding pattern, ineffective Related factors: Prematurity, neurologic impairment or delay, prolonged NPO status, anatomical abnormalities (e.g., of esophagus and stomach), *Fatigue* and difficulty breathing secondary to heart anomaly

Injury, risk for Risk factors: Meningomyelocele, omphalocele, other defects creating vulnerability

Nutrition, imbalanced: less than body requirements Related factors: Difficulty in swallowing, inadequate sucking reflex in infant, vomiting, food intolerance

Mobility: physical, impaired Related factors: *Fatigue* secondary to inadequate oxygenation, spinal cord lesions

Skin integrity, impaired Related factors: Impaired circulation, immobility (e.g., inability to move lower extremities), *Imbalanced nutritional status*

Sleep pattern, disturbed Related factor: *Sleep deprivation* secondary to frequent therapeutic interventions

Spontaneous ventilation, impaired Related factors: Metabolic factors, respiratory muscle fatigue, pulmonary immaturity

Tissue perfusion, ineffective (peripheral) Related factors: Imbalance between oxygen supply and demand secondary to high metabolic rate, *Decreased cardiac output, Impaired gas exchange*

Urinary retention Related factor: Congenital anomaly affecting spinal cord (specify)

Ventilatory weaning response, dysfunctional (DVWR) Related factors: Pulmonary immaturity, *Impaired gas exchange, Ineffective airway clearance,* ventilator dependence > one week

Drug Withdrawal

Potential Complications (Collaborative Problems)

PC of drug withdrawal: Dehydration, drug or alcohol withdrawal, electrolyte imbalances, respiratory distress syndrome, seizures, sepsis, tachypnea

Nursing Diagnoses

Aspiration, risk for Risk factor: Oral feeding of infant with CNS irritability

Breastfeeding, ineffective Related factors: Infant *Fatigue*, poor nursing secondary to alcohol or drug exposure *in utero* and growth-deficient status at birth

Breathing pattern, ineffective Related factors: Depression of respiratory center secondary to _____ (specify drug), meconium aspiration pneumonia

Coping: family, disabled Related factors: Arbitrary disregard for patient's needs, overwhelming needs of infant in the presence of poor coping skills and continued drug use by parent(s)

Family processes, dysfunctional: alcoholism Related factors: Alcohol use by parent(s), lack of support from others, lack of coping skills

Development, delayed (e.g., failure to thrive), risk for See *Growth, risk for delayed*

Diarrhea Related factor: Hyperperistalsis secondary to narcotic withdrawal

Disorganized infant behavior Related factors: Abnormal structural development and CNS dysfunction secondary to alcohol or drug exposure *in utero*, prematurity secondary to maternal drug use, fetal withdrawal *in utero*

Fluid volume, deficient Related factors: Inadequate fluid intake secondary to inadequate sucking reflex, vomiting secondary to fetal alcohol syndrome or narcotic withdrawal

Growth, risk for delayed (e.g., small for gestational age) Risk factors: Unhealthy maternal lifestyle during pregnancy, intrauterine exposure to alcohol/drugs

Home maintenance, impaired Related factors: Physical or psychologic impairment of family member other than infant, inadequate support system, insufficient family organization or planning, continued substance abuse by parent(s)

Infant feeding pattern, ineffective Related factors: Neurologic impairment or delay (see *Breastfeeding, ineffective*), lethargy, failure to thrive secondary to fetal alcohol syndrome

Injury, risk for Risk factors: Psychomotor hyperactivity, seizure activity

Nutrition, imbalanced: less than body requirements Related factors: Chemical dependence or withdrawal, inadequate sucking reflex in infant, vomiting, food intolerance, failure to thrive secondary to fetal alcohol syndrome

Parent/infant/child attachment, risk for impaired See *Parenting, impaired*

Parenting, impaired Related factors: Psychologic or developmental impairment of infant, substance abuse by parent(s), presence of stressors (e.g., legal, financial), interrupted bonding process, difficulty interacting with a child with inability to express feelings of pleasure, anger, and so forth

Sensory perception, disturbed (specify) Related factors: Hypersensitivity to environmental stimuli, inability to maintain alertness and attentiveness to environment, difficulty with attending to and engaging in auditory and visual stimuli

Skin integrity, impaired Related factors: Excoriated buttocks, knees, elbows; facial scratches; pressure point abrasions—all secondary to intrauterine or newborn withdrawal or abstinence syndrome; diaphoresis; *Diarrhea*

Sleep pattern, disturbed Related factors: Sleep deprivation secondary to _____ (specify), effect of depressants or stimulants on CNS *in utero*, newborn withdrawal

Feeding Problems

Include but are not limited to food allergies or intolerances, malabsorption, or motor problems that affect the infant's ability to consume food

Nursing Diagnoses

Breastfeeding, ineffective Related factors: Inadequate sucking reflex in infant, infant *Fatigue* secondary to illnesses such as respiratory distress syndrome or heart anomalies, inability of infant to latch-on, CNS anomalies, prematurity

Diarrhea Related factor: Food intolerance

Disorganized infant behavior Related factors: Abnormal structural development and CNS dysfunction, prematurity

Family processes, interrupted Related factors: Illness or disability of family member, separation of family members

Fluid volume, deficient Related factors: Inadequate fluid intake, psychomotor immaturity (e.g., poor suck-swallow response), inadequate milk production, *Diarrhea*

Infant feeding pattern, ineffective Related factors: Prematurity, neurologic impairment or delay, oral hypersensitivity, prolonged NPO status, anatomical abnormalities

Nutrition, imbalanced: less than body requirements Related factors: Difficulty in swallowing, inadequate sucking reflex in the infant, vomiting, food intolerance, failure to thrive, insufficient maternal milk production

Swallowing, impaired Related factor: Motor problem (specify)

High-Risk Infant

Includes but is not limited to birth asphyxia, meconium aspiration, prematurity, postmaturity, large for gestational age (LGA), small for gestational age (SGA), premature rupture of membranes, maternal infection, infant of diabetic mother, intrauterine growth retardation, infant of adolescent mother, infant of chemically dependent mother, and lack of prenatal care

Potential Complications (Collaborative Problems)

PC of *in utero* infections: Anemia, cataracts, congenital heart disease, deafness, hepatosplenomegaly, hydrocephalus, hyperbilirubinemia, mental retardation, microcephaly, seizures, septicemia, thrombocytopenic purpura

PC of prematurity: Acidosis, apnea, bradycardia, cold stress, hyperbilirubinemia, hypocalcemia, hypoglycemia, pneumonia, respiratory distress syndrome, seizures, sepsis

PC of postmaturity: Birth asphyxia, birth trauma secondary to LGA status, CNS depression, cerebral edema, hypoglycemia, intestinal absorption problems, meconium aspiration, polycythemia (due to SGA status), renal tubular necrosis

Nursing Diagnoses

Activity intolerance Related factors: Inadequate oxygenation secondary to respiratory insufficiency, *Ineffective airway clearance*, respiratory distress syndrome

Airway clearance, ineffective Related factors: Meconium aspiration, tracheobronchial secretions

Aspiration, risk for Risk factors: Immobility, increased secretions, presence of enteral or tracheal tubes

Body temperature, risk for imbalanced See *Thermoregulation, ineffective*

Breastfeeding, ineffective Related factors: Infant *Fatigue*, inadequate sucking reflex, interrupted or infrequent feeding

Breastfeeding, interrupted Related factors: Infant illness, prematurity, maternal obligations outside the home, abrupt weaning of infant

Breathing pattern, ineffective Related factors: Decreased energy or *Fatigue* secondary to illness (e.g., sepsis, respiratory distress syndrome), medication side effects, immature respiratory center, metabolic imbalances

Cardiac output, decreased Related factors: Increased ventricular workload, hypovolemia, cardiac anomaly (specify)

Caregiver role strain Related factors: Illness severity of the infant; premature birth or congenital defect; unpredictable illness course; situational stressors within the family; chronicity of caregiving; caregiver's health; lack of developmental readiness, knowledge, skills, or experience; competing role commitments; ineffective coping styles; isolation; limited opportunity for respite and recreation

Constipation Related factors: Decreased activity and decreased motility secondary to prematurity

Diarrhea Related factor: Increased intestinal motility secondary to inflammation

Disorganized infant behavior Related factors: Immature CNS and excess environmental stimulation

Development, risk for delayed See *Growth, risk for delayed.*

Family processes, interrupted Related factors: Illness or disability of family member, separation of family members

Fear (parental) Related factor: Threat to child

Fluid volume, deficient Related factors: Abnormal blood loss, abnormal fluid loss (specify, e.g., *Diarrhea*, diaphoresis), inadequate fluid intake secondary to _____ (specify, e.g., poor sucking reflex)

Fluid volume excess Related factor: Decreased urinary output secondary to heart failure

Gas exchange, impaired Related factors: Decreased functional lung tissue secondary to pneumonia, chronic lung disease, atelectasis, alveolar capillary membrane changes secondary to inadequate surfactant, cold stress, immature CNS

Grieving, anticipatory (parental) Related factor: Imminent loss of child

Growth, risk for delayed Risk factors: Congenital anomaly, fetal distress, prematurity, unhealthy maternal lifestyle during pregnancy, serious illness

Home maintenance, impaired Related factors: Inadequate support system, insufficient family organization or planning, complex needs of infant

Infant feeding pattern, ineffective Related factors: Prematurity, neurologic impairment or delay, prolonged NPO status, anatomical abnormalities, lethargy

Infection, risk for Risk factors: Inadequate immune system; lack of normal flora; insufficient family knowledge, organization, or planning; invasive treatments or lines; open wounds (e.g., circumcision, umbilical cord), *in utero* infection

Infection (transmission), risk for Risk factor: Contagious nature of organism acquired *in utero*

Nutrition, imbalanced: less than body requirements Related factors: Inadequate sucking reflex in the infant, vomiting, food intolerance, high metabolic rate

Skin integrity, impaired Related factors: Fragility of skin, immobility, susceptibility to infections, and lack of normal skin flora secondary to prematurity; absence of vernix and prolonged exposure to amniotic fluid secondary to postmaturity and LGA status

Spontaneous ventilation, impaired Related factors: Metabolic factors, respiratory muscle fatigue, pulmonary immaturity

Thermoregulation, ineffective Related factors: Prematurity (immature CNS, decreased body-mass to body-surface ratio, minimal subcutaneous fat, limited brown fat, inability to shiver or sweat), transition to extrauterine environment, exposure to environment secondary to need for frequent treatments or interventions

Ventilatory weaning response, dysfunctional (DVWR) Related factors: Pulmonary immaturity, *Impaired gas exchange, Ineffective airway clearance*, ventilator dependence > one week

<u>Hyperbilirubinemia</u>

Potential Complications (Collaborative Problems)

PC of hyperbilirubinemia: Anemia, hepatosplenomegaly, hydrops fetalis (including hepatosplenomegaly, anasarca, hydrothorax, ascites, thrombocytopenia, hypoglycemia secondary to adrenal and pancreatic hyperplasia), kernicterus, renal failure

PC of kernicterus: Athetosis, hearing loss, intellectual deficits

PC of phototherapy: Dehydration, diarrhea, hyperthermia, hypothermia, weight loss, retinal damage, corneal abrasions)

Nursing Diagnoses

Breastfeeding, ineffective Related factor: Poor sucking reflex secondary to kernicterus

Breastfeeding, interrupted Related factor: Infant illness

Diarrhea Related factors: Dietary changes, phototherapy

Family processes, interrupted Related factor: Separation of family members

Fluid volume, deficient Related factors: Abnormal fluid loss (specify, e.g., *Diarrhea* and insensible loss secondary to phototherapy), inadequate fluid intake secondary to _____ (specify)

Injury, risk for Risk factor: Reabsorption of bilirubin secondary to decreased defecation

Nutrition, imbalanced: less than body requirements Related factors: Lethargy, inadequate sucking reflex in infant

Parent/infant/child attachment, risk for impaired Risk factors: Lack of visual stimulation and contact secondary to phototherapy, *Fear* of hurting infant or displacing tubes or lines

Parenting, impaired Related factor: Interruption in bonding process

Sensory perception, disturbed (visual, tactile) Related factor: Sensory deficit secondary to use of eye patches for protection of eyes during phototherapy, lack of tactile stimulation

Skin integrity, impaired Related and risk factors: *Diarrhea*, drying of skin secondary to phototherapy, pruritus, excretion of bilirubin in urine and feces, exposure to phototherapy

Sleep pattern, disturbed Related factors: *Sleep deprivation* secondary to frequent assessment and treatments, discomfort, environmental stimuli

Tissue integrity, impaired (corneal) Related factors: Phototherapy, continuous wearing of eye pads

Hypoglycemia

Potential Complications (Collaborative Problems)

PC of hypoglycemia: Apnea, CNS damage, respiratory distress, seizures, tremors, jerkiness

Nursing Diagnoses

Cardiac output, decreased Related factor: Poor cardiac contractility

Family processes, interrupted Related factors: Illness of infant, separation of family members, *Ineffective coping, Deficient knowledge*

Injury, risk for Risk factor: Seizure activity

Nutrition, imbalanced: less than body requirements Related factors: Inadequate sucking reflex in infant, high metabolic rate or physiologic stress, vomiting, loss of swallowing reflex

Hypothermia

Potential Complications (Collaborative Problems)

PC of hypothermia: Atelectasis, hyperbilirubinemia, hypoglycemia, hypoxemia, metabolic acidosis

Nursing Diagnoses

Breathing pattern, ineffective Related factor: Decreased energy or *Fatigue*, atelectasis

Cardiac output, decreased Related factor: Bradycardia

Family processes, interrupted Related factor: Separation of family members, *Anxiety, Ineffective coping*

Nutrition, imbalanced: less than body requirements Related factor: Loss of or decreased appetite

Tissue perfusion, ineffective (peripheral) Related factors: Imbalance between oxygen supply and demand, hypoxemia secondary to atelectasis and pulmonary vasoconstriction

Low Birth Weight/Small for Gestational Age

Potential Complications (Collaborative Problems)

PC of SGA: Aspiration syndrome; hypocalcemia; hypoglycemia, causing CNS abnormalities, and mental retardation; hypothermia; perinatal asphyxia; polycythemia

Nursing Diagnoses

Activity intolerance Related factor: Weakness or *Fatigue*

Airway clearance, ineffective Related factors: Decreased energy or *Fatigue*, meconium aspiration

Body temperature, risk for imbalanced Risk factors: Diminished subcutaneous fat, large body surface compared to body mass, decreased brown fat stores

Breastfeeding, ineffective Related factors: Infant *Fatigue*, inadequate sucking reflex, interrupted or infrequent feeding

Breastfeeding, interrupted Related factor: Illness of infant

Breathing pattern, ineffective Related factor: Decreased energy or *Fatigue*

Family processes, interrupted Related factors: Illness or disability of family member, separation of family members, feelings of guilt, blame

Fatigue Related factors: Decreased energy, high metabolic rate, poor oxygenation

Fluid volume, deficient Related factor: Inadequate fluid intake

Gas exchange, impaired Related factors: Decreased pulmonary blood supply secondary to respiratory distress syndrome; decreased functional lung tissue secondary to atelectasis, respiratory distress syndrome, and meconium aspiration

Grieving, dysfunctional Related factor: Anticipated or perceived loss of the perfect child

Home maintenance, impaired Related factors: Inadequate support system, insufficient family organization or planning, lack of resources, lack of support

Infant feeding pattern, ineffective See *Imbalanced nutrition: less than body requirements*

Nutrition, imbalanced: less than body requirements Related factors: Inadequate sucking reflex in infant, food intolerance, high metabolic rate, decreased glycogen stores

Parent/infant/child attachment, risk for impaired Risk factors: Infant's illness, need for technologic support, long hospitalization

Parenting, impaired Related factor: Prolonged separation of newborn and parents

Skin integrity, impaired Related factors: Fragile, dry, desquamating skin; lack of subcutaneous fat

Sleep pattern, disturbed Related factor: *Sleep deprivation* secondary to frequent therapeutic interventions

Tissue perfusion, ineffective (peripheral) Related factors: Imbalance between oxygen supply and demand, increased blood viscosity

Normal Newborn

Potential Complications (Collaborative Problems)

PC of adjustment to extrauterine life: Bleeding secondary to circumcision, cold stress, hemorrhagic disease of newborn, hyperbilirubinemia, hypoglycemia, meconium aspiration pneumonia

Nursing Diagnoses

Airway clearance, ineffective Related factors: Oropharynx secretions, obligatory nose breather, apnea

Body temperature, risk for imbalanced Risk factors: Large body surface-to-mass ratio, inability to shiver, extrauterine transition

Fluid volume, deficient Related factors: Inadequate oral intake, increased metabolic rate secondary to excessive handling of newborn

Infection, risk for Risk factors: Lack of acquired immunity, inadequate primary defenses (e.g., open wound such as circumcision) and secondary defenses (e.g., altered phagocytosis), lack of normal flora, exposure to pathogens (e.g., *Neisseria gonorrhoeae*) during passage through birth canal

Nutrition, imbalanced: less than body requirements Related factors: *Ineffective breastfeeding*, inadequate breast milk production, inadequate glucose stores, parental *Deficient knowledge*

Pain Related factors: Circumcision, gastroesophageal reflux, colic

Parent/infant attachment, risk for impaired Risk factors: *Anxiety* about parenting, unmet expectations of parents for labor, delivery, and infant; lack of early parent–infant contact; marital discord; lack of privacy during immediate postpartum period

Parenting, impaired Related factors: *Deficient knowledge* (e.g., related to infant care, follow-up visits), *Anxiety* over new roles, lack of support, financial problems, marital problems

Skin integrity, impaired Related and risk factors: Lack of normal skin flora, inadequate primary or secondary defenses, relative fragility of skin

Thermoregulation, ineffective See *Body temperature, risk for imbalanced*

Urinary retention Related factor: Urethral obstruction secondary to post-circumcision edema

Respiratory Distress

Includes but is not limited to bronchopulmonary dysplasia, respiratory distress syndrome and hyaline membrane disease, meconium aspiration, pneumonia, pneumothorax, and transient tachypnea

Potential Complications (Collaborative Problems)

PC of respiratory distress: Acidosis, atelectasis, cardiopulmonary shunting, hypoxemia, respiratory failure

Nursing Diagnoses

Activity intolerance Related factor: Weakness and *Fatigue* secondary to inadequate oxygenation and respiratory difficulty

Airway clearance, ineffective Related factors: Decreased energy and *Fatigue*, tracheobronchial secretions

Aspiration, risk for Risk factors: Presence of enteral or tracheal tubes, increased oropharyngeal secretions

Breastfeeding, interrupted Related factors: Prematurity, infant illness

Breathing pattern, ineffective Related factors: Decreased energy and *Fatigue*, dependence on ventilator

Cardiac output, decreased Related factors: Increased ventricular workload, cardiac anomaly (specify), hypotension

Caregiver role strain Related and risk factors: Life-threatening illness, premature birth or congenital defect; unpredictable illness course; situational stressors within the family; chronicity of caregiving; caregiver's health; lack of developmental readiness, knowledge, skills, or experience; competing role commitments; ineffective coping styles; isolation; limited opportunity for respite and recreation; financial difficulties

Constipation Related factor: Decreased fluid intake

Coping: family, compromised/disabled Related factors: Life-threatening illness, ineffective communication among family members, lack of support, lack of resources (see *Caregiver role strain*)

Family processes, interrupted Related factors: Illness or disability of family member, separation of family members (see *Caregiver role strain* and *Family Coping, Compromised/disabled)*

Fatigue Related factor: Disease process

Fear (parental) Related factor: Real threat to child

Fluid volume, deficient Related factors: Inadequate fluid intake secondary to *Fatigue* with oral feedings, prescribed fluid restrictions (e.g., to treat cerebral edema), abnormal fluid loss (insensible water loss secondary to rapid respiratory rate)

Gas exchange, impaired Related factors: Decreased pulmonary blood supply secondary to pulmonary hypertension and persistent fetal circulation, respiratory distress syndrome, decreased functional lung tissue secondary to pneumonia, atelectasis, respiratory distress syndrome, diaphragmatic hernia

Grieving, anticipatory (parental) Related factor: Anticipated or perceived loss of child

Home maintenance, impaired Related factors: Inadequate support system, insufficient family planning or organization, overwhelming demands of caregiving and maintaining usual roles

Infant feeding pattern, ineffective Related factors: Prematurity, anatomical abnormalities

Infection, risk for Risk factors: Inadequate immune system, invasive procedures, break in primary defenses (e.g., circumcision, umbilical cord)

Nutrition, imbalanced: less than body requirements Related factors: Inadequate sucking reflex in infant, food intolerance, high metabolic rate of stressed infant, lethargy

Skin integrity, impaired Related and risk factors: Decreased peripheral perfusion, fragility of skin, lack of normal skin flora

Sleep pattern, disturbed Related factor: *Sleep deprivation* secondary to frequent therapeutic interventions

Spontaneous ventilation, impaired Related factors: Metabolic factors, respiratory muscle fatigue, pulmonary immaturity

Thermoregulation, ineffective Related factors: Increased respiratory effort secondary to respiratory distress syndrome

Tissue perfusion, ineffective (peripheral) Related factors: Imbalance between oxygen supply and demand, compensatory responses

Ventilatory weaning response, dysfunctional (DVWR) Related factors: Pulmonary immaturity, *Impaired gas exchange, Ineffective airway clearance*, ventilator dependence > one week

Pediatric Conditions

Developmental problems/needs related to illness

Burns

Cancer (see Medical Conditions: Cancer, pp. 643–645)

Casts and traction

Child abuse

Cleft lip/cleft palate: surgical repair

Coagulation disorders

Congenital malformations of the central nervous system: surgical repair

Diabetes mellitus (see Medical Conditions: Diabetes Mellitus/Hypoglycemia, p. 651)

Failure to thrive

Gastroenteritis

Gastrointestinal obstruction: Surgical repair

Infection of CNS

Ingestion or accidental poisoning

Juvenile rheumatoid arthritis (see Medical Conditions: Arthritis, pp. 638–639)

Obese child

Osteomyelitis

Pregnancy in adolescence

Renal failure, Acute (see Medical Conditions: Renal failure, Acute, p. 660)

Renal failure, Chronic (see Medical Conditions: Renal failure, Chronic, pp. 660–662)

Respiratory disorder, chronic

Respiratory infection, acute

Rheumatic fever (see Medical Conditions: Pericarditis/endocarditis, p. 648)

Seizure disorders

Sepsis

Sickle cell crisis

Suicidal adolescent (see Psychiatric Conditions: Suicide,
  pp. 686–687)

Tonsillectomy

Developmental Problems/Needs Related to Illness

The following nursing diagnoses (as well as *Deficient knowledge*) should be considered for all pediatric medical/surgical conditions. For nursing diagnoses specific to a medical condition (e.g., burns, gastroenteritis), add the nursing diagnoses in that section to the following general illness and development-related diagnoses that apply.

Nursing Diagnoses

Activity intolerance Related factors: Decreased strength and endurance, weakness and *Fatigue*, imbalance between oxygen supply and demand, *Pain (acute or chronic), Imbalanced nutrition: less than body requirements*, limited mobility, frail or debilitated state, chronic illness, decreased hemoglobin

Adjustment, impaired Related factors: Incomplete grieving, *Dysfunctional grieving*, necessity for major lifestyle or behavior change, pattern of dependence, inadequate support systems, failure to accomplish developmental tasks

Anxiety Related factors: Threat to or change in role functioning and interaction patterns, unmet needs, separation anxiety

Caregiver role strain Related factors: Illness severity of the child, premature birth or congenital defect, developmental delay or retardation of the child or caregiver, marginal caregiver coping patterns, duration of caregiving required, caregiver's competing role commitments, complexity and amount of caregiving tasks, lack of respite and recreation for caregiver

Coping: family, compromised/disabled Related factors: Arbitrary disregard for child's needs, conflicting coping styles, highly ambivalent relationships (see *Interrupted family processes* and *Caregiver role strain*)

Decisional conflict Related factors: Necessity to make choices about treatments or interventions, weighing needs of ill child against those of healthy siblings

Development, risk for delayed See *Growth and development, delayed*

Diversional activity, deficient Related factors: Separation from school, friends, and family secondary to hospitalization or disability, *Pain*, illness

Family processes, interrupted Related factors: Change in family roles, illness or disability of family member, unmet expectations for child, inadequate support systems, overwhelming stressors, emotional and physical exhaustion, financial problems, separation of family members, prolonged illness

Fear Related factors: *Powerlessness*, threat to well-being of self/child

Grieving, anticipatory/dysfunctional Related factors: Loss (actual or anticipated) secondary to the particular condition, chronic illness

Growth and development, delayed Related factors: Inability to achieve developmental tasks secondary to serious illness, prescribed dependence or limitations

Home maintenance, impaired Related factors: Home environment obstacles, inadequate support system, insufficient family organization or planning, insufficient finances, lack of familiarity with community resources, developmental disability of caregivers, physical and psychologic impairment of family member other than patient, *Deficient knowledge*

Hopelessness Related factor: Failing or deteriorating physical condition of child

Noncompliance Related factors: Denial of illness, negative consequence of treatment regimen, perceived benefits of continued illness, lack of parental supervision or support

Parental role conflict Related factors: Separation of family members secondary to hospitalization(s) of child, inability to maintain usual role demands (e.g., work, spouse), intimidation with invasive or technical procedures

Parenting, impaired Related factors: Interruption in bonding process; treatment-imposed separation; abuse, rejection, or overprotection secondary to inadequate coping skills; lack of knowledge or skill necessary to address the child's special needs; inadequate supports and resources

Powerlessness Related factor: Chronic illness

Role performance, ineffective Related factors: Chronic illness, *Chronic pain*

Self-care deficit: (specify) Related factors: Specific to illness (e.g., depression, *Pain* and discomfort, *Activity intolerance*, decreased strength and endurance)

Self-esteem, low (chronic, situational) Related factors: Chronic illness, *Chronic pain*

Social interaction, impaired Related factors: Self-concept disturbance, limited physical mobility

Social isolation Related factors: Actual or perceived reactions of others to child's disability, intensity of caregiving demands (e.g., lack of time, energy)

Spiritual distress Related factor: Test of spiritual beliefs

Therapeutic regimen management, ineffective Related factors: *Deficient knowledge* (e.g., illness or surgical procedure, signs and symptoms of complications, medications, home care and treatments, dietary modifications), complex treatments and medication regimens

Burns

Nursing Diagnoses

See Medical Conditions: Burns, pp. 642–643, and Pediatric Conditions: Developmental Problems/Needs Related to Illness, pp. 707–708.

Body image, disturbed Related factors: Burns, scarring

Body temperature, risk for imbalanced Risk factors: Dehydration secondary to impairment in skin integrity, infection

Constipation Related factors: Decreased GI motility, dehydration

Coping, ineffective Related factors: Multiple stressors (e.g., severe injury, *Pain*, repeated painful procedures, *Fear* of disfigurement), prolonged treatment period

Fear Related factors: Painful therapeutic procedures, environmental stressors secondary to hospitalization, separation from family

Fluid volume, deficient Related factor: Abnormal fluid loss secondary to loss of skin integrity

Infection, risk for Risk factors: Malnutrition, loss of primary defense (i.e., *Impaired skin integrity*)

Nutrition, imbalanced: less than body requirements Related factors: High metabolic needs, loss of appetite secondary to *Fear* and *Pain*

Pain Related factors: Injury, *Fear*

Skin integrity, impaired Related factors: Burns, immobility

Social interaction, impaired Related factor: Fear of rejection

Social isolation Related factor: Reactions of others to disfigurement

Casts and Traction

Includes but is not limited to orthopedic trauma and congenital hip dysplasia. See Surgical Conditions: Musculoskeletal Surgery, pp. 671–672, and Pediatric Conditions: Developmental Problems/Needs Related to Illness, pp. 707–708.

Nursing Diagnoses

Body image, disturbed Related factors: Surgery, appliances, congenital defects

Infection, risk for Risk factors: *Impaired tissue integrity* secondary to trauma or surgery, broken skin (e.g., secondary to pins)

Mobility: physical, impaired Related factors: *Pain* and discomfort, medically imposed restrictions, musculoskeletal impairment, casts, traction

Pain Related factors: *Pain* secondary to injury, *Pain* secondary to surgery, muscle cramps secondary to immobilization, muscle soreness (e.g., from walking with crutches)

Peripheral neurovascular dysfunction, risk for Risk factors: Immobilization, tissue trauma

Skin integrity, impaired Related factors: Altered circulation, prescribed immobility, *Impaired mobility* secondary to pain, broken skin (e.g., secondary to external pins)

Tissue perfusion, ineffective (peripheral) Related factors: Interruption of venous flow to _____ (specify) secondary to constriction pressure, interruption of arterial flow to _____ (specify) secondary to compartmental syndrome, tissue trauma

Urinary Incontinence, Functional Related factor: Mobility deficits

Child Abuse

Nursing Diagnoses

See Pediatric Conditions: Developmental Problems/Needs Related to Illness, pp. 707–708.

Coping: family, compromised/disabled Related factors: Chronically unresolved feelings (specify), lack of extended family, financial problems, highly ambivalent family relationships, unwanted child, unwanted characteristics of child (e.g., appearance, mental retardation, hyperactivity), substance-abusing family member, emotionally disturbed family member, use of violence to manage conflict, child sexual or physical abuse

Coping (abuser), ineffective Related factors: History of abuse by own family, lack of love from own family, *Social isolation*, lack of support system, *Situational low self-esteem*, mental illness, emotional immaturity, unrealistic expectations of child

Coping (child), ineffective Related factor: Personal vulnerability in situational crisis

Fear (child) Related factors: Real threat to own well-being, *Powerlessness*, possibility of placement in a foster home

Fear (parent) Related factors: Possibility that abuse will be discovered, anticipated reactions of others, loss of child, criminal prosecution

Hopelessness Related factors: Long-term stress or abuse, inability to escape

Injury, risk for Risk factors: Physical or psychologic abuse, parental neglect

Nutrition, imbalanced: less than body requirements Related factor: Parental neglect

Pain Related factor: Trauma

Parenting, impaired Related factors: Absent or ineffective role model; interruption in bonding process; lack of knowledge or skill; lack of or inappropriate response of child to parent; lack of support for nurturing figure(s); psychologic impairment; physical illness; unrealistic expectations of self, child, or partner; dysfunctional relationship between parents or nurturing figures; situational crisis (specific to family)

Post-trauma response Related factors: Abuse, assault, torture, accidents, and incest

Self-esteem, low (chronic, situational) Related factors: Abuse, negative feedback from family members, feelings of abandonment

Sleep pattern, disturbed Related factors: *Anxiety*, emotional state

Social interaction, impaired Related factors: *Chronic or situational low self-esteem*, isolation enforced by parents

Social isolation See *Social interaction, impaired*

Trauma (specify; e.g., poisoning, physical injury), risk for Risk factors: Vulnerability secondary to congenital problems or chronic illness; lack of support system for caregivers; dysfunctional family interactions

Violence: directed at others, risk for Risk factor: History of physical or mental abuse by others

Cleft Lip/Cleft Palate: Surgical Repair

See Pediatric Conditions: Developmental Problems/Needs Related to Illness, pp. 707–708.

Potential Complications (Collaborative Problems)

PC of cleft lip/palate: Failure to thrive, otitis media, excessive scar formation, poor cosmetic effect secondary to sloughing of sutures

PC of cleft lip/palate, surgical repair: Hypostatic pneumonia

Nursing Diagnoses

Airway clearance, ineffective Related factor: Edema secondary to surgery

Aspiration, risk for Risk factors: Aspiration of feedings through congenital defect in palate, postoperative aspiration of mucus and blood

Body image, disturbed Related factor: Obvious congenital anomaly

Communication, impaired verbal Related factors: Incomplete palate repair, delayed muscle development, dental problems, hearing loss

Fear Related factors: Environmental stressors or hospitalization, separation from parent, parental *Fear* that child will aspirate or suture line will be harmed

Fluid volume, deficient Related factor: Deviation affecting access to or intake of fluids secondary to difficult handling of oral fluids

Infant feeding pattern, ineffective Related factors: Anatomical abnormalities, oral hypersensitivity

Infection, risk for Risk factors: Trauma secondary to surgery, aspiration of feedings, difficulty cleaning sutures

Injury, risk for (disruption of surgical site) Risk factors: Limitations of maturational age; tension on suture line secondary to crying, feeding, or cleansing the area, sucking or blowing

Nutrition, imbalanced: less than body requirements Related factors: Difficulty in chewing, difficulty in swallowing secondary to *Acute pain*, postoperative *Nausea* and vomiting, prescribed diet modifications (e.g., liquids)

Oral mucous membrane, impaired Related factor: Surgery in oral cavity

Pain Related factors: Surgical repair of cleft lip and palate, restraints

Mobility: physical, impaired Related factors: Use of restraints to protect surgical repair

Self-care deficit: feeding Related factors: Age of child and need for adapted feeding

Swallowing, impaired Related factors: *Pain*, unfamiliar method of feeding

Coagulation Disorders

These include but are not limited to hemophilia, von Willebrand disease, and idiopathic thrombocytopenic purpura. See Pediatric Conditions: Developmental Problems/Needs Related to Illness, pp. 707–708, and Medical Conditions: Blood Disorders, pp. 641–642.

Potential Complications (Collaborative Problems)

PC of coagulation disorders: Hemorrhage

Nursing Diagnoses

Coping, ineffective Related factors: Chronic illness and limitations

Fear Related factors: Risks associated with diagnosis (e.g., uncontrollable bleeding, potential joint degeneration, transfusion-acquired diseases)

Mobility: physical, impaired Related factors: Joint hemorrhage, swelling, or degenerative changes; muscle atrophy

Pain Related factors: Joint hemorrhage, swelling

Protection, ineffective Related factors: Abnormal blood profile, medication therapy (e.g., corticosteroids)

Congenital Malformations of the Central Nervous System: Surgical Repair

These include but are not limited to spina bifida, meningocele, myelomeningocele, and hydrocephalus. See Pediatric Conditions: Developmental Problems/Needs Related to Illness, pp. 707–708.

Potential Complications (Collaborative Problems)

PC of hydrocephalus Increased intracranial pressure

PC of myelomeningocele: Hydrocephalus

PC of congenital malformation or surgery of the CNS Neurovascular insufficiency, sepsis, urinary tract infections

Nursing Diagnoses

Incontinence, bowel Related factors: Effects of spinal cord anomaly on anal sphincter

Incontinence, urinary, total Related factors: Effects of spinal cord anomaly on bladder

Infection, risk for Risk factor: Loss of intact skin secondary to congenital anomaly or surgery

Injury, risk for Risk factors: Increased intracranial pressure or seizures secondary to shunt malfunction in hydrocephalus, inability to support large head

Mobility: physical, impaired Related factor: Neuromuscular impairment secondary to spinal cord involvement

Nutrition, imbalanced: less than body requirements Related factor: Vomiting secondary to increased intracranial pressure

Pain Related factor: Surgery

Sensory perception, disturbed (kinesthetic, tactile) Related factors: Sensory deficits secondary to spinal cord involvement

Skin integrity, risk for impaired Risk factors: Immobility (e.g., related to limbs, head and neck), incontinence of stool or urine

Failure To Thrive

See Pediatric Conditions: Developmental Problems/Needs Related to Illness, pp. 707–708.

Potential Complications (Collaborative Problems)

PC of failure to thrive: Dehydration, metabolic disorders

Nursing Diagnoses

Activity intolerance Related factor: Weakness and *Fatigue* secondary to malnutrition

Fluid volume, deficient Related factors: Inadequate fluid intake secondary to disinterest in eating or drinking, parental neglect, abnormal fluid loss (loose stools)

Infection, risk for Risk factors: Weakened defenses secondary to malnutrition, parental neglect (e.g., hygiene)

Nutrition, imbalanced: less than body requirements Related factors: Food intolerance, malabsorption, loss of appetite, parental neglect, lack of emotional and sensory stimulation, parental *Deficient knowledge*, metabolic disorders, organ dysfunction

Sensory perception, disturbed (specify) Related factor: Lack of sensory stimulation from caregiver or parents

Skin integrity, impaired Related factors: Impaired nutritional status, parental neglect (e.g., hygiene)

Sleep pattern, disturbed Related factors: *Anxiety*, parental emotional deprivation

Social interaction, impaired Related factors: Developmental disability, limited physical mobility, *Low self-esteem*

Gastroenteritis

See Pediatric Conditions: Developmental Problems/Needs Related to Illness, pp. 707–708.

Potential Complications (Collaborative Problems)

PC of gastroenteritis: Fluid and electrolyte imbalance

Nursing Diagnoses

Diarrhea Related factors: Food intolerance, infection and inflammation, stress, dietary changes, increased intestinal motility

Fluid volume, deficient Related factors: Abnormal fluid loss (*Diarrhea*, vomiting) secondary to infection, food intolerance, malabsorption

Nutrition, imbalanced: less than body requirements Related factors: Loss of appetite, *Nausea* and vomiting

Oral mucous membrane, impaired Related factor: Dehydration, vomiting

Pain Related factor: *Diarrhea*, abdominal cramps secondary to inflammation, distention, and hyperperistalsis

Sensory perception, disturbed (specify) Related factor: Electrolyte imbalance

Skin integrity, impaired Related and risk factor: Incontinence of stool secondary to *Diarrhea*

Gastrointestinal Obstruction: Surgical Repair

This includes but is not limited to gastroschisis, omphalocele, intestinal atresia, meconium ileus, imperforate anus, Hirschsprung disease, pyloric stenosis, intussusception, inguinal hernia, and hydrocele. See Surgical Conditions, Abdominal Surgery, pp. 665–667, and Pediatric Conditions: Developmental Problems/Needs Related to Illness, pp. 707–708.

Potential Complications (Collaborative Problems)

PC of GI obstruction/surgery: Hemorrhage, ileus, sepsis

Nursing Diagnoses

Body image, disturbed Related factors: Effects of condition or surgery on body

Breathing pattern, ineffective Related factor: *Acute Pain*

Fluid volume, deficient Related factors: Abnormal blood loss, abnormal fluid loss, NPO status

Nausea Related factors: *Pain*, abdominal distention, obstruction

Nutrition, imbalanced: less than body requirements Related factors: Loss of appetite, *Nausea* and vomiting, dietary changes

Pain Related factor: Surgery

Skin integrity, impaired Related and risk factors: Altered nutritional status, surgical wound

Infection of Central Nervous System (CNS)

This includes but is not limited to meningitis, encephalitis, rabies, Reye syndrome, and Guillain-Barré, syndrome. See Pediatric Conditions: Developmental Problems/Needs Related to Illness, pp. 707–708, and Medical Conditions: Neurologic Disorders, pp. 657–658.

Potential Complications (Collaborative Problems)

PC of CNS infection: Atelectasis, coma, fluid and electrolyte imbalance, hepatic failure, increased intracranial pressure, pneumonia, renal failure, respiratory distress, seizures, sepsis

PC of Reye syndrome: Diabetes insipidus

Nursing Diagnoses

Airway clearance, ineffective Related factors: Impaired gag reflex, Impaired swallowing, Fatigue, weakness or paralysis of respiratory muscles, tracheobronchial obstruction, aspiration pneumonia

Breathing patterns, ineffective See *Airway clearance, ineffective*

Communication, impaired verbal Related factors: Inability to speak secondary to coma, dysarthrias secondary to weakness of speech muscles

Confusion, acute See *Memory, impaired*

Disuse syndrome, risk for Risk factors: Paralysis, coma

Fluid volume, deficient Related factors: Inadequate fluid intake secondary to *Nausea*, abnormal fluid loss secondary to vomiting, failure of regulatory mechanisms (e.g., diabetes insipidus)

Hyperthermia Related factors: Illness, dehydration, increased metabolic rate secondary to infectious process

Infection, risk for (transmission) Risk factor: Contagious pathogen

Injury, risk for Risk factors: Seizure activity, generalized weakness, reduced coordination, cognitive deficits, sensory deficits, unsteady gait

Memory, impaired Related factors: Decreased cerebral tissue perfusion secondary to edema, hypovolemia, or increased intracranial pressure

Mobility: physical, impaired Related factors: Neuromuscular impairment, coma, *Pain*, partial or complete paralysis, loss of muscle strength and control, muscle rigidity or tremors

Nutrition, imbalanced: less than body requirements Related factors: *Impaired swallowing*, dysphagia or chewing difficulties secondary to cranial nerve involvement

Pain Related factors: *Nausea* and vomiting, headache secondary to meningeal irritation or inflammation, muscle spasms (neck, shoulders), paresthesia

Sensory perception, disturbed (specify) Related factors: Sensory deficits secondary to coma; sleep deprivation; altered sensory reception, transmission, and integration; electrolyte imbalance; hypoxia; emotional stress

Skin integrity, impaired Related factor: Impaired physical mobility

Suffocation, risk for Risk factors: Decreased level of consciousness, seizures, muscle weakness or paralysis

Swallowing, impaired Related factor: Cerebellar lesions

Tissue perfusion, ineffective (cerebral) Related factors: Cerebral edema, increased intracranial pressure pressure, hypovolemia, acidosis

Ingestion/Accidental Poisoning

See Pediatric Conditions: Developmental Problems/Needs Related to Illness, pp. 707–708.

Potential Complications (Collaborative Problems)

PC of lead poisoning: Anemia, aspiration, blindness, burns (e.g., acid, alkaline), hemorrhage, metabolic acidosis, respiratory alkalosis (Carpenito 1997b, p. 536)

Nursing Diagnoses

Anxiety Related factors: Emergency nature of situation, concern about parents' reactions, guilt feelings

Breathing pattern, ineffective Related factor: Depression of respiratory center secondary to _____ (specify drug)

Fluid volume excess Related factors: Decreased urine output secondary to renal dysfunction, vomiting, *Diarrhea*, decreased intake

Injury (e.g., falls), risk for Risk factors: Seizures secondary to lead poisoning, aspirin toxicity, seizures, loss of coordination, decreased level of consciousness

Nutrition, imbalanced: less than body requirements Related factors: Chemically induced changes in GI, anorexia, abdominal *Pain*, anemia secondary to lead poisoning

Pain, chronic Related factor: Deposits of lead in soft tissues and bone

Sensory perception, disturbed (specify) Related factors: Decreased consciousness, encephalopathy

Thought processes, disturbed Related factor: Deposit of lead in brain tissue and central nervous system

Obese Child

See Pediatric Conditions: Developmental Problems/Needs Related to Illness, pp. 707–708.

Nursing Diagnoses

Activity intolerance Related factors: Sedentary lifestyle, difficulty exercising because of extra weight, exertional discomfort

Body image, disturbed Related factors: Eating disorder (i.e., obesity), view of self in contrast to cultural values

Coping, ineffective Related factor: Use of food to cope with stressors

Family processes, interrupted Related factors: Effects of therapy (e.g., food restriction) on parent–child relationship

Health maintenance, ineffective Related factors: Cultural beliefs, lack of social supports, inability to make deliberate and thoughtful judgments secondary to maturational age, lack of exercise

Mobility: physical, impaired Related factor: Strain on muscles and joints because of weight

Nutrition, imbalanced: more than body requirements Related factors: Psychologic impairment; sedentary lifestyle; lack of basic nutritional knowledge; ethnic or cultural norms; eating as a way of coping; control, sex, or love issues

Self-esteem, low (chronic, situational) Related factors: Obesity, appearance not culturally valued, response of others to obesity

Social interaction, impaired Related factor: Inability to initiate relationships because of self-concept disturbance, embarrassment, and fear of others' negative responses

Social isolation Related factors: Obesity, reactions of others

Osteomyelitis

See Pediatric Conditions: Developmental Problems/Needs Related to Illness, pp. 707–708.

Potential Complications (Collaborative Problems)

PC of osteomyelitis: Infective emboli, pathologic fractures

PC of antibiotic therapy: Hematologic, hepatic, and renal problems; anaphylactic shock

Nursing Diagnoses

Constipation Related factors: Immobility, narcotic medications

Hyperthermia Related factors: Infectious process, increased metabolic rate

Injury, risk for Risk factor: Pathologic fractures related to disease process

Mobility: physical, impaired Related factors: *Pain* and discomfort, musculoskeletal impairment, prescribed immobility

Nutrition, imbalanced: less than body requirements Related factors: High metabolic rate, anorexia secondary to infectious process and *Pain*

Pain Related factors: Inflammation, swelling, hyperthermia, tissue necrosis, fractures

Skin integrity, impaired Related factors: Immobility, irritation from cast or splint

Tissue perfusion, ineffective Related factors: Inflammatory reaction with thrombosis of vessels, edema, abscess formation, tissue destruction

Pregnancy in Adolescence

This includes pregnancy, antepartum and postpartum periods, and parenting. See Pediatric Conditions: Developmental Problems/Needs Related to Illness, pp. 707–708. See also Antepartum and Postpartum Conditions, pp. 688–696.

Nursing Diagnoses

Body image, disturbed Related factors: Pregnancy and developmental stage

Coping, ineffective Related factors: Adolescent pregnancy, adolescent parenthood

Health maintenance, ineffective Related factors: Lack of social supports, lack of material resources, cultural beliefs, lack of ability to make deliberate and thoughtful judgments secondary to maturational age

Deficient knowledge (specify) Related factors: Limited exposure to information (e.g., about birth control, parenting), limited practice of skills, information misinterpretation

Nutrition, imbalanced: less than body requirements Related factors: High metabolic needs secondary to both adolescence and pregnancy, lack of basic nutritional knowledge, limited access to food, *Nausea* and vomiting

Nutrition, imbalanced: more than body requirements Related factors: Ethnic or cultural norms, lack of basic nutritional knowledge, "fast" food, "junk" food

Parent/infant/child attachment, risk for impaired See *Parenting, impaired*

Parenting, impaired Related factors: Lack of knowledge or skill; lack of support for nurturing figure from own parents; alienation from own parents; unrealistic expectations of self, infant, and partner; situational crisis

Social interaction, impaired Related factors: Sociocultural conflict, self-concept disturbance, embarrassment, withdrawal from school

Social isolation Related factors: Alteration in physical appearance, lifestyle changes

Violence: directed at others (child), risk for Risk factors: Rage reaction, history of physical or mental abuse by others, ineffective coping skills, substance abuse

Respiratory Disorder, Chronic

This includes but is not limited to asthma, bronchopulmonary dysplasia, and cystic fibrosis. See Pediatric Conditions: Developmental Problems/Needs Related to Illness, pp. 707–708. See also Medical Conditions: Acute respiratory disorders (e.g., pneumonia, pulmonary edema, pulmonary embolism), and Chronic respiratory disorders, pp. 662–664.

Potential Complications (Collaborative Problems)

PC of chronic respiratory disorder: Hypoxemia, respiratory acidosis

PC of corticosteroid therapy: Hypertension, hypokalemia, hypoglycemia, immunosuppression, osteoporosis, ulcers

Nursing Diagnoses

Activity intolerance Related factors: Inadequate oxygenation secondary to bronchospasm or increased pulmonary secretions

Airway clearance, ineffective Related factors: Tracheobronchial secretions, spasms of the bronchi and bronchioles, ineffective cough secondary to *Fatigue* or weakness

Anxiety Related factors: Air hunger, difficulty breathing, *Fear* of suffocation or dying

Breathing pattern, ineffective Related factors: *Anxiety*, pulmonary infection, decreased energy or *Fatigue*

Fear Related factors: Dyspnea, fear of recurrences

Fluid volume, deficient, risk for Risk factors: Inadequate fluid intake secondary to difficulty in breathing, abnormal fluid loss secondary to increased insensible water loss from rapid respirations

Gas exchange, impaired Related factor: Decreased functional lung tissue secondary to fibrotic, nonventilated areas of lung parenchyma in bronchopulmonary dysplasia

Infection, risk for Risk factors: Malnutrition, stasis of respiratory secretions

Nutrition, imbalanced: less than body requirements Related factors: Loss of appetite with chronic illness, high metabolic needs secondary to pulmonary infection, malabsorption of nutrients secondary to cystic fibrosis

Respiratory Infection, Acute

This includes but is not limited to tonsillitis, pharyngitis, croup, laryngotracheobronchitis, epiglottitis, bronchitis, and pneumonia. See Pediatric Conditions: Developmental Problems/Needs Related to Illness, pp. 707–708. See also Medical Conditions: Acute respiratory disorders (e.g., pneumonia, pulmonary edema, pulmonary embolism) and Chronic respiratory disorders, pp. 662–664.

Potential Complications (Collaborative Problems)

PC of acute respiratory infection: Hypoxemia, respiratory acidosis, respiratory insufficiency, sepsis

PC of corticosteroid therapy: Hypertension, hypokalemia, hypoglycemia, immunosuppression, osteoporosis, ulcers

Nursing Diagnoses

Airway clearance, ineffective Related factors: Edema, increased or viscous tracheobronchial or pulmonary secretions, bronchospasm, tracheobronchial inflammation, pleuritic pain, ineffective cough secondary to *Fatigue*

Anxiety Related factors: *Fear* of dying, dyspnea, inadequate oxygenation

Fear Related factors: Real threat to well-being, environmental stressors or hospitalization, separation from parent, dyspnea, *Fear* of recurring attacks

Fluid volume, deficient Related factors: Inadequate fluid intake secondary to difficulty in breathing, abnormal fluid loss secondary to increased insensible water loss from rapid respirations or fever

Gas exchange, impaired Related factors: Decreased functional lung tissue secondary to pneumonia, air trapping, impaired exchange of oxygen in alveoli secondary to collected secretions, hypoventilation (see *Airway clearance, ineffective*)

Nutrition, imbalanced: less than body requirements Related factors: Loss of appetite secondary to dyspnea and malaise, high metabolic needs

Pain Related factors: Sore throat, *Pain* with inspiration, pleural *Pain*

Sensory perception, disturbed (specify) Related factor: Sensory deficit secondary to time spent in croupette

Skin integrity, risk for impaired Risk factors: Altered nutritional status, hyperthermia, damp therapeutic environment, decreased mobility, diaphoresis

Seizure Disorders

See Pediatric Conditions: Developmental Problems/Needs Related to Illness, pp. 707–708. See also Medical Conditions: Neurologic Disorders, pp. 655–658.

Potential Complications (Collaborative Problems)

PC of seizure disorder: Status epilepticus

Nursing Diagnoses

Airway clearance, ineffective Related factors: Loss of tongue and gag reflexes during seizure activity

Injury, risk for Risk factor: Uncontrolled muscle movements during seizure activity

Self-esteem, low (chronic, situational) Related factors: Chronic illness, feelings of being out of control, stigma associated with seizures, perceived "weakness"

Social interaction, impaired Related factors: Embarrassment, fear of having a seizure in public

Suffocation, risk for Risk factors: Weakness, altered level of consciousness, cognitive limitations

Sepsis

See Pediatric Conditions: Developmental Problems/Needs Related to Illness, pp. 707–708.

Potential Complications (Collaborative Problems)

PC of sepsis: Anemia, edema, hemorrhage, hypotension, hypothermia or hyperthermia, meningitis, respiratory distress, seizures

Nursing Diagnoses

Cardiac output, decreased Related factors: Decreased circulating volume and venous return, increased systemic vascular resistance, effects of hypoxia

Constipation Related factor: Decreased fluid intake

Diarrhea Related factors: Increased intestinal motility, intestinal irritation secondary to infectious process

Fluid volume, deficient Related factors: Decreased fluid intake, fever, widespread vasodilation and intercompartmental fluid shifts

Injury, risk for Risk factor: Seizure activity secondary to high fever

Nutrition, imbalanced: less than body requirements Related factors: Inadequate sucking reflex in infant, vomiting, food intolerance, increased metabolic rate, lethargy

Skin integrity, impaired Related factors: Decreased peripheral perfusion, hyperthermia, edema, immobility

Sleep pattern, disturbed Related factors: Frequent therapeutic interventions, discomfort secondary to fever, difficulty breathing, diaphoresis

Tissue perfusion, ineffective (specify) Related factors: Selective vasoconstriction, presence of microemboli, hypovolemia

Sickle Cell Crisis

See Pediatric Conditions: Developmental Problems/Needs Related to Illness, pp. 707–708.

Potential Complications (Collaborative Problems)

PC of sickle cell crisis: Vaso-occlusive crisis, causing infarctions of vital organs (e.g., liver, kidneys, central nervous system); infections (e.g., pneumonia, osteomyelitis); aplastic crisis (rapidly developing severe anemia); splenic sequestration, causing circulatory collapse

PC of repeated transfusions: Hemosiderosis

Nursing Diagnoses

Body image, disturbed Related factors: Delayed onset of puberty, swelling of the hands and feet, prominence of the bones of the face and skull, *Pain,* need to avoid strenuous activities

Fluid volume, deficient Related factor: Increased need for fluid volume in blood to prevent sickling and thrombosis. (**NOTE:** This is a relative deficit. Enough fluid must be ingested to create hemodilution.)

Gas exchange, impaired Related factors: Susceptibility to pneumonia and pulmonary infarctions, decreased oxygen-carrying capacity of the blood

Infection, risk for Risk factors: Chronic illness, defects in immunologic system

Pain Related factors: Sickle cell crisis, causing tissue hypoxia and impaired peripheral circulation

Tissue perfusion, ineffective (peripheral) Related factors: Imbalance between oxygen supply and demand secondary to anemia, thrombosis secondary to clumping of red blood cells in sickle cell crisis, increased blood viscosity, arteriovenous shunts in peripheral and pulmonary circulation

Tonsillectomy

See Pediatric Conditions: Developmental Problems/Needs Related to Illness, pp. 707–708.

Potential Complications (Collaborative Problems)

PC of tonsillectomy: Airway obstruction, aspiration, hemorrhage

Nursing Diagnoses

Airway clearance, ineffective Related factors: Trauma, edema, *Pain,* tracheobronchial secretions, collection of blood in oropharynx, vomiting, sedation

Fluid volume, deficient Related factors: Blood loss secondary to surgery of highly vascular site, decreased intake secondary to painful swallowing

Nutrition, imbalanced: less than body requirements Related factors: Loss of appetite secondary to sore throat and blood swallowing

Pain Related factors: Surgery, packing, edema

BIBLIOGRAPHY

Aaronson, L. S., Teel, C. S., Cassmeyer, V., Neuberger, G. B., Pallikkathayil, L., Pierce, J., Press, A. N., Williams, P, D., & Wingate, A. (1999). Defining and measuring fatigue. Image: *Journal of Nursing Scholarship, 31*(1), 45–50.

Abraham, I., & Reel, S. (1993). Cognitive nursing interventions with long-term care residents: Effects on neurocognitive dimensions. *Archives of Psychiatric Nursing, 6*(6), 356–365.

Ackerman, L. L. (1992). Interventions related to neurological care. In G. M. Bulechek & J. C. McCloskey (Eds.), *Symposium on Nursing Interventions. Nursing Clinics of North America, 27*(2), 325–346.

Acute Pain Management Guideline Panel. (1992, Feb.). *Acute pain management: Operative or medical procedures and trauma. Clinical practice guideline.* (AHCPR Publication No. 92-0032). Rockville, MD: Agency for Health Care Policy and Research, Public Health Service, U.S. Department of Health and Human Services.

Agency for Health Care Policy and Research (1996). *Smoking cessation. Clinical practice guideline.* Washington, DC: U.S. Government Printing Office.

Agostinelli, B., Demers, K., Garrigan, D., & Waszynski, C. (1994). Targeted interventions: Use of the mini-mental state exam. *Journal of Gerontological Nursing, 20*(8), 15–23.

Ahrens, T. (1993). Changing perspectives in the assessment of oxygenation. *Critical Care Nurse, 13*(4), 78–83.

Ahrens, T. S. (1993). Respiratory disorders. In M. R. Kinney, D. R. Packa, & S. B. Dunbar (Eds.), *AACN's clinical reference for critical-care nursing* (pp. 701–704). St. Louis: Mosby.

American Academy of Pediatrics & American College of Obstetricians and Gynecologists (1992). Postpartum and follow-up care. In *Guidelines for perinatal care* (3rd ed.), (pp. 91–116). Evanston, IL: Authors.

American Association of Critical-Care Nurses. (1990). *Outcome standards for nursing care of the critically ill.* Laguna Niguel, CA: Author.

American Association of Post-Anesthesia Nurses. (1992). *Standards of post-anesthesia nursing.* Resource 18. Richmond, VA: Author.

American College of Allergy & Immunology (1992). *Interim recommendations to health professionls and organizations regarding latex allergy precautions.* Milwaukee, WI: Author.

American Nurses Association (2002). *ANA brochure. Latex Allergy: Protect yourself, protect your patients.* Retrieved December 10, 2002: www.nursingworld.org/dlwa/osh/wp7.htm.

American Psychiatric Association Practice Guidelines (1993). *American Journal of Psychiatry, 150*(2), 207–228.

American Public Health Association and the American Academy of Pediatrics. (1992). *Caring for our children: National health and performance standards: Guidelines for out-of-home child care programs.* Washington, DC: Author.

Andrews, M., & Boyle, J. (1998). *Transcultural concepts in nursing* (3rd ed.). Philadelphia: J. B. Lippincott.

Arnold, E. (1997). The stress connection. *Critical Care Nursing Clinics of North America, 9*(4): 565–575.

Arnold, E., & Boggs, K. (1999). *Interpersonal relationships: Professional communications skills for nurses* (3rd ed.). Philadelphia: Saunders.

Aronson, M. K. (Ed.). (1994). *Reshaping dementia care*. Thousand Oaks, CA: Sage Publications.

Association of Operating Room Nurses (1993). Positioning the surgical patient. In *Standards and Recommended Practices*. Denver: Author.

Association of Operating Room Nurses (1993). *Standards and recommended practices*. Denver: Author.

Association of Women's Health, Obstetric, and Neonatal Nurses (1993). *Fetal heart monitoring principles & practices*. Washington: DC: Author.

Badger, J. M. (1994). Calming the anxious patient. *American Journal of Nursing, 94*(5), 46–50.

Baer, C. L. (1993a). Acid-base balance. In M. R. Kinney, D. R. Packa, & S. B. Dunbar (Eds.), *AACN's clinical reference for critical-care nursing* (pp. 209–216). St. Louis: Mosby.

Baer, C. L. (1993b). Fluid and electrolyte balance. In M. R. Kinney, D. R. Packa, & S. B. Dunbar (Eds.), *AACN's clinical reference for critical-care nursing* (pp. 173–208). St. Louis: Mosby.

Baginski, Y. (1994). Roadblocks to home care. *Caring, 13*(12), 18–20, 22, 24.

Baker, D. M. (1993). Assessment and management of impairments in swallowing. *Nursing Clinics of North America, 28*(4), 793–806.

Bakker, R. H., Kastermans, M. C., & Dassen, T. W. N. (1995). An analysis of the nursing diagnosis "ineffective management of therapeutic regimen" compared to "noncompliance" and Orem's self-care deficit theory of nursing. *Nursing Diagnosis, 6*(4), 161–166.

Bank, L. J. (1992). Counseling. In G. M. Bulechek & J. C. McCloskey (Eds.), *Nursing interventions: Essential nursing treatments* (pp. 279–291). Philadelphia: Saunders.

Barry, K. (1993). Patient self-medication: An innovative approach to medication teaching. *Journal of Nursing Care Quality, 8*(1), 75–82.

Bates, B. (1998). *A guide to the physical examination and history taking* (7th ed.). Philadelphia: Lippincott.

Bear, K., & Tigges, B. B. (1993). Management strategies for promoting successful breastfeeding. *Nurse Practitioner: American Journal of Primary Health Care, 18*, 50, 53–54, 56–58, 60.

Beck, C. F. (1994). Malignant hyperthermia: Are you prepared? *AORN Journal, 59*(2), 367–390.

Beck, A. T., Steer, R. A., & Brown, G. (1993). Dysfunctional attitudes and suicidal ideation in psychiatric outpatients. *Suicide and Life-Threatening Behavior, 23*(1), 11–20.

Bendorf, K., & Lyman, B. (1993). Transition from the hospital to the home for the infant requiring total parenteral nutrition. *Journal of Perinatal and Neonatal Nursing, 6*(4), 80–90. (Publication No. 95–0652).

Bergstrom, N., Bennett, M., Carlson, C., et al. (1994). *Treatment of pressure ulcers.* Clinical Practice Guideline No. 15. Rockville, MD: U. S. Department of Health and Human Services, Public Health Service, Agency for Health Care Policy and Research.

Bernthal, E. (1999). Inadvertent hypothermia prevention: The anaesthetic nurses' role. *British Journal of Nursing, 8*(1): 17–18, 20–25.

Bines, A. S., & Landron, S. L. (1993). Cardiovascular emergencies in the post anesthesia care unit. In K. L. Saleh & V. Brinsko (Eds.), *Nursing Clinics of North America, 28*(3), 493–506.

Blackburn, S. (1993). Assessment and management of neurologic dysfunction. In C. Kenner, A. Brueggemeyer, & L. Gunderson (Eds.), *Comprehensive neonatal nursing.* Philadelphia: Saunders.

Blackburn, S., & Vandenberg, K. (1993). Assessment and management of neonatal neurobehavioral development. In C. Kenner, A. Brueggemeyer, & L. Gunderson (Eds.), *Comprehensive neonatal nursing.* Philadelphia: Saunders.

Bliss-Holtz, J. (1992). Temperature relationships in cold-stressed infants. *Neonatal Network, 11*(2), 72.

Boggs, R. L., & Woolridge-Kim, M. (1993). *AACH procedural manual for critical care* (3rd ed.). Philadelphia: Saunders.

Bolton, P. J., & Kline, K. A. (1994). Understanding modes of mechanical ventilation. *American Journal of Nursing, 94*(6), 36–43.

Bossert, E., Holaday, B., Harkins, A., & Turner-Henson, A. (1990). Strategies of normalization used by parents of chronically ill school age children. *Journal of Child and Adolescent Psychiatric and Mental Health Nursing, 3*(2), 57–61.

Bowers, B. (1987). Intergenerational caregiving: Adult caregivers and their aging parents. *Advances in Nursing Science, 9*(2), 20–31.

Boyes, R. J., & Kruse, J. A. (1992). Nasogastric and nasoenteric intubation. *Critical Care Clinics, 8*(4), 865–878.

Bozzette, M. (1993). Observations of pain behavior in the NICU: An exploratory study. *Journal of Perinatal and Neonatal Nursing, 7*(1), 76–87.

Breslin, E. H. (1992). Dyspnea-limited response in chronic obstructive pulmonary disease: Reduced unsupported arm activities. *Rehabilitation Nursing, 17*, 12–20.

Bricker, D. (Ed.). (1993). *AEPS measurement for birth–three years* (Vol. 1). Baltimore: Paul H. Brookes Publishing.

Brooks-Brunn, J. A. (1995). Postoperative atelectasis and pneumonia: Risk factors. *American Journal of Critical Care, 4*, 340.

Brown, D. R., Morgan, W. P., & Raglin, J. S. (1993). Effects of exercise and rest on the state of anxiety and blood pressure of physically challenged college students. *Journal of Sports Medicine and Physical Fitness, 33*(3), 300–305.

Brukwitzki, G., Holmgren, C., & Maibusch, R. M. (1996). Validation of the defining characteristics of the nursing diagnosis "ineffective airway clearance." *Nursing Diagnosis, 7*(2), 63–69.

Brundage, D. J., & Linton, A. D. (1997). Age related changes in the genitourinary system. In M. A. Matteson, E. S. McConnell, & A. D. Linton (Eds.), *Gerontological nursing: Concepts in practice* (2nd ed.). Philadelphia: Saunders.

Bull, M. J. (1994). Patients' and professionals' perceptions of quality in discharge planning. *Journal of Nursing Care Quality*, 8(2), 47–61.

Burnside, I., & Haight, B. (1994). Reminiscence and life review: Therapeutic interventions for older people. *Nurse Practitioner*, 19(4), 55–60.

Burrow, S. (1994). Nursing management of self-mutilation. *British Journal of Nursing*, 3(8), 382–386.

Caldwell, S. M. (1993). Measuring family well-being: Conceptual model, reliability, validity and use. In C. F. Waltz & O. L. Strickland (Eds.), *Measuring client outcomes*. New York: Springer.

Campbell, J., McKenna, L. S., Torres, S., Sheridan, D., & Landenburger, K. (1993). Nursing care of abused women. In J. Campbell & J. Humphreys (Eds.), *Nursing care of survivors of family violence*. St. Louis: Mosby.

Campus, R. G. (1994). Rocking and pacifiers: Two comforting interventions for heelstick pain. *Research in Nursing & Health*, 17, 321–331.

Carlson-Catalano, J. (1998). Nursing diagnosis and interventions for post-acute-phase battered women. *Nursing Diagnosis: The Journal of Nursing Language and Classification*, 9(3), 101–110.

Carlson-Catalano, J., Lunney, M., Paradiso, C., Bruno, J., Luise, B. K., Martin, T., Massoni, M., & Pachter, S. (1998). Clinical validation of ineffective breathing pattern, ineffective airway clearance, and impaired gas exchange. *Image: Journal of Nursing Scholarship*, 30(3), 243–248.

Carpenito, L. J. (1997a). *Handbook of nursing diagnosis* (7th ed.). Philadelphia: Lippincott.

Carpenito, L. J. (1997b). *Nursing diagnosis: Application to clinical practice* (7th ed.). Philadelphia: Lippincott.

Casaburi, R., & Petty, T. (1993). *Principles and practice of pulmonary rehabilitation*. Philadelphia: Saunders.

Chang, B. L., Uman, G. C., & Hirsch, M. (1998). Predictive power of clinical indicators of self-care deficit. *Nursing Diagnosis: The Journal of Nursing Language and Classification*, 9(2), 71–82.

Chilman, C., Nunnally, E., & Cox, F. (1988). *Chronic illness and disability*, (pp. 30–31). Beverly Hills, CA: Sage Publications.

Clark, C. C. (1998). Wellness self-care by healthy older adults. *Image: Journal of Nursing Scholarship*, 31(4), 351–355.

Cohen, R. K., Diegelmann, R. F., & Lindblad, W. L. (1992). *Wound healing: Biochemical and clinical aspects*. Philadelphia: Saunders.

Cole, S. L. (1992). Dress for success: A nurse's knowledge of simple clothing adaptations and dressing aids may make the difference between rehabilitation success and failure. *Geriatric Nursing*, 13(4), 217–221.

Collins, C. E., Given, B. A., & Given, C. W. (1994). Interventions with family caregivers of persons with Alzheimer's disease. *Nursing Clinics of North America*, 29(1), 127–131.

Conn, V., Talor, S., & Casey, B. (1992). Cardiac rehabilitation program participation and outcomes after myocardial infarction. *Rehabilitation Nursing*, 17(2), 58–62.

Cooley, M. E. (1992). Bereavement care: A role for nurses. *Cancer Nursing*, 15(2), 125–129.

Courtens, A. M., & Abu-Saad, H. H. (1998). Nursing diagnoses in patients with leukemia. *Nursing Diagnosis: The Journal of Nursing Language and Classification, 9*(2), 49–61.

Craft, M. J., & Willadsen, J. A. (1992). Interventions related to family. In G. M. Bulechek & J. C. McCloskey (Eds.), *Symposium on Nursing Interventions. Nursing Clinics of North America, 27*(2), 517–540.

Cullen, L. M. (1992). Interventions related to circulatory care. In G. M. Bulechek & J. C. McCLoskey (Eds.), *Symposium on Nursing Interventions. Nursing Clinics of North America, 27*(2), 445–476.

Dean, G. E., & Ferrell, B. R. (1995). Impact of fatigue on quality of life in cancer survivors. *Quality of Life—A Nursing Challenge, 4*(1), 25–28.

Dean-Barr, S. L. (1994). Standards and guidelines: How do they assure quality? In J. McCloskey & H. K. Grace (Eds.), *Current issues in nursing* (4th ed.). St. Louis: Mosby.

DeMarco-Sinatra, J. (2000). Relaxation training as a holistic nursing intervention. *Holistic Nursing Practice, 14*(3): 30–39.

Denehy, J. A. (1990). Anticipatory guidance. In M. J. Craft & J. A. Denehy (Eds.), *Nursing interventions for infants and children* (pp. 53–68). Philadelphia: Saunders.

Denehy, J. A. (1992). Interventions related to parent-infant attachment. In G. M. Bulechek & J. C. McCloskey (Eds.), *Symposium on Nursing Interventions. Nursing Clinics of North America, 27*(2), 425–444.

Donnelly, A. J. (1994). Malignant hyperthermia: Epidemiology, pathophysiology, treatment. *AORN Journal, 59*(2), 393–405.

Dougherty, C. (1997). Reconceptualization of the nursing diagnosis "decreased cardiac output." *Nursing Diagnosis: The Journal of Nursing Language and Classification, 8*(1), 29–36.

Dougherty, C. M. (1992). Surveillance. In G. M. Bulechek & J. C. McCloskey (Eds.), *Nursing interventions: Essential nursing treatments* (2nd ed., pp. 500–511). Philadelphia: Saunders.

Doughty, D. (Ed.). (1991). *Urinary and fecal incontinence: Nursing management.* St. Louis: Mosby-Year Book.

Dyckoff, D., Goldstein, L., & Levine-Schacht, L. (1996). The investigation of behavioral contracting in patients with borderline personality disorder. *Journal of the American Psychiatric Nurses Association, 2*(3), 71–76.

Eakes, G. G., Burke, M. L., & Hainsworth, M. A. (1998). Middle-range theory of chronic sorrow. *Image: Journal of Nursing Scholarship, 30*(2), 179–184.

El Camino Hospital Clinical Practice Council. (1992). *Management of the adult patient being weaned.* Mountain View, CA: El Camino Hospital.

Elek, S. M., Hudson, D. B., & Fleck, M. L. (1997). Expectant parents' experience with fatigue and sleep during pregnancy. *Birth, 24*, 49–54.

Elsen, J., & Blegen, M. (1991). Social isolation. In M. Maas, K. Buckwalter, & M. Hardy (Eds.), *Nursing diagnoses and interventions in the elderly* (pp. 519–529). Redwood City, CA: Addison-Wesley.

Fearing, M. O., & Hart, L. K. (1992). Dialysis therapy. In G. M. Bulechek & J. C. McCloskey (Eds.), *Nursing interventions: Essential nursing treatments* (2nd ed., pp. 587–601). Philadelphia: Saunders.

Ferrell, B. R., Dow, K. H., Leigh, S., Ly, J., & Gulaskekaram, P. (1995). Quality of life in long-term cancer survivors. Part 1. *Oncology Nursing Forum, 22*(6), 915–922.

Finkelman, A. (2000). Self-management for psychiatric patients at home. *Home Care Provider 5*(6): 95–101.

Fischman, S. (1993). Self-care: Practical periodontal care in today's practice. *International Dental Journal, 43,* 179–183.

Flanagan, M. (1994). Assessment criteria. *Nursing Times, 90*(35), 76–88.

Flaskerud, J., Carter, P., & Lee, P. (2000). Distressing emotions in female caregivers of people with AIDS, age-related dementials and advanced stage cancers. *Perspectives in Psychiatric Care, 36*(4): 121–130.

Folden, S. L. (1993). Definitions of health and health goals of participants in a community-based pulmonary rehabilitation program. *Public Health Nursing, 10*(1), 31–35.

Fontaine, K. L., & Fletcher, J. S. (1998). Mental health nursing (4th ed). Menlo Park, CA: Addison-Wesley Nursing.

Fowler, S. B. (1997). Impaired verbal communication during short-term oral intubation. *Nursing Diagnosis: The Journal of Nursing Language and Classification, 8*(3), 93–98.

Frieberg, K. (1992). *Human development: A life span approach* (4th ed.). Boston: Jones and Bartlett.

Friedman, M. M. (1992). *Family nursing: Theory and practice.* Norwalk, CT: Appleton & Lange.

Gabbe, S., Niebyl, J., & Simpson, J. (2002). *Obstetrics: Normal and problem pregnancies* (4th ed.). New York: Churchill Livingstone.

Gardner, D. L., & Campbell, B. (1991). Assessing postpartum fatigue. *Maternal Child Nursing Journal, 16*(5), 264–266.

Geissler, E. (1991). Transcultural nursing and nursing diagnoses. *Nursing and Health Care, 12*(4), 190–192, 203.

Gianino, S., & St. John, R. E. (1993). Nutritional assessment of the patient in the intensive care unit. *Critical Care Nursing Clinics of North America, 5*(1), 1–16.

Giger, J., & Davidhizar, R. (1999). *Transcultural nursing: Assessments and interventions* (3rd ed.). St. Louis: Mosby-Year Book.

Gill, L., & Flenstein, A. R. (1994). A critical appraisal of the quality of quality-of-life measurements. *Journal of the American Medical Association, 272,* 619–626.

Gillis, A. J. (1993). Determinants of health promoting lifestyle: An integrative review. *Journal of Advanced Nursing, 18,* 345–353.

Giuliano, K., Giuliano, A., Scott, S., et al., (2000), Temperature measurement in critically ill adults: A comparison of tympanic and oral methods. *American Journal of Critical Care, 9*(4): 254–261.

Glennon, S. (1993). Mechanical support of ventilation. In M. R. Kinney, D. R. Backa, & S. B. Dunbar (Eds.), *AACN's clinical reference for critical-care nursing* (pp. 828–840). St. Louis: Mosby.

Glick, D., Kronenfeld, J., & Jackson, K. (1993). Safety behaviors among parents of preschoolers. *Health Values, 17*(1), 18–27.

Glick, O. J. (1992). Interventions related to activity and movement. In G. M. Bulechek & J. C. McCloskey (Eds.), *Symposium on Nursing Interventions. Nursing Clinics of North America, 27*(2), 541–568.

Gordon, M. (1985). Practice based data set for a nursing information system. Journal of Medical Systems, 9:43–55.

Gordon, M. (1987). *Nursing Diagnosis: process and application* (2nd ed.). New York: McGraw-Hill.

Gordon, M. (1994). *Nursing Diagnosis: process and application* (3rd ed.). New York: McGraw-Hill.

Grancola, P. R., & Zeichner, A. (1993). Aggressive behavior in the elderly: A critical review. *Clinical Gerontologist, 13*(2), 3–22.

Greaves, P., Glik, D. C., Kronenfeld, J. J., & Jackson, K. (1994). Determinants of controllable in-home child safety hazards. *Health Education Research, 9*(3), 307–315.

Green, M. (Ed.). (1994). *Bright futures: Guidelines for health supervision of infants, children and adolescents*. Arlington, VA: National Center for Education in Maternal and Child Health.

Griffin, T., Wishba, C., & Kavanaugh, K. (1998). Nursing interventions to reduce stress in parents of hospitalized preterm infants. *Journal of Pediatric Nursing, 13*(5), 290–295.

Guyton, A. C. (1992). *Human physiology and mechanisms of disease*. Philadelphia: Saunders.

Gyulay, J. (1989). Grief responses. *Issues in Comprehensive Pediatric Nursing, 12*(1), 1–31.

Haber, J., McMahon, A. L., Price-Hoskins, P., & Sideleau, B. F. (1992). *Comprehensive psychiatric nursing* (4th ed.). St. Louis: Mosby.

Halm, M. (1990). The effect of support groups on anxiety of family members during critical illness. *Heart and Lung, 11*(6), 571–576.

Halpern, J. S. (1989). Clinical notebook: Lower extremity peripheral nerve assessment. *Journal of Emergency Nursing, 15*(4), 333–337.

Hartford, M., Karlson, B. W., Sjolin, M., Holmber, S., & Herlitz, J. (1993). Symptoms, thoughts, and environmental factors in suspected acute myocardial infarction. *Heart and Lung, 22*(1), 64–70.

Hawkins-Walsh, E. (1988). Breastfeeding the premature infant. *Pediatric Nursing Forum, 3*(4), 3–13.

Hayden, R. (1992). What keeps oxygenation on track? *American Journal of Nursing, 92*(12), 32–40.

Healthy people 2000: National health promotion and disease prevention objectives. (1990). DHHS Publication (PHS) 91-50213. Washington, DC: U.S. Department of Health and Human Services, Public Health Service.

Hegyvary, S. T. (1993). Patient care outcomes related to management of symptoms. In J. J. Fitzpatrick & J. J. Stevenson (Eds.), *Annual Review of Nursing Research, 11* (pp. 145–168). New York: Springer.

Henneman, E. A. (1991). The art and science of weaning from mechanical ventilation. *AACN Focus on Critical Care, 18*(6), 490–501.

Herr, K. A., & Mobily, P. R. (1992). Interventions related to pain. In G. M. Bulechek & J. C. McCloskey (Eds.), *Symposium on Nursing Interventions. Nursing Clinics of North America, 27*(2), 347–370.

Hickey, J. V. (1992). *The clinical practice of neurological and neurosurgical nursing.* Philadelphia: Lippincott.

Hoff, L. A. (1993). Battered women—intervention and prevention: A psychosocial cultural perspective. Part 2. *Journal of the American Academy of Nurse Practitioners, 4,* 148–155.

Hogstel, M. O., & Nelson, M. (1992). Anticipation and early detection can reduce bowel elimination complications. *Geriatric Nursing,* January/ February, 28–33.

Howells, K., & Hollin, C. R. (1992). *Clinical approaches to violence.* New York: Wiley.

Hurley, M. (Ed.). (1986). *Classification of nursing diagnoses: Proceedings of the Sixth Conference, North American Nursing Diagnosis Association.* St. Louis: Mosby.

Innerarity, S. A., & Stark, J. L. (1994). *Fluids and electrolytes* (2nd ed.). Springhouse, PA: Springhouse.

Jacox, A., Ferell, B., Heidrich, G., Hester, N., & Miaskowski, C. (1992). A guideline for the nation: Managing acute pain. *American Journal of Nursing, 92*(5), 49–55.

Janson-Bjerklie., S. (1993). Predicting the outcomes of living with asthma. *Research in Nursing and Health, 16*(4), 241–249.

Jenny, J. (1987). Deficient knowledge: Not a nursing diagnosis. *Image, 19*(4), 184–185.

Jenny, J., & Logan, J. (1991). Analyzing expert nursing practice to develop a new nursing diagnosis: Dysfunctional ventilatory weaning response. In R. M. Carroll-Johnson (Ed.), *Classification of nursing diagnoses: Proceedings of the Ninth Conference* (pp. 133–140). Philadelphia: Lippincott.

Jensen, L., & Allen, M. (1993). Wellness: The dialect of illness. *Image: The Journal of Nursing Scholarship, 25*(3), 220–224.

Jirevec, M. M., Wyman, J. F., & Wells, T. J. (1998). Addressing urinary incontinence with educational continence-care competencies. *Image: Journal of Nursing Scholarship, 30*(4), 375–378.

Johnson, M., Bulechek, G., Dochterman, J., Maas, M., and Moorhead, S. (2001). *Nursing Diagnoses, Outcomes, & Interventions: NANDA International, NOC, and NIC Linkages.* St. Louis: Mosby.

Johnson, M., & Maas, M. (Eds.). (1997). *Nursing Outcomes Classification (NOC).* St. Louis: Mosby.

Johnson, M., Maas, M., and Moorhead, S. (Eds.). (2000). *Nursing Outcomes Classification (NOC)* (2nd ed.). St. Louis: Mosby

Kalbach, L. R. (1991). Unilateral neglect: Mechanisms and nursing care. *Journal of Neuroscience Nursing, 23*(2), 125–129.

Kanak, M. F. (1992). Interventions relted to safety. In G. M. Bulechek & J. C. McCloskey (Eds.), *Symposium on Nursing Interventions. Nursing Clinics of North America, 27*(2), 371–396.

Kavchak-Keyes, M. (2000). Autonomic hyperreflexia. *Rehabilitation Nursing, 25*(1): 31–35.

Keegan, L. (2000). Protocols for practice: Applying research at the bedside. Alternative and complementary modalities for managing stress and anxiety. *Critical Care Nurse, 20*(3): 93–96.

Kelley, M. P., & Henry, P. (1993). Open discussion can lead to acceptance: The psychosocial effects of stoma surgery. *Professional Nurse, 9*(2), 101–110.

King, C. (1998). Enteral feeding for preterm infants: Nutrition and therapy. *Journal of Neonatal Nursing, 4*(5), 6, 8–10.

King, C. (1998). Parenteral nutrition for the preterm infant: Optimal levels of key nutrients. *Journal of Neonatal Nursing, 4*(4), 12–15.

Kluger, M. (1978). Fever versus hyperthermia. *New England Journal of Medicine, 299*(10), 555.

Knebel, A. F. (1991). Weaning from mechanical ventilation: Current controversies. *Heart and Lung, 20*(4), 321–333.

Krieger, D. (1979). *The therapeutic touch: How to use your hands to help or to heal.* Englewood Cliffs, NJ: Prentice Hall.

Kulbok, P., & Baldwin, J. (1992). From preventive health behavior to health promotion: Advancing a positive construct of health. *Advances in Nursing Science, 14*(4), 50–64.

Kunz, D., & Krieger, D. (1975–1990). Annual invitational workshops on therapeutic touch. Graysville, NY: Pumpkin Hollow Foundation.

Kus, R. J. (1992). Crisis intervention. In G. M. Bulechek & J. C. McCloskey (Eds.), *Nursing interventions: Essential nursing treatments* (2nd ed.), (pp. 179–190). Philadelphia: Saunders.

Lambert, M. A., & Jones, P. E. (1989). Nursing diagnoses recorded in nursing situations encountered in a department of public health. In R. M. Carroll-Johnson, (Ed.), *Classification of nursing diagnoses: Proceedings of the Eighth Conference.* Philadelphia: Lippincott.

Lane, G. H. (1990). Pulmonary therapeutic management. In L. A. Thelan, J. K. Davie., & L. D. Urden (Eds.), *Textbook of critical care nursing* (pp. 444–471). St. Louis: Mosby.

Larson, C. (2000). Evidence-based practice. Safety and efficacy of oral rehydration therapy for treatment of diarrhea and gastroenteritis in pediatrics. *Pediatric Nursing, 26*(2): 177–179.

LeMone, P. (1991). Analysis of a human phenomenon: Self-concept. *Nursing Diagnosis, 2*(3), 129–130.

LeMone, P., & Jones, D. (1997). Nursing assessment of altered sexuality: A review of salient factors and objective measures. *Nursing Diagnosis: The Journal of Nursing Language and Classification, 8*(3), 120–128.

LeMone, P., & Weber, J. (1995). Validating gender-specific defining characteristics of altered sexuality. *Nursing Diagnosis, 6*(2), 64–69.

Lepshy, M. S., & Michael, A. (1993). Chronic diarrhea: Evaluation and treatment. *American Family Physician, 48*(8), 1461–1466.

Lewis, S., Heitkemper, M., & Dirksen, S. (2000). *Medical-Surgical Nursing: Assessment and management of clinical problems.* St. Louis: Mosby.

Lindeman, M., Hokanson, J., & Batek, J. (1994). The alcoholic family. *Nursing Diagnosis, 5*(2), 65–73.

Lindgren, C. L. (1993). The caregiver career. *Image: The Journal of Nursing Scholarship, 25*(3), 214–219.

Loening-Baucke, V. (1994). Management of chronic constipation in infants and toddlers. *American Family Physician, 46*(2), 397–406.

Loeper, J. M. (1992). Positioning. In G. M. Bulechek & J. C. McCloskey (Eds.), *Nursing interventions: Essential nursing treatments* (2nd ed., pp. 86–93). Philadelphia: Saunders.

Logan, J., & Jenny, J. (1991). Interventions for the nursing diagnosis "dysfunctional ventilatory weaning response": A qualitative study. In R. M. Carroll-Johnson (Ed.), *Classification of nursing diagnoses: Proceedings of the Ninth Conference* (pp. 141–147). Philadelphia: Lippincott.

London, M., Ladewig, P., Ball, J., & Bindler, R. (2003). *Maternal-newborn & child nursing: Family-centered care.* Upper Saddle River, NJ: Pearson Education, Inc.

Longo, M. B. (1993). Facilitating acceptance of a patient's decision to stop treatment. *Clinical Nurse Specialist, 7*(3), 233–243.

Low, M. B. (1993). Women's body image: The nurse's role in promotion of self-acceptance. *AWHONN's Clinical Issues, 4*(2), 213–219.

Lowe, N. K. (1993). Maternal confidence for labor: Development of the childbirth self-efficacy inventory. *Research in Nursing and Health, 10*, 357–365.

Lowenstein, A. J., & Hoff, P. S. (1994). Discharge planning: A study of nursing staff involvement. *Journal of Nursing Administration, 24*(4), 45–40.

Luiselli, J. K. (1993). Training self-feeding skills in children who are deaf and blind. *Behavior Modification, 17*(4), 457–473.

McCaffrey, M., & Beebe, A. (1989). *Pain: Clinical manual for nursing practice.* St. Louis: Mosby.

McCance, K. L., & Huether, S. E. (1994). *Pathophysiology: The biologic basis for disease in adults and children* (2nd ed.). St. Louis: Mosby.

McCloskey, J. C., & Bulechek, M. C. (Eds.). (1996). *Nursing Interventions Classification (NIC)* (2nd ed.). St. Louis: Mosby.

McCloskey, J. C. & Bulechek, M. C. (Eds.). (2000). *Nursing Interventions Classification (NIC)* (3rd ed.). St. Louis: Mosby.

McFarland, G. K., & McFarlane, E. A. (1993). *Nursing diagnosis and intervention: Planning for patient care* (2nd ed.). St. Louis: Mosby.

McHaffie., H. (1992). The assessment of coping. *Clinical Nursing Research, 1*(1), 67–79.

McHale, J. M., Phipps, M. A., Horvath, K., & Schmelz, J. (1998). Expert nursing knowledge in the care of patients at risk of impaired swallowing. *Image: Journal of Nursing Scholarship, 30*(2), 137–141.

McLane, A. (Ed.). (1987). *Classification of nursing diagnoses: Proceedings of the Seventh Conference, North American Nursing Diagnosis Association.* St. Louis: Mosby.

McLane, A. M., & McShane, R. E. (1992). Bowel management. In G. M. Bulechek & J. C. McCloskey (Eds.), *Nursing interventions: Essential nursing treatments* (2nd ed., pp. 73–85). Philadelphia: Saunders.

Maas, M. (1991). Impaired physical mobility. In M. Maas, K. Buckwalter, & M. Hardy (Eds.), *Nursing diagnosis and interventions for the elderly* (pp. 263–284). Redwood City, CA: Addison-Wesley Nursing.

Maier-Lorentz, M. (2000). Effective nursing interventions for the management of Alzheimer's disease. *Journal of Neuroscience Nursing, 32*(2): 117–125.

Marshall-Baker, A., Lickliter, R., & Cooper, R. (1998). Prolonged exposure to a visual pattern may promote behavioral organization in preterm infants. *Journal of Perinatal and Neonatal Nursing, 12*(2), 50–62.

Maxfield, M. C., Lewis, R. E., & Connor., S. (1996). Training staff to prevent aggressive behavior of cognitively impaired elderly patients during bathing and grooming. *Journal of Gerontological Nursing, 22*(1), 37–43.

Meehan, T. C. (1991). Therapeutic touch. In G. Bulechek & J. McCloskey (Eds.), *Nursing interventions: Essential nursing treatments.* Philadelphia: Saunders.

Meiner, S. (2000). Wandering problems need ongoing nursing planning: A case study. *Geriatric Nursing, 21*(2): 101–106.

Miller, C. (1999) *Nursing care of older adults* (3rd ed.). Philadelphia: Lippincott Williams & Wilkins.

Mitchell, M. (1999). The effects of relocation of elderly. *Perspectives in Gerontological Nursing, 23*(1): 2–7.

Moss, A. B. (1992). Are the elderly safe at home? *Journal of Community Health Nursing, 9*(1), 13–19.

Murphy, T. G., & Bennett, E. J. (1992). Low-tech, high-touch perfusion assessment. *American Journal of Nursing, 92*(5), 36–46.

Murray, M., & Blaylock, B. (1994). Maintaining effective pressure ulcer prevention programs. *Medsurg Nursing, 3*(2), 85–92.

NANDA International nursing diagnoses: Definitions and classification 1999–2000. (1999). Philadelphia, PA: NANDA International.

NANDA International nursing diagnoses: Definitions and classification 2001–2003. (2001). Philadelphia, PA: NANDA International.

NANDA International nursing diagnoses: Definitions and classification 2003–2004. (2003). Philadelphia, PA: NANDA International.

National Institute for Occupational Safety and Health (1997). NIOSH alert—*Preventing allergic reactions to rubber latex in the workplace.* DHHS (NIOSH) Publication No. 97-135. Retrieved on December 10, 2002. www.cdc.gov/niosh/latexalt.html.

National Pressure Ulcer Advisory Pannel (1992). *Monograph on pressure ulcer prevention.* Buffalo: NPUAP.

Nease, R. (1994). Risk attitudes in gambles involving length of life: Aspirations, variations, and ruminations. *Medical Decision Making, 14*(2), 210–213.

Nelson, D. M. (1992). Interventions related to respiratory care. In G. M. Bulechek & J. C. McCloskey (Eds.), *Symposium on Nursing Interventions. Nursing Clinics of North America, 27*(2), 301–324.

NIC interventions linked to NANDA International diagnoses. (1993). Iowa City: IA: Iowa Intervention Project.

Norris, J. (1992). Nursing intervention for self-esteem disturbances. *Nursing Diagnosis, 3*(2), 48–53.

North American Nursing Diagnosis Association. (1986). *Seventh Conference on Classification of Nursing Diagnoses. Syllabus of Conference Proceedings.* St. Louis: Author.

North American Nursing Diagnosis Association. (1988). *Eighth Conference on Classification of Nursing Diagnoses. Syllabus of Conference Proceedings.* St. Louis: Author.

North American Nursing Diagnosis Association. (1999). *NANDA International nursing diagnoses: Definitions and classification* 1999–2000. Philadelphia: Author.

Occupational Safety & Health Administration (1999). OSHA Technical Information Bulletin. *Potential for allergy to natural rubber latex gloves and other natural rubber products.* Retrieved December 10, 2002. 222.osha-slc.gov/dts/tib/tib_data/tib19990412.html.

Olson, E. V., Johnson, B. J., Thompson, L. F., McCarthy, J. S., Edmonds, R. E., Schroeder, L. M., & Wade, M. (1967). The hazards of immobility. *American Journal of Nursing, 67*(4), 780–797.

Pack, R. (2000). The "ins and outs" of wandering. *Nursing Homes, 49*(8): 55–59.

Palmer, M. H., McCormick, K. A., Langford, A., Langlais, J., & Alvaran, M. (1992). Continence outcomes: Documentation on medical records in the home environment. *Journal of Nursing Care Quality, 6*(3), 36–43.

Palmer, S. J. (1993). Care of sick children by parents: A meaningful role. *Journal of Advanced Nursing, 18*, 85–191.

Panel for the Prediction and Prevention of Pressure Ulcers in Adults. (1992, May). *Pressure ulcers in adults: Prediction and prevention. Clinical Practice Guideline Number 3.* (AHCPR Publication No. 92-0047.) Rockville, MD: Agency for Health Care Policy and Research, Public Health Service, U.S. Department of Health and Human Services.

Pawlicki, C. M., & Gaumer, C. (1993). Nursing care of the self-mutilating patient. *Bulletin of the Menninger Clinic, 57*(3), 380–389.

Pehler, S. (1997). Children's spiritual response: Validation of the nursing diagnosis "spiritual distress." *Nursing Diagnosis: The Journal of Nursing Language and Classification, 8*(2), 55–66.

Pender, N. (1996). *Health promotion in nursing practice* (3rd ed.). Stamford, CT: Appleton & Lange.

Peruzzi, W. T., & Smith, B. (1995). Bronchial hygiene therapy. *Critical Care Clinics, 13*, 47.

Pomeroy, V. (1990). Development of an ADL-oriented assessment-of-mobility scale suitable for use for elderly people with dementia. *Physiotherapy, 76*(8), 446–448.

Potempa, K. M. (1992). Chronic fatigue. In J. J. Fitzpatrik, R. L. Taunton, & A. K. Jacox (Eds.), *Annual review of nursing research* (Vol. 10, pp. 57–76). New York: Springer.

Pridham, K., Brown, R., Sondel, S., Green, C., Wedel, N., & Lai, H. (1998). Transition time to full nipple feeding for premature infants with a history of lung disease. *Journal of Obstetric, Gynecologic, and Neonatal Nursing, 27*(5), 533–545.

Pugh, L. C., & Milligan, R. (1993). A framework for the study of child-bearing fatigue. *Advances in Nursing Science, 15*(4), 60–70.

Puntillo, K., & Weiss, S. J. (1994). Pain: Its mediators and associated morbidity in critically ill cardiovascular surgical patients. *Nursing Research,* 43(1), 31–36.

Rakel, B. A. (1992). Interventions related to patient teaching. In G. M. Bulechek & J. C. McCloskey (Eds.). *Symposium on Nursing Interventions. Nursing Clinics of North America, 27*(2), 397–424.

Rakel, B. A., & Bulechek, G. M. (1990). Development of alterations in learning: Situational learning disabilities. *Nursing Diagnosis 1*(4), 134–146.

Rantz, M. J., & McShane, R. E. (1995). Nursing interventions for chronically confused nursing home residents. *Geriatric Nursing, 16*(1), 22–27.

Rasin, J. (1990). Confusion. *Nursing Clinics of North America, 25*, 909–918.

Redman, B. K. (1993). *The process of patient education* (7th ed.). St. Louis: Mosby.

Rhodes, A., & McDaniel, R. (1995). Fatigue and advanced illness. *Quality of Life—A Nursing Challenge, 4*(1), 14–19.

Riordan, J., & Auerbach, K. (1993). *Breastfeeding and human lactation.* Boston: Jones and Bartlett.

Ruzevich, S. (1993). Cardiac assist devices. In J. M. Clochesy, C. Breu, S. Cardin, E. B. Rudy, & A. A. Whittaker (Eds.), *Critical care nursing* (pp. 183–192). Philadelphia: Saunders.

Sachs, B., Hall, L. A., Lutenbacher, M., & Rayens, M. K. (1999). Potential for abusive parenting by rural mothers with low birth weight children. *Image: Journal of Nursing Scholarship, 31*(1), 21–25.

Salazar, M. K., & Primomo, J. (1994). Taking the lead in environmental health. *American Association of Occupational Health Nurses (AAOHN), 42*(7), 317–324.

Sapala, S. (1994). Pediatric management problems. *Pediatric Nursing, 20*(1), 54–55.

Schainen, J. S. (1991). Environments for nursing care of the older client. In W. C. Chenitz, J. T. Stone, & S. A. Salisbury, *Clinical gerontological nursing.* Philadelphia: Saunders.

Schibler, K. D., & Fay, S. A. (1990). Sleep promotion. In M. J. Craft & J. A. Denehy (Eds.), *Nursing interventions for infants and children* (pp. 285–303). Philadelphia: Saunders.

Schuiling, K. D., & Sampselle, C. M. (1999). Comfort in labor and midwifery art. *Image: Journal of Nursing Scholarship, 31*(1), 77–81.

Schumacher, K. L., Stewart, B. J., & Archbold, P. G. (1998). Conceptualization and measurement of doing family caregiving well. *Image: Journal of Nursing Scholarship, 30*(1), 63–69.

Shaker, C. (1990). Nipple feeding premature infants: A different perspective. *Neonatal Network, 8*(5), 9–17.

Sheppard, M. (1993). Client satisfaction, extended intervention and interpersonal skills in community mental health. *Journal of Advanced Nursing, 18*, 246–259.

Silver, J. (2000). Early autonomic dysreflexia. *Spinal Cord, 38*, 229–233.

Sime, M. (1992). Decisional control. In M. Snyder (Ed.), *Independent nursing interventions* (2nd ed.) (pp. 110–114). Albany: Delmar.

Simon, J. M., Bauman, M. A., & Nolan, L. (1995). Differential diagnosis validation: Acute and chronic pain. *Nursing Diagnosis, 6*(2), 73–79.

Simons, M. R. (1992). Interventions related to compliance. In G. M. Bulechek & J. C. McCloskey (Eds.). *Symposium on Nursing Interventions. Nursing Clinics of North America, 27*(2), 477–494.

Simons-Morton, D. G., Mullen, P. D., Mains, D. A., Tabak, E. R., & Green, L. W. (1992). Characteristics of controlled studies of patient education and counseling for preventive health behaviors. *Patient Education and Counseling, 19*, 174–204.

Smith, J. E., Early, J. A., Green, P. T., Lauck, D. L., Oblaczynski, C., Smochek, M. R., & Wright, G. (1997). Risk for suicide and risk for violence: A case for separating the current violence diagnoses. *Nursing Diagnosis: The Journal of Nursing Language and Classification, 8*(2), 67–77.

Smith, M. (1993). Pediatric sexuality: Promoting normal sexual development in children. *Nurse Practitioner, 18*(8), 37–44.

Snyder, M. (1992). Exercise. In M. Snyder (Ed.), *Independent nursing interventions* (2nd ed., pp. 67–77). Albany: Delmar.

Specht, J., Tunink, P., Maas, M., & Bulecheck, G. (1991). Urinary incontinence. In M. Maas, K. C. Buckwalter, & M. A. Hardy (Eds.). *Nursing diagnoses and interventions for the elderly* (pp. 181–204). Redwood City, CA: Addison-Wesley.

Specht, J. P., Maas, M. L., Willett, S., & Myers, N. (1992). Intermittent catheterization. In G. M. Bulechek & J. C. McCloskey (Eds.), *Nursing interventions: Essential nursing treatments* (2nd ed., pp. 61–72). Philadelphia: Saunders.

Sprague-McRae, J. M., Lamb, W., & Homer, D. (1993). Encopresis: A study of treatment alternatives and historical behavioral characteristics. Nurse Practitioner, *18*(10), 52–63.

Starling, B. P., & Martin, A. C. (1990). Adult survivors of parental alcoholism: Implications for primary care. *Nurse Practitioner, 15*(7), 16–24.

Stephenson, C. (1991). The concept of hope revisited for nursing. *Journal of Advanced Nursing, 16*, 1456–1461.

Stevens, P., & Hall, J. (1993). Environmental health in community health nursing. In J. F. Swanson & M. Albrecht (Eds.), *Community health nursing: Promoting the health of aggregates* (pp. 567–596). Philadelphia: Saunders.

Streitmatter, J. (1993). Gender differences in identity development: An examination of longitudinal data. *Adolescence, 28*(109), 55–66.

Stuart, G. W., & Sundeen, S. J. (1999). *Principles and practice of psychiatric nursing* (6th ed.). St. Louis: Mosby.

Stuifbergen, A. K., & Rogers, S. (1997). The experience of fatigue and strategies of self-care among persons with multiple sclerosis. *Applied Nursing Research, 10*, 2–10.

Sullivan, P., & Markos, P. (1993). *Clinical procedures in therapeutic exercise*. Norwalk, CT: Appleton & Lange.

Szabo, V., & Strang, V. R. (1999). Experiencing control in caregiving. *Image: Journal of Nursing Scholarship, 31*(1), 71–75.

Talashek, M. L., Gerace, L. M., & Starr, K. L. (1994). The substance abuse pandemic: Determinants to guide interventions. *Public Health Nursing, 11*(2), 131–139.

Taylor, C., Lillis, C., & LeMone, P. (2001). *Fundamentals of nursing: The art & science of nursing care* (4th ed.). Philadelphia: Lippincott.

Thelan, L. A., & Urden, L. D. (1993). *Critical care nursing: Diagnosis and management* (2nd ed.). St. Louis: Mosby.

Thompson, E. H., Futterman, A. M., Gallagher-Thompson, D., Rose, J. M., & Lovett, S. B. (1993). Social support and caregiving burden in family caregivers of frail elders. *Journal of Gerontology, 48*, S245–S254.

Tiesinga, L. J., Dassen, T. W. N., & Ruud, J. G. H. (1996). Fatigue: A summary of the definitions, dimensions, and indicators. *Nursing Diagnosis, 7*(2), 51–62.

Titler, M. G. (1992). Interventions related to surveillance. In G. M. Bulechek & J. C. McCloskey (Eds.), *Symposium on Nursing Interventions. Nursing Clinics of North America, 27*, 2, 495–516.

Titler, M. G., & Jones, G. (1992). Airway Management. In G. M. Bulechek & J. C. McCloskey (Eds.), *Nursing interventions: Essential nursing treatments* (2nd ed., pp. 512–530). Philadelphia: Saunders.

Titler, M. G., & Walsh, S. M. (1992). Visiting critically ill adults: Strategies for practice. *Critical Care Nursing Clinics of North America, 4*(4), 623–633.

Turner, J., & Lovvorn, M. (1992). Communicable diseases and infection control practices in community health nursing. In M. Stanhope and J. Lancaster (Eds.), *Community health nursing* (3rd ed., pp. 312–331). St. Louis: Mosby.

U.S. Department of Health and Human Services. (1992). *Pressure ulcers in adults: Prediction and prevention*. Rockville, MD: Public Health Service, Agency for Health Care Policy and Research.

U.S. Department of Health and Human Services. (1994a). *Clinicians handbook of preventive services: Put prevention into practice*. Washington, DC: U.S. Government Printing Office.

U.S. Department of Health and Human Services. (1994b). *Heart failure: Evaluation and care of patients with left-ventricular systolic dysfunction*. (AHCPR Publication No. 94-0612). Rockville, MD: Public Health Service, Agency for Health Care Policy and Research.

U.S. Department of Health and Human Services. (1994c). *Treatment of pressure ulcers*. (AHCPR Publication No. 95-0047). Rockville, MD: Public Health Service, Agency for Health Care Policy and Research.

U.S. Department of Health and Human Services. (1994d). *Unstable angina: Diagnosis and management* (AHCPR Publication No. 94-0602). Rockville, MD: Public Health Service, Agency for Health Care Policy and Research.

U.S. Public Health Services (1998). *Clinician handbook of preventative services* (2nd ed.). Washington, DC: USPHS

Umbreit, A. (2000) Healing touch: Applications in the acute care setting. *ACCN Clinical Issues of Advanced Practice in Acute Critical Care, 11*(1): 105–119.

Urinary Incontinence Guideline Panel. (1992, March). *Urinary incontinence in adults: Clinical practice guideline.* (AHCPR Publication No. 92-0038). Rockville, MD: Public Health Service, Agency for Health Care Policy and Research.

Van Wynsberghe, D., Noback, C. R., & Carola, R. (1995). *Human anatomy and physiology* (3rd ed.). New York: McGraw-Hill.

Walker, C. (1995). When to wean: Whose advice do mothers find helpful? *Health Visitor, 68*, 109–111.

Wallhagen, M. I., & Kagan, S. H. (1993). Staying within bounds: Perceived control and the experience of elderly caregivers. *Journal of Aging Studies, 7*(2), 197–213.

Wasson, D., & Anderson, M. A. (1995). Chemical dependency and adolescent self-esteem. Clinical Nursing Research, 4(3), 274–289.

Watson, D. L., & Tharp, R. G. (1993). *Self-directing behavior: Self-modification for personal adjustment* (2nd ed.). Monterey, CA: Brooks/Cole.

Weeks, S., Hubbartt, E., & Michaels, T. (2000) Keys to bowel success. *Rehab Nursing 25*(2), 66–69.

Weitzel, E. A. (1991). Unilateral neglect. In M. Maas, K. Buckwalter, & M. Hardy (Eds.), *Nursing diagnoses and interventions for the elderly* (pp. 387–395). Redwood City, CA: Addison-Wesley.

Whitley, G. G. (1994). Expert validation and differentiation of the nursing diagnoses anxiety and fear. *Nursing Diagnosis, 5*(4), 143–149.

Whitley, G. G., & Tousman, S. A. (1996). A multivariate approach for validation of anxiety and fear. *Nursing Diagnosis, 7*(8), 116–123.

Whitman, G. (1993). Shock. In M. R. Kinney, D. R. Packa, & S. B. Dunbar (Eds.), *AACN's clinical reference for critical-care nursing* (pp. 133–172). St. Louis: Mosby.

Whitney, E., Cataldo, C., & Rolfes, S. (1998). Understanding normal and clinical nutrition (5th ed.). Belmont, CA: Wadsworth Publishing.

Wilkinson, J. (2001). *Nursing process & critical thinking* (3rd ed.). Upper Saddle River, NJ: Prentice Hall.

Winslow, E. H., Lane, L. D., & Woods, R. J. (1995). Dangling: A review of relevant physiology, research, and practice. *Heart and Lung, 24*, 263.

Wong, D. L., & Whaley, L. F. (Eds). (1998). *Nursing care of infants and children* (6th ed.). St. Louis: Mosby-Year Book.

Woodtli, A. (1995a). Mixed incontinence: A new nursing diagnosis? *Nursing Diagnosis, 6*(4), 135–142.

Woodtli, A. (1995b). Stress incontinence: Clinical identification and validation of defining characteristics, *Nursing Diagnosis, 6*(3), 115–122.

Wooldridge, J., Herman, J., Garrison, D., Haddock, S., Massey, J., & Tavakoli, A. (1998). A validation study using the case-control method of the nursing diagnosis "Risk for aspiration." *Nursing Diagnosis: The Journal of Nursing Language and Classification, 9*(1), 5–13.

Workman, M. L. (1993). The immune system: Your defensive partner and offensive foe. *AACN Clinical Issues in Critical Care Nursing, 4*(3), 453–570.

Wright, K. B. (1998). Professional, ethical, and legal implications for spiritual care in nursing. *Image: Journal of Nursing Scholarship, 30*(1), 81–83.

Yang, K. L., & Tobin, M. J. (1991). A prospective study of indexes predicting the outcome of trials of weaning from mechanical ventilation. *New England Journal of Medicine, 324*, 1445–1451.

Young, C. K., & While, S. (1992). Preparing patients for tube feedings at home. *American Journal of Nursing, 92*(4), 46–53.

Ziegler, D. B., & Prior, M. M. (1994). Preparation for surgery and adjustment to hospitalization. *Nursing Clinics of North America, 29*(4), 655–669.

APPENDIX A

2003–2004 NANDA International-Approved Nursing Diagnoses

Grouped by Gordon's Functional Health Patterns

Nutritional/Metabolic

Autonomic dysreflexia, risk for
Body temperature, risk for imbalanced
Breastfeeding, effective
Breastfeeding, ineffective
Breastfeeding, interrupted
Dentition, impaired
Dysreflexia, autonomic
Dysreflexia, autonomic, risk for
Failure to thrive, adult
Fluid balance, readiness for enhanced
Fluid volume, deficient
Fluid volume, deficient, risk for
Fluid volume, risk for imbalance
Fluid volume excess
Fluid volume imbalance, risk for
Growth, risk for disproportionate
Hyperthermia
Hypothermia
Infant feeding pattern, ineffective
Nutrition, imbalanced: less than body requirements
Nutrition, imbalanced: more than body requirements
Nutrition, imbalanced: more than body requirements, risk for
Nutrition, readiness for enhanced
Oral mucous membrane, impaired
Skin integrity, impaired
Skin integrity, risk for impaired
Sudden infant death syndrome, risk for
Swallowing, impaired
Thermoregulation, ineffective
Tissue integrity, impaired

Health-perception/Health Management

Aspiration, risk for
Denial, ineffective
Falls, risk for
Health maintenance, ineffective
Health seeking behaviors (specify)
Infection, risk for
Injury, risk for

Latex allergy response
Latex allergy response, risk for
Management of therapeutic regimen, effective
Management of therapeutic regimen: community, ineffective
Management of therapeutic regimen: family, ineffective
Management of therapeutic regimen, ineffective
Management of therapeutic regimen, readiness for enhanced
Noncompliance (specify)
Poisoning, risk for
Protection, ineffective
Sudden infant death syndrome, risk for
Suffocation, risk for
Surgical recovery, delayed
Trauma, risk for

Sleep/Rest

Sleep deprivation
Sleep pattern, disturbed
Sleep, readiness for enhanced

Activity/Exercise

Activity intolerance
Activity intolerance, risk for
Adaptive capacity: intracranial, decreased
Airway clearance, ineffective
Breathing pattern, ineffective
Cardiac output, decreased
Development, risk for delayed
Disorganized infant behavior
Disorganized infant behavior, risk for
Disuse syndrome, risk for
Diversional activity, deficient
Energy field disturbed
Fatigue
Gas exchange, impaired
Home maintenance, impaired
Mobility: bed, impaired
Mobility: physical, impaired
Mobility: wheelchair, impaired
Organized infant behavior, readiness for enhanced
Perioperative positioning injury, risk for
Peripheral neurovascular dysfunction, risk for
Self-care deficit: bathing and hygiene, dressing and grooming, feeding,
    toileting, total
Spontaneous ventilation, impaired
Tissue perfusion, ineffective (specify): cardiopulmonary, cerebral,
    gastrointestinal, peripheral, renal

Transfer ability, impaired
Ventilatory weaning response, dysfunctional
Walking, impaired

Elimination

Constipation
Constipation, perceived
Constipation, risk for
Diarrhea
Incontinence: bowel
Incontinence: urinary, functional
Incontinence: urinary, reflex
Incontinence: urinary, stress
Incontinence: urinary, total
Incontinence: urinary, urge
Incontinence: urinary, urge, risk for
Urinary elimination, impaired
Urinary elimination, readiness for enhanced
Urinary retention

Value/Belief

Decisional conflict (specify)
Grieving, anticipatory
Grieving, dysfunctional
Sorrow, chronic
Spiritual distress
Spiritual distress, risk for
Spiritual well-being, readiness for enhanced

Sexuality–Reproductivity

Sexual dysfunction
Sexuality patterns, ineffective

Self-perception/Self-concept

Anxiety
Anxiety, death
Body image, disturbed
Environmental interpretation syndrome, impaired
Fear
Hopelessness
Personal identity, disturbed
Powerlessness
Powerlessness, risk for
Self-concept, readiness for enhanced
Self esteem, chronic low
Self esteem, situational low
Self esteem, risk for situational low

Cognitive/Perceptual

Communication, impaired verbal
Communication, readiness for enhanced
Confusion, acute
Confusion, chronic
Knowledge, deficient (specify)
Knowledge of (specify), readiness for enhanced
Memory, impaired
Nausea
Pain, acute
Pain, chronic
Sensory perception, disturbed (specify): auditory, gustatory, kines-
    thetic, olfactory, tactile, visual
Thought processes, disturbed
Wandering
Unilateral neglect

Coping/Stress Tolerance

Adjustment, impaired
Coping: community, ineffective
Coping: community, readiness for enhanced
Coping, defensive
Coping: family, compromised
Coping: family, disabled
Coping: family, readiness for enhanced
Coping: Individual, readiness for enhanced
Coping, ineffective
Denial, ineffective
Post-trauma syndrome
Post-trauma syndrome, risk for
Rape-trauma syndrome
Rape-trauma syndrome, compound reaction
Rape-trauma syndrome, silent reaction
Relocation stress syndrome
Relocation stress syndrome, risk for
Self-mutilation
Self-mutilation, risk for
Suicide, risk for
Violence, risk for self-directed

Role-relationship

Caregiver role strain
Caregiver role strain, risk for
Family processes, interrupted
Family processes, dysfunctional: alcoholism
Family processes, readiness for enhanced

Home maintenance, impaired
Loneliness, risk for
Parent/infant/child attachment, risk for impaired
Parenting, impaired
Parenting, readiness for enhanced
Parenting, risk for impaired
Role conflict, parental
Role performance, ineffective
Social interaction, impaired
Social isolation
Violence, risk for other-directed

Note: The diagnoses, Risk for delayed development, Delayed growth and development, and Risk for disproportionate growth, can occur in any of the Functional Health Patterns.

Used by permission of NANDA International.

Adapted from Functional Health Patterns, Gordon, M. (1994). *Nursing diagnosis: Process and application,* 3rd ed. St. Louis: Mosby.

APPENDIX B

NANDA International-Approved Nursing Diagnoses (2003–2004), Taxonomy II: Domains, Classes, and Diagnoses

This taxonomically organized list represents the NANDA International-approved nursing diagnoses for clinical use and testing.

Domain 1. Health Promotion

The awareness of well-being or normality of function and the strategies used to maintain control of and enhance that well-being or normality of function

Class 1. Health Awareness. Recognition of normal function and well-being

Class 2. Health Management. Identifying, controlling, performing, and integrating activities to maintain health and well-being

Approved Diagnoses

00082	Effective therapeutic regimen management
00078	Ineffective therapeutic regimen management
00080	Ineffective family therapeutic regimen management
00081	Ineffective community therapeutic regimen management
00084	Health-seeking behaviors (specify)
00099	Ineffective health maintenance
00098	Impaired home maintenance
00162	Readiness for enhanced management of therapeutic regimen
00163	Readiness for enhanced nutrition

Domain 2. Nutrition

The activities of taking in, assimilating, and using nutrients for the purposes of tissue maintenance, tissue repair, and the production of energy

Class 1. Ingestion. Taking food or nutrients into the body

Approved Diagnoses

00107	Ineffective infant feeding pattern
00103	Impaired swallowing
00002	Imbalanced nutrition: less than body requirements
00001	Imbalanced nutrition: more than body requirements
00003	Risk for imbalanced nutrition: more than body requirements

Class 2. Digestion. The physical and chemical activities that convert foodstuffs into substances suitable for absorption and assimilation

Class 3. Absorption. The act of taking up nutrients through body tissues.

Class 4. Metabolism. The chemical and physical processes occurring in living organisms and cells for the development and use of protoplasm and production of waste and energy, with the release of energy for all vital processes

Class 5. Hydration. The taking in and absorption of fluids and electrolytes

Approved Diagnoses

00027	Deficient fluid volume
00028	Risk for deficient fluid volume
00026	Excess fluid volume
00025	Risk for fluid volume imbalance
00160	Readiness for enhanced fluid balance

Domain 3. Elimination

Secretion and excretion of waste products from the body

Class 1. Urinary System. The process of secretion and excretion of urine

Approved Diagnoses

00016	Impaired urinary elimination
00023	Urinary retention
00021	Total urinary incontinence
00020	Functional urinary incontinence
00017	Stress urinary incontinence
00019	Urge urinary incontinence
00018	Reflex urinary incontinence
00022	Risk for urge urinary incontinence
00166	Readiness for enhanced urinary elimination

Class 2. Gastrointestinal System. Excretion and expulsion of waste products from the bowel

Approved Diagnoses

00014	Bowel incontinence
00013	Diarrhea
00011	Constipation
00015	Risk for constipation
00012	Perceived constipation

Class 3. Integumentary System. Process of secretion and excretion through the skin

Class 4. Pulmonary System. Removal of byproducts of metabolic products, secretions, and foreign material from the lungs or bronchi

Approved Diagnoses

00030	Impaired gas exchange

Domain 4. Activity/Rest

The production, conservation, expenditure, or balance of energy resources

Class 1. Sleep/Rest. Slumber, repose, ease, or inactivity

Approved Diagnoses

00095	Disturbed sleep pattern
00096	Sleep deprivation
00165	Readiness for enhanced sleep

Class 2. Activity/Exercise. Moving parts of the body (mobility), doing work, or performing actions often (but not always) against resistance

Approved Diagnoses

00040	Risk for disuse syndrome
00085	Impaired physical mobility
00091	Impaired bed mobility
00089	Impaired wheelchair mobility
00090	Impaired transfer ability
00088	Impaired walking
00097	Deficient diversional activity
00109	Dressing/grooming self-care deficit
00108	Bathing/hygiene self-care deficit
00102	Feeding self-care deficit
00110	Toileting self-care deficit
00100	Delayed surgical recovery

Class 3. Energy Balance. A dynamic state of harmony between intake and expenditure of resources

Approved Diagnoses

00050	Disturbed energy field
00093	fatigue

Class 4. Cardiovascular/Pulmonary Responses. Cardiopulmonary mechanisms that support activity or rest

Approved Diagnoses

00029	Decreased cardiac output
00033	Impaired spontaneous ventilation
00032	Ineffective breathing pattern
00092	Activity intolerance
00094	Risk for activity intolerance
00034	Dysfunctional ventilatory weaning response
00024	Ineffective tissue perfusion (specify type: renal, cerebral, cardiopulmonary, gastrointestinal, peripheral)

Domain 5. Perception/Cognition

The human information processing system including attention, orientation, sensation, perception, cognition, and communication

Class 1. Attention. Mental readiness to notice or observe

Approved Diagnoses

00123	Unilateral neglect

Class 2. Orientation. Awareness of time, place, and person

Approved Diagnoses

00127	Impaired environmental interpretation syndrome
00154	Wandering

Class 3. Sensation/Perception. Receiving information through the senses of touch, taste, smell, vision, hearing, and kinesthesia and the comprehension of sense data resulting in naming, associating, or pattern recognition

Approved Diagnoses

00122	Disturbed sensory perception (specify: visual, auditory, kinesthetic, gustatory, tactile, olfactory)

Class 4. Cognition. Use of memory, learning, thinking, problem solving, abstraction, judgment, insight, intellectual capacity, calculation, and language

Approved Diagnoses

00126	Deficient knowledge (specify)
00161	Readiness for enhanced knowledge (specify)
00128	Acute confusion
00129	Chronic confusion
00131	Impaired memory
00130	Disturbed thought processes

Class 5. Communication. Sending and receiving verbal and nonverbal information

Approved Diagnoses

00051	Impaired verbal communication
00157	Readiness for enhanced communication

Domain 6. Self-Perception

Awareness about the self

Class 1. Self-Concept. The perception(s) about the total self

Approved Diagnoses

00121	Disturbed personal identity
00125	Powerlessness
00152	Risk for powerlessness
00124	Hopelessness
00054	Risk for loneliness
00167	Readiness for enhanced self-concept

Class 2. Self-esteem. Assessment of one's own worth, capability, significance, and success

Approved Diagnoses

00119	Chronic low self-esteem
00120	Situational low self-esteem
00153	Risk for situational low self-esteem

Class 3. Body Image. A mental image of one's own body

Approved Diagnoses

00118	Disturbed body image

Domain 7. Role Relationships

The positive and negative connections or associations between persons or groups of persons and the means by which those connections are demonstrated

Class 1. Caregiving Roles. Socially expected behavior patterns by persons providing care who are not health care professionals

Approved Diagnoses

00061	Caregiver role strain
00062	Risk for caregiver role strain
00056	Impaired parenting
00057	Risk for impaired parenting
00164	Readiness for enhanced parenting

Class 2. Family Relationships. Associations of people who are biologically related or related by choice

Approved Diagnoses

00060	Interrupted family processes
00159	Readiness for enhanced family processes
00063	Dysfunctional family processes: Alcoholism
00058	Risk for impaired parent/infant/child attachment

Class 3. Role Performance. Quality of functioning in socially expected behavior patterns

Approved Diagnoses

00106	Effective breastfeeding
00104	Ineffective breastfeeding
00105	Interrupted breastfeeding
00055	Ineffective role performance
00064	Parental role conflict
00052	Impaired social interaction

Domain 8. Sexuality

Sexual identity, sexual function, and reproduction

Class 1. Sexual Identity. The state of being a specific person in regard to sexuality or gender

Class 2. Sexual Function. The capacity or ability to participate in sexual activities

Approved Diagnoses

00059	Sexual dysfunction
00065	Ineffective sexuality patterns

Class 3. Reproduction. Any process by which new individuals (people) are produced

Domain 9. Coping/Stress Tolerance

Contending with life events and life processes

Class 1. Post-Trauma Responses. Reactions occurring after physical or psychological trauma

Approved Diagnoses

00114	Relocation stress syndrome
00149	Risk for relocation stress syndrome
00142	Rape-trauma syndrome
00144	Rape-trauma syndrome: Silent reaction
00143	Rape-trauma syndrome: Compound reaction
00141	Post-trauma syndrome
00145	Risk for post-trauma syndrome

Class 2. Coping Responses. The process of managing environmental stress

Approved Diagnoses

00148	Fear
00146	Anxiety
00147	Death anxiety
00137	Chronic sorrow
00072	Ineffective denial
00136	Anticipatory grieving
00135	Dysfunctional grieving
00070	Impaired adjustment
00069	Ineffective coping
00073	Disabled family coping
00074	Compromised family coping
00071	Defensive coping
00077	Ineffective community coping
00158	Readiness for enhanced coping
00075	Readiness for enhanced family coping
00076	Readiness for enhanced community coping

Class 3. Neurobehavioral Stress. Behavioral responses reflecting nerve and brain function

Approved Diagnoses

00009	Autonomic dysreflexia
00010	Risk for autonomic dysreflexia
00116	Disorganized infant behavior
00115	Risk for disorganized infant behavior
00117	Readiness for enhanced organized infant behavior
00049	Decreased intracranial adaptive capacity

Domain 10. Life Principles

Principles underlying conduct, thought and behavior about acts, customs, or institutions viewed as being true or having intrinsic worth

Class 1. Values. The identification and ranking of preferred modes of conduct or end states

Class 2. Beliefs. Opinions, expectations, or judgments about acts, customs, or institutions viewed as being true or having intrinsic worth

Approved Diagnoses

00068	Readiness for enhanced spiritual well-being

Class 3. Value/Belief/Action Congruence. The correspondence or balance achieved between values, beliefs, and actions

Approved Diagnoses

00066	Spiritual distress
00067	Risk for spiritual distress
00083	Decisional conflict (specify)
00079	Noncompliance (specify)

Domain 11. Safety/Protection

Freedom from danger, physical injury or immune system damage, preservation from loss, and protection of safety and security

Class 1. Infection. Host responses following pathogenic invasion

Approved Diagnoses

00004	Risk for infection

Class 2. Physical Injury. Bodily harm or hurt

Approved Diagnoses

00045	Impaired oral mucous membrane
00035	Risk for injury
00087	Risk for perioperative positioning injury
00155	Risk for falls
00038	Risk for trauma
00046	Impaired skin integrity
00047	Risk for impaired skin integrity
00044	Impaired tissue integrity
00048	Impaired dentition
00036	Risk for suffocation
00039	Risk for aspiration
00031	Ineffective airway clearance
00086	Risk for peripheral neurovascular dysfunction
00043	Ineffective protection
00156	Risk for sudden infant death syndrome

Class 3. Violence. The exertion of excessive force or power so as to cause injury or abuse

Approved Diagnoses

00139	Risk for self-mutilation
00151	Self-mutilation
00138	Risk for other-directed violence
00140	Risk for self-directed violence
00150	Risk for suicide

Class 4. Environmental Hazards. Sources of danger in the surroundings

Approved Diagnoses

00037	Risk for poisoning

Class 5. Defensive Processes. The proceses by which the self protects itself from the nonself

Approved Diagnoses

00041	Latex allergy response
00042	Risk for latex allergy response

Class 6. Thermoregulation. The physiologic process of regulating heat and energy within the body for the purposes of protecting the organism

Approved Diagnoses

00005	Risk for imbalanced body temperature
00008	Ineffective thermoregulation
00006	Hypothermia
00007	Hyperthermia

Domain 12. Comfort

Sense of mental, physical, or social well-being or ease

Class 1. Physical Comfort. Sense of well-being or ease

Approved Diagnoses

00132	Acute pain
00133	Chronic pain
00134	Nausea

Class 2. Environmental Comfort. Sense of well-being or ease in or with one's environment

Class 3. Social Comfort. Sense of well-being or ease with one's social situations

Approved Diagnoses

00053	Social isolation

Domain 13. Growth/Development

Age-appropriate increases in physical dimensions, organ systems, or attainment of developmental milestones

Class 1. Growth. Increases in physical dimensions or maturity of organ systems

Approved Diagnoses

00113	Risk for disproportionate growth
00101	Adult failure to thrive

Class 2. Development. Attainment, lack of attainment, or loss of developmental milestones

Approved Diagnoses

00111	Delayed growth and development
00112	Risk for delayed development

APPENDIX C

Selected NANDA International Axis Descriptors

Axis 2 Descriptors: Time (formerly called Diagnosis Qualifiers) (NANDA International)

Acute	Less than 6 months
Chronic	More than 6 months
Intermittent	Stopping or starting again at intervals, periodic, cyclic
Continuous	Uninterrupted, going on without stop

Axis 3 Descriptors: Unit of Care (formerly called Qualifiers) (NANDA International)

Individual	A single human being distinct from others, a person
Family	Two or more people having continuous or sustained relationships, perceiving reciprocal obligations, sensing common meaning, and sharing certain obligations toward others; related by blood or choice
Group	Individuals gathered, classified, or acting together
Community	"A group of people living in the same locale under the same government. Examples include neighborhoods, cities, census tracts, and populations at risk." (Craft-Rosenberg, as cited in NANDA International, 2001, p. 218.)

Axis 6 Descriptors (formerly called Diagnosis Qualifiers) (NANDA International)

(Suggested but not limited to the following)

Descriptor	Definition
Ability	Capacity to do or act
Anticipatory	To realize beforehand, foresee
Balance	State of equilirium
Compromised	To make vulnerable to threat
Decreased	Lessened; lesser in size, amount, or degree
Deficient	Inadequate in amount, quality, or degree; defective; not sufficient; incomplete
Delayed	To postpone, impede, and retard
Depleted	Emptied wholly or in part; exhausted of
Disproportionate	Not consistent with a standard
Disabling	To make unable or unfit, to incapacitate

Disorganized	To destroy the systematic arrangement
Disturbed	Agitated; interrupted, interfered with
Dysfunctional	Abnormal, incomplete functioning
Excessive	Characterized by an amount or quantity that is greater than necessary, desirable, or useful
Functional	Normal complete functioning
Imbalanced	State of disequilibrium
Impaired	Made worse, weakened; damaged, reduced; deteriorated
Inability	Incapacity to do or act
Increased	Greater in size, amount, or degree
Ineffective	Not producing the desired effect
Interrupted	To break the continuity or uniformity
Organized	To form as into a systematic arrangement
Perceived	To become aware of by means of the senses; assignment of meaning
Readiness for Enhanced	To make greater, to increase in quality, to attain the more desired (for use with wellness diagnoses)

NOTE. From *NANDA International Nursing Diagnoses: Definitions and Classification 2003–2004* by the North American Nursing Diagnosis Association, 2003, Philadelphia: Author.

APPENDIX D
MULTIDISCIPLINARY (COLLABORATIVE) PROBLEMS ASSOCIATED WITH DISEASES AND OTHER PHYSIOLOGIC DISORDERS

Cancer

*Potential Complications of cancer: Anemia, bowel obstruction, cachexia, clotting disorders, electrolyte imbalance, pathologic fractures, hemorrhage, obstructive uropathy, metastasis to vital organs (e.g., brain, lungs), pericardial effusions, tamponade, sepsis→septic shock, spinal cord compression, superior vena cava syndrome, tissue anoxia→necrosis

Potential Complications of antineoplastic medications: Specify for each drug (e.g., anemia, bone marrow depression, cardiac toxicity, CNS toxicity, congestive heart failure, electrolyte imbalance, enteritis, leukopenia, necrosis at IV site, pneumonitis, renal failure, thrombocytopenia)

Potential Complications of narcotic medications: Depressed respirations, consciousness, and BP; cardiovascular collapse, biliary spasm

Potential Complications of radiation therapy: Increased intracranial pressure, myelosuppression, inflammation, fluid and electrolyte imbalances

Cardiac Function Disorders

Potential Complications of angina/coronary artery disease: Myocardial infarction

Potential Complications of congestive heart failure: Ascites, severe cardiac decompensation, cardiogenic shock, deep vein thrombosis, gastrointestinal congestion→malabsorption, hepatic failure, acute pulmonary edema, renal failure

Potential Complications of digitalis administration: Toxicity

Potential Complications of dysrhythmias: Decreased cardiac output→decreased myocardial perfusion→heart failure, severe atrioventricular conduction blocks, thromboemboli formation→ stroke, ventricular fibrillation

Potential Complications of myocardial infarction: Cardiogenic shock, dysrhythmia, infarct extension or expansion, myocardial

---

*Also see specific disorders, such as Gastrointestinal Function Disorders, for effects of cancer on those patterns.

rupture, pulmonary edema, pulmonary embolism, pericarditis, thromboembolism, ventricular aneurysm

Potential Complications of pericarditis/endocarditis: Cardiac tamponade, congestive heart failure, emboli (pulmonary, cerebral, renal, splenic, cardiac), valvular stenosis

Potential Complications of rheumatic fever/rheumatic heart disease: Congestive heart failure, decreased ventricular function, endocarditis, pericardial effusion, valvular changes

Endocrine Function Disorders

Potential Complications of adrenal gland disorders:

Potential Complications of Addison disease: Addisonian crisis (shock, coma), diabetes mellitus, thyroid disease

Potential Complications of Cushing disease: Congestive heart failure, hyperglycemia, hypertension, pancreatic tumors, potassium and sodium imbalance, psychosis

Potential Complications of diabetes mellitus: Coma, coronary artery disease, hypoglycemia, infections, ketoacidosis, nephropathy, peripheral vascular disease, retinopathy

Potential Complications of parathyroid gland disorders:

Potential Complications of hyperparathyroidism: Hypercalcemia→cardiac dysrhythmias, hypertension, metabolic acidosis, pathologic fractures, peptic ulcers, psychosis, renal calculi, renal failure

Potential Complications of hypoparathyroidism: Hypocalcemia→Cardiac dysrhythmias, convulsions, malabsorption, psychosis, tetany

Potential Complications of pituitary gland disorders:

Potential Complications of anterior pituitary disorders: Acromegaly, congestive heart failure, seizures

Potential Complications of posterior pituitary disorders: Loss of consciousness, hypernatremia, seizures

Potential Complications of thyroid gland disorders:

Potential Complications of hyperthyroidism: Exophthalmos, heart disease, negative nitrogen balance, thyroid crisis

Potential Complications of hypothyroidism: Adrenal insufficiency, cardiovascular disorders, myxedema coma, psychosis

Gastrointestinal (GI) Function Disorders

Potential Complications of esophageal disorders:

Potential Complications of esophageal diverticula: Obstruction, pulmonary aspiration of regurgitated food

Potential Complications of esophageal surgery: Reflux esophagitis, stricture formation

Potential Complications of hiatal hernia: Incarceration, necrosis→hemorrhage

Potential Complications of gallbladder, liver, and pancreatic disorders

Potential Complications of cirrhosis: Ascites, anemia, diabetes mellitus, disseminated intravascular coagulation (DIC), esophageal varices, GI bleeding or hemorrhage, hepatic encephalopathy, hyperbilirubinemia, hypokalemia, splenomegaly, peritonitis, renal failure

Potential Complications of cholelithiasis and cholecystitis: Fistula, gallbladder perforation, intestinal ileus or obstruction, obstruction of common bile duct→liver damage, pancreatitis, peritonitis

Potential Complications of hepatic abscess: Fluid and electrolyte, imbalance, hyperbilirubinemia

Potential Complications of metronidazole or iodoquinol administration: Bone marrow suppression

Potential Complications of hepatitis: Cirrhosis, hepatic encephalopathy, hepatic necrosis

Potential Complications of pancreatitis: Ascites, cardiac failure, coma, delirium tremens, diabetes mellitus, hemorrhage, hypovolemic shock, hypocalcemia, hyperglycemia or hypoglycemia, pancreatic abscess, pancreatic pseudocyst, pleural effusion or respiratory failure, psychosis, renal failure, tetany

Potential Complications of GI infections

Potential Complications of appendicitis: Abscess, gangrenous appendicitis, perforated appendix, peritonitis, pylephlebitis

Potential Complications of bacterial or viral infections (e.g., food poisoning): Bowel perforation, dehydration, hemolytic uremic syndome, hypokalemia, hypovolemic shock, metabolic acidosis, metabolic alkalosis, peritonitis, respiratory muscle paralysis, thrombotic thrombocytopenic purpura

Potential Complications of helminthic infections: Anemia; bowel, biliary, or pancreatic duct obstruction; migration to liver or lungs

Potential Complications of peritonitis: Hypovolemic shock, septicemia, septic shock

Potential Complications of GI inflammatory diseases (e.g., diverticulitis, gastritis, peptic ulcer, ulcerative colitis):

Abscess, anal fissure, anemia, colorectal carcinoma, fistula, fluid and electrolyte imbalances, GI bleeding or hemorrhage, intestinal obstruction, intestinal perforation, peritonitis, pyloric obstruction, toxic megacolon

Potential Complications of gastrectomy, pyloroplasty: Dumping syndrome

Potential Complications of structural and obstructive GI disorders:

Potential Complications of hemorrhoids and anorectal lesions: Anemia, infection, thrombosed hemorrhoid, sepsis

Potential Complications of hernias: Bowel infarction, bowel perforation, hernia incarceration and strangulation, peritonitis

Potential Complications of intestinal obstruction: Bowel wall necrosis, gangrene, fluid and electrolyte imbalance, hypovolemic or septic shock, intestinal perforation, peritonitis

Potential Complications of malabsorption syndromes:

Anemia, bleeding, delayed maturity, lack of growth, muscle wasting, rickets (and other nutrient deficiencies), tetany

Hematologic Disorders

Potential Complications of aplastic anemia: Congestive heart failure, hemorrhage, infections

Potential Complications of coagulation disorders: Hemorrhage (specific effects are determined by site of bleeding, for example, increased intracranial pressure in the brain, adult respiratory distress syndrome in the cardiovascular system), joint deformity or disability

Potential Complications of leukemias: Anemia, bleeding difficulties or internal hemorrhage, bone infarctions, coma, hepatomegaly, infections, renal failure, seizures, splenomegaly, tachycardia

Potential Complications of nutritional anemias: Impaired neurologic function (e.g., problems with proprioception), impaired cardiac function

Potential Complications of iron therapy: Hypersensitivity, toxicity (cardiovascular collapse, liver necrosis, metabolic acidosis)

Potential Complications of cyanocobalamin therapy: Hypersensitivity, hypokalemia, peripheral vascular thrombosis, pulmonary edema

Potential Complications of polycythemia: Bone marrow fibrosis, GI bleeding and ulcers, splenomegaly, thrombosis (various organs)

Potential Complications of sickle cell anemia: Multisystem organ failure (e.g., congestive heart failure, hyperuricemia, hepatomegaly, hepatic abscesses and fibrosis, hyperbilirubinemia, gallstones, bone marrow aplasia, osteomyelitis, aseptic bone necrosis, skin ulcers, vitreous hemorrhage, retinal detachment), sickle cell crisis

Potential Complications of sickle cell crisis: Aplastic crisis, CVA, hemosiderosis (from repeated transfusions), infections (e.g., pneumonia), seizures, splenic sequestration→circulatory collapse

Immune Function Disorders

Potential Complications of altered immune function: Allergic reactions→anaphylaxis, autoimmune disorders (e.g., systemic lupus erythematosus), delayed wound healing, infections (e.g., nosocomial, opportunistic), sepsis→septicemia, acute or chronic tissue inflammation (e.g., granulomas), transplant or graft rejection

Potential Complications of autoimmune deficiency syndrome (AIDS): HIV wasting syndrome; malignancies (cervical cancer, Kaposi sarcoma, lymphomas); neurologic (dementia complex, meningitis); opportunistic infections (e.g., candidiasis, cytomegalovirus infection, herpes infection, Mycobacterium avium infection, Pneumocystis carinii pneumonia, toxoplasmosis, tuberculosis)

Immobilized Patient

Potential Complications of immobility: Contractures, decreased cardiac output, decubitus ulcers, embolus, hypostatic pneumonia, joint ankylosis, orthostatic hypotension, osteoporosis, renal calculi, thrombophlebitis

Musculoskeletal Disorders and Trauma

Potential Complications of amputation: Contracture, delayed healing, edema of the stump, infection

Potential Complications of fractures: Compartment syndrome, deep vein thrombosis, delayed union, fat embolism, infection, necrosis, reflex sympathetic dystrophy, shock

Potential Complications of gout: Nephropathy, uric acid stones →renal failure

Potential Complications of osteoarthritis: Contractures, herniated disk

Potential Complications of osteomyelitis: Cutaneous sinus tract formation, necrosis, soft tissue abscesses

Potential Complications of osteoporosis, osteomalacia: Fractures, neuropathies, post-traumatic arthritis

Potential Complications of Paget disease: Bone tumors, cardiovascular complications (e.g., arteriosclerosis, hypertension, congestive heart failure), degenerative osteoarthritis, dementia, fractures, renal calculi

Potential Complications of rheumatoid arthritis: Anemia, bony or fibrous ankylosis, carpal tunnel syndrome, contractures, episcleritis or scleritis of the eye, Felty syndrome, muscle atrophy, neuropathy, pericarditis, pleural disease, vasculitis

Potential Complications of corticosteroid intra-articular injections: Intra-articular infection, joint degeneration

Potential Complications of corticosteroid systemic administration: Atherosclerosis, cataract formation, congestive heart failure, Cushing syndrome, delayed wound healing, depressed immune response, edema, growth retardation (children), hyperglycemia, hypertension, hypokalemia, muscle wasting, osteoporosis, peptic ulcers, psychotic reactions, renal failure, thrombophlebitis

Potential Complications of nonsteroidal anti-inflammatory medications: Gastric ulcers or bleeding, nephropathy

Neurologic Disorders

Potential Complications of organic brain diseases (e.g., Alzheimer disease): Aspiration pneumonia, dehydration, delusions, depression, falls, malnutrition, paranoid reactions, pneumonia

Potential Complications of brain injury and intracranial hemorrhage: Brain ischemia, herniation, increased intracranial pressure

Potential Complications of brain tumor: Hyperthermia, increased intracranial pressure, paralysis, sensorimotor changes

Potential Complications of cerebrovascular accident (CVA): Behavioral changes, brain stem failure, cardiac dysrhythmias, coma, elimination disorders, increased intracranial pressure, language disorders, motor deficits, respiratory infection, seizures, sensory-perceptual deficits (**NOTE:** The manifestations and complications of a CVA vary according to the area of the brain affected. Also, it is difficult to determine which effects are manifestations and symptoms and which are actually complications. Furthermore, many of the complications of CVA are due to the resulting immobility rather than to the pathophysiology of the CVA itself. Refer to Immobilized Patient on page 757.)

Potential Complications of increased intracranial pressure (e.g., cerebral edema, hydrocephalus): CNS ischemic response (increased mean arterial pressure, increased pulse pressure, and bradycardia), coma, failure of autoregulation of cerebral blood flow, hyperthermia resulting from impaired hypothalamic function, motor impairment (decorticate or decerebrate posturing)

Potential Complications of intracranial aneurysm: Hydrocephalus, hypothalamic dysfunction, rebleeding, seizures, vasospasm

Potential Complications of meningitis and encephalitis: Arthritis, brain infarction, coma, cranial nerve damage, hydrocephalus, increased intracranial pressure, seizures

Potential Complications of multiple sclerosis: Pneumonia; dementia; sudden progression of neurologic symptoms (convulsions, coma), urinary tract infection

Potential Complications of myasthenia gravis: Aspiration, cholinergic crisis, dehydration, myasthenic crisis, pneumonia

Potential Complications of Parkinson disease: Depression and social isolation, falls, infections related to immobility (e.g., pneumonia), malnutrition related to dysphagia and immobility, oculogyric crisis, paranoia and hallucinations, pressure ulcers

Potential Complications of seizure disorder: Accidental trauma (e.g., burns, falls), aspiration, head injury, status epilepticus→ acidosis, hyperthermia, hypoglycemia, hypoxia

Potential Complications of spinal cord injury: Autonomic dysreflexia, cardiac dysrhythmias, complications due to immobility (see Immobilized Patient), hypercalcemia, necrosis of spinal cord tissue, paralytic ileus, respiratory infection secondary to decreased cough reflex, spinal shock

Peripheral Vascular and Lymphatic Disorders

Potential Complications of aortic aneurysm: Dissection, hemiplegia and lower extremity paralysis (with dissection), rupture→hypovolemic shock

Potential Complications of femoral and popliteal aneurysms: Embolism, gangrene, rupture, thrombosis

Potential Complications of hypertension: Aortic dissection, CVA, congestive heart failure, hypertensive crisis, malignant hypertension, myocardial ischemia, papilledema, renal insufficiency, retinal damage

Potential Complications of lymphedema: Cellulitis, lymphangitis

Potential Complications of peripheral arterial disease: Arterial thrombosis, cellulitis, CVA, hypertension, ischemic ulcers, tissue necrosis→gangrene

Potential Complications of thrombophlebitis: Chronic leg edema, pulmonary embolism, stasis ulcers

Potential Complications of varicose veins: Cellulitis, hemorrhage, vascular rupture, venous stasis ulcers

Respiratory Function Disorders

Potential Complications of asthma: Atelectasis, cor pulmonale, dehydration, pneumothorax, respiratory infection, status asthmaticus

> *Potential Complications of corticosteroid therapy:* Hypertension, hypokalemia, hypoglycemia, immunosuppression, osteoporosis, ulcers

> *Potential Complications of methylxanthine therapy:* Toxicity (seizures, circulatory failure, respiratory arrest)

Potential Complications of chronic obstructive pulmonary disease (COPD): Hypoxemia, respiratory acidosis, respiratory failure, respiratory infection, right-sided heart failure, spontaneous pneumothorax

Potential Complications of pneumonia: Bacteremia→endocarditis, meningitis, peritonitis; lung abscess and empyema; lung tissue necrosis; pleuritis

Potential Complications of pulmonary edema: Cerebral hypoxia, multisystem organ failure, right-sided heart failure

Potential Complications of pulmonary embolism: Pulmonary infarction with necrosis, right ventricular heart failure, sudden death

Potential Complications of tuberculosis: Bacteremia→extrapulmonary tuberculosis (e.g., genitourinary tuberculosis, meningitis, peritonitis, pericarditis), bronchopleural fistula, empyema

Potential Complications of medications for tuberculosis: Hepatotoxicity, hypersensitivity, nephrotoxicity, peripheral neuropathy (isoniazid), optic neuritis (ethambutol)

Sexually Transmitted Disease

Potential Complications of chlamydial infections:

Females: Abortion, infertility, pelvic abscesses, pelvic inflammatory disease, postpartum endometritis, spontaneous abortion, stillbirth

Males: Epididymitis, prostatitis, urethritis

Neonates: Ophthalmia neonatorum, pneumonia

Potential Complications of genital herpes:

All: Herpes keratitis

Females: Cervical cancer

Males: Ascending myelitis, lymphatic suppuration, meningitis, neuralgia, urethral strictures

Neonates: Potentially fatal infections; infections of eyes, skin, mucous membranes, and CNS.

Potential Complications of genital warts:

All: Urinary obstruction and bleeding

Females: Increased risk of cancer of the cervix, vagina, vulva, and anus; obstruction of the birth canal during labor; transmission to neonate

Neonates: Respiratory papillomatosis

Potential Complications of gonorrhea:

All: Secondary infection of lesions; fistulas; chronic ulcers; sterility

Females: Abdominal adhesions, ectopic pregnancy, pelvic inflammatory disease

Males: Epididymitis, nephritis, prostatitis, urethritis

Neonates: Ophthalmia neonatorum

Potential Complications of syphilis: Blindness, paralysis, heart failure, liver failure, mental illness

Shock

Potential Complications of shock: Cerebral hypoxia→coma, multiple organ system failure, paralytic ileus, pulmonary emboli, renal failure

Skin Integrity Disorders

Potential Complications of burns: Airway obstruction (inhalation injury), Curling ulcer, hypothermia, hypovolemic shock, hypervolemia, infection secondary to suppression of immune system, negative nitrogen balance, paralytic ileus, renal failure, sepsis, stress ulcers

Potential Complications of skin lesions/dermatitis/acne: Cyst formation, malignancy, infection

Potential Complications of herpes zoster: Dissemination→visceral lesions, encephalitis, loss of vision

Potential Complications of pressure ulcer: Necrotic damage to muscle, bone, tendons, joint capsule; infection, sepsis

Urinary Elimination Disorders

Potential Complications of cystitis: Bladder ulceration, bladder wall necrosis, renal infection

Potential Complications of polycystic kidney disease: Renal calculi, urinary tract infection, renal failure

Potential Complications of pyelonephritis: Bacteremia, chronic pyelonephritis, renal insufficiency, renal failure

Potential Complications of acute renal failure: Electrolyte imbalance, fluid overload, metabolic acidosis, pericarditis, platelet dysfunction, secondary infections

Potential Complications of chronic renal failure: Anemia, cardiac tamponade, pericarditis, congestive heart failure, fluid and electrolyte imbalance, GI bleeding, hyperparathyroidism, infections, medication toxicity, metabolic acidosis, pleural effusion, pulmonary edema, uremia

Potential Complications of urolithiasis: Hydronephrosis, hydroureter, infection, pyelonephritis, renal insufficiency

APPENDIX E
MULTIDISCIPLINARY (COLLABORATIVE) PROBLEMS ASSOCIATED WITH TESTS AND TREATMENTS

Test or Treatment	Potential Complications (Collaborative Problems)
Arteriogram	Allergic reaction, embolism, hemorrhage; hematoma, paresthesia, renal failure, thrombosis at site
Bone marrow studies	Bleeding, infection
Bronchoscopy	Airway obstruction or bronchoconstriction, hemorrhage
Cardiac catheterization	Cardiac dysrhythmias, infarction, perforation, embolism, thrombus formation, hypervolemia, hypovolemia, paresthesia, site hemorrhage or hematoma
Casts and traction	Bleeding, edema, impaired circulation, misalignment of bones, neurologic compromise
Chest tubes	Bleeding→hemothorax, blockage or displacement→pneumothorax, septicemia
Foley catheter	Bladder distention (tube not patent), urinary tract infection
Hemodialysis	Air embolism, bleeding, dialysis dementia, electrolyte imbalance, embolism, fluid shifts, hepatitis B, infection or septicemia, shunt clotting; fistulas, transfusion reactions
Intravenous therapy	Fluid overload, infiltration, phlebitis
Medications	Allergic reactions, side effects (specify), toxic effects or overdose (specify)
Nasogastric suction	Electrolyte imbalance, gastric ulceration→ hemorrhage
Radiation therapy	Fistulas, tissue necrosis, hemorrhage, radiation burns, radiation pneumonia
Tracheal suctioning	Bleeding, hypoxia
Ventilation, assisted	Acid–base imbalance, airway obstruction (tube plugged or displaced), ineffective O_2–CO_2 exchange, pneumothorax, respirator dependence, tracheal necrosis

Adapted from *Nursing Process & Critical Thinking* (3rd ed., p. 157) by J. Wilkinson, 2001, Upper Saddle River, NJ: Prentice Hall.

APPENDIX F
MULTIDISCIPLINARY (COLLABORATIVE) PROBLEMS ASSOCIATED WITH SURGICAL TREATMENTS

Format for problem statement:

"Potential Complication of [*column 1*]: [*column 2*],"

For example, Potential Complication of general surgery: *Atelectasis, bronchospasm, and so forth.*

Column 1 **Type of Surgery "Potential Complication of"**	*Column 2* **Potential Complications (Multidisciplinary Problems)**
General surgery (complications that can occur regardless of type of surgery)	Atelectasis, bronchospasm or laryngospasm on extubation (with general anesthesia), electrolyte imbalance, excessive bleeding→ shock, fluid imbalance, headache from leakage of cerebrospinal fluid (with regional anesthesia), hypotension (with regional anesthesia), ileus, infection, stasis pneumonia, urinary retention→bladder distention, venous thrombosis→pulmonary embolism, wound dehiscence→evisceration

Instructions: Choose complications from General surgery above; then choose those that apply to patient's particular type of surgery. Potential complications of various types of surgery follow; these complications are in addition to those of General surgery.

Abdominal surgery	Dehiscence, fistula formation, paralytic ileus, peritonitis, renal failure, surgical trauma (e.g., to ureter, bladder, or rectum)
Breast surgery	Cellulitis, hematoma, lymphedema, seroma
Chest surgery: coronary artery bypass graft	Cardiovascular insufficiency, renal insufficiency, respiratory insufficiency
Chest surgery: thoracotomy	Adult respiratory distress syndrome, bronchopleural fistula, cardiac dysrhythmias, empyema of the chest cavity, hemothorax, infection at chest tube sites, mediastinal shift, myocardial infarction, pneumothorax, pulmonary edema, subcutaneous emphysema

Craniotomy	Cardiac dysrhythmias, cerebral or cerebellar dysfunction, cerebrospinal fluid leaks, cranial nerve impairment, gastrointestinal bleeding, hematomas, hydrocephalus, hygromas, hyperthermia or hypothermia, hypoxemia, increased intracranial pressure, meningitis or encephalitis, residual neurologic defects, seizures
Eye surgery	Endophthalmus, hyphema, increased intraocular pressure, lens implant dislocation, macular edema, retinal detachment, secondary glaucoma
Musculoskeletal surgeries	Bone necrosis, fat embolus, flexion contractures, hematoma, joint dislocation or displacement of prosthesis, nerve damage, sepsis, synovial herniation
Neck surgeries	Airway obstruction, aspiration, cerebral infarction, cranial nerve damage, fistula formation (e.g., between hypopharynx and skin), flap rejection (in radical neck dissection), hypertension or hypotension, hypoparathyroidism (in thyroidectomy or parathyroidectomy), local nerve damage (e.g., to the laryngeal nerve), respiratory distress, tetany (in thyroidectomy), thyroid storm, tracheal stenosis, vocal cord paralysis
Rectal surgery	Fistula formation, stricture formation
Skin grafts	Edema, flap necrosis, graft rejection, hematoma
Spinal surgery	Displacement of bone graft (in laminectomy or spinal fusion), bladder or bowel dysfunction, cerebrospinal fistula, hematoma, nerve root injury, paralytic ileus, sensorineural impairments, spinal cord edema or injury
Urologic surgery	Bladder neck constriction, bladder perforation (intraoperative), epididymitis, paralytic ileus, retrograde ejaculation (in prostate resection or prostatectomy) stomal necrosis, stenosis, obstruction (in urostomy or nephrostomy), urethral stricture, urinary tract infection
Vascular surgery: Aortic aneurysm resection	Congestive heart failure, myocardial infarction, renal failure, rupture of the suture line→hemorrhage, spinal cord ischemia
Vascular surgery: Other	Cardiac dysrhythmia, compartmental syndrome, failure of anastomosis, lymphocele, occlusion of graft

APPENDIX G
NURSING DIAGNOSES ACCEPTED FOR
FURTHER DEVELOPMENT, LEVEL 1.4
(NANDA INTERNATIONAL)

NOTE: These diagnoses require further development for future submission, and should be used advisedly for other than developmental purposes.

Activities of Daily Living, Readiness for Enhanced
Definition: A pattern of executing the tasks of daily living that is adequate for meeting health-related goals and can be strengthened

Defining Characteristics

Evidence of balance between activity and rest, work and leisure; achieves self-care as appropriate for developmental stage and ability; demonstrates moderation in behaviors; manages a home as indicated; expresses satisfaction with lifestyle; demands of daily living are normally achievable; support systems are available for meeting demands of daily living; no unusual barriers to achieving activities of daily living

Bowel Elimination, Readiness for Enhanced
Definition: A pattern of bowel function that is adequate for meeting elimination needs and can be strengthened

Defining Characteristics

Regular bowel elimination; stool is formed and soft; intake of foods and fluids is adequate to meet daily needs; no excessive straining for expulsion of stool; little or no abdominal pain, discomfort, distention, nausea, belching, or expulsion of gas; occasional or infrequent use of laxatives, stool softeners, and antidiarrheal medications; activity is adequate to promote peristalsis

Comfort, Readiness for Enhanced
Definition: A pattern of contentment that is sufficient for well-being and can be strengthened

Defining Characteristics

Expresses feelings of contentment; relaxed expression and posture; few to no complaints

Decision Making, Readiness for Enhanced
Definition: A pattern of choosing courses of action that is sufficient for meeting short- and long-term goals and can be strengthened

Defining Characteristics

Expresses feelings about choices objectively; explains possible choices in specific situation; makes decisions that are congruent with values and goals

Exercise, Readiness for Enhanced

Definition: A pattern of physical activity that is sufficient to meet health-related goals and can be strengthened

Defining Characteristics

Describes interest and motivation to start or maintain a regular pattern of exercise; expresses knowledge of the relationship of regular activity to health-related goals; activities are appropriate for age, physical abilities, and other factors; muscle size, muscle strength, and motor skill performance are adequate for meeting daily needs and health goals; joint flexibility is adequate; cardiovascular status is within normal limits for age and other factors

Grieving, Readiness for Enhanced

Definition: A pattern of feelings and behaviors pertaining to loss that is sufficient for recovery and can be strengthened

Defining Characteristics

Able to describe source of grief and the grief process; reports grief feelings and behaviors as expected for loss; able to maintain health behaviors; resumes activities of daily living; makes plans for the future

Hope, Readiness for Enhanced

Definition: A pattern of expectations and desires that is sufficient for mobilizing energy on one's own behalf and can be strengthened

Defining Characteristics

Expresses expectations that are congruent with desires; sets goals; active participant in meeting goals; expresses optimism' expresses belief in possibilities; expresses willingness to build on strengths

Immunization Status, Readiness for Enhanced

Definition: A pattern of conforming to local, national, and/or international standards of immunization to prevent infectious disease(s) that is sufficient to protect a person, family, or community and can be strengthened

Defining Characteristics

Obtains immunizations appropriate for age and health status; expresses knowledge of immunization standards; exhibits behavior to prevent infectious diseases; keeps records of immunizations; identifies providers of immunizations; values immunizations as a health priority; describes possible problems associated with immunizations

Power, Readiness for Enhanced

Definition: A pattern of participating knowingly in change that is sufficient for well being and can be strengthened

Defining Characteristics

Describes awareness of possible changes to be made; explains choices that can be made for change; discusses freedom to act intentionally for change; involved in creating change; explains knowledge for participating in change; participates in choices for daily living and health

Self-Care, Readiness for Enhanced

Definition: A pattern of performing activities for oneself that is sufficient for meeting health-related goals and can be strengthened

Defining Characteristics

Independent as capable in bathing or hygiene, toileting, feeding, dressing, mobility, and maintaining continence; expresses knowledge of strategies for self-care; accepts responsibility for self-care

Recreation and/or Leisure, Readiness for Enhanced

Definition: A pattern of planned activities and responses to spontaneous events that is sufficient for pleasure and growth and can be strengthened

Defining Characteristics

Activities for pleasure are planned; expresses intrinsic motivation for planning and responding to pleasurable events; strives for balance between work and leisure; includes pleasurable activities in daily or weekly schedule; uses humor

Values/Beliefs, Readiness for Enhanced

Definition: A pattern of disposition toward persons, objects, or ideas that is sufficient for giving direction and meaning to life and can be strengthened

Defining Characteristics

Chooses freely; chooses from possible alternatives; considers outcomes of alternatives; happy with personal beliefs and actions; affirming choices to others; acts on choices; extablishes a pattern of actions that is congruent with values and beliefs

CREDITS

INDEX